Useful Units in Radiology

SI Prefixes

Factor	Prefix	Symbol
10^{18}	Exa	E
10^{15}	Peta	P
10^{12}	Tera	T
10^{9}	Giga	G
10^{6}	Mega	M
10^{3}	Kilo	k
10^{2}	Hecto	h
10^{1}	Deca	da
10^{-1}	Deci	d
10^{-2}	Centi	c
10^{-3}	Milli	m
10^{-6}	Micro	μ
10^{-9}	Nano	n
10^{-12}	Pico	p
10^{-15}	Femto	f
10^{-18}	Atto	a

SI Base Units

Quantity	Name	Symbol
Length	Meter	m
Mass	Kilogram	kg
Time	Second	s
Electric current	Ampere	A

SI Derived Units Expressed in Terms of Base Units

Quantity	SI Unit Name	SI Unit Symbol
Area	Square meter	m^2
Volume	Cubic meter	m^3
Speed, velocity	Meter per second	m/s
Acceleration	Meter per second squared	m/s^2
Density, mass density	Kilogram per cubic meter	kg/m^3
Current density	Ampere per square meter	A/m^2
Concentration (of amount of substance)	Mole per cubic meter	$mole/m^3$
Specific volume	Cubic meter per kilogram	m^3/kg

Special Quantities of Radiologic Science and Their Associated Special Units

Quantity	Customary Unit Name	Customary Unit Symbol	SI Unit Name	SI Unit Symbol
Exposure	roentgen	R	air kerma	Gy_a
Absorbed dose	rad	rad	gray	Gy_1
Effective dose	rem	rem	seivert	Sv
Radioactivity	curie	Ci	becquerel	Bq

Multiply	R	by	0.01	to obtain	Gy_a
Multiply	rad	by	0.01	to obtain	Gy_t
Multiply	rem	by	0.01	to obtain	Sv
Multiply	Ci	by	3.7×10^{10}	to obtain	Bq
Multiply	R	by	2.58×10^{-4}	to obtain	C/kg

RADIOLOGIC SCIENCE for TECHNOLOGISTS

Physics, Biology, and Protection

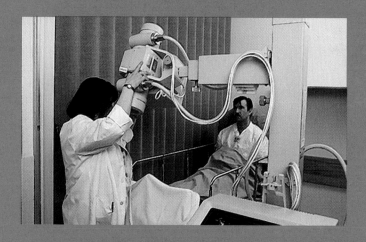

Seventh Edition

RADIOLOGIC SCIENCE for TECHNOLOGISTS

Physics, Biology, and Protection

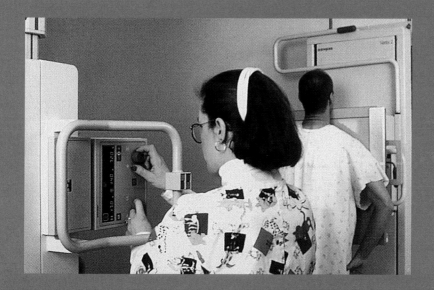

STEWART C. BUSHONG, Sc.D., FACR, FACMP

Professor of Radiologic Science
Baylor College of Medicine
Houston, Texas

with 756 illustrations, 616 in color

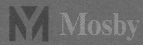 Mosby

An Affiliate of Elsevier Science
St. Louis   London   Philadelphia   Sydney   Toronto

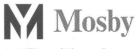

An Affiliate of Elsevier Science

Executive Editor: Jeanne Wilke
Developmental Editors: Jennifer Moorhead
Editorial Assistant: Melissa Kuster
Project Manager: Carol Sullivan Weis
Designer: Mark Oberkrom
Cover Art: Radiograph courtesy Alex Backus; photograph from
Mosby's radiographic instructional series: radiographic imaging,
St. Louis, 1998, Mosby.

Mosby, Inc.
An Affiliate of Elsevier Science
11830 Westline Industrial Drive
St. Louis, Missouri 63146

Printed in the United States of America

International Standard Book Number 0-323-01337-6

02 03 04 05 TG/KPT 9 8 7 6 5 4 3

Reviewers

Rachel Bailey, B.S., R.T. (R)
Program Director
Columbia/St. Mary's Hospitals
School of Radiologic Technology
Milwaukee, Wisconsin

Alberto Bello, Jr., M.Ed., R.T., (R) (CV)
Associate Professor
Department of Medical Imaging
Oregon Institute of Technology
Klamath Falls, Oregon

Deanna Butcher, B.S., R.T. (R)
Program Director
St. Luke's College
Sioux City, Iowa

Henry Y. Cashion, B.S., R.T. (R)
Program Director
Mineral Area Regional Medical Center
School of Radiologic Technology
Farmington, Missouri

John H. Clouse, M.S.R., R.T. (R)
Associate Professor of Radiography
Owensboro Community College
Owensboro, Kentucky

Blake Daley, B.S., R.T.
Instructor/Clinical Coordinator
Department of Radiologic Technology
South Arkansas Community College
El Dorado, Arkansas

Richard Hone, ME.d., R.T. (R)
Professor
Department of Medical Imaging Technology
Oregon Institute of Technology
Klamath Falls, Oregon

Debbie Hornbacher, B.S., R.T. (R)
Program Director
Trinity Hospital School of Radiologic Technology
Minot, North Dakota

Michael O. Loomis, M.H.A., R.T. (R)
Education Coordinator
Huntington Hospital
Pasadena, California

Mahadevappa Mahesh, Ph.D., D.A.B.R.
Chief Physicist and Research Associate
Johns Hopkins University
Baltimore, Maryland

Starla L. Mason, M.S., R.T. (R) (QM)
Radiography Coordinator
Laramie County Community College
Cheyenne, Wyoming

Gloria Strickland, M.H.S., R.T. (R) (M) (QM)
Assistant Professor
Armstrong Atlantic State University
Savannah, Georgia

Elwin R. Tilson, Ed.D., R.T. (R) (M) (QM) (CT)
Professor of Radiologic Sciences
Department of Radiologic Sciences
Armstrong Atlantic University
Savannah, Georgia

Bonnie Young, B.A., R.T. (R)
Radiographer
Academic Support Services
Clark State Community College
Springfield, Ohio

Dedicated to

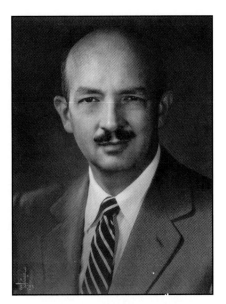

Vincent P. Collins, M.D.
First Chairman of the Department of Radiology,
Baylor College of Medicine
1952 to 1968

and

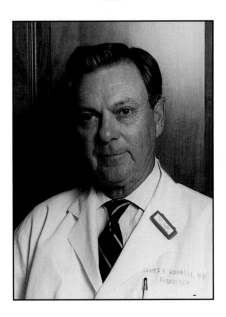

James E. Harrell, Sr., M.D.
Chairman, Department of Radiology,
Baylor College of Medicine
1976 to 2000

Two outstanding academic radiologists who encouraged me, supported me, and allowed me the freedom
to do science, lecture and write . . . and we became good personal friends.

To:
Bettie,
Leslie,
Stephen,
Andrew,
Butterscotch,†
Jemimah,†
Geraldine,†
Casper,†
Ginger,†
Sebastian,†
Buffy,†
Brie,†
Linus,†
Midnight,†
Boef,†
Cassie,†
Lucy,†
Toto,†
Choco,†
Molly,†
Maxwell† and my lenses,
Bandit,†
Kate,†
Misty,†
Chester,†
Petra,†
Travis,†
Brutus,†
and Ebony†

†R.I.P.

Preface

PURPOSE AND CONTENT

The purpose of *Radiologic Science For Technologists: Physics, Biology, and Protection* is threefold: to convey a working knowledge of radiologic physics, to prepare radiography students for the certification examination by the ARRT, and to provide a base of knowledge from which practicing radiographers can make informed decisions about technical factors and diagnostic image quality. To these ends, this text provides a solid presentation of radiologic science, including the fundamentals of radiologic physics, imaging, radiobiology, and radiation protection. Special topics include mammography, fluoroscopy, cardiovascular and interventional procedures, and multislice spiral computed tomography.

The fundamentals of radiologic science cannot be divorced from mathematics, but this textbook does not assume a mathematics background for its readers. Mathematical equations are always followed by sample problems with direct clinical application whenever possible. As a further aid to learning, all mathematical formulas are highlighted with their own icon in a colorful box:

Likewise, the most important ideas under discussion are presented with their own colorful icon and box:

The seventh edition improves this popular feature by including even more key concepts and definitions in each chapter. This edition also continues to present learning objectives, chapter overviews, and chapter summaries that encourage students and make the text user-friendly for all its readers. Challenge Questions at the end of each chapter include definition exercises, short-answer questions, and calculations. These questions can be used for homework assignments, for review sessions, or for self-directed testing and practice. Answers to the odd-numbered questions are provided in the back of the book. A full answer key can be obtained by contacting the publisher directly.

HISTORICAL PERSPECTIVE

For 7 decades after Roentgen's discovery of x-rays in 1895, diagnostic radiology remained a relatively stable field of study and practice. Truly great changes during that time can be counted on one hand: the Crookes tube, the Potter-Bucky diaphragm, and image intensification.

Since the publication of the first edition of this textbook in 1975, however, more and more innovative types of examinations have come into routine use in medical imaging: computed tomography, computed radiography, digital fluoroscopy, spiral computed tomography, and most recently, multislice spiral computed tomography. Truly spectacular advances in computer technology and x-ray tube and image receptor design have made these innovations possible, and they continue to transform the imaging sciences.

NEW TO THIS EDITION

The seventh edition presents many updates in the areas of special imaging, where the greatest advances in technology have occurred. There is an important new section on multislice spiral CT. Another recent innovation described in this textbook is direct-capture radiography. There is a new discussion of charge-coupled devices and their advantages for cardiovascular and interventional procedures. Also discussed are advances in target composition, compression, and digital imaging for mammography.

The seventh edition also includes more in-text definitions and chapter cross-references. All bolded terms are defined when first introduced and are collected in an expanded glossary. New radiographs and line drawings keep this text fresh and fun.

ANCILLARIES
Student Workbook and Laboratory Manual

This three-part resource has been updated to reflect the changes in the text and the rapid advancements in the field of radiologic science. Part One offers a complete selection of worksheets organized by textbook chapter. Part Two, the Math Tutor, provides an outstanding refresher for any student. Part Three, Laboratory Experiments, collects experiments designed to demonstrate important concepts in radiologic science.

Related Multimedia

Instructional materials to support teaching and learning radiologic physics have been developed by Mosby and may be obtained by contacting the publisher directly. Multimedia presentations of basic physics, imaging, radiobiology, and radiation protection are available in both slide/audiotape and CD-ROM formats.

A NOTE ON THE TEXT

Although the United States has not formally adopted the International System of Units (SI units), they are presented in this textbook. With this system come the corresponding units of radiation and radioactivity. The roentgen, the rad, and the rem are being replaced by the coulomb/kilogram (C/kg), the gray (Gy), and the sievert (Sv), respectively. Radioactivity is expressed in becquerels (Bq). A summary of special quantities and units in radiologic science can be found on the inside front cover of the text.

Radiation in air may be quantified in terms of exposure, measured in SI units of C/kg, or in terms of air kerma, measured in units of mGy. Because mGy is also a unit of dose, a measurement of air kerma is distinguished from tissue dose by applying a subscript a or t to mGy, according to the recommendation of Archer and Wagner (*Minimizing Risk from Fluoroscopic X-Rays*, PRM, 1999). Therefore, when the SI is used, air kerma is measured in mGy_a and tissue dose in mGy_t.

ACKNOWLEDGMENTS

For the preparation of this edition, I am indebted to the many readers of the earlier editions who submitted suggestions, criticisms, corrections, and compliments. And for this edition, I am particularly indebted to the following radiologic science educators for their suggestions for change and clarification. Many supplied radiographic illustrations, and they are additionally acknowledged with the illustration.

Nancy Adams, Itawamba Community College, Mississippi; **Ken Carson,** Itawamba Community College, Mississippi; **Donna Deos,** Portland Community College, Oregon; **Pat Duffy,** Sunny Upstate Medical University, New York; **Evelyn Engler,** New Mexico State University, New Mexico; **Mike Enriquez,** Merced College, California; **Pamela Eugene,** Delgado Community College, California; **Richard Fischer,** Baylor College of Medicine, Texas; **Richard Geise,** University of Minnesota; Minnesota; **Lee Goldman,** Hartford, Connecticut; **Edward Goldschmidt, Jr.,** University Medical Center, New Jersey; **Art Haus,** Columbus, Ohio; **Vincent Hinck,** Medford, Oregon; **Lee Kitts,** Hendersonville, North Carolina; **Dan Larkin,** Portland Community College, Oregon; **Charles Mistretta,** University of Wisconsin, Wisconsin; **Patrick Monahan,** Bloomington School of Radiography, Indiana; **Bill Mulky,** Midlands Technical College, South Carolina; **Cindy Murphy,** Halifax, Canada; **Satish Prasad,** SUNY Upstate Medical University, New York; **Hobie Shackford,** Roger Williams Medical Center, Rhode Island; **Bette Schans,** Mesa State University, Colorado; **Barbara Smith Pruner,** Portland Community College, Oregon; **Sandy Strickland,** Community College of Southern Nevada, Nevada; **Dawn Sturk,** Hurley School of Radiologic Technology, Michigan; **Rees Stuteville,** Oregon Institute of Technology, Oregon; and **Patti Ward,** Mesa State University, Colorado.

Special thanks to my colleagues **Benjamin Archer,** Baylor College of Medicine, and **Louis Wagner,** University of Texas Health Science Center, for their introduction of the radiologic terms mGy_a and mGy_t.

I am deeply indebted to my associates **Sharon Glaze, Robert Parry, David Hearne, Gary Isenhower,** and **Carol Walsh** who have assisted me with this revision. The illustrations are the work of many people who worked exceptionally hard to render all illustrations in full color. The cartoons by **Kraig Emmert** help ease any pain associated with medical physics.

I am also particularly indebted to **Judy Matteau Faldyn, Linda Sumpter,** and especially **Yvonne Young** for the many times they had to struggle through my handwritten notes and unfamiliar symbols and equations. I appreciate their hard work and conscientious approach to preparing the manuscript.

As you, student or educator, use this text and have questions or comments, I hope you will e-mail me at sbushong@bcm.tmc.edu so that together we can strive to make this very difficult material easier to learn.

"Physics is fun" is the motto of my radiologic science courses, and I believe this text will help make physics enjoyable for the student radiologic technologist.

Stewart C. Bushong

Contents

RADIOLOGIC SCIENCE for TECHNOLOGISTS

Physics, Biology, and Protection

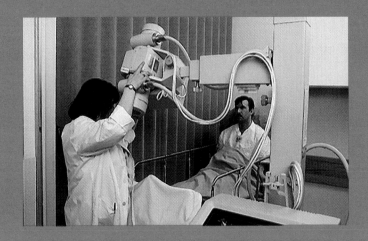

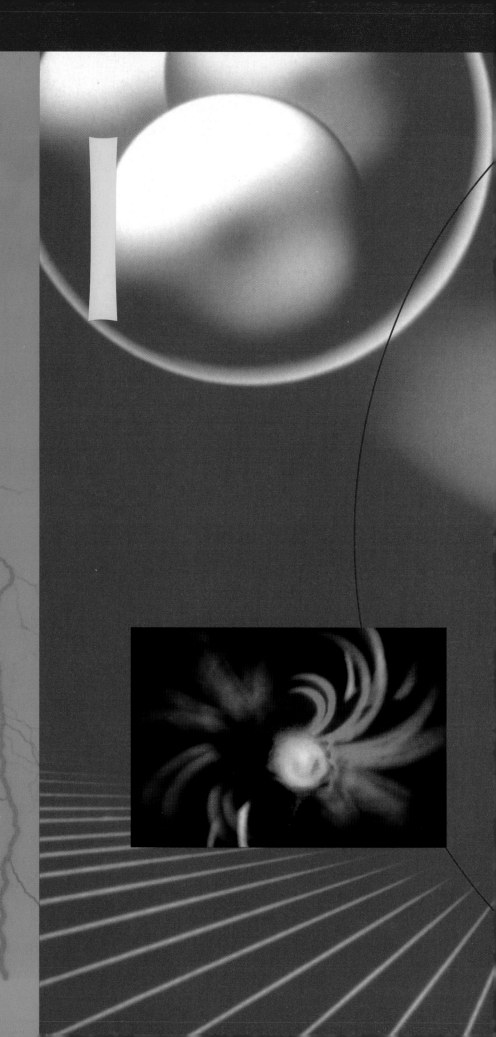

PART

I

RADIOLOGIC PHYSICS

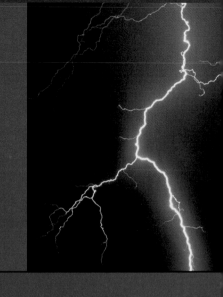

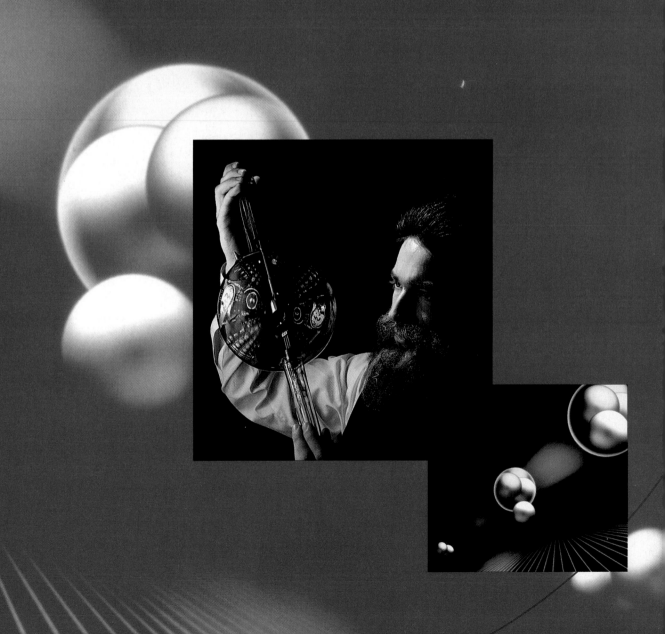

Concepts of Radiologic Science

OBJECTIVES

At the completion of this chapter, the student should be able to:

1. Describe the characteristics of matter and energy
2. Identify the various forms of energy
3. Define *electromagnetic radiation* and specifically *ionizing radiation*
4. State the relative intensity of ionizing radiation from various sources
5. Relate the accidental discovery of x-rays by Roentgen
6. Discuss examples of human injury caused by radiation
7. List the concepts of basic radiation protection

OUTLINE

This chapter explores the basic concepts of the science and technology of x-ray imaging. These include the study of matter, energy, the electromagnetic spectrum, and ionizing radiation. The production of ionizing radiation and its use as a diagnostic tool are the bases of radiography. Radiologic technologists who deal specifically with x-ray imaging are radiographers or radiologic technologists. Radiographers have a great responsibility in performing medical x-ray examinations using established radiation-protection standards to maintain the safety of patients and medical personnel. Radiography is a career choice with great, yet diverse opportunities. Welcome to the field of diagnostic imaging.

NATURE OF OUR SURROUNDINGS

In a physical analysis, all things visible can be classified as matter or energy. Matter is anything that occupies space and has form or shape. Energy is the ability to do work. All matter is composed of fundamental building blocks called *atoms*, which are arranged in complex ways. These atomic arrangements are considered at length in Chapter 4.

Matter and Mass

Matter is anything that occupies space. It is the material substance of which physical objects are composed and that gives them form and shape. A primary, distinguishing characteristic of matter is **mass**, the quantity of matter contained in any physical object. The **kilogram** is the scientific unit of mass and is unrelated to gravitational effects. The prefix **kilo-** stands for "1000"; a kilogram (kg) is equal to 1000 grams (g).

We generally use the term *weight* to describe the mass of an object in a gravitational field. For our purposes, we may consider mass and weight to be the same, but they are not the same in the strictest sense because weight is the force exerted by a body under the influence of gravity, whereas mass remains constant.

Mass is the constant quantity of matter within a physical object.

For example, on earth a 200-lb (91-kg) man weighs more than a 120-lb (55-kg) woman. The difference in weight occurs because of the mutual attraction, called *gravity*, between the earth's mass and the mass of an object, in this case a man or a woman. The moon, on the other hand, has about one sixth of the Earth's mass, so on the moon, the man and the woman each weigh only about one sixth of what they weigh on earth. However, the mass of the man and the mass of the woman remain unchanged at 91 kg and 55 kg, respectively.

Although mass remains unchanged regardless of its surroundings, it can be transformed from one size, shape, and form to another. Consider a 1-kg block of ice, whose shape changes as the ice melts into a puddle of water. If the puddle is allowed to dry, the water apparently disappears entirely. We know, however, that the ice is transformed from a solid to a liquid state and that liquid water becomes water vapor suspended in the air. If we could gather all the molecules making up the ice, the water, and the water vapor and measure their masses, we would find that each form has the same mass.

Energy

Energy is the ability to do work.

Energy is the ability to do work. It is measured in an International System (SI) unit called the *joule (J)*, which is also the unit of work. Like matter, energy can exist in several forms.

Potential energy is the ability to do work by virtue of position. A guillotine blade held aloft by a rope and pulley is an example of an object that possess potential energy (Figure 1-1). If the rope is cut, the blade descends and does its ghastly task. Work is required to get the

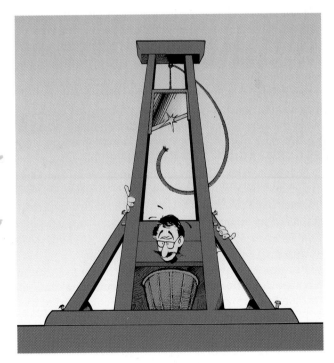

FIGURE 1-1 The blade of a guillotine offers a dramatic example of both potential and kinetic energy. When the blade is pulled to its maximum height and locked in place, it has potential energy. When the blade is allowed to fall, the potential energy is released as kinetic energy.

blade to its high position, and because of this position the blade is said to possess potential energy. Other examples of objects that possess potential energy include a roller coaster on top of the incline and the stretched spring of an open screen door.

Kinetic energy is the energy of motion. It is possessed by all matter in motion: a moving automobile, a turning windmill wheel, a falling guillotine blade. These systems can all do work because of their motion.

Chemical energy is the energy released by a chemical reaction. An important example is the type of energy provided to our bodies through chemical reactions involving the food we eat. At the molecular level, this area of science is called **biochemistry.** The energy released when dynamite explodes is a more dramatic example.

Electrical energy represents the work that can be done when an electron or an electronic charge moves through an electric potential. The most familiar form of electrical energy is normal household electricity, which involves the movement of electrons through a copper wire by an electric potential of 110 volts (V). All electric apparatus, such as motors, heaters, and blowers, function through the use of electrical energy.

Thermal energy (heat) is the energy of motion at the molecular level. It is the kinetic energy of molecules. Thermal energy is measured by temperature. The faster the molecules of a substance are moving, the more thermal energy the substance contains and the higher its temperature is.

Nuclear energy is the energy contained in the nucleus of atom. We control the release and use of this type of energy in nuclear electric power plants. An example of the uncontrolled release of nuclear energy is the atomic bomb.

Electromagnetic energy is perhaps the least familiar form of energy. It is the most important for our purposes, however, because it is the type of energy in an x-ray. In addition to x-rays, electromagnetic energy includes radio waves, microwaves, and visible light.

Just as matter can be transformed from one size, shape, and form to another, energy can be transformed from one type to another. In radiology, for example, electrical energy in the x-ray tube is used to produce electromagnetic energy (the x-ray), which then is converted to chemical energy in the radiographic film.

Reconsider now the statement that all things can be classified as matter or energy. Look around and think of absolutely anything, and you should be convinced of this statement. You should be able to classify anything as matter, energy, or both. Frequently, matter and energy exist side by side: a moving automobile has mass and kinetic energy, and boiling water has mass and thermal energy; the Leaning Tower of Pisa has mass and potential energy.

Perhaps the strangest property associated with matter and energy is that they are interchangeable, a char-acteristic first described by Albert Einstein in his famous theory of relativity. Einstein's **mass-energy equivalence** equation is a cornerstone of that theory.

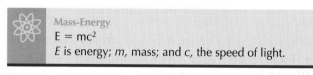

Mass-Energy
$$E = mc^2$$
E is energy; m, mass; and c, the speed of light.

This mass-energy equivalence is the basis for the atomic bomb, nuclear power plants, and certain nuclear medicine imaging techniques.

Energy emitted and transferred through space is called **radiation.** When a piano string vibrates, it is said to radiate sound, which is a form of radiation. Ripples, or waves, radiate from the point where a pebble is dropped into a still pond. Visible light, a form of electromagnetic energy, is radiated by the sun and often is called **electromagnetic radiation.** In fact, electromagnetic energy usually is referred to as *electromagnetic radiation* or simply *radiation.*

 Radiation is the transfer of energy.

Matter that intercepts radiation and absorbs part or all of it is said to be **exposed** or **irradiated.** Spending a day at the beach exposes you to ultraviolet light. Ultraviolet light is the kind of radiation that causes sunburn. During a radiographic examination, the patient is exposed to x-rays. The patient is said to be *irradiated.*

Ionizing radiation is a special type of radiation that includes x-rays. **Ionizing radiation** is any kind of radiation capable of removing an orbital electron from the atom with which it interacts (Figure 1-2). This type of

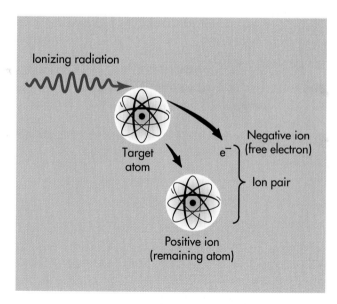

FIGURE 1-2 Ionization is the removal of an electron *(e⁻)* from an atom. The ejected electron and the resulting positively charged atom are called an *ion pair.*

interaction between radiation and matter is called **ionization.** Ionization occurs when an x-ray passes close enough to an orbital electron of an atom to transfer sufficient energy to the electron to cause it to escape from its atom. This free electron may ionize surrounding atoms by transferring energy to them. The orbital electron and the atom from which it was separated are called an **ion pair.** The free electron is a negative ion. The atom is a positive ion.

 Ionization is the removal of an electron from an atom.

Thus any type of energy capable of ionizing matter is known as *ionizing radiation.* X-rays and gamma rays (γ-rays) are the only form of electromagnetic radiation with sufficient energy to ionize. Some fast-moving particles (particles with high kinetic energy) are also capable of ionization. Examples of particle-type ionizing radiation are alpha and beta particles. Although alpha and beta particles are sometimes called *rays,* such designation is incorrect.

SOURCES OF IONIZING RADIATION

Many types of radiation are harmless, but ionizing radiation can seriously injure humans. We are exposed to many sources of ionizing radiation (Figure 1-3). These sources can be divided into two main categories: those that are naturally occurring and those that are made by humans.

There are three components to natural environmental radiation: **cosmic rays, terrestrial radiation,** and naturally occurring radionuclides in the human body, which can be called **internally deposited radionuclides.** Cosmic rays are particulate and electromagnetic radiated by the sun and the stars. On Earth th' cosmic rays increases with altitude and increase. the poles. Terrestrial radiation is emitted from depos.. of uranium, thorium, and other radionuclides in the Earth. The intensity of the terrestrial radiation depends on the geology of the area where deposits are located.

The largest component of natural environmental radiation is **radon.** Radon is a radioactive gas produced by the natural decay of uranium, which is present in trace quantities in the Earth. All Earth-based materials, such as concrete, bricks, and gypsum wallboard, contain radon. Radon is an alpha emitter that principally delivers radiation dose to lung tissue.

Internally deposited radionuclides, mainly potassium −40, are natural metabolites; that is, they are part of the human metabolism. As such, they have been part of environmental radiation for as long as humans have been on the Earth. Human evolution has undoubtedly been influenced by this natural environmental radiation. Some genetic scientists contend that evolution, or changes in the genetic substance of organisms, was influenced by the ionization of deoxyribonucleic acid (DNA). If this is true, it is one more reason to follow radiation-control measures, especially considering the increase in medical applications for radiation over the past century.

Diagnostic x-rays constitute the largest source of man-made ionizing radiation (39 mrem/yr). A millirem (mrem) is 1/1000 of a **rem.** The rem is the unit of *radiation equivalent man;* it is used to express the quantity of radiation received by humans. The approximate average annual dose resulting from medical applications of ionizing radiation (diagnostic x-ray and nuclear medicine studies [see Figure 1-3]) is 53 mrem. Unlike the natural radiation dose of 295 mrem, this level takes into account the people not receiving a radiologic examination and those receiving several examinations within a year.

Question: What percentage of our average annual radiation exposure is due to diagnostic x-ray studies? (See Figure 1-3.)

Answer: $\dfrac{39 \text{ mrem}}{360 \text{ mrem}} = 0.108 \cong 11\%$

Other sources of man-made radiation include nuclear power generation, research applications, industrial sources, and consumer items. Nuclear power stations and other industrial applications contribute very little to our average annual radiation dose. Consumer products such as watch dials, exit signs, smoke detectors, camping lantern mantles, and airport surveillance systems contribue a few millirads to our average annual dose.

DISCOVERY OF X-RAYS

X-rays were not developed; they were discovered and quite by accident. During the 1870s and 1880s, many

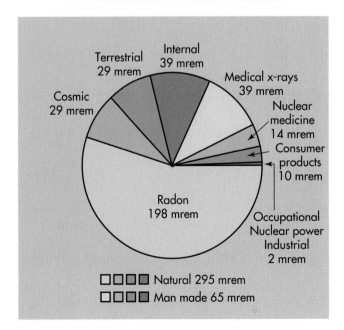

FIGURE 1-3   The contribution of various sources to the average U.S. population radiation dose.

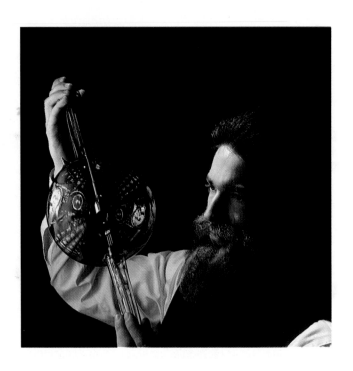

FIGURE 1-4 The type of Crookes tube Roentgen used when he discovered x-rays. Cathode rays (electrons) leaving the cathode are attracted to the anode by the high voltage where x-rays are produced. *(Courtesy Gary Leach.)*

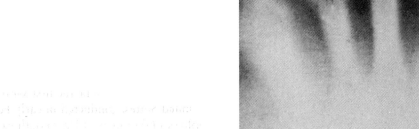

FIGURE 1-5 The hand shown in this radiograph is Mrs. Roentgen's. This was the first indication of the possible medical applications of x-rays and was made within a few days of the discovery. *(Courtesy Deutsches Roentgen Museum.)*

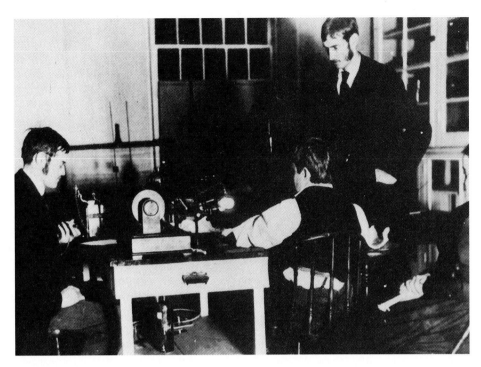

FIGURE 1-6 This photograph records the first medical x-ray examination in the United States. A young patient, Eddie McCarthy of Hanover, New Hampshire, broke his wrist while skating on the Connecticut River and submitted to having it photographed by the X-light. With him are *(left to right)* Professor E.B. Frost, Dartmouth College; his brother, Dr. G.D. Frost, Medical Director, Mary Hitchcock Hospital; and Mrs. G.D. Frost, the hospital's first head nurse. The apparatus was assembled by Professor F.G. Austin in his physics laboratory in Reed Hall, Dartmouth College, on February 3, 1896. *(Courtesy Mary Hitchcock Hospital.)*

university physics laboratories were investigating the conduction of **cathode rays,** or electrons, through a large, partially evacuated glass tube known as a **Crookes tube.** Sir William Crookes was an Englishman from a rather humble background who was a self-taught genius. The tube that bears his name was the forerunner of modern fluorescent lamps and x-ray tubes. There were many different types of Crookes tubes; the majority were capable of producing x-rays. Wilhelm Roentgen was experimenting with a type of Crookes tube when he discovered x-rays (Figure 1-4).

On November 8, 1895, Roentgen was working in his physics laboratory at Würzburg University in Germany. He had darkened his laboratory and completely enclosed his Crookes tube with black photographic paper so that he could better visualize the effects of the cathode rays in the tube. A plate coated with **barium platinocyanide,** a fluorescent material, happened to be lying on a bench several feet from the Crookes tube. No visible light escaped from the Crookes tube because of the black paper enclosing it, but Roentgen noted that the barium platinocyanide glowed regardless of its distance from the Crookes tube. The intensity of the glow increased as the plate was brought closer to the tube. This glow is called **fluorescence.**

There was little doubt about the origin of fluorescence, but the kind of light was unclear. Roentgen called the rays *X-light* because it was an unknown ray. His immediate approach to investigating this "X-light" was to interpose various materials—wood, aluminum, his hand(!)—between the Crooke's tube and the fluorescing plate. He feverishly continued these investigations for weeks.

These initial investigations were extremely thorough, and Roentgen was able to report his experimental results to the scientific community before the end of 1895. In 1901, he received the first Nobel prize in physics for this work. Roentgen recognized the value of his discovery to medicine. He produced and published the first medical x-ray film in early 1896. It was an x-ray image of his wife's hand (Figure 1-5). Figure 1-6 is a photograph of what is reported to be the first x-ray examination in the United States, conducted in early February 1896 in the physics laboratory at Dartmouth College.

There are many amazing features about the discovery of x-rays that cause it to rank high in the events of human history. First, the discovery was accidental. Second, probably no fewer than a dozen contemporaries of Roentgen had previously observed x-radiation, but none of these other physicists had recognized its significance or investigated it. Third, Roentgen followed his discovery with such scientific vigor that within little more than a month he had described x-radiation with nearly all the properties we recognize today.

DEVELOPMENT OF MODERN RADIOLOGY

There are two general types of x-ray examinations: **radiography** and **fluoroscopy**. Radiography uses x-ray film and usually an x-ray tube mounted from the ceiling on a track that allows the tube to be moved in any direction. Such examinations provide the radiologist with fixed, or immovable, images. Fluoroscopy is usually conducted with an x-ray tube located under the examination table. The radiologist is provided with moving or dynamic images on a television monitor. There are many variations of these two basic types of examinations, but in general the x-ray equipment is similar.

To provide an x-ray satisfactory for imaging, one must supply the x-ray tube with sufficient high-voltage electric current. X-ray voltages are measured in **kilovolt peak (kVp)**. One kilovolt (kV) is equal to 1000 volts (V) of electrical potential. X-ray currents are measured in milliamperes (**mA**), where the ampere (A) is a measure of electric current. The prefix **milli-** stands for 1/1000, or 0.001.

Question: The usual x-ray source-to-image receptor distance (SID) is 1 m. How many millimeters is that?

Answer: 1 mm = 1/1000 m or 10^{-3}; therefore 1000 mm = 1 m.

Today, voltage and current are supplied to an x-ray tube through rather complicated electric circuits, but in Roentgen's time, only simple static generators were available. These units could provide currents of only a few milliamperes and voltages to perhaps 50 kVp.

Radiographic procedures using equipment with these limitations of electric current and potential often required exposure times of 30 minutes or more for a satisfactory examination. One development that helped reduce this exposure time was the use of a fluorescent **intensifying screen** in conjunction with the glass photographic plates. Michael Pupin is said to have demonstrated this technique in 1896, but only several years later did it receive adequate recognition and use. Radiographs during Roentgen's time were made by exposing a glass plate with a layer of photographic emulsion coated on one side.

Charles L. Leonard found that by exposing two glass x-ray plates with the emulsion surfaces together, exposure time was halved and the image was considerably enhanced. This demonstration of double-emulsion radiography was conducted in 1904, but **double-emulsion film** did not become commercially available until 1918.

During World War I, radiologists began to make use of film rather than glass plates. Much of the high-quality glass used in radiography came from Belgium and other European countries. This supply was interrupted during World War I. The demands of the army for increased radiologic services made a substitute for the glass plate necessary. The substitute was cellulose nitrate, and it quickly became apparent that the substitute was better than the original glass plate.

The **fluoroscope** was developed in 1898 by the American inventor Thomas A. Edison (Figure 1-7). Edison's original fluorescent material was barium platinocyanide, a widely used laboratory material. He investigated the fluorescent properties of over 1800 other materials, including zinc cadmium sulfide and calcium tungstate, two materials in use today. There is no telling what further inventions Edison might have developed had he continued his x-ray research, but he abandoned it when his assistant and long-time friend, Clarence Dally, suffered a severe x-ray burn that eventually required amputation of both arms. Daily died in 1904 and is counted as the first x-ray fatality in the United States.

Two devices designed to reduce the exposure of patients to x-rays and thereby minimize the possibility of x-ray burn were introduced before the turn of the twentieth century by a Boston dentist, William Rollins. Rollins used x-rays to image teeth and found that restricting the x-ray beam with a sheet of lead having a hole in the center, or a diaphragm, and inserting a leather or aluminum filter improved the diagnostic quality of his

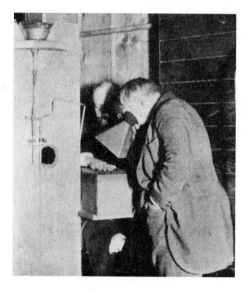

FIGURE 1-7 Thomas Edison is seen viewing the hand of his unfortunate assistant, Clarence Dally, through a fluoroscope of his own design. Dally's hand rests on the box containing the x-ray tube.

radiographs. This first application of **collimation** and **filtration** was followed very slowly by general adoption of these techniques. It was later recognized that these devices reduce the hazard associated with x-rays.

Two developments that occurred at approximately the same time transformed the use of x-rays from a novelty in the hands of a few physicists into a valuable, large-scale medical specialty. In 1907, H.C. Snook introduced a substitute high-voltage power supply, an interrupterless transformer, for the static machines and induction coils then in use. Although the Snook transformer was far superior to these other devices, its capability greatly exceeded the capability of the Crookes tube. It was not until the introduction of the Coolidge tube that the Snook transformer was widely adopted.

 Radiology emerged as a medical specialty because of the Snook transformer and the Coolidge x-ray tube.

The type of Crookes tube that Roentgen used in 1895 had existed for a number of years. Although some modifications were made by x-ray workers, it remained essentially unchanged into the second decade of the twentieth century. After considerable clinical testing, William D. Coolidge unveiled his hot-cathode x-ray tube to the medical community in 1913. It was immediately recognized as far superior to the Crookes tube. It was a vacuum tube and allowed x-ray intensity and energy to be selected separately and with great accuracy. This had not been possible with gas-filled tubes, which made standards for techniques difficult to obtain. X-ray tubes in use today are refinements of the Coolidge tube.

The era of modern radiography is dated from the matching of the Coolidge tube with the Snook transformer; only then did acceptable levels of voltage and current become possible. Few developments since that time have had such a major influence on diagnostic radiology. In 1921 the Potter-Bucky grid, which greatly increased image contrast, was developed. In 1946 the light amplifier tube was demonstrated at the Bell Telephone Laboratories. This device was adapted for fluoroscopy by 1950. Today, image-intensified fluoroscopy is universal.

Each recent decade has seen remarkable improvement in diagnostic imaging. Diagnostic ultrasound appeared in the 1960s; positron emission tomography (PET) and x-ray computed tomography (CT) were developed in the 1970s. Magnetic resonance imaging (MRI) became an accepted modality in the 1980s, and now magnetoencepholography (MEG) is being investigated. Box 1-1 chronologically summarizes some of the more important developments.

BOX 1-1   Some Important Dates in the Development of Modern Radiology

1895:	Roentgen discovers x-rays.
1896:	First medical application of x-rays in diagnosis and therapy are made.
1900:	The American Roentgen Society, the first American radiology organization, is founded.
1901:	Roentgen receives the first Nobel Prize in physics.
1905:	Einstein introduces his theory of relativity and the famous equation, $E = mc^2$.
1907:	The Snook interrupterless transformer is introduced.
1913:	Bohr theorizes his model of the atom, featuring a nucleus and planetary electrons.
1913:	The Coolidge hot-filament x-ray tube is developed.
1917:	Cellulose nitrate film base is widely adopted.
1920:	Several investigators demonstrate the use of soluble iodine compounds as contrast media.
1920:	The American Society of Radiologic Technologists (ASRT) is founded.
1921:	The Potter-Bucky grid is introduced.
1922:	Compton describes the scattering of x-rays.
1923:	Cellulose acetate "safety" x-ray film is introduced (Eastman Kodak).
1925:	The First International Congress of Radiology is convened in London.
1928:	The roentgen is defined as the unit of x-ray intensity.
1929:	Forssmann demonstrates cardiac catherization...on himself!
1929:	The rotating anode tube is introduced. *3400 rpm*
1930:	Tomographic devices are shown by several independent investigators.
1932:	Blue tint is added to x-ray film (Dupont).
1932:	The U.S. Committee on X-Ray and Radium Protection (now the National Council on Radiation Protection and Measurements [NCRP]) issues the first radiation dose limits.
1942:	Morgan exhibits an electronic phototiming device.
1942:	The first automatic film processor (Pako) is introduced.
1948:	Coltman develops the first fluoroscopic image intensifier.

Continued

BOX 1-1   Some Important Dates in the Development of Modern Radiology—cont'd

1951:	Multidirectional tomography (polytomography) is introduced.
1953:	The rad is officially adopted as the unit of absorbed dose.
1956:	Xeroradiography is demonstrated.
1956:	The first automatic-roller-transport film processing (Eastman Kodak) is introduced.
1960:	Polyester-based film is introduced (Dupont).
1963:	Kuhl and Edwards demonstrate single-photon emission computed tomography (SPECT).
1965:	A 90-second rapid processor is introduced (Eastman Kodak).
1966:	Diagnostic ultrasound enters routine use.
1972:	Single-emulsion film and one-screen mammography become available (Dupont).
1973:	Hounsfield completes the development of the first computed tomographic imager (EMI).
1973:	Damadian and Lauterbur produce the first MR images.
1974:	Rare-earth radiographic intensifying screens are introduced.
1979:	Mistretta demonstrates digital fluoroscopy.
1980:	The first commercial superconducting MR imager is introduced.
1981:	The International System (SI) of units is adopted by the International Commission on Radiation Units and Measurements (ICRU).
1982:	Picture archiving and communications systems (PACS) become available.
1983:	The first tabular grain film emulsion (Eastman Kodak) is developed.
1984:	Laser-stimulable phosphors for direct digital radiographs appear (Fuji).
1988:	A superconducting quantum interference device (SQUID) is first used for magnetoencepholography (MEG).
1990:	The last xeromammography system is produced.
1990:	Spiral CT is introduced (Toshiba).
1991:	Twin CT is developed (Elscint).
1992:	The Mammography Quality Standard Acts (MQSA) are passed.
1996:	Direct digital radiography is developed using a flat panel array of thin-film transistors (TFTs).
1998:	Multislice CT is developed by General Electric.
1998:	Amorphous silicon and amorphous selenium are demonstrated for digital radiology.
2000:	The first direct digital mammographic imaging system is made available by General Electric.

REPORTS OF RADIATION INJURY

The first x-ray fatality in the United States occurred in 1904. Unfortunately, radiation injuries occurred rather frequently in the early years. These injuries usually took the form of skin damage (sometimes severe), loss of hair, and anemia. Physicians and more commonly, patients were injured, primarily because of the low energy of radiation available at the time, resulting in the long exposure times required for an acceptable radiograph.

By approximately 1910, reports of radiation-induced injury to patients and physicians decreased. Years later, it was discovered that radiologists were developing blood disorders such as aplastic anemia and leukemia at a much higher rate than others. Because of these observations, radiation-protection devices and apparel, such as lead gloves and aprons, were developed for use by radiologists. X-ray workers were routinely observed for any effects of their occupational exposure and were provided with personnel radiation-monitoring devices. This attention to radiation safety in radiology has been effective.

 Because of effective radiation-protection practices, radiology is now considered a safe occupation.

BASIC RADIATION PROTECTION

Today the emphasis on radiation control in diagnostic radiology has shifted back to protection of the patient. Current studies suggest that even the low doses of x-radiation used in routine diagnostic procedures may result in a small incidence of latent harmful effects. It is also well established that the human fetus is sensitive to x-radiation early in pregnancy.

The National Council on Radiation Protection and Measurements (NCRP) recommends limits of radiation exposure for both radiation workers and the general public. The goal of these recommendations is to minimize the potential for harm to all individuals exposed to man-made sources of radiation.

Another group concerned with radiation safety, the International Committee of Radiation Protection (ICRP) also recommends dose limits. The ICRP was first to introduce the goal of **ALARA** for all radiation workers.

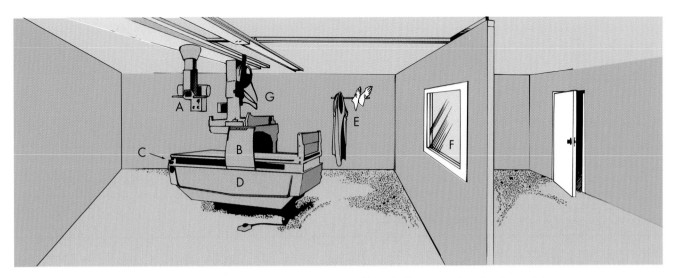

FIGURE 1-8 The general-purpose x-ray room usually includes an overhead radiographic tube (**A**) and a fluoroscopic examining table with an x-ray tube under the table (**D**). Some of the more common radiation-protection devices are a lead curtain (**B**), Bucky slot cover (**C**), leaded apron and gloves (**E**), and protective viewing window (**F**). The location of the image intensifier (**G**) and associated imaging equipment is also shown.

The acronym stands for *as low as reasonably achievable.* ALARA is a concept that recommends some basic rules about radiation exposure but offers no specific quantitative guidelines:

1. Radiation exposure must have a specific benefit.
2. All exposure should be kept as low as reasonably achievable.
3. Individual dose levels should remain below the maximum allowed.

One caution is in order early in training: After working with x-ray imaging systems for a time, you will become so familiar with your work environment that you may become complacent about radiation control. Do not allow yourself to develop this attitude because it can lead to unnecessary radiation exposure. Radiation protection must be the first consideration during each x-ray procedure.

 Always practice ALARA. Keep radiation exposures as *low* as *reasonably achievable.*

Minimizing radiation exposure to the radiologic technologist and patient is easy if the radiographic and fluoroscopic imaging units designed for this purpose are recognized and understood (Figure 1-8).

Filtration. Metal filters, usually aluminum or copper, are inserted into the x-ray tube housing so that low-energy x-rays emitted are absorbed before they reach the patient. These x-rays have little diagnostic value.

Collimation. Collimation restricts the useful x-ray beam to the part of the body being imaged and thereby spares adjacent tissue from unnecessary exposure. Collimators take many different forms. Adjustable light-locating collimators are the most frequently used. Collimation also reduces scatter radiation and thus improves image contrast.

Intensifying screens. Today, most x-ray films are exposed in a cassette with radiographic intensifying screens on both sides of the film. Examinations conducted with radiographic intensifying screens reduce the exposure of the patient to x-rays by more than 95% compared with examinations conducted without radiographic intensifying screens.

Protective apparel. Lead-impregnated material is used to make aprons and gloves worn by radiologists and radiologic technologists during fluoroscopy and some radiographic procedures.

Gonadal shielding. The same lead-impregnated material used in aprons and gloves is used to fabricate gonadal shields. Gonadal shields should be used with all patients of childbearing age when the gonads are in or near the useful x-ray beam and when use of such shielding does not interfere with the diagnostic value of the examination.

Protective barriers. The radiographic control console is always located behind a protective barrier. Often the barrier is lined with lead and equipped with a leaded-glass window. Under normal circumstances, personnel remain behind the barrier during radiographic examination. Figure 1-8 is a rendering of a radiographic/fluoro-

---

BOX 1-2   The Ten Commandments of Radiology

1. Understand and apply the cardinal principles of radiation control: time, distance, and shielding.
2. Do not allow familiarity to result in false security.
3. Never stand in the primary beam.
4. Always wear protective apparel when not behind a protective barrier.
5. Always wear a radiation monitor and position it outside the protective apron at the collar.
6. Never hold a patient during radiographic examination. Use mechanical restraining devices when possible. Otherwise, have parents or friends hold the patient.
7. Always have the person holding the patient wear a protective apron and if possible, protective gloves.
8. Use gonadal shields on all people within childbearing age when such use will not interfere with the examination.
9. Examination of the pelvis and lower abdomen of a pregnant patient should, whenever possible, be avoided, especially during the first trimester.
10. Always collimate to the smallest field size appropriate for the examination.

BOX 1-3   Clinical Skills Required for Examination by the American Registry of Radiologic Technologists

Evaluate the need for and use of protective shielding.
Take appropriate precautions to minimize radiation exposure to patients.
Restrict the beam to limit the exposure area, improve image quality, and reduce radiation dose.
Set the kilovolt, milliamperage, and time or automated exposure systems to achieve optimal image quality, safe operating conditions, and minimum radiation dose.
Prevent all unnecessary people from remaining in area during x-ray exposure.
Take appropriate precautions to minimize occupational radiation exposure.
Wear a personal radiation-monitoring device while on duty.
Review and evaluate individual occupational exposure reports.
Warm-up the x-ray tube according to the manufacturer's recommendations.
Prepare and adjust the radiographic imager and accessories.
Prepare and adjust the fluoroscopic imager and accessories.
Recognize and report malfunctions in the radiographic or fluoroscopic imager and accessories.
Perform basic evaluations of radiographic equipment and accessories (for example, lead aprons, collimator accuracy).
Inspect and clean screens and cassettes.
Perform start-up or shut-down procedures on the automatic processor.
Recognize and report malfunctions in the automatic processor.
Process exposed film.
Reload cassettes by selecting film of the proper size and type.
Store the film or cassette in a manner that will reduce the possibility of artifact production.
Select the appropriate film-screen combination and grid.
Determine appropriate exposure factors using calipers, technique charts, and tube rating charts.
Modify exposure factors for circumstances such as involuntary motion, casts and splints, pathologic conditions, or patient inability to cooperate.
Use radiopaque markers to indicate anatomic side, position, or other relevant information.
Evaluate the patient and radiographs to determine whether additional projections or positions should be recommended.
Evaluate the radiographs for diagnostic quality.
Determine corrective measures if the radiograph is not of diagnostic quality and take appropriate action.
Select equipment and accessories for the examination requested.
Remove all radiopaque materials from patient or table that could interfere with the radiographic image.

---

scopic examination room. Many of the radiation safety features are illustrated.

Other procedures should be followed. Abdominal x-ray examinations of expectant mothers should never be taken during the first trimester unless absolutely necessary. Every effort should be taken to ensure that an examination will not have to be repeated because of technical error. Repeat examinations subject the patient to twice the necessary radiation.

When shielding patients for x-ray examination, one should consider the medical management of the patient. Except for screening mammography, examination of asymptomatic patients is not indicated.

Patients requiring assistance during examination

BOX 1-4 **Personal Skills Required for Examination by the American Registry of Radiologic Technologists**

Explain breathing instructions before making the exposure.
Position the patient using body landmarks to demonstrate the desired anatomic structure.
Explain patient preparation (for example, diet restrictions, preparatory medications) before an imaging procedure.
Properly sequence radiographic procedures to prevent residual contrast material from affecting future examinations.
Examine radiographic requisition to verify the accuracy and completeness of information.
Use universal precautions.
Confirm the patient's identity.
Question female patients of childbearing age about a possible pregnancy.
Explain procedures to the patient or patient's family.
Evaluate the patient's ability to comply with positioning requirements for the requested examination.
Observe and monitor vital signs.
Use proper body mechanics or mechanical transfer devices when assisting patients.
Provide for patient comfort and modesty.
Select immobilization devices, when indicated, to prevent patient movement or ensure patient safety.
Verify the accuracy of patient film identification.
Maintain the confidentiality of patient information.
Use sterile or aseptic technique to prevent the contamination of sterile trays, instruments, or fields.
Prepare contrast media for administration.
Before the administration of contrast agent, gather information to determine whether the patient is at increased risk of adverse reaction.
Perform venipuncture.
Observe the patient after the administration of contrast media to detect adverse reactions.
Recognize the need for prompt medical attention and administer emergency care.
Document required information on the patient's medical record.
Clean, disinfect, or sterilize facilities and equipment and dispose of contaminated items in preparation for next examination.
Follow appropriate procedures when in contact with a patient in reverse or protective isolation.
Monitor medical equipment attached to the patient (for example, intravenous lines, oxygen) during the radiographic procedure.
Position the patient, x-ray tube, and image receptor to produce radiographs.

should never be held by x-ray personnel. Usually, it is best for a member of the patient's family to provide the necessary assistance.

Box 1-2 lists the 10 commandments of radiology. It explains the important aspects of radiation protection.

DIAGNOSTIC IMAGING TEAM

To become part of this exciting profession, a student must complete the prescribed academic courses, obtain clinical experience, and pass the national certification examination given by the American Registry of Radiologic Technologists (ARRT). Both academic expertise and clinical skills are required of radiographers. Box 1-3 is a list of the clinical skills required by an individual who can place *RT* after his or her name. The requisite personal skills are shown in Box 1-4.

SUMMARY

Radiography offers a career in many areas of medical imaging and requires a modest knowledge of medicine, biology, and physics: radiologic science. This first chapter weaves the history and development of radiography

with an introduction to medical physics. Medical physics includes the study of matter, energy, and the electromagnetic spectrum of which x-radiation is a part. It is the production of x-radiation and its safe, diagnostic use that is the basis of radiography. As well as emphasizing the importance of radiation safety, this chapter also presents a detailed list of clinical and patient care skills required by the radiographer.

CHALLENGE QUESTIONS

1. Define or otherwise identify:
   a. Energy
   b. Einstein's mass-energy equivalence equation
   c. Ionizing radiation
   d. The millirad
   e. The average level of natural environmental radiation
   f. The Coolidge tube
   g. Fluoroscopy
   h. Collimation
   i. The term applied to the chemistry of the body
   j. Barium platinocyanide

2. Match the following dates with the appropriate event:
   a. 1901   1. Roentgen discovers x-rays
   b. 1907   2. Roentgen wins first Nobel Prize in physics
   c. 1913   3. The Snook transformer is developed
   d. 1895   4. The Coolidge hot-cathode x-ray tube is introduced

3. Describe how weight is different from mass.

4. Name four examples of electromagnetic radiation.

5. How do x-rays interact differently from other electromagnetic radiation?

6. What is the purpose of x-ray beam filtration?

7. Describe the process that results in the formation of a negative ion and a positive ion.

8. What percentage of average annual radiation exposure to a human is due to medical x-rays?

9. Why was the discovery of x-rays one of the amazing events in human history?

10. Why is radiography now considered a radiation-safe occupation?

11. For what does the acronym *ALARA* stand?

12. Name devices designed for minimizing radiation exposure to the patient and the radiologic technologist.

13. Briefly describe the history of x-ray film.

14. What are the three sources of whole-body radiation exposure from natural sources?

15. What naturally occurring radiation source is responsible for exposure to the lungs?

16. How would you describe the term *radiation?*

17. What are cathode rays?

18. Place the following in chronologic order of appearance:
    a. Digital fluoroscopy
    b. American Society of Radiologic Technologists (ASRT)
    c. Computed tomography (CT)
    d. Radiographic grids
    e. Automatic film processing

19. List five clinical skills required by the ARRT.

20. List five personal skills required by the ARRT.

Mathematics and Terminology for Radiology

OBJECTIVES

At the completion of this chapter, the student should be able to:

1. Calculate problems using fractions, decimals, exponents, and algebraic equations
2. Identify scientific exponential notation and the associated prefixes
3. List and define units of radiation and radioactivity

OUTLINE

Physics owes a great deal of its certainty to the use of mathematics, and accordingly, most of the concepts of physics can be expressed mathematically. It is therefore important in the study of radiologic science to have a solid foundation in the basic concept of mathematics. This chapter defines and illustrates the units of radiation and radioactivity used in medical imaging. A review of mathematics is offered to help with the understanding of such units. Emphasis is placed on basic mathematics topics that apply to x-ray imaging: algebra, number systems, exponents, and graphing. The first sections review fundamental mathematics. You should become proficient at working each type of problem presented in this review.

MATHEMATICS FOR RADIOLOGY
Fractions

A **fraction** is a numerical value expressed by dividing one number by another; it is also called the quotient of two numbers. A fraction has a numerator and a denominator.

> **Fraction**
> $$\text{Fraction} = \frac{x}{y} = \frac{\text{Numerator}}{\text{Denominator}}$$

If the quotient is less than 1 when the numerator is divided by the denominator, the value is a **proper fraction**. **Improper fractions** have a value greater than 1.

Question: Give examples of a proper fraction.

Answer: $\frac{1}{2}, \frac{3}{5}, \frac{5}{7}, \frac{9}{10}$

Question: Give examples of an improper fraction.

Answer: $\frac{3}{2}, \frac{6}{5}, \frac{10}{7}, \frac{13}{10}$

Addition and subtraction. First, find a common denominator and then add or subtract.

> **Adding Fractions**
> $$\frac{x}{y} + \frac{a}{b} = \frac{xb}{yb} + \frac{ay}{yb} = \frac{xb + ay}{yb}$$

Question: What is the value of $\frac{2}{3} + \frac{4}{5}$?

Answer: $\frac{2}{3} + \frac{4}{5} = \frac{10}{15} + \frac{12}{15} = \frac{22}{15}$
an improper fraction

Question: What is the value of $\frac{4}{5} - \frac{2}{3}$?

Answer: $\frac{4}{5} - \frac{2}{3} = \frac{12}{15} - \frac{10}{15} = \frac{2}{15}$
a proper fraction

Multiplication. To multiply fractions, simply multiply numerators and denominators.

> **Multiplying Fractions**
> $$\frac{x}{y} \times \frac{a}{b} = \frac{xa}{yb}$$

Question: What is the value of $\frac{2}{5} \times \frac{7}{4}$?

Answer: $\frac{2}{5} \times \frac{7}{4} = \frac{14}{20} = \frac{7}{10}$
a proper fraction

Question: What is the value of $\frac{9}{8} \times \frac{12}{7}$?

Answer: $\frac{9}{8} \times \frac{12}{7} = \frac{108}{56} = \frac{54}{28}$
an improper fraction

Division. To divide fractions, invert the second fraction and multiply.

> **Dividing Fractions**
> $$\frac{x}{y} \div \frac{a}{b} = \frac{x}{y} \times \frac{b}{a} = \frac{xb}{ya}$$

Question: What is the value of $\frac{5}{2} \div \frac{7}{4}$?

Answer: $\frac{5}{2} \div \frac{7}{4} = \frac{5}{2} \times \frac{4}{7} = \frac{20}{14} = \frac{10}{7}$
an improper fraction

Question: What is the value of $\frac{3}{10} \div \frac{7}{2}$?

Answer: $\frac{3}{10} \div \frac{7}{2} = \frac{3}{10} \times \frac{2}{7} = \frac{6}{70} = \frac{3}{35}$
a proper fraction

A special application of fractions to radiology is the **ratio**. Ratios express the mathematical relationship between similar quantities such as feet to the mile or pounds to the kilogram.

Question: What is the ratio of feet to a mile?

Answer: There are 5260 feet in a mile; therefore the ratio is $\frac{5260 \text{ ft}}{1 \text{ mi}} = 5260 \text{ ft/mi}$.

Question: What is the ratio of kilograms to the pound?

Answer: There are 2.2 kilograms in a pound; therefore the ratio is $\frac{2.2 \text{ kg}}{1 \text{ lb}} = 2.2 \text{ kg/lb}$.

Decimals

Fractions in which the denominator is a power of 10 may easily be converted to decimals.

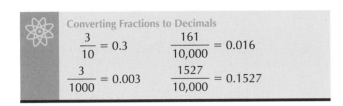

Converting Fractions to Decimals

$$\frac{3}{10} = 0.3 \qquad \frac{161}{10,000} = 0.016$$

$$\frac{3}{1000} = 0.003 \qquad \frac{1527}{10,000} = 0.1527$$

If the denominator is not a power of 10, the decimal equivalent can be found by dividing or by using a calculator.

$$\frac{5}{12} = \text{(long division equation)}$$

$$\begin{array}{r} 0.41\overline{6} \\ 12\,\overline{)5.000} \\ \underline{48} \\ 20 \\ \underline{12} \\ 80 \\ \underline{72} \\ 8 \end{array}$$

The bar above the 6 indicates that this digit is repeating. When one divides 5 by 12, the answer is 0.416666.

Rarely do we convert fractions to decimals without a hand calculator or computer. Depending on the calculator, it is simply a matter of keying numbers in the proper sequence.

Question: What is the decimal equivalent of the proper fraction ³⁄₇?

Answer: ³⁄₇ = 0.429

Question: What is the decimal equivalent of the improper fraction ¹²³⁄₆₉?

Answer: ¹²³⁄₆₉ = 1.78

Significant Figures

Students often wonder how many decimal places to report in an answer. For example, suppose you were asked to find the area of a circle.

Question: What is the area of a circle with radius of 1.25 cm?

Answer: A = πr²
= (3.14) (1.25 cm)²
= (3.14) (1.5625 cm²)
= 4.90625 cm²

This answer is unsuitable, however, since it implies much greater precision in the measurement of the area than we actually have. This result must be rounded off according to specific rules.

 In addition and subtraction, round to the same number of decimal places as the entry with the least number of decimal places to the right of the decimal point.

Question: Add 5.0631, 117.2, and 21.42 and round off the answer.

Answer:
5.0631
117.2
+ 21.42
143.6831
Since 117.2 has one digit, 2, to the right of the decimal point, the answer is 143.7.

Question: Solve the following and round off the answer: 42.8 − 7.614.

Answer:
42.83
− 7.6147
35.2153
Since 42.83 has two digits, 83, to the right of the decimal point, the answer is 35.22.

 In multiplication and division, round to the same number of digits as the entry with the least number of significant figures.

Question: What is the product of 17.24 and 0.382?

Answer:
17.24
× 0.382
6.58568
Since 0.382 has three significant figures and 17.24 has four, the answer must have three digits. The answer is 6.59.

Question: How would you report the area of the circle discussed previously?

Answer: 4.91 cm²

Question: What is the quotient of 3.1416 by 1.05?

Answer: $\frac{3.1416}{1.05} = 2.992$
Since 1.05 has three significant digits and 3.1416 has five significant digits, the answer must have three digits. The answer is 2.99.

Algebra

The rules of algebra provide definite ways to manipulate fractions and equations to solve for unknown quantities. Usually, the unknowns are designed by an alphabetic symbol such as x, y, or z. Three principal rules of algebra are used to solve problems in diagnostic radiology.

 1. When an unknown, x, is multiplied by a number, divide both sides of the equation by that number. ax = c
$$\frac{ax}{a} = \frac{c}{a}$$
$$x = \frac{c}{a}$$

Question: Solve the equation 5x = 10 for *x*.

Answer:
$$5x = 10$$
$$\frac{5x}{5} = \frac{10}{5}$$
$$x = 2$$

2. When numbers are added to an unknown, *x*, subtract that number from both sides of the equation.

$$x + a = b$$
$$x + a - a = b - a$$
$$x = b - a$$

Question: Solve the equation x + 7 = 10.

Answer:
$$x + 7 - 7 = 10 - 7$$
$$x = 3$$

3. When an equation is presented in fractional form, cross-multiply and then solve for the unknown, *x*.

$$\frac{x}{a} = \frac{b}{c}$$
$$\frac{x}{a} \diagdown\!\!\!\!\diagup \frac{b}{c}$$
$$cx = ab$$
$$x = \frac{ab}{c}$$

The crossed arrows show the direction of cross-multiplication.

Question: Solve the equation $\frac{x}{5} = \frac{3}{8}$ for *x*.

Answer:
$$\frac{x}{5} = \frac{3}{8}$$
$$8x = 3 \times 5$$
$$8x = 15$$
$$\frac{8x}{8} = \frac{15}{8}$$
$$x = 1\tfrac{7}{8}$$

Often, it may be necessary to use all three rules to solve a particular problem.

Question: Solve 6x + 3 = 15 for the value of *x*.

Answer:
$$6x + 3 = 15$$
$$6x + 3 - 3 = 15 - 3$$
$$6x = 12$$
$$\frac{6x}{6} = \frac{12}{6}$$
$$x = 2$$

Question: Solve $\frac{4}{x} = \left(\frac{3}{4}\right)^2$ for the value of *x*.

Answer:
$$\frac{4}{x} = \left(\frac{3}{4}\right)^2$$
$$\frac{4}{x} = \frac{9}{16}$$
$$64 = 9x$$
$$\frac{64}{9} = \frac{9x}{9}$$
$$7.1 = x$$

Question: Solve ABx + C = D for *x*.

Answer:
$$ABx + C = D$$
$$ABx + C - C = D - C$$
$$ABx = D - C$$
$$\frac{ABx}{AB} = \frac{D - C}{AB}$$
$$x = \frac{D - C}{AB}$$

Note that the first and third examples are nearly identical in form. Symbols are often used in physics equations instead of numbers.

A special application of fractions and rules of algebra to radiology is the **proportion**. A proportion expresses the relationship of one ratio to another ratio. The ratio of a radiographic grid is directly proportional to the quotient of the height to the interspace (space between grid lines).

Question: If the grid height is 800 μm and the interspace 80 μm, what is the grid ratio?

Answer: $\frac{800 \ \mu m}{80 \ \mu m} = \frac{10}{1}$ the grid ratio

Sometimes this is written 10:1 and expressed as a *10-to-1 ratio.*

The statement, "Gas mileage is inversely proportional to automobile weight," can be used as a numerical proportion to solve for an unknown quantity.

Question: A 1650-lb compact car can go 34 miles per gallon (mpg) of gas. What is the expected mileage for a 3600-lb luxury car?

Answer: Set up the inverse proportion as follows:

$$\frac{x}{1650 \ lb} = \frac{34 \ mpg}{3600 \ lb}$$

and use the rules of algebra to solve for *x*:

$$x = \frac{(34 mpg)(1650 \ lb)}{3600 \ lb}$$
$$x = 15.6 \ mpg$$

Radiation output is directly proportional to the milliampere-seconds (mAs) of an x-ray imaging system.

Question: At 50 mAs the entrance skin exposure (ESE) is 240 mR. What will be the ESE if the mAs is increased to 60 mAs?

TABLE 2-1	Various Ways to Represent Numbers in the Decimal System			
Fractional Form	**Decimal Form**	**Exponential Form**	**Logarithmic Form**	
10,000	10,000	10^4	4.000	
1000	1000	10^3	3.000	
100	100	10^2	2.000	
10	10	10^1	1.000	
1	1	10^0	0.000	
1/10	0.1	10^{-1}	−1.000	
1/100	0.01	10^{-2}	−2.000	
1/1000	0.001	10^{-3}	−3.000	
1/10,000	0.0001	10^{-4}	−4.000	

Answer:
$$\frac{x}{60 \text{ mAs}} = \frac{240 \text{ mR}}{50 \text{ mAs}}$$
$$x = \frac{(240 \text{ mR})(60 \text{ mAs})}{50 \text{ mAs}}$$
$$x = 288 \text{ mR}$$

Number Systems

We use a system of numbers that is based on multiples of 10, called the **decimal system.** The origin of this system is unknown, but there are theories (Figure 2-1). Numbers in this system can be represented in various ways, four of which are shown in Table 2-1. The logarithmic form, although particularly useful in some areas of physics and mathematics, has little application in radiology except in the description of some characteristics of radiographic film.

The superscript on 10 in the exponential form column of Table 2-1 is called the **exponent.** The **exponential form,** often referred to as **power-of-10 notation** or **scientific notation,** is particularly useful in radiology. Note that very large and very small numbers are difficult to write in decimal and fractional form. In radiology, many numbers are either very large or very small. Scientific notation allows these numbers to be written and manipulated with relative ease.

To express a number is scientific notation, first write the number in decimal form. If there are digits to the left of the decimal point, the exponent is positive. To determine the value of this positive exponent, position the decimal point after the first digit and count the number of digits the decimal point was moved. For example, the national debt of the United States was approximately 7 trillion dollars on January 1, 2000. To express this in scientific notation, position the decimal point after the first 7 and count the number of digits moved. This indicates that the exponent will be +12. The U.S. National Debt on Jan. 1, 2000, was $7,327,644,102,329 = 7.3 \times 10^{12}$.

If there are no nonzero digits to the left of the decimal point, the exponent is negative. The value of this negative exponent is found by positioning the decimal point to the right of the first nonzero digit and count-

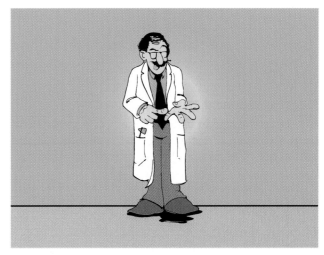

FIGURE 2-1 Probable origin of the decimal number system.

ing the number of digits the decimal point was moved. For example, a string on Robert Earle Keene's guitar has a diameter of 0.00075 m. What is its diameter in scientific notation? First, position the decimal point between the 7 and the 5. Next, count the number of digits the decimal point has moved and express this quantity as the negative exponent: 0.00075 m = 7.5×10^{-4} m.

Another example from physics is a number called **Planck's constant,** symbolized by h. Planck's constant is related to the energy of an x-ray. Its decimal form is:

h = 0.000000000000000000000000000000000663 J s

Obviously, this form is too cumbersome to write each time. Thus Planck's constant is always written in scientific notation:

$$h = 6.63 \times 10^{-34} \text{ J s}$$

Question: Express 4050 in scientific notation.

Answer: $4050 = 4.05 \times 10^3$

Question: Express ½₀₀₀ in scientific notation.

Answer: First convert ½₀₀₀ to decimal form:
$$1/2000 = 0.0005$$
$$0.0005 = 5 \times 10^{-4}$$

Question: X-rays have a velocity of 300,000,000.0 m/s. Express this in scientific notation.

Answer: $300,000,000.0 = 3 \times 10^8$ m/s

Question: Dedicated chest x-ray imaging units were once installed with a 10-ft source-to-image receptor distance (SID). Express this in centimeters in scientific notation.

Answer: $10 \text{ ft} \times \dfrac{12 \text{ in}}{\text{ft}} \times \dfrac{2.54 \text{ cm}}{\text{in}} = 304.8 \text{ cm}$
$$304.8 \text{ cm} = 3.05 \times 10^2 \text{ cm}$$

Actually, today's dedicated chest units are installed at a 3-m SID.

Rules for Exponents

Another advantage of handling numbers in exponential form is evident in operations other than addition and subtraction. The general rules for these types of numerical operations are shown in Table 2-2.

The following examples should sufficiently emphasize the principles involved.

Question: Simplify $2^3/2^5$.

Answer: $2^3/2^5 = 2^{3-5} = 2^{-2} = 1/2^2 = 1/4$

Question: Simplify $(3 \times 10^{10})^2$.

Answer: $(3 \times 10^{10})^2 = 3^2 \times (10^{10})^2$
$$= 9 \times 10^{20}$$

Question: Simplify $(2.718 \times 10^{-4})^3$.

Answer: $(2.718 \times 10^{-4})^3 = (2.718)^3 \times (10^{-4})^3$
$$= 20.08 \times 10^{-12}$$
$$= 2.008 \times 10^{-11}$$

Question: Simplify $2^3/3^2$.

Answer: $2^3/3^2 = \dfrac{2 \times 2 \times 2}{3 \times 3} = \dfrac{8}{9}$

Note, as the last example indicates, that the rules for exponents apply only when the numbers raised to a power are the same.

Question: Given $a = 6.62 \times 10^{-27}$ and $b = 3.766 \times 10^{12}$, what is $a \times b$?

Answer: $a \times b = 6.62 \times 10^{-27} \times 3.766 \times 10^{12}$
$$= (6.62 \times 3.766) \times 10^{-27} \times 10^{12}$$
$$= 24.931 \times 10^{-27 + 12}$$
$$= 24.93 \times 10^{-15}$$
$$= 2.49 \times 10^{-14}$$

Graphing

Knowledge of graphing is essential to the study of radiologic science. It is important not only to be able to read information from graphs but also to graph data obtained from measurements or observations.

Most graphs are based on two axes: a horizontal or **x-axis** and a vertical or **y-axis**. The point where the two axes meet is called the **origin** (labeled 0 in Figure 2-2). Co-

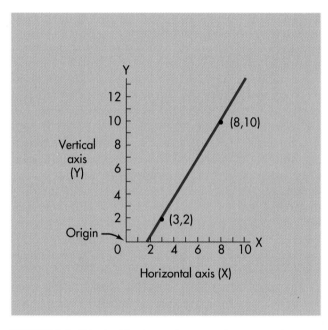

FIGURE 2-2 Principal features of any graph are x- and y-axes that intersect at the origin. Points of data are entered as ordered pairs.

TABLE 2-2	Rules for Handling Numbers in Exponential Form		
	Operation	**Rule**	**Example**
	Multiplication	$10^x \times 10^y = 10^{x+y}$	$10^2 \times 10^3 = 10^{2+3} = 10^5$
	Division	$10^x \div 10^y = 10^{x-y}$	$10^6 \div 10^4 = 10^{6-4} = 10^2$
	Raising to a power	$(10^x)^y = 10^{xy}$	$(10^5)^3 = 10^{5 \times 3} = 10^{15}$
	Inverse	$10^{-x} = 1/10^x$	$10^{-3} = 1/10^3 = 1/1000$
	Unity	$10^0 = 1$	$3.7 \times 10^0 = 3.7$

ordinates have the form of **ordered pairs** (x,y), where the first number of the pair represents a distance along the x-axis and the second number indicates a distance up the y-axis. For example, the ordered pair (3,2) represents a point three units over on the x-axis and two units up on the y-axis. How does it differ from the point (2,3)? If the value of one additional ordered pair is known (e.g., [8,10]), a straight-line graph can be constructed.

In radiologic science the axes of graphs are not usually labeled x and y. Generally, the relationship between two specific quantities is desired. Suppose, for example, that you were asked to graph the effect of mAs on optical density (OD), the darkening of a radiograph.

mAs vs. OD	
mAs	Optical Density
0	0.20
10	0.25
20	0.46
30	0.70
40	0.91
60	1.24
80	1.45
100	1.60

The first step would be to draw the axes. In this example the data are recorded in ordered pairs, where mAs represents the x-value and optical density represents the y-value. Next, note the range of each quantity and choose a convenient scale that allows the data to adequately fill the graph. Very small graphs should generally be avoided. Then label the axes and carefully plot each point. Finally, draw the best smooth curve through the points. The

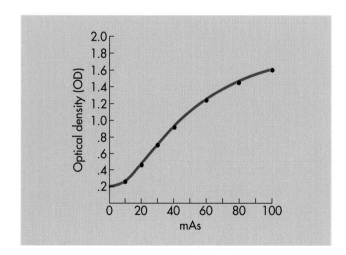

FIGURE 2-3 Relationship of optical density and mAs from the data presented in the text.

curve need not touch each of the plotted points. A completed graph of these data is shown in Figure 2-3.

Question: The following data were obtained from an experiment to determine how much x-radiation it takes to kill 50% of irradiated mice in 30 days ($LD_{50/30}$). Plot this data and estimate the $LD_{50/30}$.

Radiation dose (rad)	No. of mice irradiated	No. of mice dead within 30 days	Percentage lethality
700	36	0	0
750	36	2	6
800	46	5	11
850	36	13	36
900	46	29	64
950	36	31	86
1000	40	37	93

Answer: The columns of data to be plotted are the first and the last. Label the axes so that the range of data is covered. Now plot the ordered pairs of data and connect them with a smooth curve.

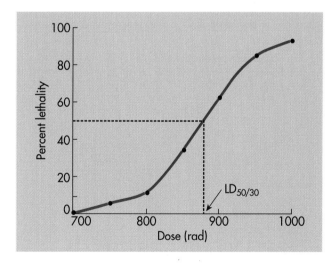

Finally, draw a horizontal line at the 50% lethality level, and when it intersects the smooth curve, drop to the dose axis. This is the $LD_{50/30}$ for the mice in this experiment (approximately 880 rad). The $LD_{50/30}$ for humans is approximately 350 rad.

Often, the data to be plotted are in scientific notation and therefore extend over a very large range of values. In these situations a linear scale is not adequate; a logarithmic scale must be used (Figure 2-4).

Radiologic data frequently require a graph on semilogarithmic paper (Figure 2-5). The y-axis on semilogarithmic paper is a logarithmic scale used to accommodate a wide range of values. The x-axis is a linear scale.

Question: The following data were obtained to determine how much lead (Pb) would be required to reduce x-ray intensity from 330 to 10 mR.

Lead thickness (mm)	0	2	4	6	8
X-ray intensity (mR)	330	140	58	25	11

Plot this data on linear and semilogarithmic graph paper and estimate the thickness of Pb required.

Answer: See Figure 2-5. From the semilogarithmic plot, it is easy to see that the answer is 8.2 mm Pb. The linear plot is not so easy to read.

TERMINOLOGY FOR RADIOLOGY

Every profession has its own language. Radiologic technology is no exception. Several words and phrases characterstic of radiologic technology already have been identified; many more are defined and used throughout this book. For now, an introduction to this terminology should be sufficient.

Numeric Prefixes

In radiologic technology, we must describe very large or very small multiples of standard units. Two units, mil-

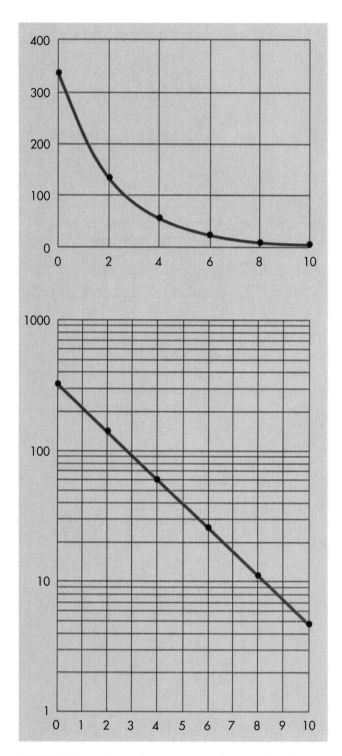

FIGURE 2-5 Semilogarithmic paper is often used for plotting radiologic data.

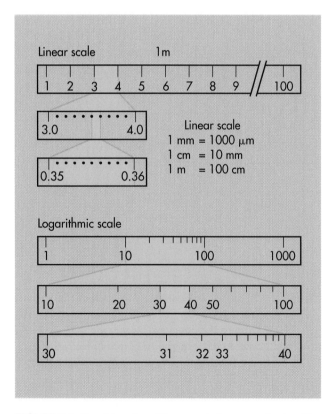

FIGURE 2-4 Equal lengths of linear scale have equal value. The logarithmic scale allows a large range of values to be plotted.

liampere (mA) and kilovolt peak (kVp), have already been discussed. By writing 70 kVp instead of 70,000 volt peak, we can understandably express the same quantity with fewer characters. For such economy of expression, scientists have devised a system of prefixes and symbols (Table 2-3).

Question: How many kilovolts equal 37,000 volts?

Answer: $37,000 \text{ V} = 37 \times 10^3 \text{ V}$
$$= 37 \text{ kV}$$

Question: The diameter of a blood cell is about 10 micrometers (μm). How many meters is that?

Answer: $10 \, \mu\text{m} = 10 \times 10^{-6} \text{ m}$
$$= 10^{-5} \text{ m}$$
$$= 0.00001 \text{ m}$$

Radiologic Units

The four units used to measure radiation should become a familiar part of your vocabulary. Figure 2-6 relates them to a hypothetical situation in which they would be used. Table 2-4 shows the relationship of the customary radiologic units to their international equivalents.

In 1981, the International Commission on Radiologic Units (ICRU) issued standard units that have since been adopted by all except the United States. Most U.S. scien-

TABLE 2-3	Standard Scientific and Engineering Prefixes	
Multiple	**Prefix***	**Symbol**
10^{18}	exa-	E
10^{15}	peta-	P
10^{12}	tera-	T
10^{9}	giga-	G
10^{6}	**mega-**	**M**
10^{3}	**kilo-**	**k**
10^{2}	hecto-	h
10^{1}	deka-	da
10^{-1}	deci-	d
10^{-2}	**centi-**	**c**
10^{-3}	**milli-**	**m**
10^{-6}	**micro-**	μ
10^{-9}	nano-	n
10^{-12}	pico-	p
10^{-15}	femto-	f
10^{-18}	atto-	a

*Boldfaced prefixes are those frequently used in radiologic science.

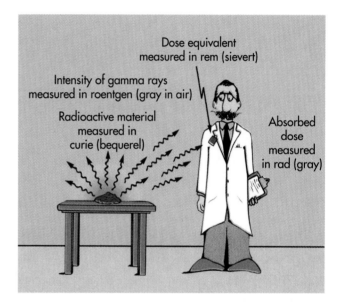

FIGURE 2-6 Radiation is emitted by radioactive material. The quantity of radioactive material is measured in becquerels. Radiation quantity is measured in roentgens, rads, or rems, depending on precise use. In diagnostic imaging, we may consider 1 R = 1 rad = 1 rem.

TABLE 2-4	Special Quantities of Radiologic Science and Their Associated Special Units				
	CUSTOMARY UNIT			**SI UNIT**	
Quantity	**Name**		**Symbol**	**Name**	**Symbol**
Exposure	roentgen		R	air kerma	Gy_a
Absorbed dose	rad		rad	gray	Gy_t
Effective dose	rem		rem	seivert	Sv
Radioactivity	curie		Ci	becquerel	Bq
Multiply	R	by	0.01	to obtain	Gy_a
Multiply	rad	by	0.01	to obtain	Gy_t
Multiply	rem	by	0.01	to obtain	Sv
Multiply	Ci	by	3.7×10^{10}	to obtain	Bq

tific journals and societies have adopted Le Systéme Internationale des Unites (The International System of Units, or SI), but regulatory agencies and the American Registry of Radiologic Technologists (ARRT) have not. Consequently, this book uses the customary radiologic units followed by the SI equivalent in parentheses throughout.

Roentgen (R) or coulomb/kilogram (C/kg) (Gy_a). The roentgen is equal to the radiation intensity that will create 2.08×10^9 ion pair in a cubic centimeter of air; that is, $1 R = 2.08 \times 10^9$ ip/cm³. The official definition, however, is in terms of electric charge per unit mass of air (1 R = 2.58×10^{-4} C/kg). The charge refers to the electrons liberated by ionization. The roentgen was first defined as a unit of radiation quantity in 1928. Since then, the definition has been revised many times. Radiation monitors usually are calibrated in roentgens. The output of x-ray imaging systems usually is specified in milliroentgen (mR). The roentgen applies only to x-rays and gamma rays and their interactions with air. In keeping with the adoption of the Wagner/Archer method described in the preface, the SI unit of air kerma (mGy_a) is used.

 The roentgen is the unit of radiation exposure or intensity.

Question: The output intensity of an x-ray imaging system is 100 mR. What is this value in SI units?

Answer: 100 R = 1 Gy_a
100 mR = 0.001 Gy_a
100 mR = 1 mGy_a

Rad (rad) (Gy_t). Biologic effects usually are related to the radiation *absorbed dose*, and therefore the rad is the unit most often used when describing the quantity of radiation received by a patient. The rad is used for any type of ionizing radiation and any exposed matter, not just air. One rad is equal to 100 erg/g (10^{-2} Gy_t), where the **erg (joule)** is a unit of energy and the **gram (kilogram)** is a unit of mass.

 The rad is the unit of *r*adiation *a*bsorbed *d*ose.

Rem (rem) (Sv). Occupational radiation-monitoring devices, such as film badges, are analyzed in terms of rem (*r*ad *e*quivalent in *m*an). The rem is used to express the quantity of radiation received by radiation workers and populations. *Effective dose* or *effective dose equivalent* is a term used to specify the relative risk of biologic effect caused by radiation exposure. Some types of radiation produce more damage than x-rays. The rem accounts for these diffferences in biologic effectiveness. This is particularly important to people working near nuclear reactors or particle accelerators or with x-rays.

 The rem is the unit of occupational radiation exposure expressed as effective dose (E).

Curie (Ci) (Bq). The curie is the unit of the quantity of radioactive material and not the radiation emitted by that material. One curie is that quantity of radioactivity in which 3.7×10^{10} nuclei disintegrate every second (3.7×10^{10} Bq). The millicurie (mCi) and microcurie (μCi) are common quantities of radioactive material. Radioactivity and the curie have nothing to do with x-rays.

 The curie is a unit of radioactivity.

Question: 0.05 μCi ^{125}I is used for radioimmunoassay. What is this radioactivity in becquerel?

Answer: 0.05 μCi = 0.05×10^{-6} Ci
= $(5 \times 10^{-8}$ Ci$)(3.7 \times 10^{10}$ Bq/Ci$)$
= 1.85×10^3 Bq = 1850 Bq

Diagnostic radiology is concerned primarily with x-rays. For x-ray exposure to humans, we may consider that 1 R is equal to 1 rad is equal to 1 rem (1 mGy_a = 1 mGy_t = 1 mSv). With other types of ionizing radiation, this generalization is not true.

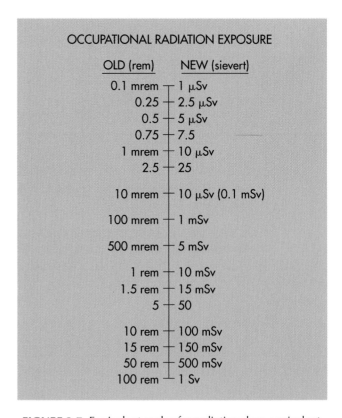

FIGURE 2-7 Equivalent scales for radiation dose equivalent.

SUMMARY

The technical aspects of radiography are complex. A basic knowledge of mathematics, as well as identification and proper use of the units of radiation measurements, is required. As you review this chapter, consider again fraction/decimal conversion, algebraic relationships, numeric prefixes and exponents, and graphing. All are important for understanding the principles of radiologic science related to x-ray imaging. Figure 2-7 summarizes the conversion from conventional units of occupational radiation exposure to SI units.

CHALLENGE QUESTIONS

1. Define or otherwise identify the following:
   a. Linear scale
   b. Significant figure
   c. Radiologic unit
   d. Ordered pair
   e. Units of Planck's constant
   f. Ratio
   g. Logarithmic scale
   h. y in the fraction x/y
   i. Scientific notation

2. Determine your height in the SI system.

3. Simplify the fraction $2^2/2^5$.

4. Solve the following:
   a. $\dfrac{7}{8} + \dfrac{5}{32} =$
   b. $\dfrac{4}{9} \times \dfrac{3}{8} =$
   c. $\dfrac{16}{2} \div \dfrac{4}{9} =$

5. Write the following as decimals:
   a. $\dfrac{7}{10} =$
   b. $\dfrac{81}{1000} =$
   c. $\dfrac{7}{15} =$

6. Write the following in scientific notation:
   a. 1,480,000
   b. 711,000

7. Write the following in scientific notation:
   a. 0.0042
   b. 0.01067

8. Solve the following:
   a. $(2 \times 10^6) \times (4 \times 10^4) =$
   b. $(8 \times 10^{15}) \div (2 \times 10^5) =$

9. Solve the following:
   a. $3x - 9 = 12; x =$
   b. $\dfrac{x}{3} = \dfrac{5}{7}; x =$

10. Given $a = 6.62 \times 10^{-27}$ and $b = 3.766 \times 10^{12}$, what is $a \times b$?

11. Find the decimal equivalent of 3/1000.

12. What is the decimal equivalent of 5/12?

13. What is the first step when adding or subtracting fractions?

14. What sequence of steps should be taken when dividing fractions?

15. What does the phrase *directly proportional to* mean?

16. Which number system is easiest for you to understand?

17. What is the product of 17.24 and 0.382? Round off to the appropriate decimal place.

18. In the equation $x/5 = 3/8$, $x =$

19. If gas mileage were inversely proportional to automobile weight, what would be the expected mileage for a 1600-kg car if a 750-kg car gets 14 km/L?

20. Radiation exposure is directly proportional to the technical factor mAs. At 50 mAs the entrance skin exposure (ESE) is 240 mR. What will be the ESE if the exposure technique is increased to 60 mAs?

Fundamentals of Physics

OBJECTIVES

At the completion of this chapter, the student should be able to:

1. Discuss the derivation of scientific systems of measurement
2. List the three systems of measurement
3. Identify nine categories of mechanics

OUTLINE

In Chapter 1, *matter* and *energy* are defined. Mechanics, which involves matter in motion, is discussed in this chapter. This chapter also includes a discussion of the standard units of measurement needed to describe matter, energy, and mechanics.

Physics is traditionally grouped into fields such as thermodynamics, optics, acoustics, mechanics, electromagnetism, and atomic and nuclear physics. In radiography, however, physics is limited principally to mechanics and electromagnetism.

STANDARD UNITS OF MEASUREMENT

Physics is the study of interactions of matter and energy in all their diverse forms. Like all scientists, physicists strive for exactness or certainty in describing these interactions. Consider, for example, the act of kicking a football. If several observers were asked to describe this event, each would give a description based on his or her perception. One might describe the stature of the kicker and the kicking stance. Another might simply conclude that "a football was kicked about 30 yards" or "the kick was wide left." There could be as many different descriptions as observers.

Physicists, however, try to remove uncertainty by eliminating subjective descriptions such as these. A physicist describing this event might determine quantities such as the mass of the football, the initial velocity of the ball, the wind velocity, and the exact distance the football travels. Each of these requires a measurement that ultimately can be represented by a number. Assuming that all measurements are correctly made, each observer using the methods of physics obtains exactly the same results.

In addition to seeking certainty, physicists strive for simplicity. There are three measurable quantities that are considered basic. These base quantities are **length, mass,** and **time,** and they are the building blocks of all other quantities. Figure 3-1 indicates the roles that these base quantities play in supporting some of the other quantities used in radiologic science. The secondary quantities are called **derived quantities,** since they are derived from a combination of one or more of the three base quantities. For example, volume is length cubed (l^3), density is mass divided by volume (m/l^3), and velocity is length divided by time (l/t). Additional quantities are designed to support measurement in specialized areas of science and technology. These additional quantities are called **special quantities;** in radiology the special quantities are **exposure, dose, effective dose,** and **radioactivity,** which are discussed in Chapter 2.

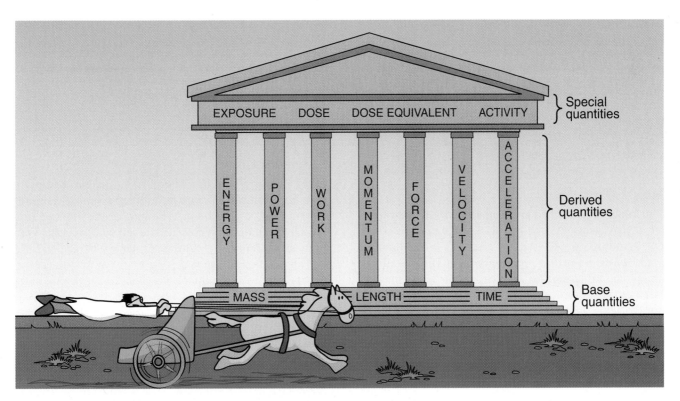

FIGURE 3-1 Base quantities support derived quantities, which in turn support the special quantities of radiologic science.

TABLE 3-1	System of Units			
	SI Units*	**MKS**	**CGS**	**British**
Length	Meter (m)	Meter (m)	Centimeter (cm)	Foot (ft)
Mass	Kilogram (kg)	Kilogram (kg)	Gram (g)	Pound (lb)†
Time	Second (s)	Second (s)	Second (s)	Second (s)

*The SI includes four additional base units. See Table 3-2.
†The pound is actually a unit of force but is related to mass.

Whether a physicist is studying something large, such as the universe, or something small, such as an atom, meaningful measurements must be reproducible. Therefore once the fundamental quantities are established, it is essential that they be related to a well-defined and invariable standard. Standards are normally defined by international organizations and usually redefined when the progress of science requires greater precision.

Length

For many years the standard unit of length was accepted to be the distance between two lines engraved on a platinum-iridium bar kept at the International Bureau of Weights and Measures in Paris. This distance was defined to be exactly one meter (1 m).

The English-speaking countries also base their standards of length on the meter.

$$1 \text{ yd} = 0.9144 \text{ m}$$
$$1 \text{ in} = 2.54 \text{ cm} = 0.0254 \text{ m}$$

In 1960, the need for a more accurate standard of length led to the redefinition of the meter in terms of the wavelength of orange light emitted from an isotope of krypton (^{86}Kr). One meter is now defined as 1,650,763.73 wavelengths of this light.

The meter (m) is based on the wavelength of light emitted by ^{86}Kr.

Mass

The kilogram is defined as the mass of 1000 cm³ of water at 0° Celsius (°C). In the same vault in Paris where the standard meter is kept, there is a cylinder of platinum-iridium that represents the standard unit of mass—the **kilogram (kg)**, which has the same mass as 1000 cm³ of water. As discussed in Chapter 1, mass is not the same quantity as weight. The kilogram is a unit of mass, whereas the newton or the pound, a British unit, are units of weight.

The kilogram (kg) is the mass of 1000 cm³ of water at 0° C.

TABLE 3-2	Four Aditional Base SI Units	
Radiologic Quantities	**Special Units**	**SI Units**
Exposure	C/kg	Air kerma (Gy$_a$)
Dose	J/kg	Gray$_t$ (Gy$_t$)
Effective Dose	J/kg	Seivert (Sv)
Radioactivity	s^{-1}	Becquerel (Bq)

Time

The standard unit of time is the **second (s)**. Originally, the second was defined as a fraction of the rotation of the earth on its axis—the mean solar day. In 1956, it was redefined as a fraction of the tropical year 1900. In 1964, the need for a better standard of time led to another definition. Now, time is measured by an atomic clock and is based on the vibration of cesium (Cs) atoms. The atomic clock is capable of keeping time correctly to about 1 s in 5000 years. The accuracy of future hydrogen maser clocks promises to be even greater—perhaps to 1 s in several million years.

The second (s) is based on the vibration of atoms of Cs.

Systems of Units

Every measurement has two parts: a **magnitude** and a **unit**. For example, the standard source-to-image receptor distance (SID) is 100 cm. The magnitude, 100, is not meaningful unless a unit is also designated. Here the unit of measurement is the centimeter (cm).

Table 3-1 shows that there are four systems of units to represent the base quantities. The MKS (meters, kilograms, seconds) and the CGS (centimeters, grams, seconds) systems are more widely used in science and in most countries of the world than the British system. Le Système Internationale des Unites (International System of Units, or SI) is an extension of the MKS system and represents the present state of units. SI includes the three base units of the MKS system plus an additional four. (Table 3-2). There are derived units and special units of SI to represent derived quantities and special quantities.

> The same system of units must always be used when working on problems or reporting answers.

The following would be unacceptable because of improper units: Mass density = 8.1 g/ft³ and pressure = 700 lb/cm².

Mass density should be reported with units of grams per cubic centimeter (g/cm³), kilograms per cubic meter (kg/m³), or pounds per cubic foot (lb/ft³). Pressure should be given in pounds per square inch (lb/in²) or newtons per square meter (N/m²).

Question: The dimensions of a box are 30 cm × 86 cm × 4.2 m. Find the volume.

Answer: The formula for the volume of a rectangle is given by:
$$V = \text{Length} \times \text{Width} \times \text{Height}$$
OR
$$V = lwh$$
Since the dimensions are given in different systems of units, however, we must choose only one system. Therefore:
$$V = (0.30 \text{m})(0.86 \text{ m})(4.2 \text{m})$$
$$= 1.1 \text{ m}^3$$

Note that the units are multiplied also: m 3 m 3 m 5 m³.

Question: Find the mass density of a ball with a volume of 200 cm³ and a mass of 0.4 kg.

Answer: D = Mass/Volume   (change 0.4 kg to 400 g)
$$= 400 \text{ g}/200 \text{ cm}^3$$
$$= 2 \text{ g/cm}^3$$
OR
$$D = \frac{0.4 \text{ kg}}{200 \text{ cm}^3 \times \frac{1 \text{m}^3}{10^6 \text{ cm}^3}} \quad \text{(change 200 cm}^3 \text{ to } 2 \times 10^{-4} \text{m}^3\text{)}$$
$$= \frac{0.4 \text{ kg}}{2 \times 10^{-4} \text{m}^3}$$
$$= \frac{0.4 \text{ kg}}{2 \text{ m}^3} \times 10^4$$
$$= 4000 \text{ kg}/2 \text{ m}^3$$
$$= 2000 \text{ kg/m}^3$$

Question: The area marked for imaging on a patient measures 9 inches thick. The SID is 100 cm. What will be the magnification of the skin marker?

Answer: The formula for magnification is as follows:
$$M = \frac{SID}{SOD} = \frac{\text{Source-to-image receptor distance}}{\text{Source-to-object distance}}$$
$$M = \frac{SID}{SOD} = \frac{100 \text{ cm}}{100 \text{ cm} - 9 \text{ inches}}$$
The 9 inches must be converted to centimeters so that the units are consistent.
$$M = \frac{SID}{SOD} = \frac{100 \text{ cm}}{100 \text{ cm} - (9 \text{ inches} \times 2.54 \text{ cm/in})}$$
$$= \frac{100 \text{ cm}}{100 \text{ cm} - (23 \text{ cm})}$$
$$= \frac{100 \text{ cm}}{77 \text{ cm}}$$
$$= 1.3$$

MECHANICS

Mechanics is a segment of physics that deals with the motion of objects. Many of the quantities studied in mechanics depend on the direction of motion and are known as *vectors*. A **vector** is a quantity that has both **magnitude** and **direction**. Quantities that have magnitude only are called **scalars**. A vector description of a distance might be 36 km, North. This distance reported as a scalar would be 36 km.

Velocity

The motion of an object can be described by the use of two terms: **velocity (v)** and **acceleration (a)**. Velocity, sometimes called **speed**, is a measure of how fast something is moving or more precisely, the rate of change of its position with time. The velocity of a car is measured in miles per hour (kilometer per hour). Units of velocity in SI are meters per second (m/s). The equation for velocity (v) is:

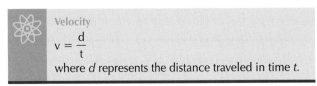

> **Velocity**
> $$v = \frac{d}{t}$$
> where *d* represents the distance traveled in time *t*.

Question: What is the velocity of a ball that travels 60 m in 4 s?

Answer: v = d/t
$$= 60 \text{ m}/4 \text{ s}$$
$$= 15 \text{ m/s}$$

Question: Light is capable of traveling 669 million miles in 1 hr. What is its velocity in SI units?

Answer: $$v = \frac{d}{t}$$
$$= \frac{6.69 \times 10^8 \text{ miles}}{1 \text{ hr}} \times \frac{1609 \text{ m/mile}}{3600 \text{ s/hr}}$$
$$= 2.99 \times 10^8 \text{ m/s}$$

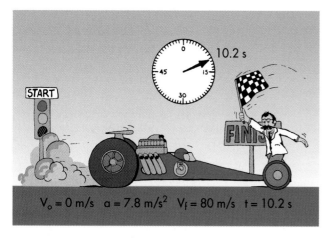

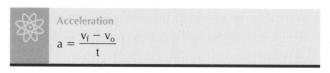

$V_o = 0$ m/s $a = 7.8$ m/s^2 $V_f = 80$ m/s $t = 10.2$ s

FIGURE 3-2 Drag racing provides a familiar example for the relationships among initial velocity, final velocity, acceleration, and time.

Velocity of Light
The velocity of light is constant. It is symbolized by c: $c = 3 \times 10^8$ m/s.

Often the velocity of an object changes as its position changes. For example, a dragster running a race starts from rest and finishes with a velocity of 80 m/s. The initial velocity designated by v_o is zero (Figure 3-2). The final velocity represented by v_f is 80 m/s. The average velocity can be calculated from the expression:

Average Velocity

$$\bar{v} = \frac{v_o + v_f}{2}$$

where the bar over the *v* represents average velocity.

Question: What is the average velocity of the dragster?

Answer: $\bar{v} = \dfrac{0 \text{ m/s} + 80 \text{ m/s}}{2}$
                 $= 40$ m/s

Question: A Corvette can reach a velocity of 88 mph in ¼ mile. What is its average velocity?

Answer: $\bar{v} = \dfrac{v_o + v_f}{2}$
                 $= \dfrac{0 + 88}{2}$
                 $= 44$ mi/hr

Acceleration

The rate of change of velocity with time is **acceleration (a)**. It is how "fast" the velocity is changing. Since acceleration is velocity divided by time, the unit is meters per second squared (m/s^2).

If velocity is constant, the acceleration is zero. On the other hand, a constant acceleration of 2 m/s^2 means that the velocity of an object increased by 2 m/s each second. The defining equation for acceleration is given by:

Acceleration

$$a = \frac{v_f - v_o}{t}$$

Question: What is the acceleration of the dragster?

Answer: $a = \dfrac{80 \text{ m/s} - 0 \text{ m/s}}{10.2 \text{ s}}$
                 $= 7.8$ m/s^2

Question: A 5L Mustang can accelerate to 60 mph in 5.9 s. What is the acceleration in SI units?

Answer: $a = \dfrac{v_f - v_o}{t}$
                 $= (60 \text{ mph} \times 1609 \text{ m/mi}) \div 3600 \text{ s/hr}$
                 $= 26.8$ m/s
                 $a = \dfrac{26.8 - 0}{5.9}$
                 $= 4.5$ m/s^2

Newton's Law of Motion

In 1686 the English scientist, Isaac Newton, presented three principles that even today are recognized as **fundamental laws of motion.**

Newton's First Law: Inertia
A body will remain at rest or continue to move with a constant velocity in a straight line unless acted on by an external force.

Newton's first law states that if no force acts on an object, there will be no acceleration. The property of matter that acts to resist a change in its state of motion is called **inertia**. Newton's first law is thus often referred to as the **law of inertia** (Figure 3-3). A portable x-ray imaging system obviously does not move until forced by a push. Once in motion, however, it continues to move forever, even when the pushing force is removed, unless an opposing force—friction—is present.

Newton's Second Law: Force
The force (F) acted on an object with acceleration (a) is equal to the mass (m) multiplied by the acceleration.
$F = m \times a$

The SI unit of force is the newton (N). Newton's second law is illustrated in Figure 3-4.

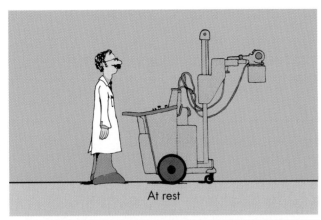

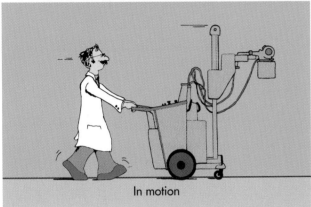

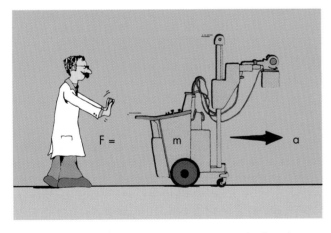

FIGURE 3-3 Newton's first law states that a body at rest remains at rest and a body in motion continues in motion until acted on by an outside force.

FIGURE 3-4 Newton's second law states that the force applied to move an object is equal to the mass of the object multiplied by the acceleration.

Question: Find the force on a 55-kg mass accelerated at 14 m/s².

Answer: $F = ma$
$= (55 \text{ kg})(14 \text{ m/s}^2)$
$= 770 \text{ N}$

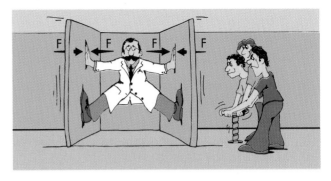

FIGURE 3-5 Crazed student technologists performing a routine physics experiment to prove Newton's third law.

Question: For a 3600-lb (1636-kg) Explorer to accelerate at 15 m/s, what force is required?

Answer: $F = ma$
$= (1636 \text{ kg})(15 \text{ m/s})$
$= 24,540 \text{ N}$

 Newton's Third Law: Action/Reaction
For every action there is an equal and opposite reaction.

According to Newton's third law, if you push on a heavy block, the block will push back on you with the same force that you apply. On the other hand, if you were the physics professor illustrated in Figure 3-5, whose crazed students had tricked him into the clamp room, no matter how hard you pushed, the walls would continue to close because the force is opposite but not equal.

Weight

Weight (Wt) is a **force** on a body caused by the downward pull of gravity (g) on it. Experiments have shown that objects falling to earth accelerate at a constant rate. This rate, termed the **acceleration of gravity (g)**, has the following values on earth:

$g = 9.8 \text{ m/s}^2$ in SI units
$g = 32 \text{ ft/s}^2$ in British units

The value of gravity on the moon is only about one sixth that on the earth. "Weightlessness" observed in outer space is due to the absence of gravity. Thus the value of gravity in space is zero. The weight of an object is equal to the product of its mass and the acceleration of gravity.

Weight
$Wt = mg$

The units of weight are the same as those for force: newtons and pounds.

Weight is the product of mass and the acceleration of gravity on earth, 1 lb = 4.5 N.

Question: A student has a mass of 75 kg. What is her weight on the earth? On the moon?

Answer: Earth: g = 9.8 m/s²
$$Wt = mg$$
$$= 75 \text{ kg } (9.8 \text{ m/s}^2)$$
$$= 735 \text{ N}$$
Moon: g = 1.6 m/s²
$$Wt = mg$$
$$= 75 \text{ kg } (1.6 \text{ m/s}^2)$$
$$= 120 \text{ N}$$

The example displays an important concept. The weight of an object can vary according to the value of gravity acting on it. Note, however, that the mass of an object does not change regardless of its location. The student's 75-kg mass remains the same on earth, on the moon, or in space.

Momentum

The product of the mass of an object and its velocity is called **momentum**, represented by **p**.

 Momentum
$$p = mv$$

The greater the velocity of an object, the more momentum the object possesses. A truck accelerating down a hill, for example, gains momentum as its velocity increases.

 Momentum is the product of mass and velocity.

The total momentum before any interaction is equal to the total momentum after the interaction. Imagine a billiard ball colliding with two other balls at rest (Figure 3-6). The total momentum before the collision is the mass multiplied by the velocity of the cue ball. After the collision, this momentum is shared by the three balls. Thus the original momentum of the cue ball is conserved after the interaction.

Work

Work, as used in physics, has specific meaning. The work done on an object is the force applied multiplied by the distance (d) over which it is applied. In mathematical terms:

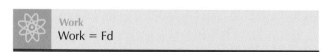 Work
Work = Fd

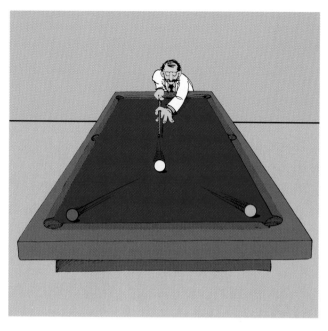

FIGURE 3-6 The conservation of momentum occurs with every pool shot.

The unit of work is the joule (J) in SI. In a diagnostic imaging department, lifting a radiographic cassette is work. As defined in physics, no work is done, however, when the cassette is held motionless.

 Work is the product of force and distance.

Question: Find the work done in lifting an infant weighing 90 N (20 lb) to a height of 1.5 m.

Answer: Work = Fd
$$= (90 \text{ N})(1.5 \text{ m})$$
$$= 135 \text{ J}$$

Power

Power (P) is the rate of doing work. Recall that the same amount of work is required to lift a cassette to a given height, whether it takes 1 second or 1 minute to do so. Power gives us a way to include the time required to perform the work. The equation for power is:

 Power
P = Work/t = Fd/t

The SI unit of power is the joule/second (J/s), which is called the **watt (W)**. The British unit of power is the **horsepower (hp)**.

1 hp = 746 W
1000 W = 1 kilowatt (kW)

Power is work divided by time.

Question: A radiographer lifts a 0.8-kg cassette from the floor to the top of a 1.5-m table with an acceleration of 3 m/s^2. What is the power exerted if it takes 1.2 s?

Answer: This is a multistep problem. We know that P = work/t; however, the value of work is not given in the problem. Recall that work = Fd and F = ma. First, find F.

F = ma
$\quad$ = (0.8 kg)(3 m/s^2)
$\quad$ = 2.4 N

Next, find work:

Work = Fd
$\quad\quad$ = (2.4 N)(1.5 m)
$\quad\quad$ = 3.6 J

Now, P can be determined:

P = Work/t
$\quad$ = 3.6 J/1.2 s
$\quad$ = 3 W

Question: A hurried radiographer pushes a 35-kg portable down a 25-m hall in 9 seconds with a final velocity of 3 m/s. How much power did this require?

Answer:

$$a = \frac{v_f - v_o}{t}$$

$$a = \frac{3 - 0}{9}$$

$\quad\quad$ = 0.33 m/s^2

F = ma
$\quad$ = 35 kg × 0.33 m/s^2
$\quad$ = 11.6 N

Work = Fd
$\quad\quad$ = 11.6 N × 25 m
$\quad\quad$ = 290 J

P = 290 J/9 s
$\quad$ = 32 W

Energy

Energy is the ability to do work. The forms of energy are discussed in Chapter 1. The **law of conservation of energy** states that energy may be transformed from one form to another but cannot be created or destroyed; the total amount of energy is constant. For example, electrical energy is converted into light energy and heat energy in an electric light bulb. The unit of energy and work is the same: the joule.

Energy
Energy is the ability to do work.

Two forms of **mechanical energy** are often used in radiologic science: kinetic energy and potential energy. **Kinetic energy (KE)** is the energy associated with the motion of an object as expressed by the following:

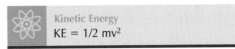
Kinetic Energy
KE = 1/2 mv^2

It is apparent that KE depends on the mass of the object and on the square of its velocity.

Question: Consider two rodeo chuck wagons, A and B, with the same mass. If B has twice the velocity of A, verify that the KE of chuck wagon B is four times that of chuck wagon A.

Answer: Chuck wagon A: KE$_A$ = ½ mv$_A^2$
Chuck wagon B: KE$_B$ = ½ mv$_B^2$
However, m$_A$ = m$_B$, v$_B$ = 2v$_A$
therefore KE$_B$ = ½ m$_A$ (2 v$_A$)^2
$\quad\quad\quad\quad$ = ½ m$_A$ (4 v$_a^2$)
KE$_B$ = 2 mv$_A^2$
$\quad\quad$ = 4 (½ mv$_A^2$)
$\quad\quad$ = 4 KE$_A$

Potential energy (PE) is the stored energy of position or configuration. A textbook on a desk has PE because of its height above the floor . . . and the potential for a better job if it is read? It has the ability to do work by falling to the ground. Gravitational PE is given by the following equation:

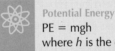
Potential Energy
PE = mgh
where *h* is the distance above the Earth's surface.

A skier at the top of a jump, a coiled spring, and a stretched rubber band are examples of other systems that have PE because of their position or configuration.

If a scientist held a ball in the air atop the Leaning Tower of Pisa (Figure 3-7), the ball would have only PE, no KE. When it is released and begins to fall, the PE decreases as the height decreases. At the same time the KE is increasing as the ball accelerates. Just before impact, the KE of the ball becomes maximum as its velocity reaches maximum. Since it now has no height, the PE becomes zero. All the initial PE of the ball has been converted into KE during the fall.

Question: A radiographer holds a 6-kg x-ray tube 1.5 m above the ground. What is its potential energy?

Answer: PE = mgh
$\quad\quad$ = 6 kg × 9.8 m/s × 1.5 m
$\quad\quad$ = 88 kg m^2/s
$\quad\quad$ = 88 J

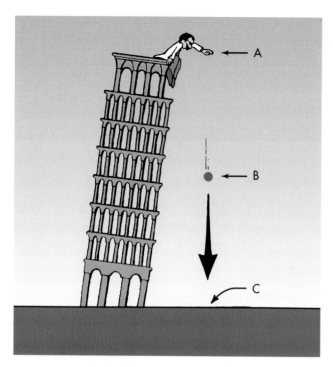

FIGURE 3-7 Potential energy results from the position of an object. Kinetic energy is the energy of motion. **A,** Maximum potential energy, no kinetic energy. **B,** Potential energy and kinetic energy. **C,** Maximum kinetic energy, no potential energy.

Heat

Heat is a form of energy that is very important to the radiologic technologist. Excessive heat is a deadly enemy of an x-ray tube and can cause permanent damage. For this reason, the technologist should be aware of the properties of heat.

> Heat is the kinetic energy of the random motion of molecules.

The more rapid and disordered the motion of molecules, the more heat matter contains. The unit of heat, the calorie (C), is defined as the energy necessary to raise the temperature of 1 g of water 1° C. The same amount of heat may have different effects on different materials. For example, the heat required to change the temperature of 1 g of silver by 1° C is approximately 0.05 C, or only one twentieth that required for a similar temperature change in water.

Heat is transferred by conduction, convection, and radiation. **Conduction** is the transfer of heat by touching. Molecular motion from a high-temperature object that touches a lower-temperature object equalizes the temperature of both. Conduction is easily observed when a hot object and cold object are placed in contact. After a short time, heat conducted to the cooler object results in equal temperatures of the two objects. Heat is

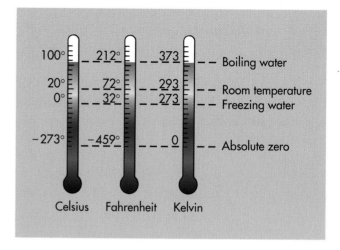

FIGURE 3-8 Three principal scales used to represent temperature. Celsius is the adopted scale for weather reporting everywhere except the United States. Kelvin is the scientific scale.

conducted from an x-ray tube anode through the rotor to insulating oil.

Convection is the mechanical transfer of rapidly moving or "hot" molecules in a gas or liquid from one place to another. A steam radiator or forced-air furnace warms a room by convection. The heat from a radiator is an example of natural convection. The air around the radiator is heated, causing it to rise. Then cooler air takes its place. A forced-air furnace blows heated air into the room, providing forced circulation to complement the natural convection. Heat is convected from the housing of an x-ray tube to air.

Thermal radiation is the transfer of heat. Generally speaking, radiation is a method of transferring energy through space. Heat is transferred by the emission of **infrared radiation,** which is a type of electromagnetic radiation. Thermal radiation is recognized by the reddish glow emitted from hot objects. An x-ray tube cools primarily by radiation.

Table 3-3 presents a summary of the quantities, equations, and units in mechanics.

Temperature is normally measured with a reproducible scale called a **thermometer.** A thermometer is usually calibrated at two reference points: the freezing and boiling points of water. The three scales that have been developed to measure temperature are Celsius (°C), Fahrenheit (°F), and Kelvin (K) (Figure 3-8).

These scales are interrelated as follows:

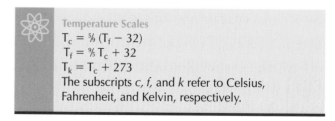
> **Temperature Scales**
> $T_c = \frac{5}{9}(T_f - 32)$
> $T_f = \frac{9}{5}T_c + 32$
> $T_k = T_c + 273$
> The subscripts c, f, and k refer to Celsius, Fahrenheit, and Kelvin, respectively.

TABLE 3-3	Summary of Quantities, Equations, and Units Used in Mechanics				
				UNITS	
Quantity	**Symbol**	**Defining Equation**		**SI**	**British**
Velocity	v	$v = d/t$		m/s	ft/s
Average velocity	$\bar{v}$	$v = \dfrac{v_o + v_1}{2}$		m/s	ft/s
Acceleration	a	$a = \dfrac{v_1 - v_o}{t}$		m/s²	ft/s²
Force	F	$F = ma$		N	lb
Weight	Wt	$Wt = mg$		N	lb
Momentum	p	$p = mv$		kg-m/s	ft-lb/s
Work	W	$W = Fd$		J	ft-lb
Power	P	$P = \text{Work}/t$		W	hp
Kinetic energy	KE	$KE = 1/2\ mv^2$		J	ft-lb
Potential energy	PE	$PE = mgh$		J	ft-lb

Question: Convert 77° F to degrees Celsius.

Answer: $T_c = \tfrac{5}{9}(T_f - 32)$
$= \tfrac{5}{9}(77 - 32) = \tfrac{5}{9}(45) = 25°\ C$

One can use the following for easy, approximate conversion:

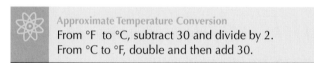

Approximate Temperature Conversion
From °F to °C, subtract 30 and divide by 2.
From °C to °F, double and then add 30.

Magnetic resonance imaging (MRI) with a superconducting magnet requires extremely cold liquids called *cryogens*. Liquid nitrogen, which boils at 77 K, and liquid helium, which boils at 4 K, are the two cryogens most often used.

Question: Liquid helium is used to cool superconducting wire in magnetic resonance imagers. What is its temperature in degrees Fahrenheit?

Answer: $T_k = T_c + 273$
$T_c = T_k - 273$
$T_c = 4 - 273$
$T_c = -269°\ C$
$T_f = \tfrac{9}{5}(-269) + 32$
$T_f = -452°\ F$

The relationship between temperature and energy is often represented by an energy thermometer (Figure 3-9). We consider x-rays to be energetic; however, on the cosmic scale they are rather ordinary.

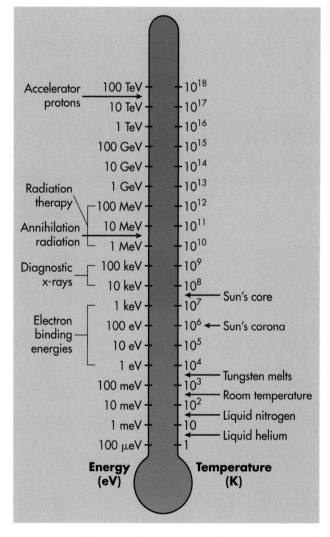

FIGURE 3-9 The energy thermometer scales temperature and energy together.

SUMMARY

This chapter introduces the various standards of measurement and applies them to concepts associated with mechanics and other areas that have an impact on radiology. Table 3-3 summarizes the concepts addressed in this chapter. Answer the Challenge Questions using that table as a reference.

CHALLENGE QUESTIONS

1. Define or otherwise identify:
   a. Base quantity
   b. Derived quantity
   c. Special quantity
   d. Inertia
   e. Acceleration
   f. Convection
   g. Work
   h. Velocity
   i. Scalar vs. vector quantity
   j. Newton's second law of motion

2. The dimensions of a box are 30 cm × 86 cm × 4.2 m. Find the volume using the formula, v (volume) = 1 (length) × w (width) × h (height).

3. What is the volume of a rectangular radiographic positioning sponge that measure 5 in × 5 in × 10 in?

4. What is the velocity of a ball that travels 50 m in 4 s?

5. What is the velocity of the mobile x-ray imaging system in the hospital elevator if the elevator travels 20 m to the next floor in 30 s?

6. A Corvette can reach a velocity of 88 mph in ¼ mile. What is the average velocity?

7. Moving down a ramp, the C-arm fluoroscope reaches a velocity of 1 ft/s every 5 s. What is the average velocity?

8. A 5L Mustang can accelerate to 60 mph in 5.9 s. What is its acceleration in SI units?

9. Find the force on a 55-kg object accelerated at 14 m/s².

10. For a 3600-lb (1636-kg) car to accelerate at 15 m/s², what force is required?

11. A professor has a mass of 75 kg. What is his weight on the earth? On the moon?

12. Find the work done lifting an infant weighing 90 N to a height of 1.5 m.

13. A radiographer lifts a 0.8-kg cassette from the floor to the top of a 1.5-m table with an acceleration of 3 m/s². What is the power exerted if it takes 1.2 s?

14. A rushed radiographer pushes a 35-kg portable down a 25-m hall in 9 s with a final velocity of 3 m/s. How much power did this require?

15. A radiographer holds a 6-kg x-ray tube 1.5 m above the ground. What is its potential energy?

16. Liquid helium with a boiling point of 4 K is used to cool superconducting magnetic resonance imagers. What is its temperature in Fahrenheit?

17. Convert 77° F to degrees Celsius.

18. Convert 80° F to degrees Celsius.

19. What are the four special quantities of radiation measurement?

20. What are the three units common to both the SI and MKS systems?

The Atom

OBJECTIVES

At the completion of this chapter, the student should be able to:

1. Relate the history of the atom
2. Identify the structure of the atom
3. Describe electron shells and instability within atomic structure
4. Discuss radioactivity and the characteristics of alpha and beta particles
5. Explain the difference between two forms of ionizing radiation: particulate and electromagnetic.

OUTLINE

This chapter diverges from the study of energy and force to return to the basis of matter itself. What composes matter? What is the magnitude of matter?

From the inner space of the atom to outer space of the universe, there is an enormous range in the size of matter. Over 40 orders of magnitude are needed to identify objects as small as the atom and as large as the universe. Because matter spans such a large magnitude, scientific notation is needed to measure objects. Figure 4-1 shows the orders of magnitude and ways that matter in our surroundings varies in size.

The atom, as the smallest unit of matter, is the building block of the radiographer's understanding of the interaction between ionizing radiation and matter. This chapter explains what happens when energy in the form of an x-ray interacts with tissue at the atomic level. Examining the structure of atoms helps you understand what happens when parts of the atom's structure are changed during ionization.

CENTURIES OF DISCOVERY
Greek Atom

One of civilization's most pronounced, continuing scientific investigations has been to precisely determine the structure of matter. The earliest recorded reference to this investigation comes from the Greeks, several hundred years BC. They thought all matter was composed of four substances: earth, water, air, and fire. According to them, all matter could be described as combinations of these four basic substances in various proportions, modified by four basic essences: wet, dry, hot, and cold. Figure 4-2 shows how this theory of matter was represented at that time.

The Greeks used the term **atom**, meaning indivisible, [*a* (not) + *temon* (cut)] to describe the smallest part of the four substances of matter. Each type of atom was represented by a symbol (Figure 4-3, *A*). Today 112 substances or **elements** have been identified; 92 are naturally occurring, and an additional 20 have been artificially produced in high-energy particle accelerators. We now know that the atom is the smallest particle of matter that has the properties of an element. Many particles are much smaller than the atom; these are called **subatomic particles**.

An atom is the smallest particle that has all the properties of an element.

Dalton Atom

The Greeks' description of the structure of matter persisted for hundreds of years. In fact, it was the theoreti-

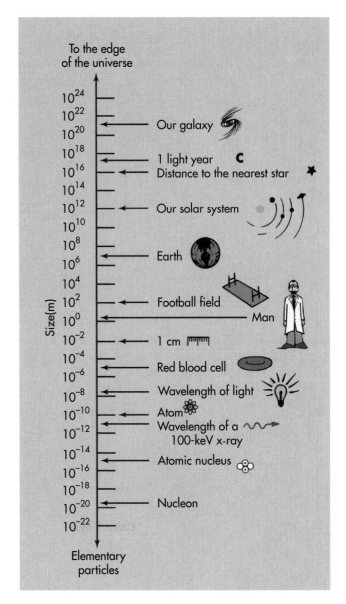

FIGURE 4-1 The size of objects varies enormously. The range of size in nature requires that scientific notation be used because over 40 orders of magnitude are necessary.

cal basis for the vain efforts by medieval alchemists to transform lead into gold. It was not until the nineteenth century that the foundation for modern atomic theory was laid. In 1808, John Dalton, an English schoolteacher, published a book summarizing his experiments, which showed that the elements could be classified according to integral values of atomic mass. According to Dalton, an element was composed of identical atoms that reacted the same way chemically. For example, all oxygen atoms were alike. They looked alike, they were constructed alike, and they reacted alike. They were, however, very different from atoms of any other element. The physical combination of one type of atom with another was visualized as being an eye-and-hook affair (Figure 4-3, *B*). The size and number of the eyes and hooks were different for each element.

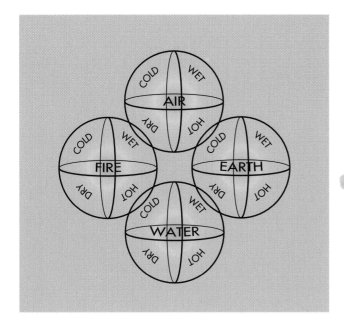

FIGURE 4-2 Symbolic representation of the substances and essences of matter as viewed by the ancient Greeks.

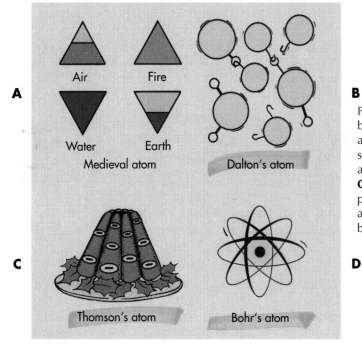

A

B

C

D

FIGURE 4-3 Through the years the atom has been represented by many symbols. **A,** The Greeks envisioned four different atoms, representing air, fire, earth, and water. These triangular symbols were adopted by medieval alchemists. **B,** Dalton's atoms had hooks and eyes to account for chemical combination. **C,** Thomson's model of the atom has been described as a plum pudding, with the plums representing the electrons. **D,** The Bohr atom has a small, dense, positively charged nucleus surrounded by electrons in precise energy levels.

Some 50 years after Dalton's work, a Russian scholar, Dmitri Mendeleev, showed that if the elements were arranged in order of increasing atomic mass, a periodic repetition of similar chemical properties occurred. At that time, about 65 elements had been identified. Mendeleev's work resulted in the first periodic table of the elements. Although there were many holes in Mendeleev's table, it showed that all the then-known elements could be placed in one of eight groups.

Figure 4-4 represents the modern periodic table of elements. Each block represents an element. The super-

script is the atomic number. The subscript is the elemental mass.

All elements in the same group (i.e., column) react chemically in a similar fashion and have similar physical properties. Except for hydrogen, the elements of group I, called the *alkali metals,* are all soft metals that combine readily with oxygen and react violently with water. The elements of group VII, called *halogens,* are gases, are easily vaporized, and combine with metals to form water-soluble salts. Group VIII elements, called the *noble gases,* are highly resistant to reaction with other elements.

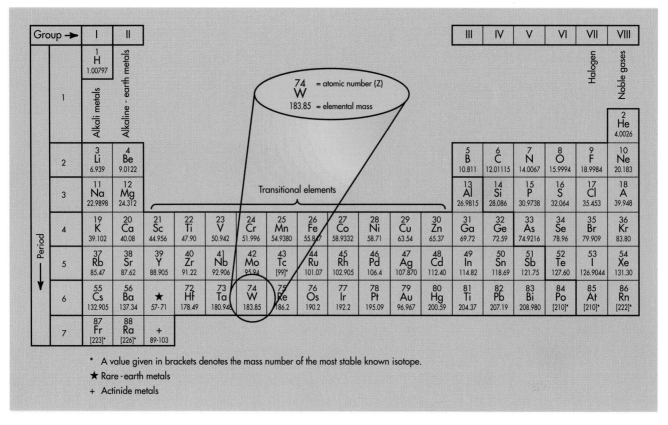

FIGURE 4-4 Periodic table of the elements.

These elemental groupings are determined by the placement of electrons in each atom. This is considered more fully later.

Thomson Atom

After the publication of Mendeleev's periodic table, additional elements were separated and identified, and the periodic table slowly became filled. Knowledge of the structure of the atom, however, remained scanty.

Before the turn of the century, atoms were considered indivisible. The only difference between the atoms of one element and the atoms of another was their mass. Through the efforts of many scientists, it slowly became apparent that there was an electrical nature to the structure of an atom.

In the late 1890s, while investigating the physical properties of cathode rays (electrons), J.J. Thomson concluded that electrons were an integral part of all atoms. He described the atom as looking something like a plum pudding, in which the plums represented negative electric charges (electrons) and the pudding was a shapeless mass of uniform positive electrification (Figure 4-3, C). The number of electrons was thought to equal the quantity of positive electrification because the atom was known to be electrically neutral.

Through a series of ingenious experiments, Ernest Rutherford in 1911 disproved Thomson's model of the atom. Rutherford introduced the nuclear model, which described the atom as containing a small, dense, positively charged center surrounded by a negative cloud of electrons. He called the center of the atom the nucleus.

Bohr Atom

In 1913, Niels Bohr improved Rutherford's description of the atom. Bohr's model was a miniature solar system in which the electrons revolved about the nucleus in prescribed orbits or **energy levels.** For our purposes, the Bohr atom (Figure 4-3, *D*) represents the best way to picture the atom, although the details of atomic structure are more accurately described by a newer model, called *quantum mechanics.* Simply put, the Bohr atom contains a small, dense, positively charged nucleus surrounded by negatively charged electrons that revolve in fixed, well-defined orbits about the nucleus. In the normal atom, the number of electrons is equal to the number of positive charges in the nucleus.

FUNDAMENTAL PARTICLES

Our understanding of the atom today is essentially that which Bohr presented nearly a century ago. With the development of high-energy **particle accelerators,** or *atom smashers* as some call them, the structure of the nucleus of an atom is slowly being mapped and identified.

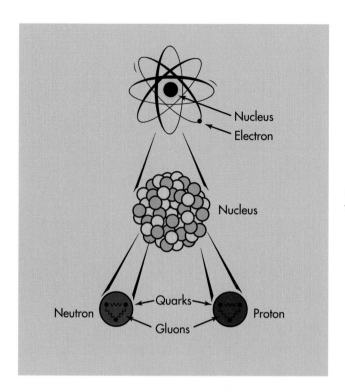

FIGURE 4-5 The nucleus consists of protons and neutrons, which are made of quarks bound together by gluons.

TABLE 4-1	Important Characteristics of the Fundamental Particles					
Particle	Location	Relative	Mass Kilograms	amu	Charge	Symbol
Electron	Shells	1	9.109×10^{-31}	0	−1	⊖
Proton	Nucleus	1836	1.673×10^{-27}	1	+1	⊕
Neutron	Nucleus	1838	1.675×10^{-27}	1	0	○

Nearly 100 subatomic particles have been detected and described by physicists working with these accelerators.

Nuclear structure is now well defined (Figure 4-5). Nucleons—protons and neutrons—are composed of quarks that are held together by gluons. These particles, however, are of little consequence to radiology. Only the three primary constituents of an atom, the **electron**, the **proton**, and the **neutron**, are considered here. They are the **fundamental particles** (Table 4-1).

 The fundamental particles of an atom are the electron, the proton, and the neutron.

The atom can be viewed as a miniature solar system whose sun is the nucleus and whose planets are the electrons. The arrangement of the electrons around the nucleus determines the manner in which atoms interact. Electrons are very small particles carrying one unit of negative electric charge. Their mass is only 9.1×10^{-31} kg. They can be pictured as revolving about the nucleus at nearly the speed of light in precisely fixed orbits, like the planets in our solar system revolve around the sun.

Because an atomic particle is extremely small, its mass is expressed in **atomic mass units** (**amu**) for convenience.

One amu is equal to one twelfth the mass of a ^{12}C atom. The electron mass is 0.000549 amu. When precision is not necessary, a system of whole numbers called **atomic mass units** (amu) is used. The atomic mass number is the amu rounded to the nearest whole number. The atomic mass number of an electron is zero.

The nucleus contains particles called **nucleons,** of which there are two types: **protons** and **neutrons.** Both have nearly 2000 times the mass of an electron. The mass of a proton is 1.673×10^{-27} kg, and the neutron is just slightly heavier at 1.675×10^{-27} kg. The atomic mass number of each is 1. The primary difference between a proton and a neutron is electric charge. The proton carries one unit of positive electric charge. The neutron carries no charge; it is electrically neutral.

ATOMIC STRUCTURE

You might be tempted to visualize the atom as a beehive of subatomic activity, since classical representations of it generally appear like that shown in Figure 4-3, *D*. Because of the space limitations of the printed page, Figure 4-3, *D*, is greatly oversimplified. In fact, the atom is mostly empty space, like our solar system. The nucleus of an atom is very small but contains nearly all the mass of the atom.

The atom is essentially empty space.

If a basketball, whose diameter is 9.6 in (0.23 m), represented the size of the uranium nucleus, the largest naturally occurring atom, the path of the orbital electrons would take them over 8 miles (12.8 km) away. Since it contains all the neutrons and protons, the nucleus of the atom contains most of its mass. For example, the nucleus of an uranium atom contains 99.998% of the entire mass of the atom.

The possible electron orbits are grouped into different "shells." The arrangement of these shells helps determine how an atom reacts chemically (that is, how it combines with other atoms to form molecules). Since a neutral atom has the same number of electrons in orbits as protons in the nucleus, the number of protons ultimately determines the chemical behavior of an atom. Therefore the number of protons determines the chemical element. Atoms that have the same number of protons but differ in the number of neutrons are called **isotopes** and behave in the same way in chemical reaction.

The periodic table of the elements (Figure 4-4) lists matter in order of increasing complexity beginning with hydrogen (H). An atom of hydrogen contains one proton in its nucleus and one electron outside the nucleus. Helium (He), the second atom in the table, contains two protons, two neutrons, and two electrons. The third atom, lithium (Li), contains three protons, four neutrons, and three electrons. Two of these electrons are in the same orbital shell, the K shell, as are the electrons of hydrogen and helium. The third electron is in the next-farther orbital shell from the nucleus, the L shell.

Electrons can exist only in certain **shells,** which represent different **electron binding energies** or **energy levels.** For identification purposes, the electron orbital shells are given the code K, L, M, N, and so forth, to represent the relative binding energies of electrons from closest to farthest from the nucleus. The closer an electron to the nucleus, the higher its binding energy.

The next atom on the periodic table, beryllium (Be), has four protons and five neutrons in the nucleus. Two electrons are in the K shell, and two are in the L shell. The complexity of the electron configuration of atoms increases as you progress through the periodic table to the most complex naturally occurring element, uranium (U). Uranium has 92 protons and 146 neutrons. The electron distribution is as follows: 2 in the K shell, 8 in the L shell, 18 in the M shell, 32 in the N shell, 21 in the O shell, 9 in the P shell, and 2 in the Q shell.

Figure 4-6 is a schematic representation of four atoms. Although these atoms are mostly empty space, they have been diagrammed on one page. If the actual size of the helium nucleus were that in Figure 4-6, the K-shell electrons would be several city blocks away.

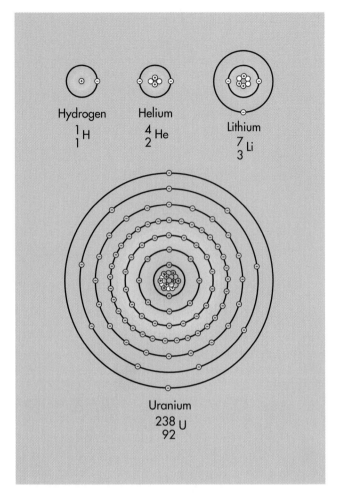

FIGURE 4-6 Atoms are composed of neutrons and protons in the nucleus and electrons in specific orbits surrounding the nucleus. Shown here are the three smallest atoms and the largest naturally occurring atom, uranium.

 In their normal state, atoms are electrically neutral; the electric charge on the atom is zero.

The total number of electrons in the orbital shells is exactly equal to the number of protons in the nucleus. If an atom has an extra electron or has had an electron removed, it is said to be *ionized*. **Ionization** is the removal of an orbital electron from an atom. An ionized atom is not electrically neutral but carries a charge equal in magnitude to the difference between the number of electrons and protons.

You might assume that atoms can be ionized by changing the number of positive charges as well as the number of negative charges. Atoms, however, cannot be ionized by the addition or subtraction of protons, since that changes the atom from one element to another. An alteration in the number of neutrons does not ionize an atom because the neutron is electrically neutral.

Figure 4-7 represents the interaction between an x-ray and a carbon atom, a primary constituent of tissue. The

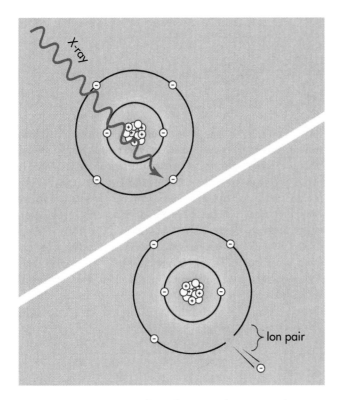

FIGURE 4-7 Ionization of a carbon atom by an x-ray leaves the atom with a net electric charge of +1. The ionized atom and the released electron are called an *ion pair*.

x-ray transfers its energy to an orbital electron and ejects that electron from the atom. This process requires approximately 34 eV of energy. The x-ray may cease to exist, and an ion pair is formed. The remaining atom is now a positive ion, since it contains one more positive charge than negative charge.

Ionization
Ionization is the removal of an orbital electron from an atom.

In all except for the lightest atoms the number of neutrons is always greater than the number of protons. The larger the atom, the greater the abundance of neutrons over protons.

Electron Arrangement

The maximum number of electrons that can exist in each shell (Table 4-2) increases with the distance of the shell from the nucleus. These numbers need not be memorized, since the electron limit per shell can be calculated from the expression:

Electrons per Shell
$2n^2$
where *n* is the shell number.

TABLE 4-2	Maximum Number of Electrons That Can Occupy Each Electron Shell	
Shell No.	Shell Symbol	No. of Electrons
1	K	2
2	L	8
3	M	18
4	N	32
5	O	50
6	P	72
7	Q	98

Question: What is the maximum number of electrons that can exist in the O shell?

Answer: The O shell is the fifth shell from the nucleus, therefore:
$n = 5$
$2n^2 = 2(5)^2$
$\quad\quad = 2(25)$
$\quad\quad = 50$ electrons

Physicists call the shell number *n* the **principal quantum number.** Every electron in every atom can be precisely identified by a set of four quantum numbers, the most important of which is the principal quantum number. The other three quantum numbers represent the existence of subshells, which are not important to radiology.

The observant reader may have noticed a relationship between the number of shells in an atom and the atom's position on the periodic table of the elements. Oxygen has eight electrons; two occupy the K shell, and six occupy the L shell. Oxygen is in the second period and the sixth group of the periodic table (Figure 4-4). Aluminum has the following electron configuration: K shell, two electrons; L shell, eight electrons; and M shell, three electrons. Therefore aluminum is in the third period (M shell) and third group (three electrons) of the periodic table.

Electron Arrangement
The number of electrons in the outermost shell of an atom is equal to its group in the periodic table. The number of electrons in the outermost shell is the valence of an atom. The number of the outermost electron shell of an atom is equal to its period in the periodic table.

Question: What are the period and group for the gastrointestinal contrast agent, barium? (Refer to Figure 4-4).

Answer: Period 6 and group II.

No outer shell can contain more than eight electrons.

Why does the periodic table show elements repeating similar chemical properties in groups of eight? In addition to the limitation on the maximum number of electrons allowed in any shell, the outer shell is always limited to eight electrons. All atoms having one electron in the outer shell lie in group I of the periodic table; atoms with two electrons in the outer shell fall in group II and so on. When eight electrons are in the outer shell, the shell is filled. Atoms with filled outer shells lie in group VIII, the noble gases, and are very stable chemically.

The orderly scheme of atomic progression from smallest to largest atom is interrupted in the fourth period. Instead of electrons being added to the next outer shell, they are added to an inner shell. The atoms associated with this phenomenon are called the **transitional elements.** Even in these elements, no outer shell ever contains more than eight electrons. The chemical properties of the transitional elements depend on the number of electrons in the two outermost shells.

The shell notation of the electron arrangement of an atom not only identifies the relative distance of an electron from the nucleus but also indicates the relative energy by which the electron is attached to the nucleus. You might expect that an electron would spontaneously fly off from the nucleus, just as a ball twirling on the end of a string would if the string was cut. This type of force is called **centripetal force,** or "center-seeking" force, and

results from a basic law of electricity stating that opposite charges attract one another and like charges repel.

Centripetal Force
The force that keeps an electron in orbit is the centripetal force. _center seeking_

You might therefore expect the electrons to drop into the nucleus because of the strong electrostatic attraction. In the normal atom the centripetal force just balances the force created by the electron velocity, the **centrifugal force,** or "flying-out-from-the-center" force, so that the electrons maintain their distance from the nucleus traveling in a circular or elliptical path.

Figure 4-8 is a representation of this state of affairs for a small atom. In more complex atoms the same balance of force exists, and each electron can be considered separately.

Centrifugal Force
Centrifugal force tends to cause an electron to travel straight and leave the atom.

Electron Binding Energy

The strength of attachment of an electron to the nucleus is called the **electron binding energy,** designated E_b. The

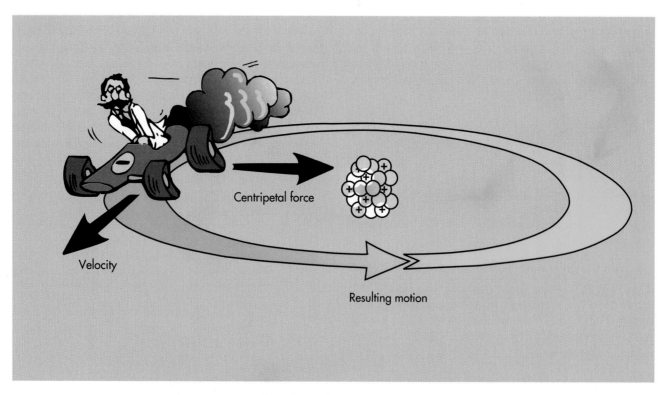

FIGURE 4-8 Electrons revolve about the nucleus in fixed orbits or shells. The electrostatic attraction produces a centripetal force that just matches the force of motion or velocity, resulting in a specific electron path about the nucleus.

closer an electron is to the nucleus, the more tightly it is bound. K-shell electrons have higher binding energies than L-shell electrons, L-shell electrons are more tightly bound to the nucleus than M shell electrons, and so on.

Not all K-shell electrons of all atoms are bound with the same binding energy. The greater the total number of electrons in an atom, the more tightly each is bound. In other words, the larger and more complex the atom, the higher the electron binding energy for electrons in any given shell. Since the electrons of large atoms are more tightly bound to the nucleus than those of small atoms, it generally takes more energy to ionize a large atom than a small one.

Figure 4-9 represents the binding energy of electrons of several atoms of radiologic importance. The metals tungsten (W) and molybdenum (Mo) are the primary constituents of the target of an x-ray tube. Barium (Ba) and iodine (I) are used extensively in radiographic and fluoroscopic contrast agents.

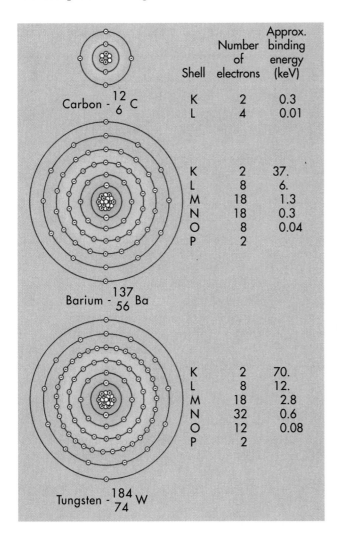

FIGURE 4-9 Atomic configurations and approximate electron binding energies for three radiologically important atoms. As atoms get bigger, the electrons in a given shell become more tightly bound.

Question: How much energy is required to ionize tungsten by the removal of a K-shell electron?

Answer: The minimum energy must equal the electron binding energy, or 70 keV. If it is less than that, the atom cannot be ionized.

Carbon (C) is an important component of human tissue. As with other tissue atoms, the electron binding energy for carbon's outer shell electrons is only about 10 eV. Yet approximately 34 eV is necessary to ionize tissue atoms, a value called the **ionization potential.** The difference, 24 eV, causes multiple electron excitations, which ultimately result in heat. The concept of ionization potential is important to the description of linear energy transfer (LET), which is discussed in Chapter 34.

Question: How much more energy is necessary to ionize barium than to ionize carbon by the removal of K-shell electrons?

Answer:
$$E_b \text{ (Ba)} = 37,000 \text{ eV}$$
$$E_b(C) = 300 \text{ eV}$$
$$\text{Difference} = 36,700 \text{ eV}$$
$$= 36.7 \text{ keV}$$

ATOMIC NOMENCLATURE

Often an element is indicated by an alphabetic abbreviation. Such abbreviations are called **chemical symbols.** Table 4-3 lists some of the important elements and their chemical symbols.

The chemical properties of an element are determined by the number and arrangement of electrons. In the neutral atom the number of electrons equals the number of protons. The number of protons is called the **atomic number,** represented by **Z.** Table 4-3 shows that the atomic number of barium is 56, indicating that 56 protons are in the barium nucleus.

The number of protons plus the number of neutrons in the nucleus of an atom is called the **atomic mass number,** symbolized by **A.** The atomic mass number is always a whole number. The use of atomic mass numbers is helpful in many areas of radiologic science.

 The atomic mass number and the precise mass of an atom are not equal.

An atom's atomic mass number is a whole number equal to the number of nucleons in the atom. The actual **atomic mass** of an atom is determined by measurement and rarely is it a whole number. ^{135}Ba has an atomic mass number of 135, since its nucleus contains 56 protons and 79 neutrons. The atomic mass of ^{135}Ba is 134.91 amu. Only one atom, ^{12}C, has an atomic mass equal to its atomic mass number. This occurs because the ^{12}C atom is the arbitrary standard for atomic measure.

Many elements in their natural state are composed of atoms with different atomic mass numbers and different

TABLE 4-3	Characteristics of Some Radiographically Important Elements					
Element	Chemical Symbol	Atomic Number (Z)	Atomic Mass Number (A)*	No. of Naturally Occurring isotopes	Elemental Mass (amu)†	K-Shell Electron Binding Energy (keV)
Beryllium	Be	4	9	1	9.01	0.1
Carbon	C	6	12	3	12.01	0.3
Oxygen	O	8	16	3	15.00	0.5
Aluminum	Al	13	27	1	26.98	1.6
Calcium	Ca	20	40	6	40.08	4.0
Iron	Fe	26	56	4	55.84	7.1
Copper	Cu	29	63	2	63.54	9.0
Molybdenum	Mo	42	98	7	95.94	20
Ruthenium	Ru	44	102	7	101.0	22
Silver	Ag	47	107	2	107.9	26
Tin	Sn	50	120	10	118.6	29
Iodine	I	53	127	1	126.9	33
Barium	Ba	56	138	7	137.3	37
Tungsten	W	74	184	5	183.8	70
Gold	Au	79	197	1	196.9	81
Lead	Pb	82	208	4	207.1	88
Uranium	U	92	238	3	238.0	116

*Most abundant isotope.
†Average of naturally occurring isotopes.

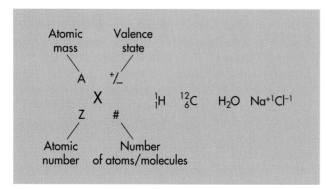

FIGURE 4-10 Protocol for representing elements in a molecule.

atomic masses but identical atomic numbers. The characteristic mass of an element, the **elemental mass,** is determined by the relative abundance of isotopes and their respective atomic masses. Barium, for example, has an atomic number of 56. The atomic mass number of its most abundant isotope is 138. Natural barium, however, consists of seven different isotopes with atomic mass numbers of 130, 132, 134, 135, 136, 137, and 138; the elemental mass is determined by the average mass of all these isotopes.

With the protocol described in Figure 4-10, the atoms of Figure 4-6 would have the following symbolic representation:

$$^1_1H, \;^4_2He, \;^7_3Li, \;^{238}_{92}U$$

Since the chemical symbol also indicates the atomic number, the subscript is often omitted.

$$^1H, \;^4He, \;^7Li, \;^{238}U$$

Isotopes
Atoms that have the same atomic number but different atomic mass numbers are isotopes.

Isotopes of a given element contain the same number of protons but varying numbers of neutrons. Most elements have more than one stable isotope. The seven natural isotopes of barium are:

$$^{130}Ba, \;^{132}Ba, \;^{134}Ba, \;^{135}Ba, \;^{136}Ba, \;^{137}Ba, \;^{138}Ba$$

Question: How many protons and neutrons are in each of the seven naturally occurring isotopes of barium?

Answer: The number of protons in each isotope is 56. The number of neutrons is equal to $A - Z$. Therefore:
$^{130}Ba: 130 - 56 = 74$ neutrons
$^{132}Ba: 132 - 56 = 76$ neutrons
$^{134}Ba: 134 - 56 = 78$ neutrons
and so on.

Isobars
Atomic nuclei that have the same atomic mass number but different atomic numbers are isobars.

Isobars are atoms that have different numbers of protons and different numbers of neutrons but the same total number of nucleons.

Isotones
Atoms that have the same number of neutrons but different numbers of protons are isotones.

TABLE 4-4	Characteristics of Various Nuclear Arrangements		
Arrangement	Atomic number	Atomic mass number	Neutron number
Isotope	Same	Different	Different
Isobar	Different	Same	Different
Isotone	Different	Different	Same
Isomer	Same	Same	Same

Isotones are atoms with different atomic numbers and different mass numbers but a constant value for the quantity A − Z.

The final category of atomic configuration is the **isomer**.

Isomers
Isomers have the same atomic number and the same atomic mass number.

In fact, isomers are identical atoms except that they exist at different energy states because of differences in nucleon arrangement. Table 4-4 is a summary of the characteristics of these nuclear arrangements.

Question: From the following list of atoms, determine which are isotopes, isobars, and isotones.
$^{131}_{54}$Xe, $^{130}_{53}$I, $^{132}_{55}$Cs, $^{131}_{53}$I

Answer: ^{130}I and ^{131}I are isotopes. ^{131}I and ^{131}Xe are isobars. ^{130}I, ^{131}Xe, and ^{132}Cs are isotones.

COMBINATION OF ATOMS

Atoms of various elements may combine to form structures called *molecules*.

Four atoms of hydrogen (H_2) and two atoms of oxygen (O_2) can combine to form two molecules of water (2 H_2O). The following equation represents this atomic combination:

$$2 H_2 + O_2 \rightarrow 2 H_2O$$

An atom of sodium (Na) can combine with an atom of chlorine (Cl) to form a molecule of sodium chloride (NaCl), which is common table salt:

$$Na + Cl \rightarrow NaCl$$

Both of these molecules are common in the human body. Molecules in turn may combine to form even larger structures: cells and tissues.

A *chemical compound* is any quantity of one type of molecule.

Although over 100 elements are known; most elements are rare. Approximately 95% of the Earth and its atmosphere consist of only a dozen elements. Similarly, hydrogen, oxygen, carbon, and nitrogen compose over 95% of the human body. Water molecules make up about 80% of the human body.

There is an organized scheme for representing elements in a molecule (Figure 4-10). This shorthand notation, which incorporates the chemical symbol with subscripts and superscripts, is used to identify atoms. The chemical symbol X is positioned between two subscripts and two superscripts. The subscript and superscript to the left of the chemical symbol represent the atomic number and atomic mass number, respectively. The subscript and superscript to the right are values for the number of atoms per molecule and the valence state of the atom, respectively. We are concerned only with the scripts to the left of X.

The formula NaCl represents one molecule of the compound sodium chloride. Sodium chloride has properties that vary more than either sodium or chloride. Atoms combine with one another to form compounds (chemical bonding) in two main ways. The examples of H_2O and NaCl can be used to describe these two types of chemical bonds.

Oxygen and hydrogen combine into water through **covalent bonds.** Oxygen has six electrons in its outermost shell. It has room for two more electrons, so in a water molecule, two hydrogen atoms share their single electrons with the oxygen. The hydrogen electrons orbit both the H and O, thus binding the atoms together. This covalent bonding is characterized by the sharing of electrons.

Sodium and chlorine combine into salt through **ionic bonds.** Sodium has one electron in its outermost shell. Chlorine has space for one more electron in its outermost shell. The sodium atom gives up its electron to the chlorine. When it does, it becomes ionized because it has lost an electron and now has an imbalance of electrical charges. The chlorine atom also becomes ionized because it has gained an electron and then has more electrons than protons. The two atoms are attracted to one another, resulting in an ionic bond because they have opposite electrostatic charge.

Sodium, hydrogen, carbon, and oxygen atoms can combine to form a molecule of sodium bicarbonate ($NaHCO_3$). A measurable quantity of sodium bicarbonate constitutes a chemical compound commonly called *baking soda.*

The smallest particle of an element is an atom; the smallest particle of a compound is a molecule.

The interrelationships among atoms, elements, molecules, and compounds are orderly. This organizational scheme is what the ancient Greeks were trying to de-

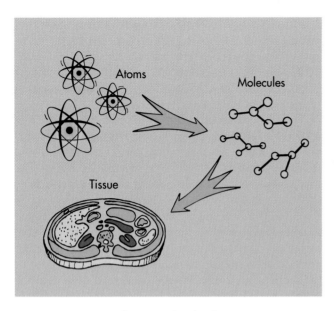

FIGURE 4-11 Matter has many levels of organization. Atoms combine to make molecules, and molecules combine to make tissues.

scribe by their substances and essences. Figure 4-11 is a diagram of this current scheme of matter.

MAGNITUDE OF MATTER

From inner space, the atom, to outer space, the universe, an enormous range of size is covered. Over 40 orders of magnitude (10^{-22} to 10^{24} m) are needed to measure objects as small as an electron and as large as the universe. Figure 4-1 shows some objects and their relative sizes and suggests the reason that scientific notation is needed.

One meter (10^0 m) is about three feet. One hundred meters (10^2 m) is about the length of a football field. One centimeter (10^{-2} m) is this long _____. Prefixes for large and small powers of 10 are shown in Table 1-3.

Question: Measured in English units, the wavelength of a 50-keV x-ray is about 0.0000000017 in. What is its value in metric units?

Answer: 0.0000000017 in = 1.7×10^{-9} in
(1.7 × 10⁻⁹ in) (0.0254 m/in) = (1.7×10^{-9} in)
(2.54×10^{-2} m/in)
= 4.3×10^{-11} m,
or 430 pm

Question: A useful calculation in x-ray physics involves dividing the speed of light (c = 3×10^8 m/s) by the x-ray wavelength. This results in the x-ray frequency. What is the result of this calculation?

Answer: $\dfrac{4 \times 10^8 \text{ m/s}}{4.3 \times 10^{-11} \text{ m}} = 0.698 \times 10^{19} \text{ s}^{-1}$
$= 6.98 \times 10^{18} \text{ Hz}$

Question: What is the approximate size of the following? (Refer to Figure 4-1 if necessary.)
  a. An atom
  b. A pencil
  c. The distance from New York to Los Angeles

Answer:
  a. The diameter of an atom is 10^{-10} m.
  b. The length of a pencil $\cong$ 6 in $\cong$ 15 cm = 0.15 m.
  c. The distance from New York to Los Angeles $\cong$ 3000 miles.
  1 mile $\cong$ 1500 m = 1.5×10^3 m

  The distance $\cong$ (1.5×10^3 m/mile) × (3×10^3 miles) = 4.5×10^6, or 4500 km

RADIOACTIVITY

Some atoms exist in an abnormally excited state characterized by an unstable nucleus. To reach stability, the nucleus spontaneously emits particles and energy and transforms itself into another atom. This process is called **radioactive disintegration** or **radioactive decay**. The atoms involved are **radionuclides**. Any nuclear arrangement is called a **nuclide;** only nuclei that undergo radioactive decay are radionuclides.

Radioactivity
Radioactivity is the emission of particles and energy by atoms to become stable.

Radioisotopes

Many factors affect nuclear stability. Perhaps the most important is the number of neutrons. When a nucleus contains either too few or too many neutrons, the atom can disintegrate radioactively, bringing the number of neutrons and protons into a stable and proper ratio. In addition to stable isotopes, many elements have radioactive isotopes, or **radioisotopes**. These may be artificially produced in machines such as particle accelerators or nuclear reactors. Seven radioisotopes of barium have been discovered, all of which are artificially produced. In the following list of barium isotopes, the radioisotopes are in boldface:

^{127}**Ba**, ^{128}**Ba**, ^{129}**Ba**, ^{130}Ba, ^{131}**Ba**, ^{132}Ba, ^{133}**Ba**, ^{134}Ba, ^{135}Ba, ^{136}Ba, ^{137}Ba, ^{138}Ba, ^{139}**Ba**, ^{140}**Ba**

Artificially produced radioisotopes have been identified for nearly all elements. A few elements have naturally occurring radioisotopes as well. There are two primary sources of these naturally occurring radioisotopes. Some originated at the time of the Earth's formation and are still decaying very slowly. An example is uranium, which decays to radium, which in turn decays to radon. These and other decay products of uranium are also radioactive. Others, such as ^{14}C are continuously produced in the upper atmosphere by the action of cosmic radiation.

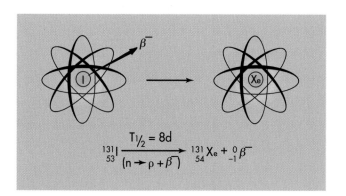

FIGURE 4-12 ^{131}I decays to ^{131}Xe to with the emission of a beta particle.

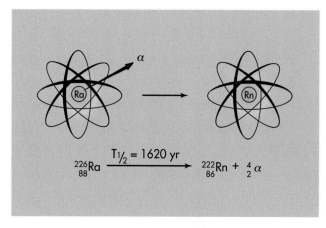

FIGURE 4-13 The decay of ^{226}Ra to ^{222}Rn is accompanied by alpha emission.

Radioisotopes can decay to stability in many ways, but only two, **beta emission** and **alpha emission,** are of particular importance here.

During beta emission, an electron-like particle created in the nucleus is ejected from the nucleus with considerable kinetic energy and escapes from the atom. The result is the loss of a small quantity of mass and one unit of negative electric charge from the nucleus of the atom. Simultaneously, a neutron undergoes conversion to a proton. The result of beta emission therefore is to increase the atomic number by one while the atomic mass number remains the same. This nuclear transformation therefore results in an atom changing from one type of element to another (Figure 4-12).

Radioactive decay by alpha emission is a much more violent process. The alpha particle consists of two protons and two neutrons bound together; its atomic mass number is 4. A nucleus must be extremely unstable to emit an alpha particle, but when it does, it loses two units of positive charge and four units of mass. The transformation is significant because the resulting atom not only is chemically different but is also lighter by 4 amu (Figure 4-13).

 Radioactive decay results in the emission of alpha particles, beta particles, and usually gamma rays.

Beta emission occurs much more frequently than alpha emission. Virtually all radioisotopes are capable of transformation by beta emission, but only heavy radioisotopes are capable of alpha emission. Some radioisotopes are pure beta emitters or pure alpha emitters, and most emit gamma rays simultaneously with the particle emission.

Question: $^{139}_{56}$Ba is a radioisotope that decays by beta emission. What will be the value of A and Z for the atom that results from this emission?

Answer: In beta emission a neutron *(n)* is converted to a proton (ρ) and a beta particle (β): n → ρ + β; therefore $^{139}_{56}$Ba → $^{139}_{57}$. Lanthanum is the element with Z = 57; thus $^{139}_{57}$La is the result of the beta decay of $^{139}_{56}$Ba.

Radioactive Half-Life

Radioactive matter is not here one day and gone the next. Rather, radioisotopes disintegrate into stable isotopes of different elements at a constant rate, but the quantity of radioactive material never quite reaches zero. Remember from Chapter 1 that radioactive material is measured in curies (Ci) and that 1 Ci is equal to 3.7 × 10^{10} atoms disintegrating each second (3.7 × 10^{10} Bq).

The rate of radioactive decay and the quantity of material present at any given time are described mathematically by a formula known as the **radioactive decay law.** From this formula we obtain a quantity known as **half-life (T½).** Half-lives of radioisotopes vary from less than a second to many years. Each radioisotope has a unique, characteristic half-life.

 Half-Life
The half-life of a radioisotope is the time required for a quantity of radioactivity to be reduced to one half its original value.

The half-life of ^{131}I is 8 days (Figure 4-13). If 100 mCi (3.7 × 10^9 Bq) of ^{131}I were present on January 1 at noon, then at noon on January 9 only 50 mCi (1.85 × 10^9 Bq) would remain. On January 17, 25 mCi (9.25 × 10^8 Bq) would remain and on January 25, 12.5 mCi (4.63 × 10^8 Bq) would remain. A plot of the radioactive decay of ^{131}I allows you to determine the amount of radioactivity remaining after any given time (Figure 4-14).

After approximately 24 days, or three half-lives, the linear-linear plot of the decay of ^{131}I becomes very difficult to read and interpret. Consequently, such graphs are

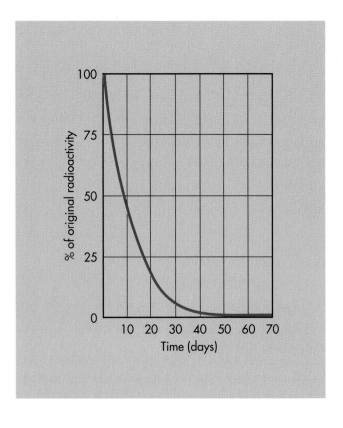

FIGURE 4-14 ^{131}I decays with a half-life of 8 days. This linear graph allows only estimation of radioactivity for a short time.

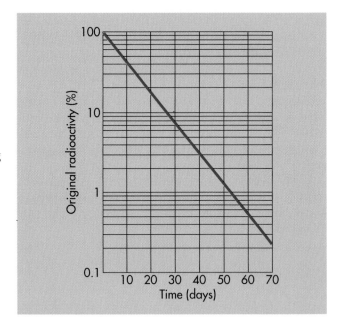

FIGURE 4-15 This semilogarithmic graph is useful for estimating the radioactivity of ^{131}I at any time.

usually presented in semilogarithmic form (Figure 4-15). With a presentation such as this, you can estimate radioactivity after a very long time.

Question: On Monday at 8 AM, 100 μCI (3.7×10^6 Bq) of ^{131}I is present. How much will remain on Friday at 5 PM?

Answer: The time of decay is 4⅓ days. According to Figure 4-15, at 4⅓ days, approximately 63% of the original activity will remain. Therefore 63 μCI (2.33×10^6 Bq) will be present on Friday at 5 PM.

Theoretically, all the radioactivity of a radioisotope never disappears. After each period equivalent to one half-

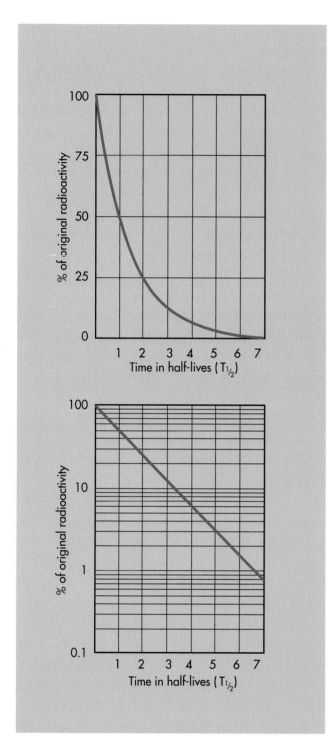

FIGURE 4-16 The radioactivity remaining after any period can be estimated from either the linear (**A**) or the semilogarithmic (**B**) graph. The original quantity is assigned a value of 100%, and the time of decay is expressed in units of half-life.

life, half the activity present at the beginning of that time remains. Therefore, although the quantity of radioisotope progressively decreases, it never quite reaches zero.

Figure 4-16 shows two similar graphs used to estimate the quantity of any radioisotope remaining after any period. In these graphs the percentage of original radioactivity remaining is plotted against time, which is measured in units of half-life. To use these graphs, you must express the initial radioactivity as 100% and convert the time of interest into units of half-life. For decay times exceeding three half-lives, the semilogarithmic form is easier to use.

Question: 65 mCi (2.4×10^9 Bq) of ^{131}I are present at noon on Wednesday. How much will remain 1 week later?

Answer: 7 days = $\frac{7}{8}$ $T_{1/2}$ = 0.875 $T_{1/2}$. Figure 4-16 shows that at 0.875 $T_{1/2}$, approximately 55% of the initial radioactivity remains; 55% $\times$ 65 mCi (2.4×10^9 Bq) = 0.55×65 = 35.8 mCi (1.32×10^9 Bq).

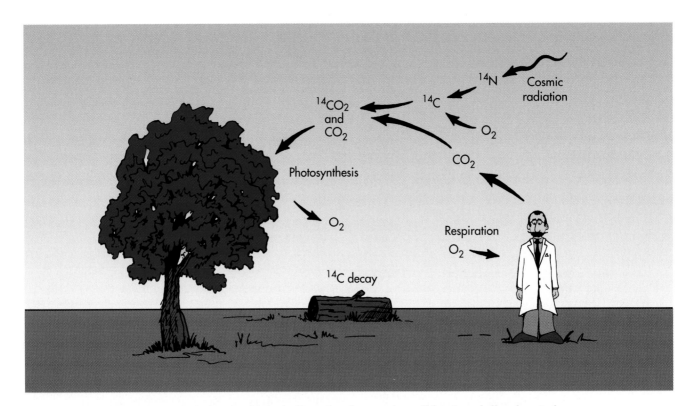

FIGURE 4-17 Carbon is a biologically active element. A small fraction of all carbon is the radioisotope ^{14}C. As a tree grows, ^{14}C is incorporated into the wood in proportion to the amount of ^{14}C in the atmosphere. When the tree dies, further exchange of ^{14}C with the atmosphere does not take place. If the dead wood is preserved by petrification, the ^{14}C content diminishes as it radioactively decays. This phenomenon is the basis for radiocarbon dating.

^{14}C is a naturally occurring radioisotope with $T_{1/2} =$ 5730 years. The concentration of ^{14}C in the environment is constant, and ^{14}C is incorporated into living material at a constant rate. Trees of the petrified forest contain less ^{14}C than living trees because the ^{14}C of living trees is in equilibrium with the atmosphere; the carbon in a petrified tree was fixed many thousands of years ago, and the fixed ^{14}C is reduced with time by radioactive decay (Figure 4-17).

Question: If a piece of petrified wood contains 25% of the ^{14}C that a tree living today contains, how old is the petrified wood?

Answer: The ^{14}C in living matter remains constant as long as the matter is alive because it is constantly exchanged with the environment. In this case the petrified wood has been dead long enough for the ^{14}C to decay to 25% of its original value. That time period represents two half-lives. Consequently, we can estimate that the petrified wood sample is approximately $2 \times 5730 = 11,460$ years old.

Question: How many half-lives are required before a quantity of radioactive material has decayed to less than 1% of its original value?

Answer: A simple approach to this type of problem is to count half-lives.

Half-life Number	Radioactivity Remaining
1	50%
2	25%
3	12.5%
4	6.25%
5	3.12%
6	1.56%
7	0.78%

A simpler approach finds the answer more precisely in Figure 4-16: 6.5 half-lives.

The concept of half-life is essential to radiology. It is used daily in nuclear medicine and has an exact parallel in x-ray terminology, the **half-value layer.** The better you understand half-life now, the better you will understand the meaning of half-value layer later.

TYPES OF IONIZING RADIATION

All ionizing radiation can be conveniently classified into only two categories: **particulate radiation** and **electromagnetic radiation** (Table 4-5). The types of radiation used in diagnostic ultrasound and in magnetic resonance imaging are **nonionizing radiation.**

TABLE 4-5	General Classification of Ionizing Radiation			
Type of Radiation *Particulate*	Symbol	Atomic Mass Number	Charge	Origin
Alpha radiation	α	4	+2	Nucleus
Beta radiation	β	0	−1	Nucleus
Electromagnetic				
Gamma rays	γ	0	0	Nucleus
X-rays	X	0	0	Electron cloud

Although all ionizing radiation acts on biologic tissue in the same manner, there are fundamental differences among various types of radiation. These differences can be analyzed according to five physical characteristics: mass, energy, velocity, charge, and origin.

Particulate Radiation

Any subatomic particle is capable of causing ionization. Consequently, electrons, protons, neutrons, and even rare nuclear fragments can all be classified as particulate ionizing radiation if they are in motion and possess sufficient kinetic energy. At rest, they cannot cause ionization. There are two types of particulate radiation: **alpha particles** and **beta particles.** Both are associated with radioactive decay.

The alpha particle is equivalent to a helium nucleus. It contains two protons and two neutrons. Its mass is approximately 4 amu, and it carries two units of positive electric charge. Compared with an electron, the alpha particle is large and exerts a great electrostatic attraction. Alpha particles are emitted only from the nuclei of heavy elements. Light elements cannot emit alpha particles, since they do not have enough excess mass (excess energy).

 An alpha particle is a helium nucleus containing two protons and two neutrons.

Once emitted from a radioactive atom, the alpha particle travels with high velocity through matter. Because of its great mass and charge, however, it easily transfers this kinetic energy to orbital electrons of other atoms. Ionization accompanies alpha radiation. The average alpha particle possesses 4 to 7 MeV of kinetic energy and ionizes approximately 40,000 atoms for every centimeter of travel through air.

Because of this amount of ionization, the energy of an alpha particle is quickly lost. It has a very short range in matter. In air, alpha particles can travel about 5 cm, whereas in soft tissue the range may be less than 100 μm. Consequently, alpha radiation from an external source is nearly harmless, since the radiation energy is deposited in the superficial layers of the skin. With an internal source of radiation, just the opposite is true. If an alpha-emitting radioisotope is deposited in the body, it can intensely irradiate the local tissue.

Beta particles differ from alpha particles in both mass and charge. They are light particles with an atomic mass number of 0 and carry one unit of negative charge. The only difference between electrons and beta particles is their origins. Beta particles originate in the nuclei of radioactive atoms, and electrons exist in shells outside the nuclei of all atoms.

 A beta particle is an electron emitted from the nucleus of a radioactive atom.

Once emitted from a radioisotope, beta particles traverse air, ionizing several hundred atoms per centimeter. The beta particle range is longer than that for the alpha particle. Depending on its energy, a beta particle may traverse 10 to 100 cm of air and about 1 to 3 cm of soft tissue.

Electromagnetic Radiation

X-rays and gamma rays are forms of electromagnetic ionizing radiation. This type of radiation is covered more completely in the next chapter; the discussion here is necessarily brief. X-rays and gamma rays are often called **photons.** Photons have no mass and no charge. They travel at the speed of light ($c = 3 \times 10^8$ m/s) and are considered energy disturbances in space.

 X-rays and gamma rays are the only forms of ionizing electromagnetic radiation.

Just as the only difference between beta particles and electrons is their origin, so the only difference between x-rays and gamma rays is their origin. Gamma rays are emitted from the nucleus of a radioisotope and are usually associated with alpha or beta emission. X-rays are produced outside the nucleus in the electron shells.

X-rays and gamma rays exist either at the speed of light or not at all. Once emitted, they have an ionization rate in air of approximately 100 ion pairs/cm, about equal to that for beta particles. Unlike beta particles, however, x-rays and gamma rays have an unlimited range in matter.

TABLE 4-6	Characteristics of Several Types of Ionizing Radiation			
		APPROXIMATE RANGE		
Type of Radiation	**Approximate Energy**	**In Air**	**In Soft Tissue**	**Origin**
Particulate				
Alpha particles	4-7 MeV	1-10 cm	Up to 0.1 mm	Heavy radioactive nuclei
Beta particles	Up to 6 MeV	Up to 10 m	Up to 3 cm	Radioactive nuclei
Electromagnetic				
X-rays	Up to 10 MeV	Up to 100 m	Up to 30 cm	Electron cloud
Gamma rays	Up to 5 MeV	Up to 100 m	Up to 30 cm	Radioactive nuclei

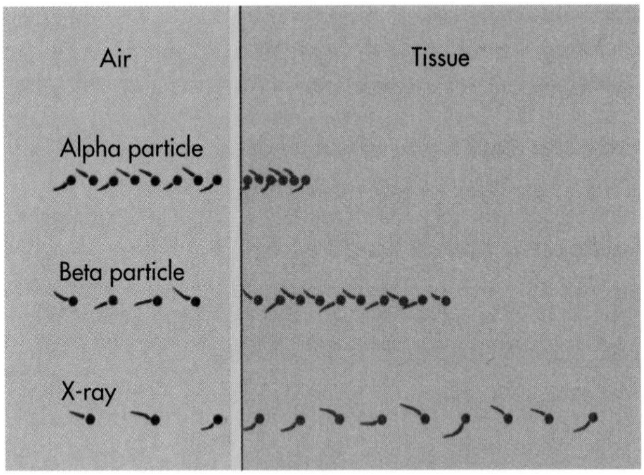

FIGURE 4-18 Different types of radiation ionize matter with different efficiency. Alpha particles are highly ionizing radiation with a very short range in matter. Beta particles do not ionize so readily and have a longer range. X-rays have low ionization rate and a very long range.

Photon radiation loses intensity with distance but theoretically never reaches zero. Particulate radiation, on the other hand, has a finite range in matter, and that range depends on the particle's energy.

Table 4-6 summarizes the more important characteristics of each of these types of ionizing radiation. In nuclear medicine, beta and gamma radiation are most important. In radiography, only x-rays are important. The penetrability and low ionization rate of x-rays make them particularly useful for medical imaging (Figure 4-18).

SUMMARY

As a miniature solar system, the Bohr atom set the stage for the modern interpretation of the structure of matter. An atom is the smallest part of an element, and a molecule is the smallest part of a compound.

The three fundamental particles of the atom are the electron, proton, and neutron. Electrons are negatively charged particles circling the nucleus in fixed orbits or shells held in place by the opposing centripetal and centrifugal forces. Chemical reactions occur when the out-ermost orbital electrons are shared or given up to other atoms. Nucleons, neutrons, and protons are each nearly 2000 times the mass of electrons. Protons are positively charged, and neutrons have no charge.

Elements are grouped in a periodic table in order of increasing complexity. The groups on the table indicate the number of electrons in the outermost shell. The elements in the periods on the periodic table have the same number orbital shells. Some atoms have the same number of protons and electrons as other elements but a different number of neutrons, giving the element a different atomic mass. These are isotopes.

Some atoms, those that contain too many or too few neutrons in the nucleus, can disintegrate. That is called *radioactivity*. Two types of particulate emission after radioactive disintegration are alpha and beta particles. The half-life of a radioactive element or a radioisotope is the time required for the quantity of radioactivity to be reduced to half its orginal value.

Ionizing radiation is either particulate or electromagnetic. Alpha and beta particles are particulate radiation. Alpha particles have four atomic mass units, are positive in charge, and originate from the nucleus of heavy elements. Beta particles have an atomic mass number of 0 and have one unit of negative charge. Beta particles originate in the nucleus of radioactive atoms.

X-rays and gamma rays are forms of electromagnetic radiation called *photons*. These rays have no mass and no charge. X-rays are produced in the electron shells, and gamma rays are emitted from the nucleus of a radioisotope.

CHALLENGE QUESTIONS

1. Define or otherwise identify:
   a. Photon
   b. The Rutherford atom
   c. Specific ionization
   d. Nucleons
   e. The arrangement of the periodic table of the elements
   f. Radioactive half-life
   g. W (chemical symbol for what element?)

h. Alpha particle
i. K shell
j. Chemical compound

2. Figure 4-1 shows the following approximate sizes: an atom, 10^{-10} m, and the Earth, 10^7 m. By how many orders of magnitude do these objects differ?

3. How many protons, neutrons, electrons and nucleons are in the following?

$$^{17}_{8}O, \quad ^{27}_{13}Al, \quad ^{60}_{27}Co, \quad ^{226}_{88}Ra$$

4. Using the data in Table 4-1, determine the mass of $^{99}_{43}Tc$ in atomic mass units and in grams.

5. Diagram the expected electron configuration of $^{40}_{20}Ca$.

6. If atoms large enough to have electrons in the *T* shell existed, what would be the maximum number allowed in that shell?

7. In Tungsten, how much more tightly bound are K-shell electrons than (a) L-shell electrons, (b) M-shell electrons, and (c) a free electron? (Refer to Figure 4-9.)

8. From the following list of nuclides, identify sets of isotopes, isobars, and isotones.

$$^{60}_{28}Ni \qquad ^{61}_{28}Ni \qquad ^{62}_{28}Ni$$
$$^{59}_{27}Co \qquad ^{60}_{27}Co \qquad ^{61}_{27}Co$$
$$^{58}_{26}Fe \qquad ^{59}_{26}Fe \qquad ^{60}_{26}Fe$$

9. $^{90}_{38}Sr$ has a half-life of 29 years. If 10 Ci (3.7×10^{11} Bq) were present in 1950, approximately how much would remain in 2010?

10. Complete the following table with relative values.

Type of Radiation	Mass	Energy	Charge	Origin
α				
β				
γ				
X				

11. For what is Mendeleev remembered?

12. Who developed the concept of the atom as a miniature solar system?

13. List the fundamental particles within an atom.

14. What property of an atom does the term *binding energy* describe?

15. Can atoms be ionized by changing the number of positive changes? Why or why not?

16. Describe how ion pairs are formed.

17. What determines the chemical reactivity of an element?

18. Why doesn't an electron spontaneously fly away from the nucleus of an atom?

19. Describe the difference between alpha emission and beta emission.

20. How does ^{14}C dating determine the age of petrified wood?

Electromagnetic Radiation

OBJECTIVES

At the completion of this chapter, the student should be able to:

1. Identify the properties of photons
2. Explain the inverse square law
3. Define *wave theory* and *quantum theory*
4. Discuss the electromagnetic spectrum

OUTLINE

Photons were first described by the ancient Greeks. Today, photons are known as *electromagnetic energy*; however, these words are commonly used interchangeably. Electromagnetic energy is present everywhere and exists over a wide energy range. X-rays and light are examples of electromagnetic photons.

The properties of photons include velocity, amplitude, frequency, and wavelength. In this chapter, discussions of visible light, radiofrequency, and ionizing radiation highlight these properties and the importance of electromagnetic radiation in radiography. The wave equation and the inverse square law are mathematical formulas that further describe how photons behave.

The wave-particle duality of electromagnetic radiation is also introduced as wave theory and quantum theory. At the end of the chapter is a summary of matter and energy and their importance to x-ray imaging.

PHOTONS

The ancient Greeks recognized the unique nature of light. It was not one of their four basic essences, but it was awarded an entirely separate status. They called an atom of light a photon. Today the term *photon* is still used.

A **photon** is the smallest quantity of any type of electromagnetic radiation, just as an atom is the smallest quantity of an element. A photon may be pictured as a small bundle of energy, sometimes called a **quantum**, traveling through space at the speed of light. We speak of x-ray photons, light photons, and other types of electromagnetic radiation as *photon radiation*.

 An x-ray photon is a quantum of electromagnetic energy.

The physics of visible light has always been a subject of investigation apart from the other areas of science. Nearly all the classic laws of optics were described hundreds of years ago. Late in the nineteenth century, James Clerk Maxwell showed that visible light has both electric and magnetic properties, hence the term **electromagnetic radiation.** By the beginning of the twentieth century, other types of electromagnetic radiation had been described, and a uniform theory evolved. Electromagnetic radiation is best explained by reference to a model in much the same way that the atom is best described by the Bohr model.

Velocity and Amplitude

Photons are energy disturbances moving through space at the speed of light (c). Some sources cite the speed of light as 186,000 miles/s but in the SI system of units it is 3×10^8 m/s.

Question: What is the value of *c* in miles per second, given that c = 3×10^8 m/s?

Answer:
$$c = \frac{3 \times 10^8 \text{ m}}{s} \times \frac{\text{mile}}{5280 \text{ ft}} \times \frac{3.2808 \text{ ft}}{m}$$
$$= \frac{3 \times 3.2808 \times 10^8 \text{ m - mile - ft}}{5.280 \times 10^3 \text{ s - ft - m}}$$
$$= 1.864 \times 10^5 \text{ miles/s}$$
$$= 186,400 \text{ miles/s}$$

 Velocity of All Electromagnetic Radiation
3×10^8 m/s.

Although photons have no mass and therefore no identifiable form, they do have electric and magnetic fields that continuously change in a **sinusoidal** fashion. The term **field** describes interactions among different energies, forces, or masses that cannot be seen but can be described mathematically. For instance, we know the gravitational field exists because we are held to the Earth by it.

Figure 5-1 shows three examples of a sinusoidal variation. This type of variation is usually called a **sine wave.** Sine waves can be described by a mathematical formula and therefore are used frequently in physics.

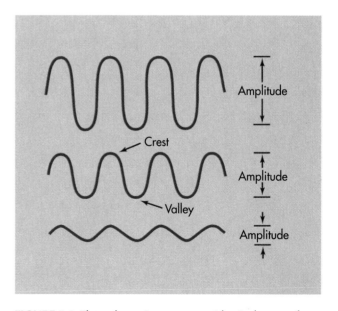

FIGURE 5-1 These three sine waves are identical except for their amplitudes.

Sine waves that exist in nature are associated with many familiar objects (Figure 5-2). Alternating electric current consists of electrons moving back and forth sinusoidally through a wire. A long rope fastened at one end vibrates as a sine wave if the free end is moved up and down in whiplike fashion. The arms of a tuning fork vibrate in sinusoidal fashion after being struck with a hard object. The weight on the end of a coil spring varies sinusoidally up and down after the spring has been stretched.

The sine waves in Figure 5-1 are identical except for their amplitude; sine wave A having the largest ampli-

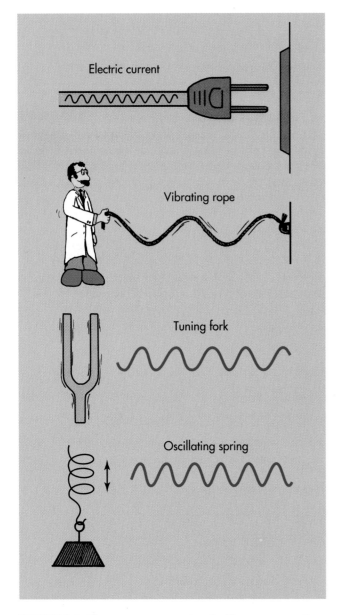

FIGURE 5-2 Sine waves are associated with many naturally occurring phenomena in addition to electromagnetic radiation.

tude and sine wave C, the smallest. Sine wave amplitude is discussed later in connection with high-voltage generation and rectification in an x-ray imaging system.

Amplitude
Amplitude is one half the range from crest to valley over which the sine wave varies.

Frequency and Wavelength

The sine-wave model of electromagnetic radiation describes the variations of the electric and magnetic fields as the photon travels with velocity (c). The important properties of this model are **frequency**, represented by **f**, and **wavelength**, represented by the Greek letter lambda (**λ**). Another interpretation of the vibrating rope in Figure 5-2 is the Texas roadside critter observing the motion of the rope from a position between the fastened end and the scientist (Figure 5-3).

What does the critter see? If he moves his field of view along the rope, he observes the crest of the sine wave traveling along the rope to the end. If he fixes his attention on one segment of the rope, such as point A, he sees the rope rise and fall harmoniously as the waves pass. The more rapidly the scientist moves the rope up and down, the faster the sequence of rise and fall that the critter sees. The number of crests or the number of valleys that pass the point of an observer (in this case, the critter) per unit time is the frequency.

Frequency is usually identified as oscillations per second or cycles per second. Its unit of measurement is the **hertz (Hz)**, which is equal to 1 cycle/s. If the critter used a stopwatch and counted 20 crests passing in 10 s, then

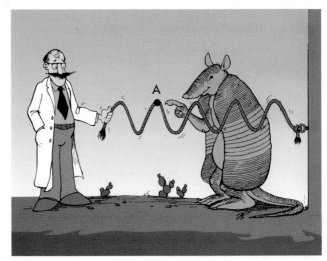

FIGURE 5-3 Moving one end of a rope in a whiplike fashion sets into motion sine waves that travel down the rope to the fastened end. An observer, midway, can determine the frequency of oscillation by counting the crests or valleys that pass a point (A) per unit time.

the frequency would be 20 cycles in 10 s, or 2 Hz. If the scientist doubles the rate at which he moves the rope up and down, the critter would count 40 crests passing in 10 s, and the frequency would be 4 Hz.

> **Frequency**
> Frequency is the number of wavelengths passing a point per second.

The distance from one crest to another, from one valley to another, or from any point on the sine wave to the next corresponding point is the **wavelength**. Figure 5-4 shows sine waves of three wavelengths. With a meter rule, you can verify that wave *A* repeats every 1 cm and therefore has a wavelength of 1 cm. Similarly, wave *B* has a wavelength of 0.5 cm and wave *C* of 1.5 mm. As the frequency is increased, the wavelength is clearly reduced. The wave amplitude is not related to wavelength or frequency.

Three wave parameters—velocity, frequency, and length—are all that is needed to describe electromagnetic radiation. The relationships among these parameters are important concepts. A change in one affects the value of one or both of the others.

Suppose a radiologic technologist is positioned to observe the flight of the sine wave of arrows to determine their frequency (Figure 5-5). The first is measured and found to have a frequency of 60 Hz; that is, 60 oscillations (wavelengths) of the sine wave passes every second. The unknown archer now puts an identical sine wave arrow into his bow and shoots it with less force so that this second arrow has only half the velocity of the first. The observer correctly measures the frequency at 30 Hz, even though the wavelength of the second arrow was the same as that of the first. In other words, as the velocity decreases, the frequency decreases proportionately. Now the archer shoots a third sine wave arrow with precisely the same velocity as the first but with a wavelength twice as long as that of the first. What should be the observed frequency? Thirty hertz is correctly observed.

> At a given velocity, wavelength and frequency are inversely proportional.

This analogy demonstrates how the three parameters associated with a sine wave are interrelated. A simple mathematical formula, called the **wave equation**, expresses the following relationship:

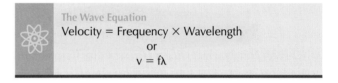

> **The Wave Equation**
> Velocity = Frequency × Wavelength
> or
> $v = f\lambda$

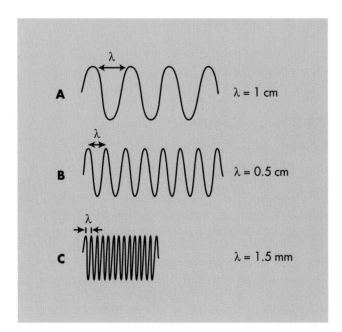

FIGURE 5-4 These three sine waves have different wavelengths. The shorter the wavelength (λ), the higher the frequency.

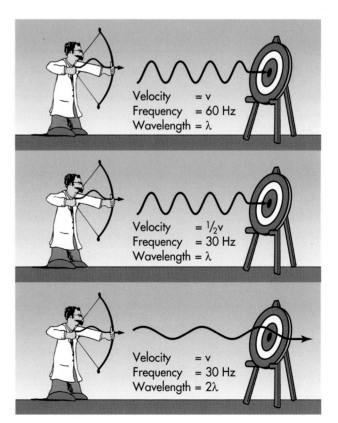

FIGURE 5-5 Relationships among velocity *(v)*, frequency *(f)*, and wavelength (λ) for any sine wave.

The wave equation is used for both sound and electromagnetic radiation. Keep in mind, however, that sound waves are very different from electromagnetic photons. The sources of sound are different, they are propagated in different ways, and their velocities vary greatly. The velocity of sound waves depends on the density of the material through which it passes. Sound cannot travel through a vacuum.

Question: The speed of sound in air is approximately 340 m/s. The highest treble tone that a person can hear is about 20 kHz. What is the wavelength of this sound?

Answer: $v = f\lambda$

$$\lambda = \frac{v}{f}$$

$$= \frac{340 \text{ m/s}}{20 \text{ kHz}}$$

$$= \frac{3.40 \times 10^2 \text{ m}}{\text{s}} \times \frac{\text{s}}{2 \times 10^4 \text{ cycle}}$$

$$= 1.7 \times 10^{-2} \text{ m}$$

$$= 1.7 \text{ cm}$$

When dealing with electromagnetic radiation, we can simplify the wave equation, as follows, because all such radiation travels with the same velocity (c):

Electromagnetic Wave Equation

$c = f\lambda$

The product of frequency and wavelength always equals the velocity of light for electromagnetic radiation. In other words, frequency and wavelength are inversely proportional for electromagnetic radiation. The electromagnetic wave equation can be expressed alternately as follows:

Electromagnetic Wave Equation

$f = \dfrac{c}{\lambda}$ and $\lambda = \dfrac{c}{f}$

As the frequency of electromagnetic radiation increases, the wavelength decreases, and vice versa.

Question: Yellow light has a wavelength of 580 nm. What is the frequency of a photon of yellow light?

Answer: $f = \dfrac{c}{\lambda}$

$$= \frac{3 \times 10^8 \text{ m/s}}{580 \text{ nm}}$$

$$= \frac{3 \times 10^8 \text{ m}}{\text{s}} \times \frac{1}{580 \times 10^{-9} \text{ m}}$$

$$= \frac{3 \times 10^8 \text{ m}}{\text{s}} \times \frac{1}{5.8 \times 10^{-7} \text{ m}}$$

$$= 0.517 \times 10^{15} \text{ cycle/s}$$

$$= 5.17 \times 10^{14} \text{ Hz}$$

Question: The highest energy x-ray produced at 100 kVp (100 keV) has a frequency of 2.42×10^{19} Hz. What is its wavelength?

Answer: $x = \dfrac{c}{f}$

$$= \frac{3 \times 10^8 \text{ m}}{\text{s}} \times \frac{\text{s}}{2.42 \times 10^{19} \text{ cycle}}$$

$$= 1.24 \times 10^{-11} \text{ m}$$

$$= 12.4 \text{ pm}$$

ELECTROMAGNETIC SPECTRUM

The frequency range of electromagnetic radiation extends from approximately 10 to 10^{24} Hz. The photon wavelengths associated with these radiations are approximately 10^7 to 10^{-16} m, respectively. This wide range of values covers many types of electromagnetic radiation, most of which are familiar to us. Grouped together, these radiations make up the **electromagnetic spectrum.**

> The electromagnetic spectrum includes the entire range of electromagnetic radiation.

The known electromagnetic spectrum has three regions most important to radiologic technology: visible light, radiofrequency, and x-radiation. Other portions of the spectrum include ultraviolet radiation, infrared light, and microwave radiation.

Photons of each of these various radiations are essentially the same. Each can be represented as a bundle of energy consisting of varying electric and magnetic fields traveling at the speed of light. The only difference among photons of these various portions of the electromagnetic spectrum is in frequency and wavelength.

Ultrasound is not produced in photon form and does not have a constant velocity. Ultrasound is a wave of moving molecules. Ultrasound requires matter; electromagnetic radiation can exist in a vacuum.

> Diagnostic ultrasound is not a part of the electromagnetic spectrum.

Measurement of the Electromagnetic Spectrum

The electromagnetic spectrum shown in Figure 5-6 contains three different scales, one each for energy, frequency, and wavelength. Since the velocity of all electromagnetic radiation is constant, the wavelength and frequency are inversely related.

Although segments of the electromagnetic spectrum are often given precise ranges, there is overlap because of the methods of producing and techniques for detecting these various radiations. For example, by definition, ultraviolet light has a shorter wavelength than violet light and cannot be sensed by the eye. What is visible violet light to one observer, however, may be ultraviolet light to another. Similarly, microwaves and infrared ra-

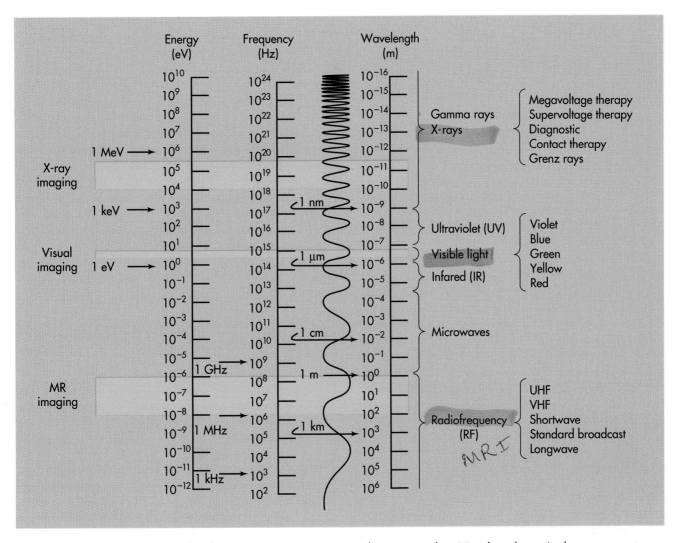

FIGURE 5-6 The electromagnetic spectrum extends over more than 25 orders of magnitude. This chart shows the values of energy, frequency, and wavelength and identifies the three imaging windows.

diation are indistinguishable in their common region of the spectrum.

The earliest studies of reflection, refraction, and diffraction showed light to be wavelike. Consequently, visible light is described by wavelength, which is measured in meters (m). In the 1880s, scientists began experimenting with the radio, which required the oscillation of electrons in a conductor. Consequently, the unit of frequency, the hertz, is used to describe radiowaves. Finally, in 1895, Roentgen discovered x-rays by applying electric potential (kilovolt) across a Crookes tube. Consequently, x-rays are described using a unit of energy, the electron volt (eV).

The three scales used to measure electromagnetic radiation are directly related mathematically. If you know the value of electromagnetic radiation of one scale, you can easily compute its value on the other two. Scientific investigation of the electromagnetic spectrum has been conducted for over 100 years, with scientists working

with radiation in one portion of the spectrum often unaware of others investigating another portion. There is therefore no generally accepted, single dimension for measuring electromagnetic radiation.

Visible Light

An optical physicist describes visible light in terms of wavelength. When sunlight passes through a prism (Figure 5-7), it emerges not as white sunlight but as the colors of the rainbow. Although photons of visible light travel in straight lines, their course can be deviated when they pass from one transparent medium to another. This deviation in line of travel, called **refraction,** is the cause of many peculiar but familiar phenomena, such as a rainbow or the apparent bending of a straw in a glass of water.

White light passing through a prism is refracted because it is composed of photons of a range of wavelengths and the prism acts to separate and group the emerging light according to wavelength. The component

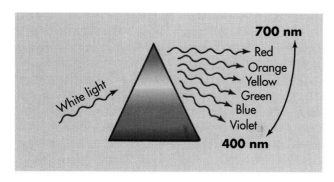

FIGURE 5-7 When it passes through a prism, white light is refracted into its component colors. These colors have wavelengths extending from approximately 400 to 700 nm.

colors of white light have wavelength values ranging from approximately 400 nm for violet to 700 nm for red.

Visible light occupies the smallest segment of the electromagnetic spectrum, and yet it is the only portion that we can sense directly. Sunlight also contains two types of invisible light: infrared and ultraviolet. **Infrared light** consists of photons with wavelengths longer than those of visible light but shorter than those of microwaves. Infrared light heats any substance on which it shines. It may be considered radiant heat. **Ultraviolet light** is located in the electromagnetic spectrum between visible light and ionizing radiation. It is responsible for molecular interactions that can result in sunburn.

Radiofrequency

A radio or television engineer describes photon emissions in terms of their frequency. For example, radio station WIMP might broadcast at 960 kHz, and its associated television station WIMP-TV might broadcast at 63.7 MHz. Communication broadcasts are usually identified by their frequency of transmission and are called **radiofrequency** emissions, or **RF.**

Radiofrequency comprises a considerable portion of the electromagnetic spectrum. Photons of radiofrequency have very low energies and very long wavelengths. Ham operators speak of broadcasting on the 10 m band or the 30 m band; these numbers refer to the approximate wavelength of emission.

A standard AM radio broadcast has a wavelength of about 100 m. Television and FM broadcasting occur at a much shorter wavelength. Because microwaves are also used for communication, considerable overlap exists between what is identified as radiofrequency and what is identified as microwave.

Short-wavelength radiofrequency is known as **microwave** radiation. Microwaves have frequencies that vary according to use but are always higher than broadcast radiofrequencies and lower than infrared. Microwaves have many uses, such as cellular telephone communication, highway speed control, and hot dog preparation.

Ionizing Radiation

Unlike radiofrequency or visible light, ionizing electromagnetic radiation is usually characterized by the energy contained in a photon. When an x-ray imager is operated at 80 kVp, the x-rays it produces contain energies varying from 0 to 80 keV. An x-ray photon contains considerably more energy than a visible light photon or a radiofrequency photon. The frequency of x-radiation is much higher and the wavelength much shorter than for other types of electromagnetic radiation.

The distinction is sometimes made that gamma ray photons have higher energy than x-ray photons. In the early days of radiology, this was true because of the limited capacity of the available x-ray equipment. Today, because of linear accelerators, it is possible to produce x-rays with energies considerably higher than those of gamma ray emissions. Consequently, the distinction by energy is not appropriate.

 The only difference between x-rays and gamma rays is their origin.

X-rays are emitted from the electron cloud of an atom that has been artificially stimulated (Figure 5-8). Gamma rays, on the other hand, come from inside the nucleus of a radioactive atom (Figure 5-9). X-rays are produced in electrical apparatus, whereas gamma rays are emitted spontaneously from radioactive material. Nevertheless, given an x-ray and a gamma ray of equal energy, you could not tell them apart.

This situation is analogous to the difference between beta particles and electrons. These particles are the same, except that beta particles come from the nucleus and electrons come from outside the nucleus.

 Visible light is identified by wavelength, radiofrequency is identified by frequency, and x-rays are identified by energy.

Three regions of the electromagnetic spectrum are particularly important to radiologic technology. Naturally, the x-ray region is fundamental to producing a high-quality radiograph. The visible light region is also important because the viewing conditions of a radiographic or fluoroscopic image are critical to diagnosis. With the introduction of magnetic resonance imaging (MRI), the radiofrequency region has taken on added importance to radiology.

WAVE-PARTICLE DUALITY

A photon of x-radiation and a photon of visible light are fundamentally the same, except that the former has a much higher frequency and hence a shorter wavelength

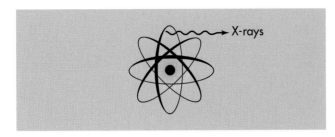

FIGURE 5-8 X-rays are produced outside the nucleus of excited atoms.

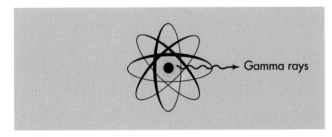

FIGURE 5-9 Gamma rays are produced inside the nucleus of radioactive atoms.

than the latter. These differences result in differences in the way these photons interact with matter. Visible light photons tend to behave more like waves than particles. The opposite is true of x-ray photons, which behave more like particles than waves. In fact, both types of photons exhibit both types of behavior, a phenomenon known as the **wave-particle duality** of radiation.

 Photons interact with matter most easily when the matter is approximately the same size as the photon wavelength.

Another general way to consider the interaction of electromagnetic radiation with matter is as a function of wavelength. Photons of radio and TV, whose wavelengths are measured in meters, interact with metal rods or wires called *antennae*. Microwaves, with wavelengths measured in centimeters, interact most easily with objects of the same size, such as hot dogs and hamburgers. Visible light, whose wavelength is measured in micrometers (μm), interacts with living cells, such as the rods and cones of the eye. Ultraviolet light interacts with molecules, and x-rays interact with atoms and electrons. All radiation with wavelengths longer than that of x-radiation interacts primarily as a wave phenomenon.

 X-rays behave as though they are particles.

Wave Model: Visible Light

One of the unique features of animal life is the sense of vision. It is interesting that we have developed organs that sense only a very narrow portion of the enormous spread of the electromagnetic spectrum. This narrow portion is called **visible light.** The visible light spectrum extends from short-wavelength violet through green and yellow radiation to long-wavelength red radiation. On either side of the visible light spectrum is ultraviolet radiation or infrared radiation. Neither can be detected by the human eye, but both can be detected by other means, such as a photographic emulsion.

Visible light interacts with matter very differently from x-rays. When a photon of light strikes an object, it sets molecules of the object into vibration. The orbital electrons of some atoms of some molecules are excited to a higher energy level than normal. This energy is immediately reirradiated as another photon of light: it is reflected.

The atomic and molecular structures of the objects determine which wavelengths of light are reflected. A leaf in the sunlight appears green because all the visible light photons are absorbed by the leaf but only photons with wavelengths in the green region are reemitted. Similarly, a balloon may appear red by absorbing all visible photons and reirradiating only the long-wavelength red photons.

Many familiar phenomena of light, such as reflection, absorption, and transmission are most easily explained by using the wave model of electromagnetic radiation. When a pebble is dropped into a still pond, ripples radiate from the center of the disturbance like miniature waves. This situation is similar to the wave nature of visible light. Figure 5-10 shows the difference in the water waves between an initial disturbance caused by a small object and one caused by a large object. The distance between the crests of the waves caused by the large object is much longer than that of those caused by the small object.

The difference in wavelength of these water waves is proportional to the energy introduced into the system. With light, the opposite is true; the shorter the photon wavelength, the greater the photon energy.

If the analogy of the pebble in the pond is extended to a continuous succession of pebbles dropped into a smooth ocean, then at the edge of the ocean the waves will appear straight rather than circular. Light waves behave as though they were straight rather than circular because the distance from the source is great. The manner in which light is reflected from or transmitted through a surface is a consequence of this straight, wavelike motion.

When the waves of the ocean crash into a vertical bulkhead (Figure 5-11), the reflected waves scatter from the bulkhead at the same angle that the incident waves struck it. When the bulkhead is removed and replaced with a beach, the water waves simply crash onto the beach, dissipate their energy and are absorbed. When an intermediate condition exists in which the bulkhead has

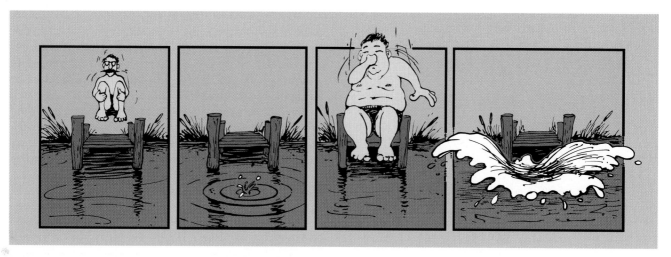

FIGURE 5-10 A small object dropped into a smooth pond creates waves of short wavelength. A large object creates waves of much longer wavelength.

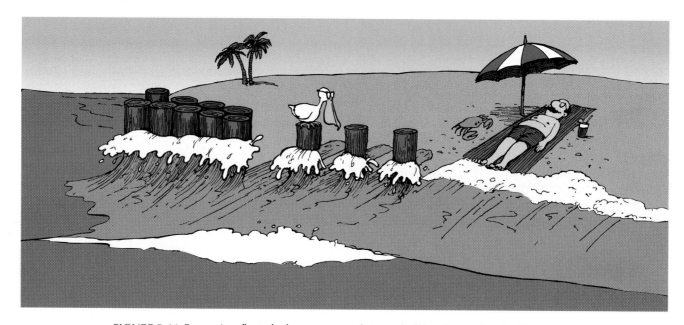

FIGURE 5-11 Energy is reflected when waves crash into a bulkhead. It is absorbed by a beach. It is partially absorbed or attenuated by a line of pilings. Light is also reflected, absorbed, or attenuated, depending on the composition of the surface on which it is incident.

been replaced by a line of pilings, the energy of the waves is scattered and absorbed.

Attenuation
Radiation attenuation is the sum of scattering and absorption.

Visible light can similarly interact with matter. **Reflection** from the silvered surface of a mirror is common. Examples of **transmission, absorption,** and **attenuation** of light are equally easy to identify. When light waves are absorbed, the energy deposited in the absorber reappears as heat. A black asphalt road re-

flects very little visible light but absorbs a considerable amount. Because of this, the road surface can become quite hot.

Just a slight modification can change the manner in which some materials transmit or absorb light. There are three degrees of interaction between light and an absorbing material: transparency, translucency, and opacity (Figure 5-12).

Window glass is **transparent;** it allows light to be transmitted almost unaltered. You can see through glass because the surface is smooth and the molecular structure is tight and orderly. Incident light waves cause molecular and electronic vibrations within the glass. These

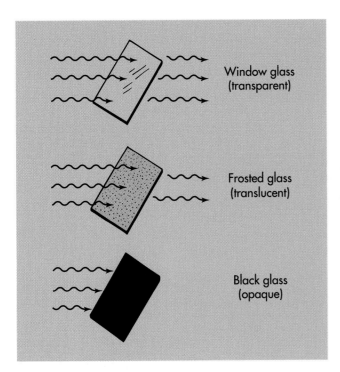

FIGURE 5-12 Objects absorb light in three degrees: not at all (transmission); partially (attenuation), and completely (absorption). The objects associated with these degrees of absorption are called *transparent, translucent,* and *opaque,* respectively.

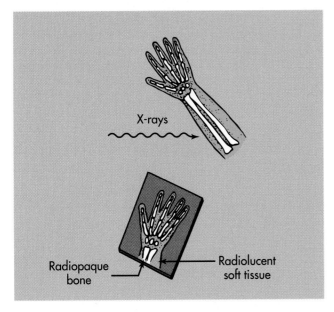

FIGURE 5-13 Structures that attenuate x-rays are described as *radiolucent* or *radiopaque,* depending on the relative degree of x-ray transmission or absorption, respectively.

vibrations are transmitted through the glass and reirradiated almost without change.

When the surface of the glass is roughened with sandpaper, light is still transmitted through the glass but is greatly altered and reduced in intensity. Instead of seeing through clearly, you see only shadows. Such glass is **translucent.**

When the glass is painted black, the characteristics of the pigment in the paint are such that no light can pass through. Any incidental light is totally absorbed in the paint. Such glass is **opaque** to visible light.

The terms **radiopaque** and **radiolucent** are used routinely in x-ray diagnosis to describe the visual appearance of anatomic structures. Structures that absorb x-rays are called *radiopaque.* Structures that attenuate x-rays are called *radiolucent* (Figure 5-13). Bone is radiopaque, whereas lung tissue and to some extent, soft tissue are radiolucent.

Inverse Square Law

When light is emitted from a source such as the sun or a light bulb, the intensity decreases rapidly with the distance from the source. X-rays exhibit precisely the same property. Figure 5-14 shows that as a book is moved farther from a light source, the intensity of light falls. This decrease in intensity is inversely proportional to the square of the distance of the object from the source. Mathematically, this is called the **inverse square law** and is expressed as follows:

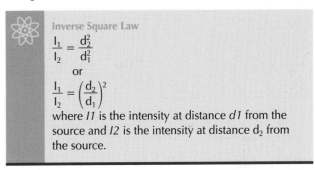

Inverse Square Law

$$\frac{I_1}{I_2} = \frac{d_2^2}{d_1^2}$$

or

$$\frac{I_1}{I_2} = \left(\frac{d_2}{d_1}\right)^2$$

where $I1$ is the intensity at distance $d1$ from the source and $I2$ is the intensity at distance d_2 from the source.

The reason for the rapid decrease in intensity with increasing distance is that the total light emitted is spread out over an increasingly larger area. The equivalent of this phenomenon in the water-wave analogy is the reduction of wave amplitude with distance from the source. The wavelength remains fixed.

 Radiation intensity is inversely related to the square of the distance from the source.

If the source of radiation is not a point but rather a line, such as a fluorescent lamp, the inverse square law does not hold at distances close to the source. At great distances from the source, the inverse square law can be applied.

 The inverse square law can be applied to distances greater than seven times the longest dimension of the source.

To apply the inverse square law, you must know three of the four parameters. The usual situation involves a

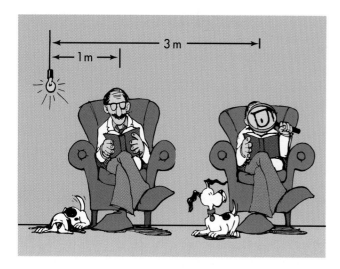

FIGURE 5-14 The inverse square law describes the relationship between radiation intensity and distance from the radiation source.

known intensity at a fixed distance from the source and an unknown intensity at a greater distance.

Question: The intensity of light from a reading lamp is 100 millilumens (mlm), I_2, at a distance of 1 m, d_2. (The lumen is a unit of light intensity.) What is the intensity, I_1, of this light at 3 m, d_1?

Answer:
$$\frac{I_1}{I_2} = \frac{d_2^2}{d_1^2}$$

$$\frac{I_1}{100 \text{ mlm}} = \frac{1 \text{ m}^2}{3 \text{ m}^2}$$

$$I_1 = (100 \text{ mlm})\left(\frac{1 \text{ m}}{3 \text{ m}}\right)^2$$

$$= (100 \text{ mlm})(1/9)$$

$$= 11 \text{ mlm}$$

This relationship between radiation intensity and distance from the source applies equally well to x-ray intensity.

Question: The exposure from an x-ray tube operated at 70 kVp, 200 mAs, is 400 mR (4 mGy$_a$), I_2, at 90 cm, d_2. What will be the exposure at 180 cm, d_1?

Answer:
$$\frac{I_1}{I_2} = \left(\frac{d_2}{d_1}\right)^2$$

$$I_1 = I_2\left(\frac{d_2}{d_1}\right)^1$$

$$= (400 \text{ mR})\left(\frac{90 \text{ cm}}{180 \text{ cm}}\right)^2$$

$$= (400 \text{ mR})(1/2)^2$$

$$= (400 \text{ mR})(1/4)$$

$$= 100 \text{ mR}$$

This example illustrates that when the distance from the source is doubled, the intensity of radiation is reduced to one fourth and conversely, when the distance is halved, the intensity is increased by a factor of four.

Question: For a given technique, the x-ray intensity at 1 m, d_2, is 450 mR (4.5 mGy$_a$), I_2. What is the intensity at the edge of the control booth, a distance of 3 m, d_1, if the useful beam is directed at the booth? (This, of course, should never be done!)

Answer:
$$\frac{I_1}{I_2} = \left(\frac{d_2}{d_1}\right)^2$$

$$I_1 = I_2\left(\frac{d_2}{d_1}\right)^2$$

$$= (450 \text{ mR})\left(\frac{1 \text{ m}}{3 \text{ m}}\right)^2$$

$$= (450 \text{ mR})(1/3)^2$$

$$= (450 \text{ mR})(1/9)$$

$$= 50 \text{ mR}$$

Often, it is necessary to determine the distance from the source at which the radiation has a given intensity. This type of problem is common in designing radiologic facilities.

Question: A temporary chest unit is to be set up in a large hall. The technique used results in an exposure of 25 mR (0.25 mGy$_a$) at 180 cm. The area behind the chest stand in which the exposure intensity exceeds 1 mR is to be cordoned off. How far from the x-ray tube will this area extend?

Answer:
$$\frac{I_1}{I_2} = \frac{d_2^2}{d_2^2}$$

$$\frac{25 \text{ mR}}{1 \text{ mR}} = \frac{(d_2)^2}{180 \text{ cm}^2}$$

$$(d_2)^2 = (180 \text{ cm})^2\left(\frac{25 \text{ mR}}{1 \text{ mR}}\right)$$

$$d_2 = \left[(180^2)\left(\frac{25}{1}\right)\right]^{1/2}$$

$$= (180)^{1/2}(25)^{1/2}$$

$$= (180)(5)$$

$$= 900 \text{ cm}$$

$$= 9 \text{ m}$$

Particle Model: Quantum Theory

Unlike other portions of the electromagnetic spectrum, x-rays are usually identified by their energy, measured in electron volts (eV). X-ray energy ranges from approximately 1 to 50 MeV. The associated wavelength for this range of x-radiation is approximately 10^{-9} to 10^{-12} m. The frequency of these photons varies from approximately 10^{18} to 10^{21} Hz. Table 5-1 describes the various types of x-rays produced and

TABLE 5-1	The Wide Range of X-Rays Produced For Application For Medicine, Research, and Industry	
Type of X-Ray	**Approximate Energy**	**Application**
Diffraction	<10 kVp	Research: structural and molecular analysis
Grenz rays*	10 to 20 kVp	Medicine: dermatology
Superficial	50 to 100 kVp	Medicine: therapy of superficial tissues
Diagnostic	30 to 150 kVp	Medicine: imaging of anatomic structures and tissues
Orthovoltage*	200 to 300 kVp	Medicine: therapy of deep tissues
Supervoltage*	300 to 1000 kVp	Medicine: therapy of deep tissues
Megavoltage	>1 MV	Medicine: therapy of deep tissues
		Industry: checking of the integrity of welded metals

*These radiation therapy modalities are no longer in use.

the general use of each. We are interested primarily in the diagnostic range of x-radiation, although what is said for that range holds equally well for other types of x-radiation.

The maximum x-ray energy possible is limited only by the voltage applied to the x-ray tube.

 The x-ray photon is a discrete bundle of energy.

An x-ray photon can be thought of as containing electric and magnetic fields that vary sinusoidally at right angles to each other and whose beginnings and ends have diminishing amplitude (Figure 5-15). The wavelength of an x-ray photon is measured like that of any electromagnetic radiation; it is the distance from any position on the sine wave to the next corresponding position. The frequency of an x-ray photon is calculated like the frequency of any electromagnetic photon, by the use of the wave equation.

X-rays are created at the speed of light and either exist with velocity (c) or do not exist at all. That is one of the substantive statements of **Planck's quantum theory.** Max Planck was a German physicist whose mathematic and physical theories synthesized our understanding of electromagnetic radiation into a uniform model; for this work he received the Nobel Prize in 1918. Another important consequence of this theory is the relationship between energy and frequency: photon energy is directly proportional to the photon frequency. The constant of proportionality, known as **Planck's constant** and symbolized by *h*, has a numerical value of 4.15×10^{-15} eVs or 6.63×10^{-34} Js. Mathematically, the relationship between energy and frequency is expressed as follows:

Planck's Quantum Equation
$E = hf$
where *E* is the photon energy, *h* is Planck's constant, and *f* is the photon frequency in hertz.

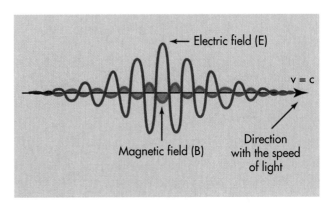

FIGURE 5-15 An x-ray can be visualized as two perpendicular sine waves traveling in a straight line at the speed of light. One of the sine waves represents an electric field and the other a magnetic field.

 The energy of a photon is directly proportional to its frequency.

Question: What is the frequency of a 70-keV x-ray?

Answer:
$$E = hf$$
$$f = \frac{E}{h}$$
$$= \frac{7 \times 10^4 \text{ eV}}{4.15 \times 10^{-15} \text{ eVs}}$$
$$= 1.69 \times 10^{19}/\text{s}$$
$$= 1.69 \times 10^{19} \text{ Hz}$$

Question: What is the energy contained in one photon of radiation from radio station WIMP-AM, which has a broadcast frequency of 960 kHz?

Answer:
$$E = hf$$
$$= (4.15 \times 10^{-15} \text{ eVs})(9.6 \times 10^5/\text{s})$$
$$= 3.98 \times 10^{-9} \text{ eV}$$

An extension of Planck's equation is the relationship between photon energy and photon wavelength; this relationship is useful in computing equivalent wavelengths of x-rays and other types of radiation.

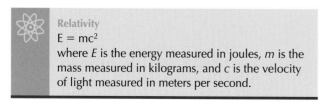

Equivalent Planck Equation

$$E = hf, \quad f = E/h, \quad E = \frac{hc}{\lambda}$$

In other words, photon energy is inversely proportional to photon wavelength. In this relationship the constant of proportionality is a combination of two constants: Planck's constant and the speed of light. The longer the wavelength of radiation, the lower the energy of each photon.

Question: What is the energy in one photon of green light whose wavelength is 550 nm?

Answer:
$$E = \frac{hc}{\lambda}$$
$$= \frac{(4.15 \times 10^{-15} \text{ eVs})(3 \times 10^8 \text{ m/s})}{550 \times 10^{-9} \text{ m}}$$
$$= \frac{12.45 \times 10^{-7} \text{ eVm}}{5.5 \times 10^{-7} \text{ m}}$$
$$= 2.26 \text{ eV}$$

MATTER AND ENERGY

We began in Chapter 1 with the statement that everything in existence can be classified as matter or energy. It was further stated that matter and energy are really manifestations of each other. According to classical physics, matter can be neither created nor destroyed, a law known as the **law of conservation of matter.** A similar law, the **law of conservation of energy,** states that energy can be neither created nor destroyed.

Planck's quantum physics and Einstein's physics of relativity greatly extended these theories. According to quantum physics and the physics of relativity, matter can be transformed into energy and vice versa. Nuclear fission, the basis for nuclear generation of electricity, is an example of converting matter into energy. In radiology, a process known as *pair production* (see Chapter 13) is an example of the conversion of energy into mass.

A simple relationship introduced in Chapter 1 allows the calculation of energy equivalence of mass and the mass equivalence of energy. This equation is a consequence of Einstein's theory of relativity and is familiar to all.

Relativity

$$E = mc^2$$
where *E* is the energy measured in joules, *m* is the mass measured in kilograms, and *c* is the velocity of light measured in meters per second.

Like the electron volt, the joule (J) is a unit of energy. One joule is equal to 6.24×10^{18} eV.

Question: What is the energy equivalence of an electron (mass = 9.109×10^{-31} kg) measured in joules and in electron volts?

Answer:
$$E = mc^2$$
$$= (9.109 \times 10^{-31} \text{ kg})(3 \times 10^8 \text{ m/s})^2$$
$$= 81.972 \times 10^{-15} \text{ J}$$
$$= (8.1972 \times 10^{-14} \text{ J})\left(\frac{6.24 \times 10^{18} \text{ eV}}{J}\right)$$
$$= 51.15 \times 10^4 \text{ eV}$$
$$= 511.5 \text{ keV}$$

The problem might be stated in the opposite direction, as follows:

Question: What is the mass equivalence of a 70-keV x-ray?

Answer:
$$E = mc^2$$
$$m = \frac{E}{c^2}$$
$$= \frac{(70 \times 10^3 \text{ eV})\left(\dfrac{J}{6.24 \times 10^{18} \text{ eV}}\right)}{(3 \times 10^8 \text{ m/s})^2}$$
$$= \frac{11.2 \times 10^{-15} \text{ J}}{9 \times 10^{16} \text{ m}^2/\text{s}^2}$$
$$= 1.25 \times 10^{-31} \text{ kg}$$

By using the relationships reported earlier, you can calculate the mass equivalence of a photon when only the photon wavelength or photon frequency is known.

Question: What is the mass equivalence of one photon of 1000-MHz microwave radiation?

Answer:
$$E = hf = mc^2$$
$$m = \frac{hf}{c^2}$$
$$= \frac{(6.626 \times 10^{-34} \text{ Js})(1000 \times 10^6 \times \text{Hz})}{(3 \times 10^8 \text{ m/s})^2}$$
$$= 0.736 \times 10^{-41} \text{ kg}$$
$$= 7.36 \times 10^{-42} \text{ kg}$$

Question: What is the mass equivalence of a 330-nm photon of ultraviolet light?

Answer:
$$E = \frac{hc}{\lambda} = mc^2$$
$$m = \left(\frac{hc}{\lambda}\right)\left(\frac{1}{c^2}\right) = \frac{h}{\lambda c}$$
$$= \frac{6.626 \times 10^{-34} \text{ Js}}{(330 \times 10^{-9} \text{ m})(3 \times 10^8 \text{ m/s})}$$
$$= 0.00669 \times 10^{-33} \text{ kg}$$
$$= 6.69 \times 10^{-36} \text{ kg}$$

Calculations of this type can be used to set up a scale of mass equivalence for the electromagnetic spectrum (Figure 5-16). This scale can be used to check the answers to these examples and to some of the problems in the companion Workbook and Laboratory Manual.

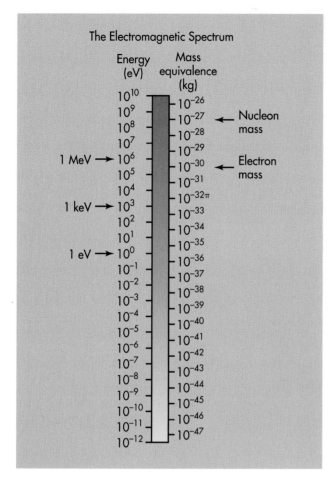

The Electromagnetic Spectrum

FIGURE 5-16 Mass and energy are two forms of the same medium. This scale shows the equivalence of mass measured in kilograms to energy measured in electron volts.

SUMMARY

Although matter and energy are interchangeable, it is energy in the form of x-ray photons interacting with tissue and an image receptor that forms the basis for x-ray imaging.

X-rays are one type of photon of electromagnetic radiation. *Velocity, amplitude, frequency,* and *wavelength* are used to describe the various imaging regions of the electromagnetic spectrum. These characteristics of electromagnetic radiation determine the manner in which such radiation interacts with matter.

CHALLENGE QUESTIONS

1. Define or otherwise identify:
   a. Photon
   b. Radiolucency
   c. The inverse square law
   d. Frequency
   e. The law of conservation of energy
   f. Gamma rays
   g. Electromagnetic spectrum
   h. Sinusoidal (sine) variation
   i. Quantum
   j. Visible light

2. Accurately diagram one photon of orange light ($\lambda =$ 620 nm) and identify its velocity, electric field, magnetic field, and wavelength.

3. A thunder clap associated with lightning has a frequency of 800 Hz. If its wavelength is 50 cm, what is its velocity? How far away is the thunder if the time interval between seeing the lightning and hearing the thunder is 6 s?

4. What is the frequency associated with a photon of microwave radiation having a wavelength of 10^{-4} m?

5. Radio station WIMP-FM broadcasts at 104 MHz. What is the wavelength of this radiation?

6. In mammography, 28-keV x-rays are used. What is the frequency of this radiation?

7. Radiography of bony structures calls for a high–kilovolt peak technique. In many of these x-rays, energy is 110 keV. What is the frequency and wavelength of this radiation?

8. What is the energy of the 110-keV x-ray of Question 7 when expressed in joules? What is its mass equivalence?

9. The output intensity of a normal radiographic unit is 3 mR/mAs at 100 cm. What is the output intensity of such a unit at 200 cm?

10. A mobile x-ray imager has an output intensity of 4 mR/mAs at 100 cm. Conditions require that a particular examination be conducted at 75 cm SID. What is the output intensity at this distance?

11. Write the wave equation.

12. How are frequency and wavelength related?

13. Write the inverse square law and describe its meaning.

14. The intensity of light from a reading lamp is 100 mlm at a distance of 1 m. What is the intensity of light at 3 m?

15. What are the three imaging windows of the electromagnetic spectrum and the unit of measure applied to each?

16. What is the energy range of diagnostic x-rays?

17. What is the difference between x-rays and gamma rays?

18. Some regions of the electromagnetic spectrum exhibit wave nature and some regions exhibit particle nature in their interaction with matter. What is this phenomenon called?

19. Define *attenuation*.

20. What is the frequency of a 70-keV x-ray photon?

Electricity

OBJECTIVES

At the completion of this chapter, the student should be able to:

1. Identify the electrical properties of subatomic particles
2. Define *electrification* and provide examples
3. List the laws of electrostatics
4. Name examples of conductors and insulators
5. Describe electric circuits and recognize circuit element symbols
6. Define *direct current* and *alternating current*
7. Identify units of electric potential and electric power

OUTLINE

This chapter on electricity introduces the basic concepts needed for further study of the x-ray imaging system and its various components.

Because the primary function of the x-ray imaging unit is to convert electric energy into electromagnetic energy—x-rays—the study of electricity is particularly important. This chapter begins by introducing some examples of familiar devices that convert electricity into other forms of energy. The fundamentals of electricity, including electrostatics and electrodynamics, are discussed in detail.

Electrostatics is the science of stationary electric charges. Electrodynamics is the science of electric charges in motion. This chapter also presents the laws governing electrostatics and electrodynamics.

ELECTRICITY

The primary function of an x-ray imaging system (Figure 6-1) is to convert electric energy into electromagnetic energy. Electric energy is supplied to the x-ray unit in the form of well-controlled electric current. A conversion takes place in the x-ray tube, where some of this electric energy is transformed into x-rays.

Figure 6-2 shows other, more familiar, examples of electric energy conversion. When an automobile battery is recharged after it runs down, an electric charge restores the chemical energy of the battery. Electric energy

is converted into mechanical energy with a device known as an *electric motor,* which can be used to drive a table saw. A kitchen toaster or electric range converts electric energy into thermal energy. There are, of course, many other examples of the conversion of electric energy into other forms of energy.

ELECTROSTATICS

Matter
Matter has mass, form, and energy equivalence. Matter may also have electric charge.

Because of the way atoms are constructed, electrons are often free to travel from the outermost shell of one atom to the next. Protons, on the other hand, are fixed inside the

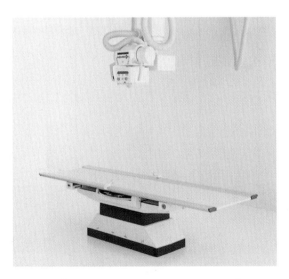

FIGURE 6-1 The x-ray imaging system converts electric energy into electromagnetic energy. *(Courtesy Toshiba.)*

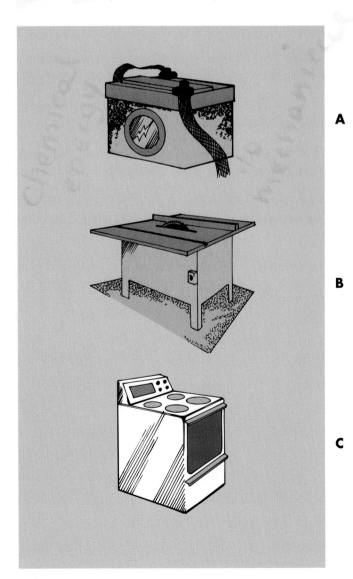

FIGURE 6-2 Electric energy can be converted from or to other forms by various devices, such as the battery **(A)** from chemical energy, motor **(B)** to mechanical energy, and kitchen range **(C)** to thermal energy.

nucleus of an atom and are not free to move. Consequently, nearly all discussions of electric charge deal with negative electric charges associated with the electron.

Electric charge comes in discrete units that are either **positive** or **negative**. The smallest units of electric charge are the electron and the proton. The electron has one unit of negative charge, and the proton has one unit of positive charge. Thus the electric charges associated with an electron and a proton have the same magnitude but opposite signs. The total net charge of all matter in the universe is neutral because the total number of negative charges equals the total number of positive charges.

Electrification

Electrification
Electrification can be created by **contact, friction,** or **induction.**

The outer-shell electrons of some types of atoms are loosely bound and can be easily removed. Removal of these electrons electrifies the substance from which they are removed and results in static electricity. **Electrostatics** is the study of stationary electric charges.

The most familiar example of static electricity might be the experience of getting a shock touching (contact) a metal doorknob after walking across a deep-pile carpet in the winter (friction). This shock occurs because electrons are rubbed off the carpet onto the shoes, which causes you to become electrified. Then the electrons are released onto the doorknob when you touch it.

An object is said to be **electrified** if it has too few or too many electrons. Electrification is an abnormal state relieved by providing some other object—the doorknob, for example—from which excess electrons can be trans-

ferred. Similarly, if you run a comb through your hair, electrons are removed from your hair and deposited onto the comb (friction). The comb becomes electrified with too many negative charges. An electrified comb can pick up tiny pieces of paper as if it were a magnet (Figure 6-3). Because the comb has excess electrons, it repels some electrons in the paper, causing the closest end of the paper to become slightly positively charged. This results in a small electrostatic attractive force. Similarly, hair is electrified because it has an abnormally low number of electrons and may stand on end because of mutual repulsion.

Electrification occurs because of the movement of negative electric charges. Positive electric charges do not move. The transfer of electrons from one object to another causes the first to be positively electrified and the second to be negatively electrified.

When a negatively electrified object is brought into contact with an electrically neutral object, the electric charges of the electrified object may be transferred to the neutral object. If the transfer is sufficiently violent, there will be a spark. One neutral object always available to accept electric charges from an electrified object is the Earth. The Earth behaves as a huge reservoir for stray electric charges. In this capacity, it is called an **electric ground**.

During a thunderstorm, wind and cloud movement can remove electrons from one cloud and deposit them on another (induction). Both clouds become electrified, one negatively and one positively. If the electrification becomes great enough, a discharge between the clouds can occur in which electrons are rapidly transported back to the cloud that is deficient. This phenomenon is called **lightning**. Although lightning can occur between clouds, it most frequently occurs between an electrified cloud and the Earth (Figure 6-4).

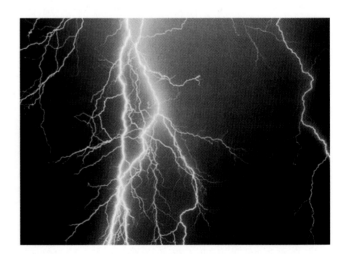

FIGURE 6-3 Running a comb briskly through your hair may cause both hair and comb to become electrified through the transfer of electrons from hair to comb. The electrified condition may make it possible to pick up small pieces of paper with the comb and may cause your hair to stand on end.

FIGURE 6-4 Electrified clouds are the source of lightning in a storm.

Another familiar example of electrification is seen in every Frankenstein movie. Usually Dr. Frankenstein's laboratory is filled with electric gadgets, wire, and large steel balls with sparks flying in every direction (Figure 6-5). The sparks are created because the various objects—wires, steel balls, and so on—are highly electrified. Eventually, the number of electric charges becomes so large that the electrification of the object is too great to be sustained. A breakdown occurs by the rapid movement of electrons through the air to an unelectrified object, resulting in the spark, which is in effect a miniature lightning bolt.

Electrostatic Charge

The smallest unit of electric charge is an electron. This charge is much too small to be useful, so the fundamental unit of electric charge is the coulomb (C), 1 C = 6.3 × 10^{18} electron charges.

Question: What is the electrostatic charge of one electron?

Answer: One coulomb (1 C) is equivalent to 6.3 × 10^{18} electron charges; therefore:

$$\frac{1\ C}{6.3 \times 10^{18}\ electron\ charges} =$$
$$1.6 \times 10^{-19}\ C/electron\ charge$$

Question: The electrostatic charge transferred between two people after one has scuffed his feet across a nylon rug is about a microcoulomb. How many electrons are transferred?

Answer: 1 C = 6.3 × 10^{18} electrons
1μC = 6.3 × 10^{12} electrons transferred

Question: mAs is a measure of what quantity?

Answer: $mAs = m\frac{C}{S}s = mC$, which is electrostatic charge

Electrostatic Laws

Four general laws of electrostatics describe the way in which electric charges interact with one another and with neutral objects.

 Unlike charges attract; like charges repel.

Associated with each electric charge is an **electric field.** The electric field radiates outward from a positive charge and into a negative charge. Uncharged particles do not have an electric field. The intensity of the electric field is illustrated in Figure 6-6 by lines associated with each charged particle.

When two similar electric charges, negative and negative or positive and positive, are brought close together, their electric fields are in opposite directions and cause the electric charges to be repelled from each other. When unlike charges, one negative and one positive, are close to each other, the electric fields radiate in the same direction and cause the two charges to be attracted to each other. The force of attraction between unlike charges or repulsion between like charges is due to the electric field.

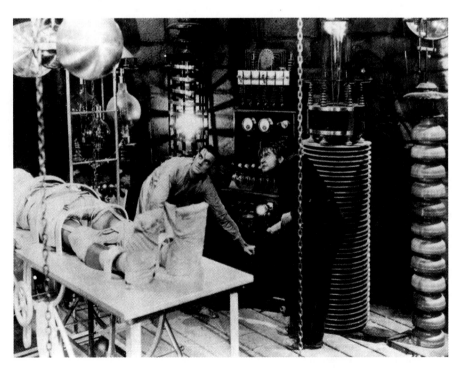

FIGURE 6-5 Early radiologic technologists are shown in this scene from the original *Frankenstein* movie (1931). *(Courtesy The Bettman Archives, Inc.)*

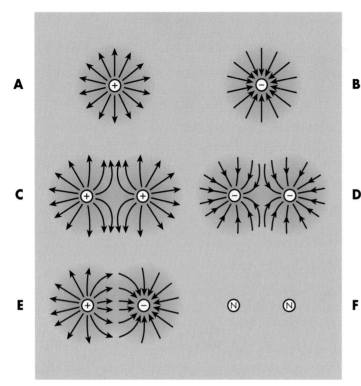

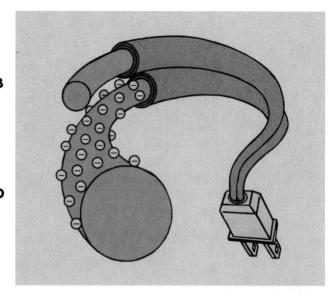

FIGURE 6-7 Cross section of electrified copper wire, showing that the electrostatic charges reside on the surface of the wire.

FIGURE 6-6 Electric fields radiate out from a positive charge **(A)** and toward a negative charge **(B)**. Like charges repel one another **(C and D)**. Unlike charges attract one another **(E)**. Uncharged particles do not have an electric field **(F)**.

It is called an *electrostatic force.* Uncharged particles exert no electrostatic force and are not acted on by charged particles.

Coulomb's Law. The magnitude of the electrostatic force is given by Coulomb's law as follows:

Coulomb's Law

$$F = k\frac{Q_A Q_B}{d^2}$$

where:
F = electrostatic force (newtons)
Q_A and Q_B = electrostatic charges (coulombs)
d = distance between the charges (m)
k = constant of proportionality

Coulomb's Law
Coulomb's law states that electrostatic force is directly proportional to the product of the electrostatic charges and inversely proportional to the square of the distance between them.

The greater the electrostatic charge on either object, the greater the electrostatic force. The electrostatic force is very strong when objects are close but decreases rapidly as objects separate. This **inverse square** relationship for electrostatic force is the same as that for x-ray intensity (see Chapter 5). The equation for electrostatic force has the same form as that for gravitational force, but electrostatic forces act only over short distances, whereas gravitational forces act over very long distances.

The electrostatic force can be attractive or repulsive, whereas the gravitational force is only attractive. The electrostatic force between two charges is unaffected by the presence of a third charge; similarly, the gravitational force between two masses is unaffected by the presence of a third mass.

When an object becomes electrified, the electric charges are uniformly distributed throughout the object or on its surface.

When a diffuse nonconductor, such as a thunder cloud, becomes electrified, the electric charges are distributed uniformly throughout. An electrified copper wire or another solid conductor has its excess electrons distributed on its outer surface (Figure 6-7).

The electric charge of a conductor is concentrated along the sharpest curvature of its surface.

An electrified cattle prod (Figure 6-8) has electric charges equally distributed on the surface of the two electrodes, except at each tip where electric charge is concentrated. "Our business is shocking," is the motto of the manufacturer of this cattle prod.

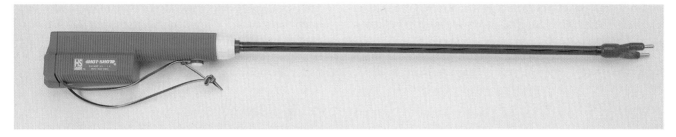

FIGURE 6-8 Electrostatic charges are concentrated on surfaces of sharpest curvature. The cattle prod is a device that takes advantage of this electrostatic law. *(Courtesy Hotshot Products Company, Inc.)*

Electric Potential

An earlier discussion of potential energy (see Chapter 1) emphasized its relationship to work. A system possessing potential energy is a system with stored energy. Such a system has the ability to do work when this energy is released. Electric charges have potential energy. When positioned close to one another, like electric charges have electric potential energy because they can do work when they fly apart. Electrons bunched up at one end of a wire possess electric potential because the electrostatic repulsive force will cause some electrons to move along the wire and work can be done.

 The unit of electric potential is the volt (V).

Electric potential is sometimes termed **electromotive force (EMF)**, or voltage; the higher the voltage, the higher the potential to do work. The electric potential in homes and offices is 110 V. X-ray imagers usually require 220 V or higher.

ELECTRODYNAMICS

 The study of electric charges in motion is electrodynamics.

We recognize electrodynamic phenomena as electricity. If an electric potential is applied to objects, such as copper wires, then electric charges move along the wire. This is called an *electric current* or *electricity*. An **electric current** is the flow of electrons. Electric currents occur in many types of objects and range from the very small currents of the human body measured by electrocardiograms to the very large currents of 440,000-V cross-country electrical transmission lines. The direction of electric current is important to remember. In his early classic experiments, Benjamin Franklin assumed that positive electric charges were conducted on his kite string. The unfortunate response of this assumption is the conventional wisdom that the direction of electric current is always opposite of electron flow.

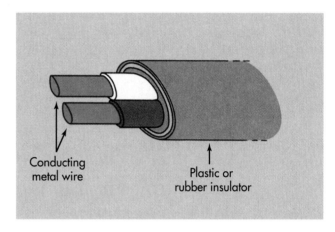

FIGURE 6-9 Conventional electric wire usually consists of two parts: the metal conductor and the insulator.

Conductors and Insulators

 Conductor
A conductor is any substance through which electrons flow easily.

A section of conventional household electric wire consists of a metal conducting wire, usually copper, coated with a rubber or plastic insulating material (Figure 6-9). The insulator confines the electron flow to the conductor. Touching the insulator does not result in a shock; touching the conductor does.

 Insulator
An insulator is any material that does not allow electron flow.

Most metals are good electric conductors, copper being the best, although aluminum is also used. Water is also a good electric conductor because of the salts and other impurities it contains. That is why everyone should avoid water when operating power tools. Glass, clay, and other earthlike materials are usually good electric insulators.

In recent years, materials have been discovered that exhibit two entirely different electric characteristics. In 1946, William Shockley demonstrated semiconduction. The prin-

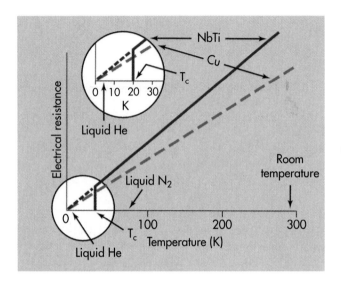

FIGURE 6-10 The electric resistance of a conductor (Cu) and a superconductor (NbTi) as a function of temperature.

cipal semiconductor materials are silicon (Si) and germanium (Ge). This development led first to the transistor and then to integrated circuits and very-large-scale integrated (VLSI) circuits and finally to microchips, which are the basis for the present explosion in computer technology.

Semiconductor
A semiconductor is a material that under some conditions behaves as an insulator, whereas under other conditions it acts as a conductor.

At room temperature, all material resists the flow of electricity. Resistance decreases as the temperature of material is reduced (Figure 6-10). **Superconductivity** is the property of some materials to exhibit no resistance below a critical temperature (T_c).

Superconductivity was discovered in 1911 but was not developed commercially until the early 1960s. Today, there is much scientific investigation resulting in the demonstration of superconductivity at increasing temperature (Figure 6-11). In 1987, the Nobel Prize in Physics was awarded to Bednorz and Muller for their work on high-temperature superconductivity in a new class of materials.

Superconducting materials such as niobium and titanium allow the flow of electrons without any resis-

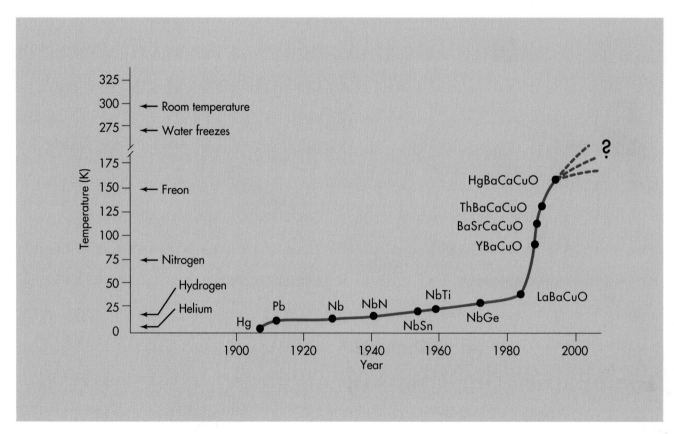

FIGURE 6-11 Recent years have shown a dramatic rise in the initial temperature for superconducting materials.

tance. Ohm's law described in the next section does not hold true for superconductors. You might view a superconducting circuit as a perpetual motion machine, since current flows without an electric potential or voltage. For material to behave as a superconductor, however, it must be made very cold, which requires energy. Table 6-1 summarizes the four electrical states of matter.

Electric Circuits

Electrons flow on the surface of a wire. Modifying the wire by reducing its diameter (wire gauge) or inserting different material (circuit elements) can increase its resistance (Figure 6-12). When this resistance is controlled and the conductor is made into a closed path, the result is an **electric circuit.**

In some respects, an electric circuit is similar to a public water system. In such a system (Figure 6-13) the first step is supplying the water with potential energy by pumping it into a water tower. As the water flows from

the water tower through pipes with successively smaller diameters, resistance to its flow increases.

Similarly, small-diameter wires resist the flow of electric current more than large-diameter wires. A defect somewhere along the water line, such as a faulty valve, creates a large resistance to flow. This is similar to resistive elements built into electric circuits. When the valve is operating properly in the water line, the resistance to the flow of water can be controlled. Similarly, variable resistors in an electric circuit allow control of the flow of electrons.

 Increasing electric resistance results in a reduction of electric current.

After the water has been distributed to homes and is used, it is conveyed along waste water pipes back into the ground. Similarly, electric currents can be conducted, after use, back to ground or the Earth.

TABLE 6-1	**Four Electrical States of Matter**		
State	**Material**	**Characteristics**
Superconductor	Niobium	Has no resistance to electron flow
	Titanium	Has no electric potential required
		Must be very cold
Conductor	Copper	Has variable resistance
	Aluminum	Obeys Ohm's law
		Requires an electric potential
Semiconductor	Silicon	Can be conductive
	Germanium	Can be resistive
		Is the basis for computer technology
Insulator	Rubber	Does not permit electron flow
	Glass	Has extremely high resistance
		Is necessary with high voltage

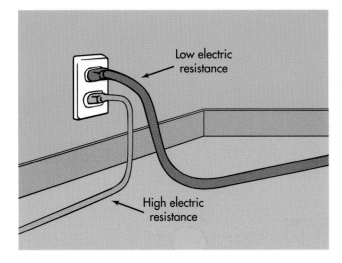

FIGURE 6-12 Electric resistance is increased with smaller wire and circuit elements.

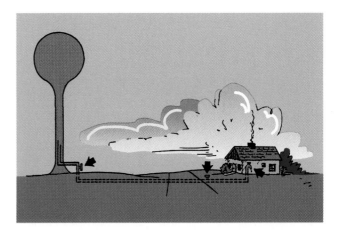

FIGURE 6-13 In some respects, a municipal water system is like an electric circuit. Water represents electric current; the water tank represents electric potential, and the valves represent electric resistors.

Electric current is measured in a unit called the *ampere (A)*. The ampere measures the number of electrons flowing in the electric circuit. One ampere is equal to an electric charge of one coulomb flowing through a conductor each second. Electric potential is measured in a unit called the *volt (V)*, and electric resistance is measured in a unit called the *ohm (Ω)*. Electrons powered by high voltage have high potential energy and a high capacity to do work. If electrons are inhibited in their flow, the circuit resistance is said to be high.

The manner in which electric currents behave in an electric circuit is described by a relationship known as *Ohm's law.*

Ohm's Law
Ohm's law states that the voltage across the total circuit or any portion of the circuit is equal to the current multiplied by the resistance.

Ohm's Law
$$V = IR$$
where *V* is the electric potential in volts, *I* is the electric current in amperes, and *R* is the electric resistance in ohms. Variations of this relationship are:
$$R = \frac{V}{I}$$
and
$$I = \frac{V}{R}$$

Question: If a current of 0.5 A flows through a conductor that has a resistance of 6 Ω, what is the voltage across the conductor?

Answer: $V = IR$
$= (0.5 \text{ A})(6 \text{ Ω})$
$= 3 \text{ V}$

Question: A kitchen toaster draws a current of 2.5 A. If the household voltage is 110 V, what is the electric resistance of the toaster?

Answer: $R = \dfrac{V}{I}$
$= \dfrac{110 \text{ V}}{2.5 \text{ A}}$
$= 44 \text{ Ω}$

Most electric circuits, such as those used in radio, television, and other electronic devices, are very complicated. X-ray circuits are also complicated and contain several types of circuit elements. Table 6-2 identifies some of these circuit elements, the functions of each, and their symbols.

Usually electric circuits can be reduced to one of two basic kinds: a series circuit (Figure 6-14) or a parallel circuit (Figure 6-15).

Series Circuit
In a series circuit, all circuit elements are connected in a line along the same conductor.

Rules for Series Circuits
1. The total resistance is equal to the sum of the individual resistances.
2. The current through each circuit element is the same and is equal to the total circuit current.
3. The sum of the voltage across each circuit element is equal to the total circuit voltage.

Parallel Circuit
A parallel circuit contains elements that bridge conductors rather than lie in a line along a conductor.

Rules for Parallel Circuits
1. The sum of the currents through each circuit element is equal to the total circuit current.
2. The voltage across each circuit element is the same and is equal to the total circuit voltage.
3. The total resistance is inversely proportional to the sum of the reciprocals of each individual resistance.

Question: A series circuit contains three resistive elements having values of 8, 12, and 15 Ω. If the voltage is 110 V, what is the total resistance and current, the current through each resistor, and the voltage across each resistor?

Answer: Refer to Figure 6-14; let $R_1 = 8 \text{ Ω }$ $R_2 = 12 \text{ Ω }$ $R_3 = 15 \text{ Ω}$
$R_T = 8 \text{ Ω} + 12 \text{ Ω} + 15 \text{ Ω} = 35 \text{ Ω}$
$I_T = I_1 = I_2 = I_3 = V/R = 110/35 = 3.14 \text{ A}$
$V_1 = (3.14 \text{ A})(8 \text{ Ω}) = 25.12 \text{ V}$
$V_2 = (3.14 \text{ A})(12 \text{ Ω}) = 37.68 \text{ V}$
$V_3 = (3.14 \text{ A})(15 \text{ Ω}) = 47.10 \text{ V}$

Question: Suppose the previous example were a parallel circuit rather than a series circuit. What would be the correct values for total resistance and current, the current through each resistor, and the voltage across each resistor?

TABLE 6-2	Electric Circuit Elements: Their Symbol and Function	
Circuit Element	**Symbol**	**Function**
Resistor	⟋⟍⟋⟍⟋⟍	Inhibits flow of electrons
Battery	+⊦⎮⎮⊦−	Provides electric potential
Capacitor (condenser)	⊦⊦	Momentarily stores electric charge
Ammeter	(A)	Measures electric current
Voltmeter	(V)	Measures electric potential
Switch	⟋	Turns circuit on or off by providing infinite resistance
Transformer		Increases or decreases voltage by fixed amount (AC only)
Rheostat	⟋⟍⟋⟍⟋⟍	Is a variable resistor
Diode	▶⎮	Allows electrons to flow in only one direction
Transistor		Is an electronic switch that can also amplify signals

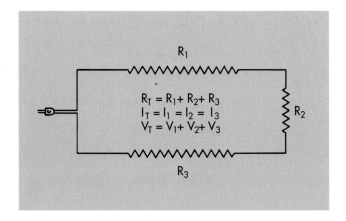

FIGURE 6-14   Series circuit and its basic rules.

$$R_T = R_1 + R_2 + R_3$$
$$I_T = I_1 = I_2 = I_3$$
$$V_T = V_1 + V_2 + V_3$$

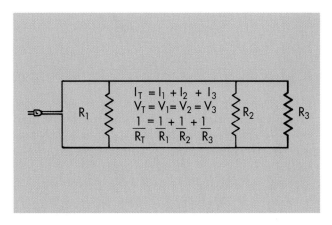

FIGURE 6-15   Parallel circuit and its basic rules.

$$I_T = I_1 + I_2 + I_3$$
$$V_T = V_1 = V_2 = V_3$$
$$\frac{1}{R_T} = \frac{1}{R_1} + \frac{1}{R_2} + \frac{1}{R_3}$$

very important

Answer: Refer to Figure 6-15.

$$\frac{1}{R_T} = \frac{1}{8\,\Omega} + \frac{1}{12\,\Omega} + \frac{1}{15\,\Omega} =$$

$$\frac{15}{120} + \frac{10}{120} + \frac{8}{120} = \frac{33}{120}$$

$$R_T = \frac{120}{33} = 3.6\,\Omega$$

$$I_t = 110\ V/3.6\,\Omega = 30.2\ A$$
$$I_1 = 110\ V/8\,\Omega = 13.6\ A$$
$$I_2 = 110\ V/12\,\Omega = 9.2\ A$$
$$I_3 = 110\ V/15\,\Omega = 7.3\ A$$
$$V_1 = V_2 = V_3 = V_T = 110\ V$$

Christmas lights are a good example of the difference between series and parallel circuits. Christmas lights wired in series have only one wire connecting each lamp; when one lamp burns out, the entire string of lights goes out. Christmas lights wired in parallel, on the other hand, have two wires connecting each lamp; when one lamp burns out, the rest remain lit.

Most electric circuits are much more complicated than this. For example, the television monitor in fluoroscopy has more than a thousand elements wired into a giant circuit consisting of many subcircuits, each of which is series or parallel or a combination of both.

Direct Current and Alternating Current

Electric current, or electricity, is the flow of electrons through a conductor. These electrons can be made to flow in one direction along the conductor, in which case the electric current is called **direct current (DC).** Most applications of electricity require that the electrons be controlled so that they flow first in one direction and then in the other. Current in which electrons oscillate back and forth is called **alternating current (AC).**

Electrons flowing in only one direction constitute DC.
Electrons flowing alternately in opposite directions constitute AC.

Figure 6-16 diagrams the phenomena of DC and shows how it can be described by a graph called a **waveform.** The horizontal axis, or x-axis, of the electronic waveform represents time; the vertical axis, or y-axis, represents the amplitude of the electric current. For DC, the electrons always flow in the same direction with the same velocity; therefore DC is represented by a horizontal line.

The vertical separation between this line and the time axis represents the magnitude of the current. If the line representing the current is above the time axis, it represents the flow of electrons in one direction. Electron flow in the opposite direction is shown by a current line below the time axis. When the current line coincides with

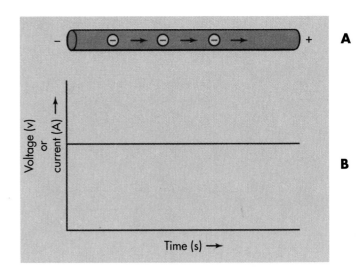

FIGURE 6-16   Representation of direct current. **A,** Electrons flow in one direction only. **B,** The graph of the associated electric waveform is a straight line.

the time axis, the magnitude of the current is zero, indicating that no electrons flow.

The waveform for AC is a sine curve (Figure 6-17). Electrons flow first in a positive direction and then in a negative direction. At one instant in time (point *0* in Figure 6-17), all electrons are at rest. Then they move, first in the positive direction with increasing velocity (segment *A*). Once they reach maximum velocity, represented by the vertical distance from the time axis (point *1*), the electrons begin to slow down (segment *B*). They come to rest again momentarily (point *2*) and then reverse motion and flow in the negative direction (segment *C*), increasing in velocity until their velocity in the negative direction is maximum (point *3*). Next, the potential is reduced to zero (segment *D*).

This oscillation in electron direction occurs in a sinusoidal fashion with each requiring $\frac{1}{60}$ second. Consequently, AC is identified as a 60 Hz-current (50 Hz in Europe and much of the rest of the world).

Electric Power

Watt
One watt is equal to one ampere of current flowing through an electric potential of 1 volt.

Electric power is measured in **watts (W).** Common household electric appliances, such as toasters, blenders, hair dryers, and radios, generally require 500 to 1500 W of electric power. Light bulbs require 30 to 150 W, and an x-ray imager may require 20 to 100 kW.

Question: If the cost of electric power is 10¢ per kilowatt hour (kW-hr), how much does it cost to operate a 100-W light bulb an average of 5 hr/day for 1 month?

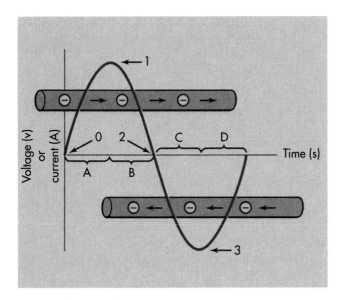

FIGURE 6-17 Representation of alternating current. Electrons flow alternately in one direction and then the other. Alternating current is represented graphically by a sinusoidal electric waveform.

Answer:

$$\text{Total on time} = (30 \text{ days/mo})$$
$$(5 \text{ hr/day})$$
$$= 150 \text{ hr/mo}$$
$$\text{Total power consumed} = (150 \text{ hr/mo}) (100 \text{ W})$$
$$= 15,000 \text{ W-hr/mo}$$
$$= 15 \text{ kW-hr/mo}$$
$$\text{Total cost} = (15 \text{ kW-hr/mo})$$
$$(10¢/\text{kW-hr})$$
$$= \$1.50/\text{mo}$$

Electric Power

$P = IV$

where *P* is the power in watts, *I* is the current in amperes, and *V* is the electric potential in volts. Alternately:

$P = I^2R$

where *R* is the resistance in ohms.

Question: An x-ray imager that draws 80 A of current is supplied with 220 V. What is the consumed power?

Answer: $P = IV$
$$= (80 \text{ A}) (220 \text{ V})$$
$$= 17,600 \text{ W}$$
$$= 17.6 \text{ kW}$$

Question: The overall resistance of a portable x-ray imager is 10 Ω. When plugged into a 110-V receptacle, how much current does it draw and how much power is consumed?

Answer: $I = \dfrac{V}{R} = \dfrac{110}{10} = 11 \text{ A}$
$$P = IV$$
$$= (11 \text{ A})(110 \text{ V})$$
$$= 1210 \text{ W}$$
$$\text{or } P = I^2R$$
$$= (11 \text{ A})^2 \ 10$$
$$= 1210 \text{ W}$$

SUMMARY

The conversion from electric energy to the electromagnetic energy of the x-ray beam involves the components of the x-ray imager. Radiography requires study of the fundamentals of electricity to understand these components. These fundamentals are summarized as follows:

Electrostatics is the study of stationary electric charges.

Electrons and protons have the same magnitude of electrostatic charge.

Electrons are negatively charged.

Protons are positively charged.

Electrons can flow from one object to another by contact, by friction, or by induction. The laws of electrostatics are:

Like charges repel.

Unlike charges attract.

Electrostatic force is directly proportional to the product of the charges and inversely proportional to the square of the distance between them.

Electric charges are distributed on the surface of a conductor.

Electric charges are concentrated along the sharpest curvature of the surface of the conductor.

Potential energy is the ability to do work when energy is released. The unit of electric potential energy is the volt (V).

Electrodynamics is the study of electrons in motion, otherwise known as *electricity*.

Conductors are materials that allow electrons to flow easily.

Insulators are materials that inhibit the flow of electrons.

Electric current is measured in amperes (A); electric potential is measured in volts (V), and electric resistance is measured in ohms (Ω).

Direct current is the flow of electrons in one direction along a conductor.

Alternating current is the flow of electrons back and forth along the conductor.

Electric power is energy produced or consumed per unit time. One watt of power is equal to one ampere of electricity flowing through an electric potential of one volt.

CHALLENGE QUESTIONS

1. Define or otherwise identify:
   a. Electric charge and its unit
   b. Electrodynamics
   c. Ohm's law
   d. Electric power
   e. Alternating current (AC)
   f. Electric circuit
   g. Insulator
   h. Electrostatics
   i. Superconductor
   j. Ammeter

2. If the distance between two charged bodies is doubled, what will be the change in the electrostatic force?

3. A lightning bolt carries about 25 C of charge. How many electrons is this?

4. What is the total circuit resistance when resistive elements of 5, 10, 15, and 20 Ω are connected in (a) series and (b) parallel?

5. If the resistive circuits in Question 4 are connected to a 110-V source, what will be the total circuit current for (a) series and (b) parallel operations?

6. If the resistive circuits in Question 4 each draw 7 A, what will be the voltage across the 10 Ω resistor for (a) series and (b) parallel operations?

7. How much electric power is consumed by the circuit in Question 6?

8. A radiographic exposure requires 100 mAs. How many electrons is this?

9. What is the fundamental unit of electric charge? What is its value?

10. What does it mean when an object is electrified?

11. What are the three ways to electrify an object?

12. Give an example of an electric ground.

13. List the four laws of electrostatics.

14. Describe an example of electrostatics.

15. Why is electrification easier in dry Phoenix than more humid Houston?

16. Why is electric potential necessary?

17. What is a semiconductor and how has it affected modern life?

18. Name the unit of electric potential.

19. What is the unit of electric power?

20. How does an electric utility company compute power consumed?

Magnetism

OBJECTIVES

At the completion of this chapter, the student should be able to:

1. Discuss the history and discovery of naturally occurring magnetic materials
2. Define *magnetic dipole*
3. List the three classifications of magnets
4. Identify the interactions between matter and magnetic fields
5. List and discuss the four laws of magnetism

OUTLINE

Magnetism has become more important in diagnostic imaging with the increased use of magnetic resonance imaging (MRI) as a medical diagnostic tool. Magnetic field safety is an issue in the modern diagnostic imaging workplace.

The nature of magnetism is described in this chapter according to the laws governing magnetic fields. These laws are similar to those governing electric fields. Knowing them is essential to understanding the function of several components of the x-ray imaging system, such as the transformer.

HISTORY OF NATURALLY OCCURRING MAGNETIC MATERIALS

Around 1000 BC, shepherds and dairy farmers of the village of Magnesia (what is now Western Turkey) discovered magnetite. **Magnetite** is a magnetic oxide of iron (Fe_3O_4). This rodlike stone rotates back and forth when suspended by a string. When it comes to rest, it allegedly points the way to water. It was called a **lodestone**, or a leading stone. Magnetites are a naturally occurring magnet and were used as a compass by ancient people.

The word **magnetism** comes from the name of that ancient village Magnesia. (It could be said that when the cows of this ancient village were milked, they produced milk of magnesia!) Magnetism is a fundamental property of some forms of matter. Ancient people observed that lodestone or magnetite attracted iron filings. They were also aware of the attraction of small, lightweight objects such as paper to an amber rod rubbed by fur. They considered both of these phenomena to be the same. We know them as *magnetism* and *electrostatics*, respectively.

NATURE OF MAGNETISM

Magnetism is perhaps more difficult to understand than other characteristic properties of matter, such as mass, energy, and electric charge, because magnetism is difficult to detect and measure. We can feel mass, visualize energy, and be shocked by electricity but we cannot sense magnetism.

 Any charged particle in motion creates a magnetic field.

The magnetic field of a charged particle, such as an electron in motion, is perpendicular to the motion of that particle. The intensity of the magnetic field is represented by imaginary lines (Figure 7-1). If the particle's motion is a closed loop, as with an electron circling a nucleus, the magnetic field lines will be perpendicular to the plane of motion (Figure 7-2).

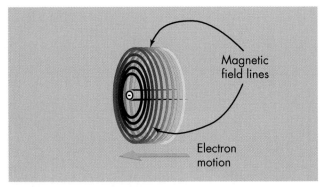

FIGURE 7-1 A moving charged particle induces a magnetic field in a plane perpendicular to its motion.

Electrons also rotate on an axis, either clockwise or counterclockwise. This rotation creates a property of electrons called **spin**. The electron spin creates a magnetic field, which is neutralized if an electron pair exists in any shell. Therefore atoms having an odd number of electrons in any shell exhibit a small magnetic field.

The lines of a magnetic field are always closed loops. They do not start or end as the lines of an electric field do. Such a field is called **bipolar** or **dipolar**; it always has a north and a south pole. The small magnet created by the electron spin is called a **magnetic dipole**. An accumulation of many such dipoles aligned creates a **magnetic domain**. If all the magnetic domains in an object are aligned, the object will act like a magnet.

In a hydrogen atom, there is a strong magnetic dipole because of the unpaired electron, but in a hydrogen molecule (H_2) the magnetic dipoles of the two electrons cancel each another, so there is no magnetic domain. Under normal circumstances, magnetic domains are randomly distributed (Figure 7-3, *A*). When acted on by an external magnetic field, however, the randomly oriented domains align with the magnetic field (Figure 7-3, *B*). The Earth creates a magnetic field because of the naturally occurring ores, mainly iron, at its core. This is why compasses align to the North Pole. Artificially induced magnetism occurs when ferromagnetic material is made into a permanent magnet.

Spinning electron charges also induce a magnetic field (Figure 7-4). This is the basis for magnetic resonance imaging (MRI).

The magnetic dipoles in a bar magnet generate imaginary lines of the magnetic field (Figure 7-5). If a nonmagnetic material is brought near such a magnet, there are no disturbances in these field lines. If ferromagnetic material, such as soft iron, is brought near the bar magnet, however, the magnet field lines are deviated and concentrated into the ferromagnetic material.

 Magnetic Permeability
Magnetic permeability is the ability of a material to attract the lines of magnetic field intensity.

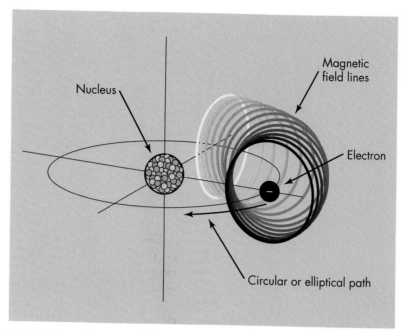

FIGURE 7-2 When a charged particle rotates, the perpendicular magnetic field also rotates.

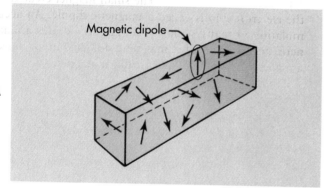

A

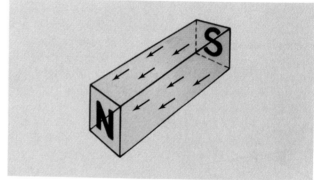

B

FIGURE 7-3 **A,** In ferromagnetic material, the magnetic dipoles are randomly oriented. **B,** This changes when they are brought under the influence of an external magnetic field.

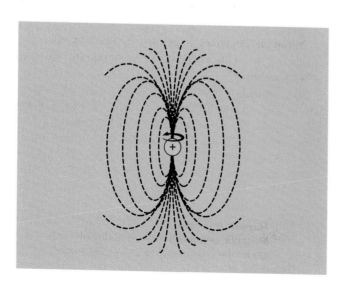

FIGURE 7-4 A spinning charged particle ind____ field along the axis of spin.

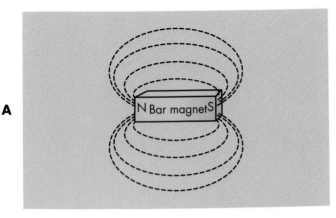

A

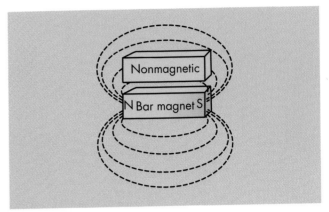

B

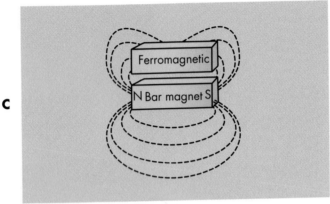

C

FIGURE 7-5 **A,** Imaginary lines of the magnified field. **B,** These lines are undisturbed by nonmagnetic material. **C,** They are deviated by ferromagnetic material. *N,* North, *S,* south.

CLASSIFICATION OF MAGNETS

 Magnets are classified according to the origin of the magnetic property.

There are three principal types of magnets: naturally occurring magnets, artificially induced permanent magnets, and electromagnets.

The best example of a **natural magnet** is the Earth itself. The Earth has a magnetic field because it spins on an axis. Lodestones of magnetite in the Earth exhibit strong magnetism, presumably because they have remained undisturbed for a long time in the Earth's magnetic field.

Artificially produced **permanent magnets** are available in many sizes and shapes but principally as bar or horseshoe-shaped magnets, usually made of iron. A compass is a prime example of an artificial permanent magnet. Permanent magnets are typically produced by placing them in the field of an electromagnet (Figure 7-6).

Permanent magnets do not necessarily stay permanent. The magnetic property of a magnet can be destroyed by heating it or even by hitting it with a hammer. Either action, which can cause the individual magnetic domains to be jarred from their alignment. They thus become randomly aligned, and magnetism is lost.

Electromagnets consist of wire wrapped around an iron core. When an electric current is conducted through the wire, a magnetic field is created. The intensity of the magnetic field is proportional to the electric current.

 All matter can be classified according to the manner in which it interacts with an external magnetic field.

Many materials are unaffected when brought into a magnetic field. Such materials are nonmagnetic and are called **diamagnetic.** They cannot be artificially magnetized, and they are not attracted to a magnet. Examples of diamagnetic materials are wood, glass, and plastic.

Ferromagnetic materials are iron, cobalt, and nickel. These are strongly attracted by a magnet and can usually be permanently magnetized by exposure to a magnetic field. An alloy of aluminum, nickel, and cobalt called **alnico** is one of the more useful magnets produced from ferromagnetic material. More recently, rare earth ceramics have been developed that are considerably stronger magnets (Figure 7-7).

Paramagnetic materials lie somewhere between ferromagnetic and nonmagnetic. They are slightly attracted to a magnet and loosely influenced by an external magnetic field. Contrast agents used in MRI are paramagnetic.

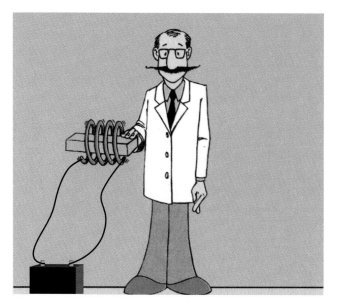

FIGURE 7-6 A method for rendering ceramic bricks magnetic with an electromagnet.

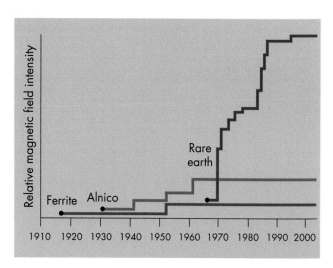

FIGURE 7-7 Developments in permanent magnet design have resulted in a great increase in magnetic field intensity.

TABLE 7-1	Three Fundamental Forces in Nature		
	Gravitational	**Electric**	**Magnetic**
The force:	Attracts only	Attracts and repels	Attracts and repels
It acts in:	A mass, m	A charge, q	A pole, p
Through an associated field:	A gravitational field, g	An electric field, E	A magnetic field, B
With intensity:	$F = m \times g$	$F = q \times E$	$F = p \times B$
The source of the field is:	A mass, M	A charge, Q	A pole, P
The intensity of the field at a distance from the source is:	$g = \dfrac{G \times M}{d^2}$	$E = \dfrac{k \times Q}{d^2}$	$B = \dfrac{kP}{d^2}$
The force between fields is given by:	Newton's law	Coulomb's law	Gauss' law
	$F = -G\dfrac{M \times m}{d^2}$	$F = k\dfrac{Q_1 \times Q_2}{d^2}$	$F = k\dfrac{P \times p}{d^2}$
Where:	$G = 6.678 \times 10^{-11}\dfrac{N \times m^2}{kg^2}$	$k = 9.0 \times 10^{9}\dfrac{N \times m^2}{C^2}$	$k = 10^{-7}\dfrac{W}{A^2}$

Magnetic Susceptibility
The degree to which various materials can be magnetized is *magnetic susceptibility*.

When wood is placed in the presence of a strong magnetic field, it does not increase the strength of the field; wood has low magnetic susceptibility. On the other hand, when iron is placed in a magnetic field, it greatly increases the strength of the field; iron has high magnetic susceptibility.

The degree of magnetism exhibited by a material is related to the number of unpaired electrons in the outer shells.

MAGNETIC LAWS

The physical laws of magnetism are similar to those of electrostatics and gravity. The forces associated with these three fields are fundamental in nature (Table 7-1). Note that the equations of force and the fields through which they act have the same form. There is considerable activity among theoretical physicists attempting to combine these fundamental forces with two others, the strong nuclear force and the weak interaction, to formulate a grand **unified field theory.**

Dipoles

Unlike the situation that exists with electricity, there is no smallest unit of magnetism. Dividing a magnet simply creates two smaller magnets, which when divided again make even smaller magnets (Figure 7-8).

How do we know that these imaginary lines of the magnetic field exist? They can be demonstrated by the action of iron filings near a magnet (Figure 7-9). If a magnet is placed on a surface with small iron filings, the filings attach most strongly and with greater concentration to the ends of the magnet. These ends are called **poles**, and every magnet has two poles. Magnetic poles exist in two forms: a **north pole** and a **south pole**, analogous to positive and negative electrostatic charges.

Attraction and Repulsion

As with electric charges, like magnetic poles repel, unlike magnetic poles attract. Also, by convention, the imaginary lines of the magnetic field leave the north pole of a magnet and return to the south pole (Figure 7-10).

Magnetic Induction

Just as an electrostatic charge can be induced from one material to another, so nonmagnetic material can be made magnetic by **induction**. The imaginary magnetic

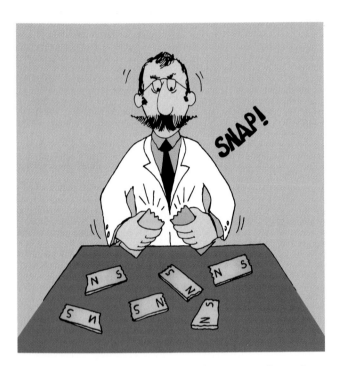

FIGURE 7-8 If a single magnet is broken into smaller and smaller pieces, smaller magnets are produced.

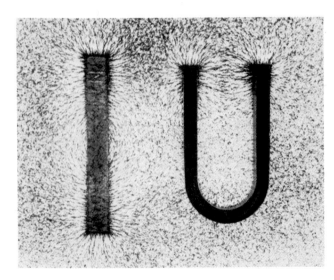

FIGURE 7-9 Demonstration of magnetic lines of force with iron filings.

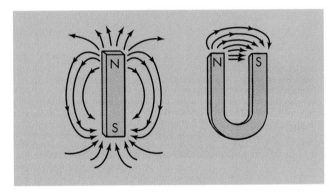

FIGURE 7-10 The imaginary lines of the magnetic field leave the north pole and enter the south pole.

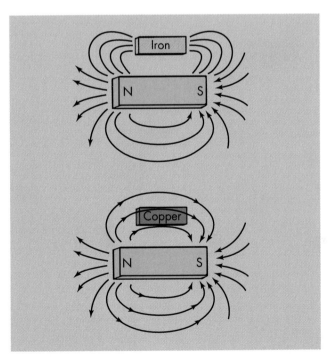

FIGURE 7-11 Ferromagnetic material such as iron attracts magnetic lines of induction, whereas nonmagnetic material such as copper does not.

field lines just described are called *magnetic lines of induction,* and the density of the lines is proportional to the intensity of the magnetic field.

 Ferromagnetic objects can be made into magnets by induction.

When ferromagnetic material, such as a piece of soft iron, is brought into the vicinity of an intense magnetic field, the lines of induction are altered by attraction to the soft iron, and the iron is temporarily made magnetic (Figure 7-11). If copper, a dimagnetic material, were to replace the soft iron, no such effect would occur.

This principle is used with many MRI units that have iron magnetic shields to reduce the level of the fringe magnetic field. Ferromagnetic material acts as a magnetic sink by drawing the lines of the magnetic field into it. This also is the basis of antimagnetic watches but does not always work, especially near the strong field of an MRI unit.

When ferromagnetic material is removed from the magnetic field, it usually does not retain its strong magnetic property. Soft iron therefore makes an excellent **temporary magnet.** It is a magnet only while its magnetism is being induced. If properly tempered by heat or exposed to an external field for a long period, however,

some ferromagnetic materials retain their magnetism when removed from the external magnetic field and become **permanent magnets.**

Magnetic Force

The electric and magnetic forces were joined by Maxwell's field theory of electromagnetic radiation, which states that the force created by a magnetic field behaves similarly to that of the electric field. This magnetic force is similar to electrostatic and gravitational forces that also are inversely proportional to the square of distance between the objects under consideration. If the distance between two bar magnets is halved, the magnetic force is increased by four times.

 Maxwell's Field Theory
The magnetic force is proportional to the product of the magnetic pole strengths divided by the square of the distance between them.

The Earth behaves as though it has a large bar magnet embedded in it. The polar convention of magnetism actually has its origin in the compass. At the equator, the north pole of a compass will point to the Earth's North Pole (which is actually the Earth's south magnetic pole). As one travels toward the North Pole, the attraction of the compass becomes more intense until the compass needle points directly into the Earth, not at the geographic North Pole but at a region in northern Canada: the magnetic pole (Figure 7-12). The magnetic pole in the southern hemisphere is in Australia. There, the compass points to the sky.

 The SI unit of magnet field strength is the tesla. An older unit is the gauss. *One tesla (T) = 10,000 gauss (G).*

The use of a compass might suggest that the Earth has a strong magnetic field, but the Earth does not. The Earth's magnetic field is approximately 50 μT at the equator and 100 μT at the poles. This is far less than the magnet on a cabinet door latch, which is about 100 mT.

SUMMARY

Lodestone, or magnetite, was observed in the ancient world as having magnetic properties. Matter has magnetic properties because some atoms and molecules have an odd number of electrons in the outer shells. The unpaired spin of these electrons produces a magnetic field in the object.

One classification of magnets is the origin of their magnetism. Natural magnets get their magnetism from the Earth, permanent magnets are artificially induced mag-

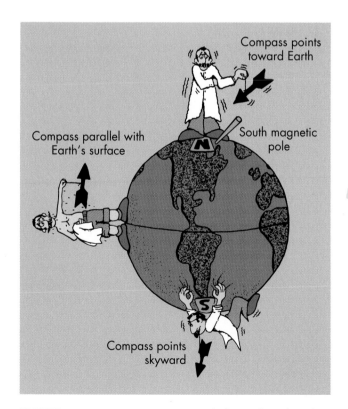

FIGURE 7-12 A compass interacts with the Earth as though it were a bar magnet.

nets, and electromagnets are produced when wire with electric current flowing are wrapped around an iron core.

Another classification of magnets is described by their interaction with an external magnetic field: ferromagnetic (easily magnetized), paramagnetic (magnetized with difficulty), and dimagnetic (cannot be magnetized). The laws of magnetism are:

Every magnet, no matter how small, has two poles: north and south.

Like magnetic poles repel, and unlike magnetic poles attract.

Ferromagnetic material can be made magnetic when it is placed in an external magnetic field.

The intensity of the magnetic field is proportional to the product of the magnetic pole strengths divided by the square of the distance between them.

The increasing use of MRI as a medical diagnostic tool emphasizes the importance of magnetism as an area of study for radiologic technologists.

CHALLENGE QUESTIONS

1. Define or otherwise identify:
   a. Dipole
   b. Magnetic pole
   c. Induction
   d. Magnetic force
   e. Magnetic domain
   f. Magnetic susceptibility
   g. Ferromagnetism
   h. Gauss vs. tesla
   i. Lodestone

2. If the distance between two magnetic poles is doubled, what will be the change in magnetic force?

3. Magnetic fields in excess of 5 G can interfere with cardiac pacemakers. How many mT is this?

4. What role does magnetism have in the study of x-ray imaging?

5. Where was lodestone discovered and how was it used?

6. How are magnets classified?

7. List the three principle types of magnets.

8. Describe an electromagnet.

9. How is matter that is not attracted to a magnet identified?

10. What is the magnetic property of MRI contrast agents?

11. Where in medical imaging is magnetic susceptibility especially important?

12. Name the SI unit of magnetic field strength.

13. Explain how a magnetic domain can cause an object to behave like a magnet.

14. Is a hydrogen atom a magnetic dipole? Explain.

15. What happens when a bar magnet is heated to a very high temperature?

16. List three dimagnetic materials.

17. Does the magnetic field obey the inverse square law of radiography?

18. Where does a compass point at the North Pole?

19. What is the range in intensity of the Earth's magnetic field?

20. An MRI unit operates at 1.5 T. How many gauss is this?

Electromagnetism

OBJECTIVES

At the completion of this chapter, the student should be able to:

1. Discuss the development of the battery as a reliable source of electric potential
2. Relate the experiments of Oersted, Lenz, and Faraday in defining the relationship between magnetism and electricity
3. Describe the solenoid and the electromagnet
4. Identify the laws of electromagnetic induction
5. Explain the design of the electric generator, the electric motor, and the transformer

OUTLINE

This chapter combines information from two previous chapters on electricity and magnetism into a discussion of electromagnetism. Electromagnetism is the force associated with electrons in motion. Electricity and magnetism are different aspects of this same force.

The chapter begins with a discussion of the electromagnetic effect, which describes how magnetism can cause electrons to acquire electric potential energy and move through a conductor. The discussion of electromagnetic induction examines how electrons flow and magnetism can cause electrons to flow in an independent conductor as in a transformer.

ELECTROMAGNETIC EFFECT

Electricity and magnetism are different aspects of the same basic force: the electromagnetic force. The electromagnetic force is one of the four fundamental forces of nature. The others are gravity, the strong nuclear force, and weak interaction. Until the nineteenth century, however, electricity and magnetism were viewed as separate effects. Although many scientists suspected a connection between the two, their research was hampered by the lack of any convenient way of producing and controlling electricity.

The study of electricity in earlier times was therefore limited to the investigation of static charges, which could be produced by friction. Charges could be induced to move but only in a sudden discharge, as with a spark jumping a gap. The development of methods for producing a steady flow of charges (that is, an electric current) during the nineteenth century stimulated investigations of both electricity and magnetism. These investigations led to an increased understanding of electromagnetic phenomena and ultimately caused the electronic revolution that is so much the basis of today's technology.

As we saw in Chapter 7, magnetic fields could be detected and generated with naturally occurring magnetic materials such as the lodestone. One of the earliest and most practical of magnetic material was found in the compass. European seafarers began using the compass as a navigational tool in the century before Christopher Columbus, but the compass was apparently known to Chinese navigators even before the fifteenth century. It is an interesting fact that the extensive migration of bees, birds, and turtles is thought to be controlled by an internal compass (Figure 8-1).

The Battery

In the late 1700s, an Italian anatomist, Luigi Galvani, made an accidental discovery. He observed that a dis-

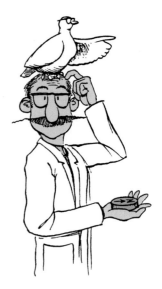

FIGURE 8-1 Magnetic deposits in the head of the pigeon allow it to know which direction is north.

sected frog leg twitched when touched by two different metals, just as if it had been touched by an electrostatic charge. This prompted a contemporary Italian physicist, Alessandro Volta, to question whether an electric current might be produced when two different metals are brought into contact with each other. Using zinc and copper plates, he succeeded in producing a feeble electric current. To increase the current, he stacked the copper-zinc plates like a Dagwood sandwich to form what was called the **Voltaic pile,** a precursor of the modern battery. Each zinc-copper sandwich is called a **battery cell.**

Modern dry cells use a carbon rod as the positive electrode surrounded by an electrolytic paste housed in a negative zinc cylindric can. The Voltaic pile, the modern battery, and the electronic symbol for the battery are shown in Figure 8-2.

These devices are examples of sources of electromotive force (EMF). Any device that converts some form of energy directly into electric energy is said to be a source of EMF. Although still commonly used, this somewhat archaic term is a little misleading. Electromotive force is not really a force, such as gravity, but rather the term refers to stored electric energy.

 Electric potential (EMF) has units of joule per coulomb or volt.

Oersted's Experiment

When scientists finally had a source of constant electric current with which to experiment, extensive investigations into the possibility of a link between electric and magnetic forces began. The first such link was discovered in 1820 by Hans Oersted, a Danish physicist. Oersted fashioned a long, straight wire, supported near a free-rotating magnetic compass (Figure 8-3). With no

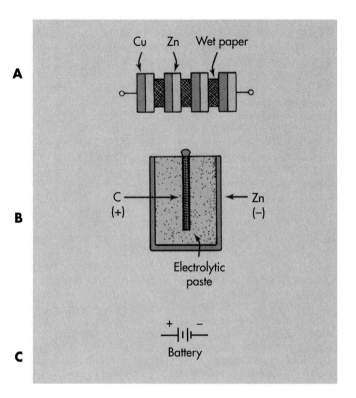

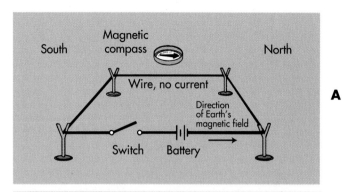

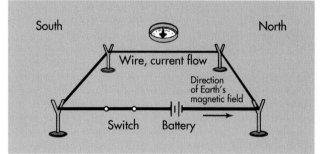

FIGURE 8-2 **A,** Original voltaic pile. **B,** Modern dry cell. **C,** Electronic symbol for a battery.

FIGURE 8-3 Oersted's experiment. **A,** With no current in the wire, the compass points north. **B,** With current flowing, the compass points toward the wire.

current flowing through the wire, the magnetic compass pointed north as expected. When a current was passed through the wire, however, the compass needle swung to point straight at the wire. Here we have evidence of a direct link between electric and magnetic phenomena. The electric current evidently produced a magnetic field strong enough to overpower the Earth's magnetic field and cause the magnetic compass to point toward the wire.

 Any charge in motion induces a magnetic field.

A charge at rest produces no magnetic field. Only electrons flowing through a wire produce a magnetic field about that wire. The magnetic field is represented by imaginary lines that form concentric circles centered on the wire (Figure 8-4). The direction of the magnetic field lines can be determined by using the **right-hand rule.** Imagine gripping the wire with the right hand. If the thumb is pointed in the direction of the current flow, the fingers of your hand will then curl in the direction of the magnetic field lines (Figure 8-5).

 A coil of wire is called a *solenoid*.

These same rules apply if the current is flowing in a circular loop. Magnetic field lines form concentric cir-

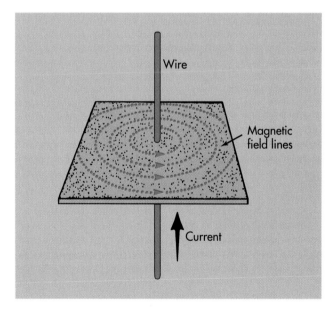

FIGURE 8-4 Magnetic field lines form concentric circles around the current-carrying wire.

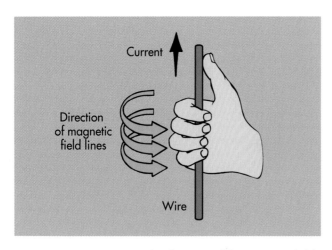

FIGURE 8-5 Determining the direction of the magnetic field around the wire using the right-hand rule.

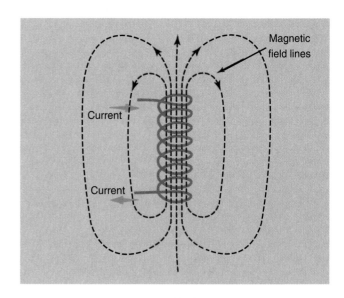

FIGURE 8-7 Magnetic field lines of a solenoid.

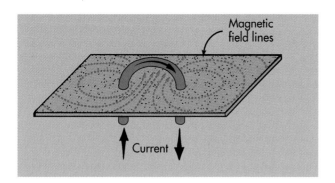

FIGURE 8-6 Magnetic field lines are concentrated on the inside of the loop.

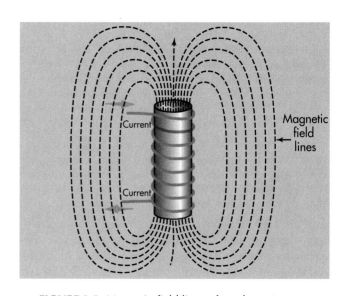

FIGURE 8-8 Magnetic field lines of an electromagnet.

cles around each tiny section of the wire. Because the wire is curved, however, these field lines overlap inside the loop. In particular, at the very center of the loop, all the field lines add together, making the magnetic field strong (Figure 8-6). Stacking more loops on top of each other increases the intensity of the magnetic field running through the center or axis of the stack of loops.

The magnetic field of a solenoid is concentrated through the center of the coil (Figure 8-7). The magnetic field can further be intensified by wrapping the coil of wire around ferromagnetic material, such as iron. The iron core concentrates and increases the strength of the magnetic field. This type of device is called an **electromagnet** (Figure 8-8).

 An electromagnet is a coil of wire wrapped around an iron core, which intensifies the magnetic field.

The magnetic field produced by an electromagnet is the same as that produced by a bar magnet. That is, if both were hidden from view behind a piece of paper, the pattern of magnetic field lines revealed by iron filings sprinkled on the paper surface would be the same. Of course, the advantage of the electromagnet is that its magnetic field can be adjusted or turned on and off simply by varying the current flow through its coil of wire.

LAWS OF ELECTROMAGNETIC INDUCTION
Faraday's Law

Oersted's experiment demonstrated that electricity can be used to generate magnetic fields. It is obvious, then, to wonder whether the reverse is true: can magnetic fields be used to generate electricity? Michael Faraday, a self-educated British experimenter, found the answer to that question.

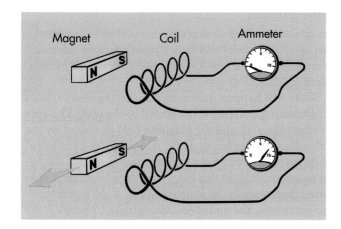

FIGURE 8-9 Schematic description of Faraday's experiment shows how a moving magnetic field induces an electric current.

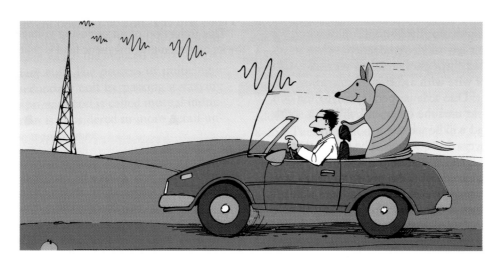

FIGURE 8-10 Radio reception is based on the principles of electromagnetic induction.

From a series of experiments, Faraday concluded that an electric current cannot be induced in a circuit merely by the presence of a magnetic field. For example, consider the situation illustrated in Figure 8-9. A coil of wire is connected to a current-measuring device called an **ammeter.** If a bar magnet were set next to the coil, the meter would indicate no current in the coil. However, Faraday discovered that if the magnet is moved, a current flows in the coiled wire, indicated by the ammeter. Therefore to induce a flow of current using a magnetic field, the magnetic field cannot be constant but must be changing.

Faraday's Law
Faraday's law states that an electric current is induced to flow in a circuit if some part of that circuit is in a changing magnetic field.

The magnitude of the induced current depends on the following factors:
1. The strength of the magnetic field
2. The velocity of the magnetic field as it moves past the conductor

3. The angle of the conductor to the magnetic field
4. The number of turns in the conductor

A changing magnetic field can be produced in many ways. For example, a bar magnet or an electromagnet can be moved near a coil of wire. Conversely, the magnet can be held stationary and the coil of wire moved near it.

Alternatively, there need be no motion. An electromagnet can be fixed near a coil of wire. If the current in the electromagnet is then either increased or decreased, its magnetic field will likewise change and induce a flow of current in the coil.

A prime example of electromagnetic induction is radio reception (Figure 8-10). Radio emission consists of waves of electromagnetic radiation. Each wave has an oscillating electric field and an oscillating magnetic field. The oscillating magnetic field induces motion in electrons in the radio antennae, resulting in a radio signal. This signal is detected and decoded to produce sound.

The essential point in all these examples is that the strength of the magnetic field at the wire must be changing to induce a current flow. If the magnetic field intensity is constant, there will be no induced current.

Electric Motor

A simple electric motor has basically the same components as an electric generator (Figure 8-16). In this case, however, electric energy is supplied to the current loop to produce a mechanical motion (that is, a rotation of the loop in the magnetic field).

When a current is passed through the wire loop, a magnetic field is produced, making the wire loop act like a tiny electromagnet. Being free to turn, the electromagnet-current loop rotates as it attempts to align itself with the stronger magnetic field produced by the external bar magnet. Just as the current loop becomes aligned with the external magnetic field, the commutator ring switches the direction of current flow through the loop and therefore reverses the coil's required alignment.

Because of the switch in current direction, the electromagnet is no longer aligned with the magnetic field of the bar magnet; it is now opposed to it. The electromagnet-current loop rotates 180 degrees in an attempt to realign itself once again with the bar magnet field. As the electromagnet again nears alignment, the commutator switches the direction of current flow and forces the loop to rotate again. This procedure repeats itself over and over.

The electromagnet-current loop is never quite able to align itself with the magnetic field of the bar magnet. The net result is that the current loop rotates continuously.

In a practical electric motor, many turns of wire are used for the current loop, and many bar magnets are used to create the external magnetic field. The principle of operation, however, is the same. This type of electric motor is called a **direct current motor.**

The type of motor used in most x-ray tubes is an **induction motor** (Figure 8-17). In this type of motor the rotating **rotor** is still a series of wire loops; however, the external magnetic field is supplied by several fixed electromagnets called **stators.**

 An induction motor powers the rotating anode of an x-ray tube.

No current is passed to the rotor. Instead, current flow is produced in the rotor windings by induction. The electromagnets surrounding the rotor are energized in sequence, producing a changing magnetic field. The induced current flow produced in the rotor windings generates a magnetic field.

Just as in a conventional electric motor, this magnetic field attempts to align itself with the magnetic field of the external electromagnets. Because these electromagnets are being energized in sequence, the rotor begins to rotate, trying to bring its magnetic field into alignment. The result is the same as in a conventional electric motor; that is, the rotor rotates continuously. The difference, however, is that the electric energy is supplied to the external magnets rather than the rotor windings.

THE TRANSFORMER

Both electric motors and generators make use of the interacting electromagnetic fields produced by electric currents. The generator converts mechanical to electric energy, and the motor converts electric to mechanical energy. Another device that makes use of the interacting magnetic fields produced by changing electric currents is the transformer. The transformer does not convert one form of energy to another but rather transforms electric potential and current into higher or lower intensities.

Recall from the discussion of mutual induction that if two coils are placed near each other and a changing current is applied to the primary coil, then a current will be induced to flow in the secondary coil. Recall also that placing a core of ferromagnetic material in the center of the coil greatly increases the strength of the magnetic field passing through its center. The magnetic field lines tend to be concentrated in the ferromagnetic material of the core.

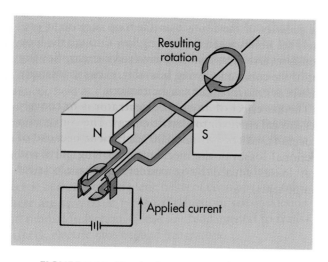

FIGURE 8-16   Simple direct current electric motor.

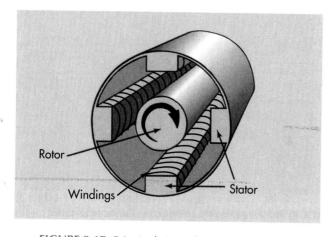

FIGURE 8-17   Principal parts of an induction motor.

A transformer changes the intensity of alternating voltage and current by mutual induction.

Imagine, however, that this ferromagnetic core is bent around so that it forms a continuous loop (Figure 8-18). There are no end surfaces from which the magnetic field lines can escape. Therefore the magnetic field tends to be confined to the loop of ferromagnetic core material.

If the secondary coil is then wound around the other side of this loop of core material, almost all the magnetic field produced by the primary coil will also pass through the center of the secondary coil. Thus there is a good **coupling** between the magnetic field produced by the primary coil and the secondary coil. A changing current in the primary coil induces a changing current in the secondary coil. This type of device is called a **transformer.**

Because it operates on the principle of mutual induction, a transformer will operate only with a changing electric current (AC). A direct current applied to the primary coil induces no current to the secondary coil.

The Transformer Law

The transformer is used to change the magnitude of voltage and current in an AC circuit. This change is directly proportional to the ratio of the number of turns (windings) of the secondary coil (N_s) to the number of turns in the primary coil (N_p). If there are 10 turns on the secondary coil for every turn on the primary coil, then the voltage generated in the secondary circuit (V_s), will be 10 times the voltage supplied to the primary circuit (V_p). Mathematically, the transformer law is represented as follows:

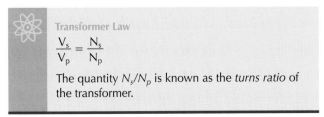

Transformer Law

$$\frac{V_s}{V_p} = \frac{N_s}{N_p}$$

The quantity N_s/N_p is known as the *turns ratio* of the transformer.

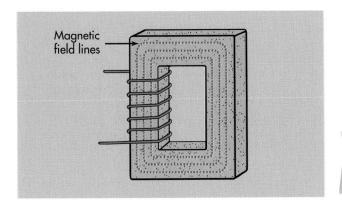

FIGURE 8-18 Electromagnet that incorporates a closed iron core produces a closed magnetic field confined primarily to the core.

Question: The secondary side of a transformer has 300,000 turns; the primary side has 600 turns. What is the turns ratio?

Answer: $N_s = 300,000$ $N_p = 600$
Turns ratio $= N_s/N_p$
$\qquad = 300,000/600$
$\qquad = 500{:}1$

The voltage change across the transformer is proportional to the turns ratio. A transformer with a turns ratio greater than 1 is a **step-up transformer** because the voltage is increased or stepped up from the primary side to the secondary side. When the turns ratio is less than 1, the transformer is a **step-down transformer.**

As the voltage changes across a transformer, the current (I) changes also. The transformer law may also be written as follows:

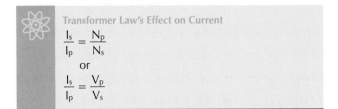

Transformer Law's Effect on Current

$$\frac{I_s}{I_p} = \frac{N_p}{N_s}$$

or

$$\frac{I_s}{I_p} = \frac{V_p}{V_s}$$

Question: The turns ratio of a filament transformer is 0.125. What will be the filament current if the current flowing through the primary winding is 0.8 A?

Answer:
$$\frac{I_s}{I_p} = \frac{N_p}{N_s}$$

$$I_s = I_p \left\{ \frac{N_p}{N_s} \right\}$$

$$= (0.8\text{ A}) \left(\frac{1}{0.125} \right)$$

$= 6.4$ A is the current flowing through the secondary winding of the filament transformer.

The change in current across a transformer is in the opposite direction from the voltage change but in the same proportion: an inverse relationship. For example, if the voltage is doubled, the current is halved. In a step-up transformer, the current on the secondary side (I_s) is smaller than the current on the primary side (I_p); in a step-down transformer, the secondary current is larger than the primary current.

 The three main causes of transformer losses or inefficiency are resistance, hysteresis, and eddy currents.

Although the transformer is not 100% efficient, losses in power from the primary side to the secondary side are considered negligible. There are three principal causes for such losses that result in power lost in the form of heat. Electric current in the copper wire experiences **resistance** that results in heat generation. The alternate reversal of the magnetic field caused by the alternating current causes an additional resistance known as **hysteresis**. Finally, **eddy currents** can be formed as predicted by Lenz's law. These currents oppose the magnetic field that induced them, creating a loss of transformer efficiency.

Question: There are 125 turns on the primary side, N_p, of a transformer and 90,000 turns on the secondary side, N_s. If 110 V AC is supplied to the primary winding, V_p, what will be the voltage induced in the secondary winding, V_s?

Answer:

$$\frac{V_s}{V_p} = \frac{N_s}{N_p}$$

$$V_s = V_p \left\{ \frac{N_s}{N_p} \right\}$$

$$= (110 \text{ V}) \left\{ \frac{90,000}{125} \right\}$$

$$= (110)(720) \text{ V}$$

$$= 79,200 \text{ V}$$

$$= 79.2 \text{ kV is the voltage induced in the secondary winding of the transformer.}$$

Types of Transformers

There are many ways to construct a transformer (Figure 8-19). The type of transformer discussed thus far, built about a square core of ferromagnetic material, is called a **closed-core transformer** (Figure 8-19, A). The core is not a single piece but rather is built up of laminated layers of iron. This layering helps reduce energy losses caused by eddy currents in the core produced by the transformer's changing magnetic field.

Another type of transformer is the **autotransformer** (Figure 8-19, B). It consists of an iron core with only one winding of wire about it. This single winding acts as both the primary and the secondary winding. The autotransformer is based on self-induction rather than mutual induction. Connections are made at different points on the coil for both the primary and secondary sides.

The autotransformer has one winding and varies voltage and current by self-induction.

An autotransformer is generally smaller, and because both the primary and the secondary sides are connected to the same wire, its use is generally restricted to those cases in which only a small step-up or step-down in voltage is required. Thus it would not be suitable for use as the high-voltage transformer in an x-ray imaging system.

The third type of transformer is the **shell-type transformer** (Figure 8-19, C). This type of transformer confines even more of the magnet field lines of the primary winding because there are essentially two closed cores. This type is more efficient than the closed-core transformer. Most transformers are shell-type.

SUMMARY

The development of the battery as a source of electric potential energy by Alessandro Volta prompted further investigations of electric magnetic fields. Hans Oersted demonstrated that electricity can be used to generate magnetic fields. It was Michael Faraday who observed

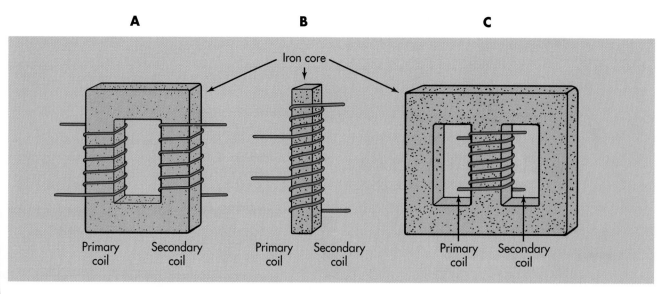

FIGURE 8-19 Type of transformers. **A,** Closed-core transformer. **B,** Autotransformer. **C,** Shell-type transformer.

the flow of current induced by a changing magnetic field and described the first law of electromagnetics (Faraday's law). Heinrich Lenz expanded on Faraday's experiments. The second law of electromagnetics is Lenz's law, which states that current flows opposite to the action that induces it.

If a steady or direct current flows through a wire, a constant magnetic field will be created around the wire. If, however, the current changes direction as in alternating current (AC) the magnetic field oscillates. Self-induction and mutual induction are the two forms of electromagnetic induction.

The practical applications of the laws of electromagnetism appear in the electric motor (electric current produces mechanical motion); the electric generator (mechanical motion produces electric current); and the transformer (alternating electric current and electric potential are transformed in intensity). The transformer law describes how electric current and voltage change from the primary coil to the secondary coil.

CHALLENGE QUESTIONS

1. Define or otherwise identify:
    a. Insulator
    b. Electromotive force
    c. Solenoid
    d. Mutual induction
    e. Commutator ring
    f. Autotransformer
    g. Ammeter
    h. Shell-type transformer
    i. Vacuum tube

2. State the two principal laws of electromagnetics.

3. How does an electric motor work?

4. A transformer has 220,000 turns on the secondary winding and 200 turns on the primary winding. If 220 V are supplied to the primary tube, what will be the voltage on the secondary side?

5. If 30 A are supplied to the primary side of the transformer in Question 4, what will be the secondary current?

6. What is the electric power resulting from the 220 V and 30 A supplied to the transformer in Question 5? From the information given, will the power be the same on the secondary side?

7. A portable x-ray imager is designed to operate on conventional 110-V AC power. Its maximum capacity is 110 kV and 100 mA. What is the high-voltage transformer turns ratio?

8. What should be the primary current in the previous question to produce a secondary current of 100 mA?

9. What is a semiconductor and how has it affected modern life?

10. State Ohm's law and describe where it is used.

11. A kitchen toaster draws a current of 2.5 A. If the household voltage is 110 V, what is the electric resistance of the toaster?

12. An x-ray imaging system draws 80 A of current and is supplied with 220 V. How much power does it consume?

13. What are the characteristics of a solenoid?

14. Where might one find an electromagnet in everyday life?

15. Describe the process of mutual induction.

16. Draw and label the parts of an electric motor.

17. Explain how an electric generator works.

18. List the components of an induction motor and describe how they work.

PART II

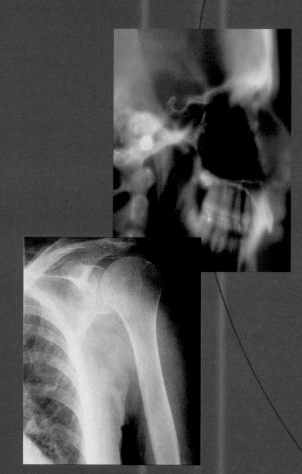

THE
X-RAY BEAM

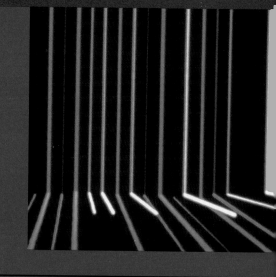

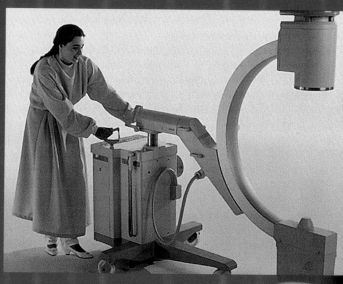

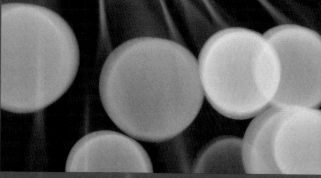

CHAPTER

9

The X-Ray Imaging System

OBJECTIVES

At the completion of this chapter, the student should be able to:

1. Identify the components of the operating console positioned outside the x-ray examination room
2. Explain the operation of the high-voltage generator, including the filament transformer and the rectifiers
3. Relate the important differences between single-phase power and three-phase power
4. Identify the voltage ripple associated with various high-voltage generators
5. Discuss the importance of voltage ripple to x-ray quantity and quality
6. Define the power rating of an x-ray imaging system

OUTLINE

When fast-moving electrons slam into a metal object, x-rays are produced because the kinetic energy of the electrons is transformed into electromagnetic energy. The purpose of the x-ray imaging system is to provide a sufficient number of electrons in controlled manner to produce the desired x-ray beam. The three main components of an x-ray imaging system are (1) the x-ray tube, (2) the operating console, and (3) the high-voltage generator. This chapter explains the components on the operating console, whereas Chapter 10 discusses the x-ray tube in detail. This chapter also discusses high-voltage generators and rectifiers.

X-RAY IMAGING SYSTEM

The many types of x-ray imaging systems are identified according to either the energy of the x-rays they produce or the purpose for which the x-rays are intended. Diagnostic x-ray units come in many shapes and sizes, some of which are shown in Figure 9-1. They are usually operated at voltage ranging from 25 to 150 kilovolt peak (kVp) and at tube currents from 100 to 1200 millampere (mA).

The general-purpose x-ray examination room usually contains a radiographic imaging system and a fluoro-scopic imaging system with an image intensifier. The fluoroscopic x-ray tube is usually located under the examining table, and the radiographic tube is attached to an overhead movable crane assembly that permits easy positioning of the tube and aiming of the x-ray beam. A room equipped in this fashion has already been described (see Figure 1-6). This type of equipment can be used for nearly all radiographic and fluoroscopic examinations. Rooms with a fluoroscope and two or more overhead radiographic tubes are used for special cardiovascular and interventional applications.

Regardless of the type of x-ray imaging system used, a patient-supporting examination table is required (Figure 9-2). The examination table may be flat or curved but must be uniform in thickness and as transparent to x-rays as possible. Carbon fiber tabletops are strong and absorb little x-radiation. This contributes to reduced patient dose because more x-rays reach and expose the film.

Most tabletops are floating: easily unlocked and moved by the radiologic technologist. Just under the tabletop is an opening to hold a thin tray for a cassette and grid (see Part III). If the table is used for fluoroscopy, the cassette tray must move to the foot of the table, and the opening is automatically shielded for radiation protection with a **Bucky slot cover** (see Chapter 39). Fluoroscopic tables tilt and are identified by their degree of tilt. For example, a 90/30 table would tilt 90 degrees to the foot side and 30 degrees to the head side (Figure 9-3).

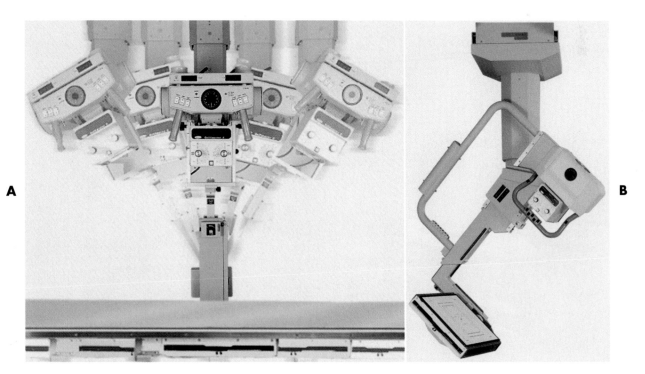

FIGURE 9-1 Types of diagnostic x-ray imaging. **A,** Tomographic. **B,** Trauma. *(Courtesy Fischer Imaging.)*

Continued

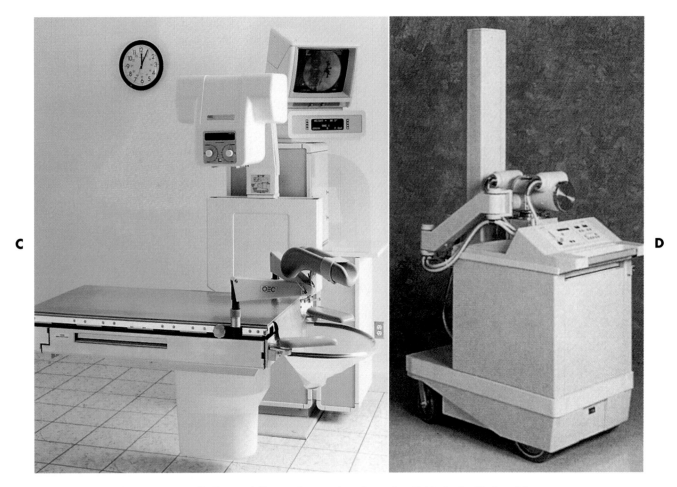

FIGURE 9-1, cont'd Types of diagnostic x-ray imaging units. **C,** Urologic. **D,** Portable. *(C courtesy Lorad Medical Systems, Inc.; D courtesy Philips Medical Systems.)*

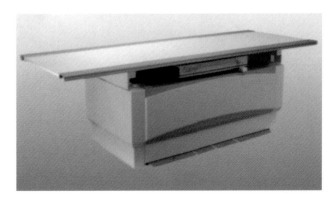

FIGURE 9-2 Patient examination table designed for bucky radiography. *(Courtesy Canon Medical Systems.)*

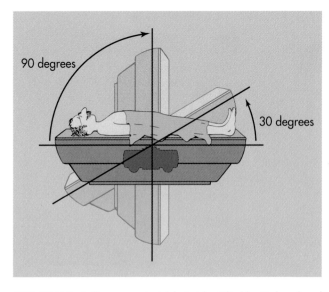

FIGURE 9-3 A fluoroscopic table is identified by its head and foot tilt.

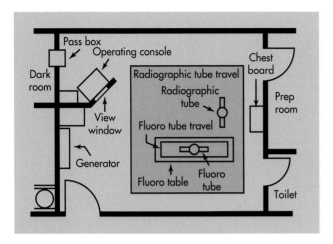

FIGURE 9-4 Floorplan of a general-purpose x-ray examination room, showing the location of the x-ray apparatus.

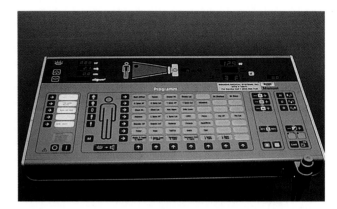

FIGURE 9-5 Typical operating console. The number of meters and controls depends on the complexity of the console.

Question: How far below horizontal will a patient's head go on a 90/15 fluoroscopic table?

Answer: 15 degrees below horizontal.

Each x-ray imaging system, regardless of its design, has three principal parts: the **x-ray tube** (which is discussed in Chapter 10), the **operating console,** and the **high-voltage generator.** In some types of x-ray apparatus, such as dental and portable imaging systems, these three components are housed compactly. In most, however, the x-ray tube is located in the examination room and the operating console in an adjoining room, with a protective barrier separating the two. The protective barrier must have a window for viewing the patient during the examination.

The high-voltage generator may be housed in an equipment cabinet positioned against a wall. The high-voltage generator is always close to the x-ray tube, usually in the examination room. A few installations take advantage of false ceilings and locate these generators out of sight above the examination room. Newer generator designs using high-frequency circuits require even less space. Figure 9-4 is a plan drawing of a conventional general-purpose x-ray examination room.

OPERATING CONSOLE

The part of the x-ray imaging system most familiar to the radiologic technologist is the **operating console.** The operating console allows the radiologic technologist to control the x-ray tube current and voltage so that the useful x-ray beam is of proper quantity and quality (Figure 9-5). *Quantity* refers to the number of x-rays or the intensity of the x-ray beam; it is usually expressed in milliroentgen (mR) or milliroentgen per milliampere-second (mAs). *Quality* refers to the penetrability of the x-ray beam and is expressed by kVp or more precisely, half-value layer (HVL) (see Chapter 12).

The operating console usually provides for control of line compensation, and exposure time. Monitors in the form of meters are usually provided for kVp and milliamperage (mA). Sometimes, an mAs meter is also provided. On equipment that incorporates phototiming, separate controls for mAs may be present.

All the electric circuits connecting the meters and controls on the operating console are at low voltage so that the possibility of hazardous shock is minimized. Figure 9-6 is a simplified schematic diagram for a typical operating console. A look inside an operating console indicates how simplified this schematic drawing is!

Many modern operating consoles are based on recent computer technology. Controls and meters are digital, and technique is selected by touching the screen. Numerical technique selection is sometimes replaced by icons indicating body part, size, and shape. Many of the features are automatic, but the radiologic technologist must know their purpose and use.

Line Compensation

Most x-ray imaging systems are designed to operate on 220-V power, although some can operate on 110 or 440 V. Unfortunately, electric power companies are not capable of providing 220 V accurately and continuously. Because of variations in power distribution to the hospital and in power consumption by the various sections of the hospital, the voltage provided to an x-ray imaging system may easily vary by as much as 5%. Such variation in supply voltage results in a large variation in the x-ray beam. This variation is unacceptable if high-quality images are to be consistently produced.

The line compensator incorporates a meter to measure the voltage provided to the x-ray imaging system and a control to adjust that voltage to precisely 220 V. The control is usually wired to the autotransformer. On

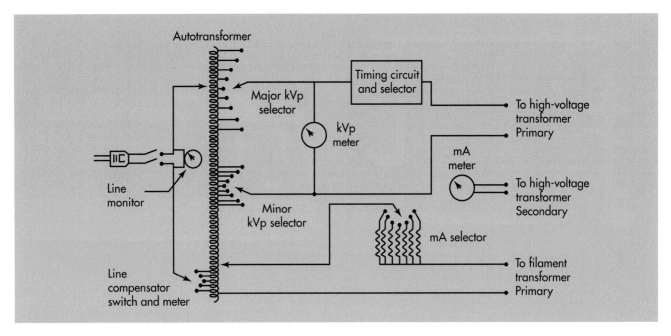

FIGURE 9-6 Circuit diagram of the operating console identifies the controls and meters.

older units, adjustment of the supply voltage while observing the line voltage meter was required. Today, line compensation is automatic, and there is no meter. The power supply to the x-ray imaging system is routed to a special transformer called an *autotransformer*.

Autotransformer

The **autotransformer** is designed to supply a precise voltage to the filament circuit and to the high-voltage circuit of the x-ray imaging system. The voltage supplied from the autotransformer to the high-voltage transformer is controlled but variable. It is much safer and easier to vary low voltage and then increase it than it is to increase a low voltage to the kilovolt level and then vary its magnitude.

The autotransformer works on the principle of electromagnetic induction but is very different from the conventional transformer. It has only one winding and one core. This single winding has a number of connections located along its length (Figure 9-7). Two of the connections, *A* and *A'*, as shown, conduct the input power to the autotransformer and are called *primary connections*. Some of the secondary connections, such as *C*, are located closer to one end of the winding than the primary connections. This allows the autotransformer to both increase and decrease voltage. The autotransformer can be designed to step up voltage to approximately twice the input voltage value.

Because the autotransformer operates as an induction device, the voltage it receives (the primary voltage) and the voltage it provides (the secondary voltage) are in direct relation to the number of turns of the transformer

enclosed by the respective connections. The **autotransformer law** is the same as the transformer law.

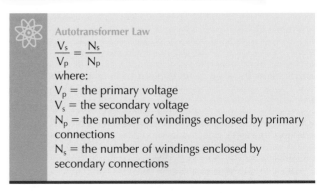

Autotransformer Law
$$\frac{V_s}{V_p} = \frac{N_s}{N_p}$$
where:
V_p = the primary voltage
V_s = the secondary voltage
N_p = the number of windings enclosed by primary connections
N_s = the number of windings enclosed by secondary connections

Question: If the autotransformer in Figure 9-8 is supplied with 220 V to the primary connections *AA'*, which enclose 500 windings, what will be the secondary voltage across *BB'* (500 windings), *CB'* (700 windings), and *DE* (200 windings)?

Answer: $BB'V_s = V_p\left(\dfrac{N_s}{N_p}\right)$

$\qquad\qquad = (220V)\left(\dfrac{500}{500}\right) = (220V)$

$\qquad CB': V_s = (220V)\left(\dfrac{700}{500}\right)$

$\qquad\qquad = (220V)(1.4) = 308V$

$\qquad DE: V_s = (220V)\left(\dfrac{200}{500}\right)$

$\qquad\qquad = (200V)(0.4) = 88V$

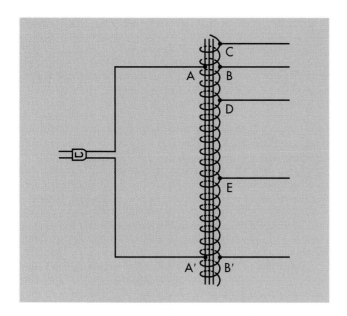

FIGURE 9-7 Autotransformer in simplified terms

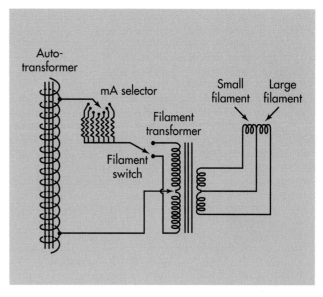

FIGURE 9-8 Filament circuit for dual-filament x-ray tube.

kVp Adjustment

Some older x-ray operating consoles have adjustments labeled *major kVp* and *minor kVp,* and by selecting a combination of these controls, the radiologic technologist can provide precisely the required kVp and thus the quality of the x-ray beam.

 kVp determines the quality of the x-ray beam.

The major and minor kVp adjustments represent two separate series of connections on the autotransformer. Selection of the appropriate connections can be made by an adjustment knob, push button, or touch screen. If the primary voltage to the autotransformer is 220 V, the output of the autotransformer is usually controllable from about 100 to 400 volts, depending on the design of the autotransformer. This low voltage from the autotransformer becomes the input to the high-voltage step-up transformer that will increase the voltage to the kilovoltage chosen.

Question: An autotransformer connected to a 440-V supply contains 4000 turns, all of which are enclosed by the primary connections. If 2300 turns are enclosed by secondary connections, what will be the voltage supplied to the high-voltage generator?

Answer: $V_s = V_p \left(\dfrac{N_s}{N_p} \right)$

$\qquad = (440 \text{ V}) \left(\dfrac{2300}{4000} \right)$

$\qquad = (440 \text{ V})(0.575)$

$\qquad = 253 \text{ V}$

The kVp meter is placed across the output terminals of the autotransformer, and therefore it reads voltage, not kilovoltage. The scale of the kVp meter, however, registers kilovolts.

On most operating consoles the kVp meter registers even though an exposure is not being made and no current is flowing in the circuit. This type of meter is known as a **prereading voltmeter.** It allows the voltage to be monitored before an exposure.

mA Control

The x-ray tube current, the number of electrons crossing from cathode to anode per second, is measured in milliamperes (mA). The number of electrons emitted by the filament is determined by the temperature of the filament. The filament temperature is in turn controlled by the filament current, which is measured in amperes (A). As filament current increases, the filament becomes hotter, and more electrons are released by thermionic emission. Filaments normally operate at currents between 3 and 6 A.

X-ray tube current is controlled through a separate circuit that is called the *filament circuit.* Voltage for the filament circuit is provided from connections on the autotransformer. This voltage is reduced by the use of precision resistors to a value corresponding to the mA station selected. X-ray tube current normally is not continuously variable. Fixed-mA stations that provide tube currents of 100, 200, and 300 mA and higher result from the precision resistors. In some units, the mA can be varied continuously during an exposure to minimize the exposure time. This is referred to as *falling load,* a feature that is found on falling-load generators (see Chapter 20).

The product of x-ray tube current (mA) and exposure (s) is electrostatic charge (C).

Question: An image is made at 400 mA and an exposure time of 100 ms. Express this as mAs, as the total number of electrons.

Answer:
$$100 \text{ ms} = 0.1 \text{ s}$$
$$(400 \text{ mA})(0.1 \text{ s}) = 40 \text{ mAs}$$
$$40 \text{ mAs} = (40 \text{ mC/s})(\text{s});$$
remember that 1 A = 1 C/s
$$= 40 \text{ mC}$$
$$= (40 \times 10^{-3} \text{ C})(6.3 \times 10^{18} \text{ e}^-/\text{C})$$
$$= 252 \times 10^{15} \text{ e}^-$$
$$= 2.52 \times 10^{17} \text{ electrons}$$

The voltage from the mA-selector switch is then delivered to the filament transformer. The filament transformer is a step-down transformer; therefore the voltage supplied to the filament is lower, by a factor equal to the turns ratio, than the voltage supplied to the filament transformer. Similarly, the current is increased across the filament transformer in proportion to the turns ratio.

Question: A filament transformer with a turns ratio of 1:10 provides 6.2 A to the filament. What is the current flowing through the primary coil of the filament transformer?

Answer:
$$\frac{I_p}{I_s} = \frac{N_s}{N_p}$$
$$I_p = I_s\left(\frac{N_s}{N_p}\right)$$
$$= (6.2)\left(\frac{1}{10}\right)$$
$$= 0.62 \text{ A}$$

X-ray tube current is monitored with an mA meter that must be placed in the tube circuit. The mA meter is connected at the center of the secondary winding of the high-voltage step-up transformer. The secondary voltage is alternating at 60 Hz such that the center of this winding is always at zero volts (Figure 9-8). In this way, no part of the meter is in contact with the high voltage, and it may safely be put on the operating console. Variations of this meter are sometimes provided so that mAs can be monitored in addition to mA.

Exposure Timers

For any given radiographic examination the number of x-rays reaching the image receptor is directly related to both the x-ray tube current and the time that the tube is energized. X-ray operating consoles provide a wide se-

lection of x-ray beam-on times and when used with the appropriate mA station, provide an even wider selection of mAs values.

Question: A KUB examination (radiography of the *k*idneys, *u*reters, and *b*ladder) calls for 62 kVp and 80 mAs. If the radiologic technologist selects the 200-mA station, what exposure time should be used?

Answer: $\dfrac{80 \text{ mAs}}{200 \text{ mA}} = 0.4 \text{ s or } \frac{2}{5} \text{ s or } 400 \text{ ms}$

Question: A lateral cerebral angiogram calls for 78 kVp and 90 mAs. If the generator has a 1000-mA capacity, what is the shortest exposure time possible?

Answer: $\dfrac{90 \text{ mAs}}{1000 \text{ mA}} = 0.09 \text{ s or } 90 \text{ ms}$

The timer circuit is separate from the other main circuits of the x-ray imaging system. It consists of a mechanical or electronic device whose action is to "make" and "break" the high voltage across the x-ray tube. This is nearly always done on the primary side of the high-voltage transformer, where the voltage is lower.

There are five types of timing circuits. Four are controlled by the radiologic technologist, and one is automatic. After studying this section, try to identify the types of timers on the equipment you use.

Mechanical timers. Mechanical timers are very simple devices now used only in some portable and dental units. The mechanical timer operates by clockwork. A preset exposure time is dialed by turning a knob that winds a spring. When the exposure button is depressed, the spring is released and unwinds. The time required to unwind corresponds to the exposure time. Mechanical timers are inexpensive but are not very accurate. They can be used only for exposure times greater than about 250 ms.

Synchronous timers. In the United States, electric current is supplied at a frequency of 60 Hz. In Europe, Latin America, and other parts of the world, the frequency is 50 Hz. A special type of electric motor, known as a *synchronous motor,* is a precision device designed to drive a shaft at precisely 60 revolutions per second (rps). In some x-ray imagers, synchronous motors are used as timing mechanisms. Machines with synchronous timers are recognizable because the minimum exposure time possible is $\frac{1}{60}$ s (17 ms) and timing intervals increase by multiples thereof (for example, $\frac{1}{30}$ s, $\frac{1}{20}$ s). Synchronous timers cannot be used for serial exposures because they must be reset after each exposure, which even when done automatically, requires too much time.

Electronic timers. Electronic timers are the most sophisticated, most complicated, and most accurate of the x-ray exposure timers. Electronic timers consist of rather complex circuitry based on the time required to charge a capacitor through a variable resistance. They allow a wide range of time intervals to be selected and are accurate to intervals as small as 1 ms. Because they can be used for rapid serial exposures, they are particularly suitable for cardiovascular and interventional procedures. Most exposure timers are electronic.

mAs timers. Most x-ray apparatus is designed for accurate control of tube current and exposure time. The product, however, of mA and time—mAs—determines the number of x-rays emitted and therefore the optical density of the image. A special kind of electronic timer, called *mAs timer,* monitors the product of mA and exposure time and terminates the exposure when the desired mAs is attained.

The mAs timer is usually designed to provide the highest safe tube current for the shortest time of exposure for any mAs selected. Since the mAs timer must monitor the actual tube current, it is located on the secondary side of the high-voltage transformer.

Automatic exposure control. Unlike the four previous timing devices, the automatic exposure control (AEC) requires no operation by the radiologic technologist. The AEC is a device that measures the quantity of radiation reaching the image receptor. It automatically terminates the exposure when sufficient radiation to provide the required optical density has reached the image receptor. Figure 9-9 shows the operation of an AEC.

The type of AEC used by most manufacturers incorporates a flat, parallel plate ionization chamber positioned between the patient and the image receptor (Figure 9-10). The chamber is made radiolucent so that it will not interfere with the radiographic image. Ionization within the chamber creates a charge calibrated to produce a given average optical density on the radiograph. When the appropriate charge has been reached, the exposure is terminated.

When a phototimed x-ray imaging system is installed, it must be calibrated. This calls for making exposures of a phantom and adjusting the AEC for the range of optical densities on the image required by the radiologist. Usually the service engineer takes care of this calibration.

Once the AEC has been placed in clinical operation, the radiologic technologist simply selects the appropriate optical density and places the exposure time in the AEC mode. When the electric charge from the ionization chamber reaches a preset level, a signal is returned to the operating console, where the exposure is terminated.

AEC is now widely used and often is provided in addition to an electronic timer. Care should be taken when using the AEC mode, especially in low-kVp examinations, such as in mammography. Because of varying tissue thickness and composition, the AEC may not respond properly at low kVp, which can result in varying optical density. When radiographs are taken in the AEC mode, the electronic timer should be set to 2 s as a backup timer in case the AEC fails to terminate. This precaution should be followed for the protection of the patient and x-ray tube. This is done automatically on many units.

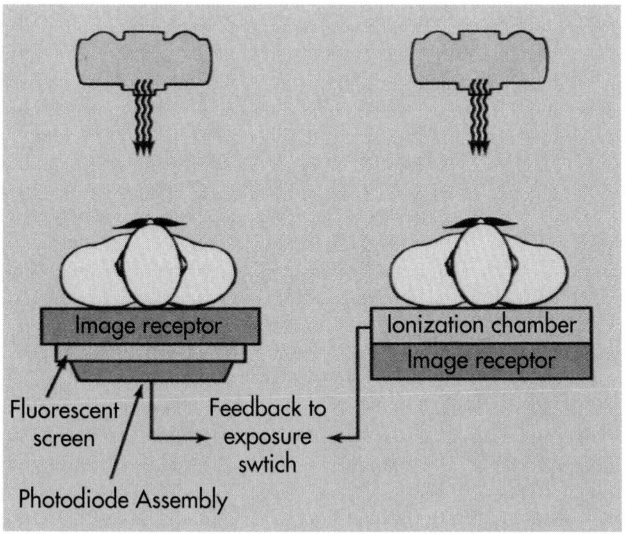

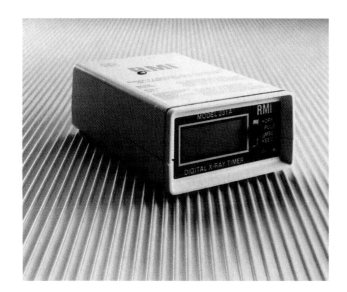

FIGURE 9-9 An automatic exposure control terminates the x-ray exposure at the desired film optical density. This is done with an ionization chamber or photodiode.

Image receptor

Ionization chamber
Image receptor

Fluorescent
screen

Feedback to
exposure
swtich

Photodiode Assembly

FIGURE 9-10 Solid-state radiation detectors are used to check timer accuracy. *(Courtesy Gammex RMI.)*

Checking the timer. It is essential that exposure timers on x-ray imaging systems function properly and accurately because inaccurate or malfunctioning exposure timers result in poor images, retakes, and unnecessary patient exposure.

Solid-state radiation detectors are now used for exposure-timer checks (Figure 9-10). These devices operate with a very accurate internal clock based on a quartz-crystal oscillator. They are capable of measuring exposure times as short as 1 ms and when used with an oscilloscope, can display radiation waveforms. Such devices, however, are highly sophisticated and are normally operated only by medical physicists and service engineers.

HIGH-VOLTAGE GENERATOR

The **high-voltage generator** of an x-ray imaging system is responsible for converting the low voltage from the electric power company into a kilovoltage of the proper waveform. A cutaway view of a typical high-voltage generator is shown in Figure 9-11. Although some heat is generated in the high-voltage section, which is conducted to oil, oil is used primarily for electric insulation. The high-voltage generator contains three primary parts: the high-voltage transformer, the filament transformer, and rectifiers.

High-Voltage Transformer

The high-voltage transformer is a step-up transformer; that is, the secondary voltage is greater than the primary voltage because the number of secondary windings is greater than the number of primary windings. The ratio of the number of secondary windings to the number of primary windings is called the **turns ratio** (see Chapter 8).

The voltage increase is proportional to the turns ratio according to the transformer law, and the current is reduced proportionally.

The turns ratio of a high-voltage transformer is usually between 500:1 and 1000:1. Since transformers operate only on alternating current, the voltage waveform on both sides of a high-voltage transformer is sinusoidal (Figure 9-12). The only difference between the primary and secondary waveforms is their **amplitude.** The primary voltage is measured in volts, and the secondary voltage is measured in kilovolts.

Question: The turns ratio of a high-voltage transformer is 700:1, and the supply voltage peaks at 120 V. What is the secondary voltage supplied to the x-ray tube?

Answer: (120 Vp)(700:1) = 84,000 Vp
                  = 84 kVp

Voltage Rectification

 Voltage rectification is the process of converting alternating current (AC) to direct current (DC).

The current from a common wall plug is alternating (AC), changing direction 60 times each second. Although transformers operate with AC, x-ray tubes require DC, or electron flow in only one direction. X-rays are produced by the acceleration of electrons from the cathode to the anode and cannot be produced by electrons flowing in the reverse direction, from anode to cathode.

It would be disastrous to the x-ray tube for electron flow to be reversed because the construction of the cathode assembly is such that it could not withstand the tremendous heat generated by such a reversal. If the elec-

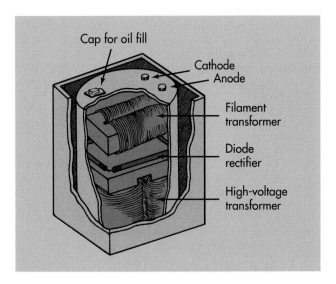

FIGURE 9-11 Cutaway view of typical high-voltage generator, showing oil-immersed diodes and transformers.

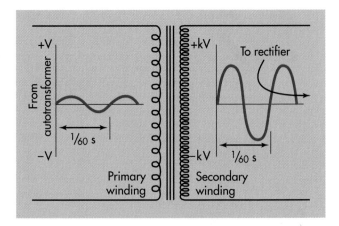

FIGURE 9-12 Voltage induced in the secondary winding of a high-voltage step-up transformer is alternating like the primary voltage but has a higher value.

tron flow is to be only in the cathode-to-anode direction, the secondary voltage of the high-voltage transformer must be rectified. This process of converting AC to DC is called **rectification,** and the electronic device that allows current flow in only one direction is a **rectifier.**

 Voltage rectification is required to ensure electron flow in one direction: from cathode to anode.

Rectification is accomplished with diodes. A diode is an electronic device containing two *(di-)* electrodes. All diode rectifiers were originally vacuum tubes called *valve tubes.* Valve tubes have been replaced in most x-ray imaging systems by solid-state rectifiers made of silicon (Figure 9-13). There are two principal types of rectifiers: (1) vacuum-tube rectifiers and (2) solid state diodes.

Vacuum-tube rectifiers. Consider an evacuated glass tube with a small coil of wire, the **filament,** at one end (Figure 9-14). If a large current is passed through this filament, it will heat up and "boil" electrons off its surface. This process is called **thermionic emission.** *Therm* refers to heat, *ion* refers to a charged particle, and *emission,* of course, means to "give off"; thus *thermionic emission* refers to giving off electrons from a heated surface.

This emitter of electrons is the filament and constitutes the **cathode,** or negative side, of the vacuum tube rectifier. A cold metallic plate is placed at the other end of the glass envelope. This is the **anode,** or positive side. This combination of hot, electron-emitting cathode and cold anode enclosed in a vacuum-sealed glass tube is the basis for most electronic tubes, including the x-ray tube.

An electric current is made up of a flow of electrons. Therefore the electrons, thermionically emitted by the hot filament of a vacuum tube, form an electric current. If the anode is connected to a positive voltage relative to

the cathode, the electrons at the cathode will be attracted to the anode. They stream across the length of the tube, causing an electron flow through the tube (Figure 9-15) from the cathode to the anode.

If, however, a higher voltage is placed on the cathode than the anode, the electrons will be attracted to the cathode. There are no free electrons at the anode available to stream across the gap. Therefore no electrons flow across the vacuum tube rectifier from the anode to the cathode, and there is no electric current.

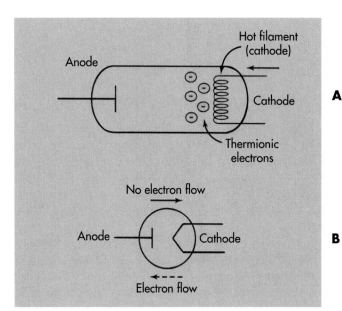

FIGURE 9-14 A, Basic vacuum tube. **B,** Its electronic symbol.

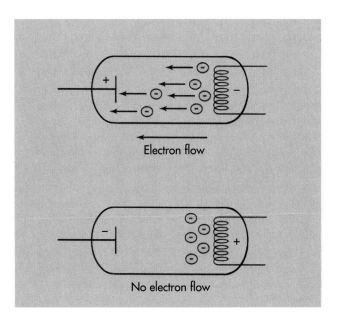

FIGURE 9-15 The vacuum-tube diode conducts electrons in only one direction: from cathode to anode.

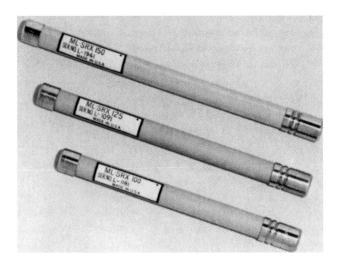

FIGURE 9-13 Rectifiers in most modern x-ray generators are the silicon, semiconductor type. *(Courtesy Varian Medical Systems.)*

A simple vacuum tube conducts electrons in only one direction: from cathode to anode, *not* from anode to cathode. This type of vacuum tube, sometimes called a *diode* because it has two *(di-)* electrodes, is therefore a rectifier.

Solid-state rectifiers. Vacuum-tube devices were first developed in the early part of the twentieth century. It had long been known that metals are good conductors of electricity and that some other materials, such as glass and plastics, are poor conductors of electricity or insulators.

In the 1950s, a third class of materials called **semiconductors,** were developed. Semiconductors lie between the range of insulators and conductors in their ability to conduct electricity. Tiny crystals of these semiconductors were found to have some useful electric properties, and they are the basis of the solid-state microchips available today.

Semiconductors are classed into two types: n-type and p-type. N-type semiconductors have loosely bound electrons that are relatively free to move about inside the material. P-type semiconductors have spaces, called *holes,* where there are no electrons. These holes are like the space between cars in heavy traffic. Holes are as mobile as electrons.

Consider a tiny crystal of n-type material placed in contact with a p-type crystal to form what is called a *p-n junction* (Figure 9-16). If a higher potential is placed on the p side of the junction, then the electrons and holes will both migrate toward the junction and wander across it. This flow of electrons and holes constitutes an electric current. If, however, a positive potential is placed on the n side of the junction, both the electrons and the holes will be swept away from the junction, and no electrons will be available at the junction surface to form an electric current. Thus, in this case, there will be no electric current through the p-n junction.

Therefore a solid-state p-n junction tends to conduct electricity in only one direction. This type of p-n junction is called a **solid-state diode.** Solid-state diodes, like tubes, are rectifiers because they pass electric current in only one direction. The arrowhead in the symbol for a diode indicates the direction of the electric current, which is opposite to the flow of the electrons (Figure 9-17).

Rectification in an x-ray imaging system is essential for the safe and efficient operation of the x-ray tube. Rectifiers are located in the high-voltage section.

Unrectified voltage. Figure 9-18 shows the unrectified voltage at the secondary side of the high-voltage step-up transformer. This voltage waveform looks like the voltage waveform supplied to the primary side of the high-voltage transformer, except its amplitude is much greater. The current passing through the x-ray tube, however, exists only during the positive half of the cycle, when the anode is positive and the cathode negative. During the negative half of the cycle, current can flow only from anode to cathode, but this does not occur because the anode is not constructed to emit electrons. The voltage across the x-ray tube during the negative half cycle is

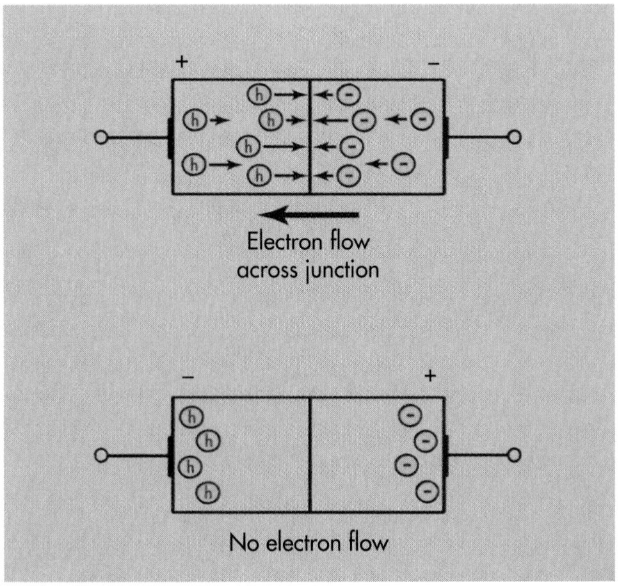

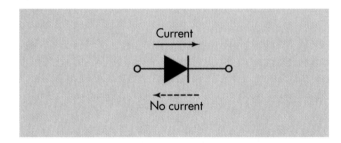

FIGURE 9-17 The electronic symbol for a solid-state diode.

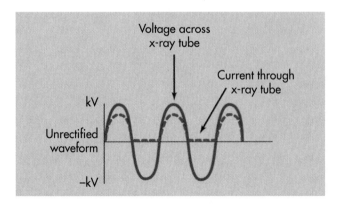

FIGURE 9-18 Unrectified voltage and current waveforms on the secondary side.

FIGURE 9-16 A p-n junction semiconductor shown as a solid-state diode.

called **inverse voltage** and can cause failure of the x-ray tube.

Half-wave rectification. The inverse voltage is removed from the supply to the x-ray tube by rectification. Half-wave rectification (Figure 9-19) represents a condition in which the voltage is not allowed to swing negatively during the negative half of its cycle.

Rectifiers are assembled into electronic circuits to convert AC into the DC necessary for the operation of an x-ray tube (Figure 9-20). During the positive portion of the AC waveform, the rectifier conducts freely and allows electric current to pass through the x-ray tube. During the negative portion of the AC waveform, however, the rectifier does not conduct, so no electric current is allowed. The resulting electric current is a series of positive pulses separated by gaps when the negative current is not conducted.

This output electric current is a rectified current, since electrons flow in only one direction. This form of rectification is called **half-wave rectification** because only half of the AC waveform appears in the output. The negative portion of the AC waveform has been removed.

In some portable and dental x-ray imaging systems, the x-ray tube serves as the vacuum-tube rectifier. Such a system is said to be **self-rectified,** and the resulting wave-

form is the same as that of half-wave rectification. Self-rectification is not used in most x-ray imaging systems because the x-ray tube cannot handle the higher power levels.

Half-wave-rectified circuits contain no diodes or only one or two. The x-ray output from a half-wave, high-voltage generator is pulsating, with 60 x-ray pulses produced each second.

Full-wave rectification. One shortcoming of half-wave rectification is that it wastes half the supply power. It also requires twice the exposure time. It is possible, however, to devise a circuit that will rectify the entire AC waveform. This form of rectification is called **full-wave rectification.** Full-wave-rectified x-ray imaging systems contain at least four diodes in the high-voltage circuit, usually arranged as in Figure 9-21. In a full-wave-rectified circuit, the negative half-cycle corresponding to the inverse voltage is reversed so that a positive voltage is always directed across the x-ray tube (Figure 9-22).

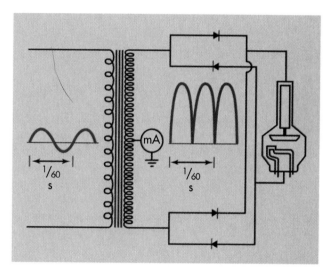

FIGURE 9-21 A full-wave-rectified circuit contains at least four diodes. Current is passed through the tube at 120 pulses in a second.

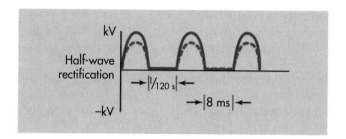

FIGURE 9-19 Half-wave rectification.

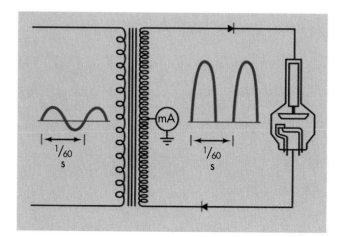

FIGURE 9-20 A half-wave-rectified circuit usually contains two diodes, although some contain one or more.

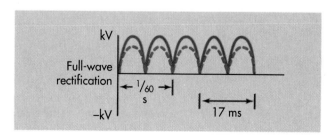

FIGURE 9-22 A positive voltage is always directed across a full-wave-rectified circuit.

The current through the circuit is shown during both the positive and negative phases of the input waveform. Note that in both cases the output voltage across the x-ray tube is positive. Also, there are no gaps in the output waveform. All of the input waveform is rectified into usable output. This is the preferred circuit for use in x-ray imaging systems, since it does not waste any of the input source.

Figure 9-23 helps explain how full-wave rectification works. During the positive half-cycle of the secondary voltage waveform, electrons flow from the negative side to diodes C and D. Diode C is unable to conduct electrons in that direction, but diode D can. The electrons flow through diode D and the x-ray tube. The electrons then abut diodes A and B. Only diode A is positioned to conduct them, and they flow to the positive side of the transformer, thus completing the circuit.

During the negative half-cycle, diodes B and C are pressed into service, but diodes A and D block electron flow. Note that the polarity of the x-ray tube remains unchanged. The cathode is always negative and the anode always positive, even though the induced secondary voltage alternates between positive and negative.

The main advantage to full-wave rectification is that the exposure time for any given technique is cut in half. The half-wave-rectified x-ray tube emits x-rays only half the time it is on. The pulsed x-ray output of a full-wave-rectified machine occurs 120 instead of 60 times per second as with half-wave rectification.

SINGLE-PHASE POWER

All the voltage waveforms discussed so far are produced by single-phase electric power. Single-phase power results in a pulsating x-ray beam. This is caused by the alternate swing in voltage from zero to maximum potential 120 times each second under full-wave rectification.

The x-rays produced when the single-phase voltage waveform has a value near zero are of little diagnostic value because of their low energy, and therefore they have low penetrability. One method of overcoming this deficiency is to use some sophisticated electrical engineering principles to generate three simultaneous voltage waveforms out of step with one another. Such a manipulation results in **three-phase electric power.**

THREE-PHASE POWER

The engineering required to produce three-phase power involves the manner in which the high-voltage step-up transformer is wired into the circuit. A discussion of precisely how this is done is unnecessary for our requirements. Figure 9-24 shows the voltage waveforms for single-phase power, for three-phase power, and for three-phase power when full-wave rectified.

When three-phase power is provided, multiple voltage waveforms are superimposed on one another, result-

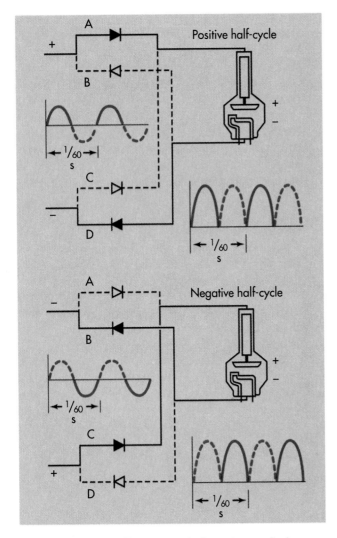

FIGURE 9-23 In a full-wave-rectified circuit, two diodes (**A** and **D**) conduct during the positive half-cycle and two (**B** and **C**) during the negative half-cycle.

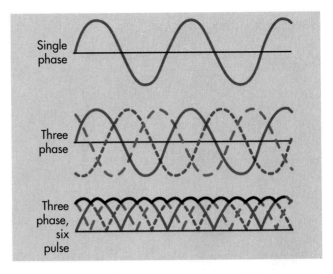

FIGURE 9-24 Three-phase power is a more efficient way to produce x-rays than single-phase power. Shown are the voltage waveforms for unrectified single-phase and three-phase power and rectified three-phase power.

ing in a waveform that maintains a nearly constant high voltage. There can be 6 pulses every 1/60 s or 12 pulses per 1/60 s, compared to the two pulses characteristic of single-phase power. With three-phase power, the voltage impressed across the x-ray tube is nearly constant, never dropping to zero during exposure.

There are limitations to the speed of starting an exposure—**initiation time**—and ending an exposure—**extinction time**—because of how the iron in the high-voltage step-up transformer responds. Additional electronic circuits and hardware are necessary to correct this deficiency and add to the additional size and cost of the three-phase generator.

HIGH-FREQUENCY GENERATOR

The newest development in high-voltage generator design uses a high-frequency circuit. Full-wave-rectified power at 60 Hz is converted to a higher frequency, usually 500 to 5,000 Hz (Figure 9-25). One advantage to the high-frequency generator is its small size; such generators can be placed within the x-ray tube housing. High-frequency generators produce a nearly constant potential voltage waveform, which results in improved image quality at lower patient dose. Portable x-ray imaging systems were the first to benefit from this technology; however, almost all stationary x-ray imaging systems use high-frequency voltage generation.

High-frequency voltage generation uses **inverter** circuits (Figure 9-26). Inverter circuits are high-speed switches or choppers, which convert DC into a series of square pulses. Many portable x-ray high-voltage generators use storage batteries and silicon-controlled rectifiers (SCRs) to generate square waves at 500 Hz, which becomes the input to the high-voltage step-up transformer. The high-voltage step-up transformer operating at 500 Hz is about one tenth the size of a 60-Hz transformer, which is rather large and heavy. At 500 Hz, one can sometimes hear the transformer "sing" during exposure.

The small time gap between square wave pulses, unlike 60-Hz sine waves, is easy to filter, producing a near-constant voltage of the anode. Such portable x-ray generators perform as well as the best three-phase generators.

High-frequency x-ray generators are sometimes grouped by frequency (Table 9-1). The principal differences are in the electric components designed as the inverter module. The real advantage to such circuits is that they are much smaller, less costly, and more efficient than three-phase circuits.

 Full-wave rectification or high-frequency voltage generation is used in almost all stationary x-ray imaging systems.

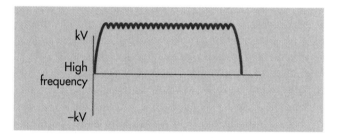

FIGURE 9-25 High-frequency voltage waveform.

TABLE 9-1	Characteristics of High-Frequency X-Ray Generators	
Frequency Range	**Inverter Features**
Up to 1 kHz	Thyristers
1 to 10 kHz	Large SCRs
10 to 100 kHz	Power-field-effect transistors

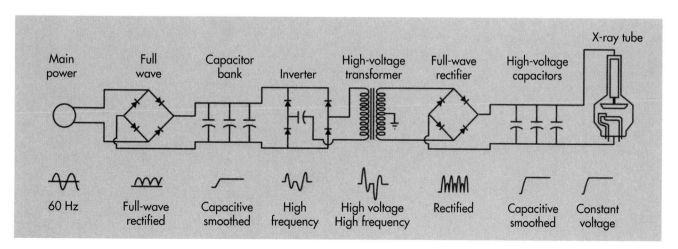

FIGURE 9-26 Inverter circuit of a high-voltage generator.

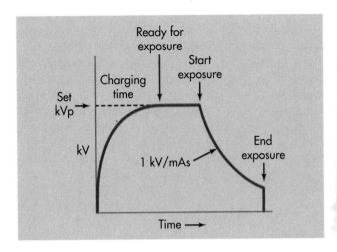

FIGURE 9-27 Tube voltage falls during exposure using a capacitor discharge generator.

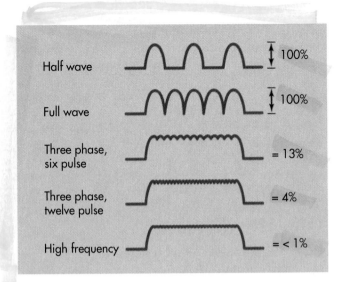

FIGURE 9-28 Voltage waveforms resulting from various power supplies.

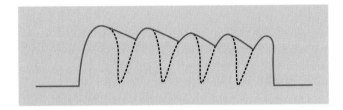

FIGURE 9-29 Voltage waveform is smoothed by the capacitance of long high-voltage cables.

CAPACITOR-DISCHARGE GENERATOR

Some portable x-ray imaging systems still use a high-voltage generator, which operates by charging a series of SCRs from the DC voltage of a nickel-cadmium (NiCd) battery. By stacking (in an electrical sense) the SCRs, the charge is stored at very high electrical potential: high voltage. During exposure, the charge is released (discharged) to form the x-ray tube current to produce x-rays. During capacitor discharge, the voltage falls approximately 1 kV/mAs (Figure 9-27).

This falling voltage limits the available x-ray tube current and results in a falling kVp during exposure. The result is the need for precise radiographic technique charts. After a given exposure time, the capacitor bank continues to discharge, which could cause continued x-ray emission. Such x-ray emission is stopped by either a grid-controlled x-ray tube, an automatic lead beam stopper, or both. A grid-controlled x-ray tube has a specially designed cathode to control x-ray current.

VOLTAGE RIPPLE

Another way to characterize these voltage waveforms is by **voltage ripple.** Single-phase power has **100% voltage ripple;** the voltage varies from zero to its maximum value. Three-phase, six-pulse power produces voltage with only approximately **14% ripple;** consequently, the voltage supplied to the x-ray tube never falls below 86% of the peak value.

A further improvement in three-phase power results in twelve rather than six pulses per cycle. Three-phase, twelve-pulse power results in only **4% ripple,** and therefore the voltage supplied to the x-ray tube does not fall below 96% of the peak value. High-frequency generators have approximately **1% ripple** and therefore higher x-ray quantity and quality.

Figure 9-28 shows the resulting voltage waveform provided to the x-ray tube by these various power sources. The approximate voltage ripple is also shown. The most efficient method of x-ray production also has the waveform with the lowest voltage ripple.

 Less voltage ripple results in higher radiation quantity and quality.

There are many advantages to x-ray tube voltage generated with less ripple. The principal advantage is the higher radiation quantity and quality resulting from the more constant voltage supplied to the x-ray tube. The radiation quantity is higher because the efficiency of x-ray production is higher when x-ray tube voltage is high. Stated differently, for any projectile electron emitted by the x-ray tube filament, more x-rays are produced when the electron energy (keV) is high than when it is low.

The radiation quality is increased with low-voltage ripple because there are fewer low-energy projectile electrons passing from cathode to anode to produce low-energy x-rays. Consequently, the average x-ray energy is increased over that resulting from high-voltage ripple modes.

Because the x-ray beam intensity and penetrability are greater for less voltage ripple than for single-phase power, technique charts developed for one cannot be used on the other. It is necessary to develop new technique charts when using three-phase or high-frequency x-ray imaging systems. Three-phase operation may require as much as a 10-kVp reduction to produce the same radio-graphic optical density when operated at the same mAs as single phase. A 12-kVp reduction may be necessary when using a high-frequency generator.

Three-phase radiographic equipment is manufactured with tube currents as high as 1200 mA; therefore exceedingly short, high-intensity exposures are possible. This capacity is particularly helpful in cardiovascular and interventional procedures.

When three-phase power is provided for a radiographic/fluoroscopic room or for cardiovascular and interventional rooms, all radiographic exposures are under three-phase control. The fluoroscopic mode, however, usually remains single phase and takes advantage of the electric capacitance of the x-ray tube cables. Fluoroscopic mA is very low compared with radiographic mA. Because the x-ray cables are long, they have considerable capacitance, resulting in smoothing of the voltage waveform (Figure 9-29). The exception is cineradiography, which is usually three-phase.

The principal disadvantage of three-phase x-ray apparatus is its initial cost. The cost of installation and operation, however, can be lower than that associated with single-phase equipment. High-frequency generators have a moderate cost. The overall capacity and flexibility provided by low-ripple generators are greater than those for single-phase equipment.

POWER RATING

Transformers and high-voltage generators are usually identified by their power rating in kilowatt (kW). Electric power for any device is specified in watt, as shown in the following equations from Chapter 6:

Power = Current × Potential
Watt = Ampere × Volt

A high-voltage generator for a basic radiographic unit would be rated at 30 to 50 kW. Generators for cardiovascular and interventional suites have power ratings up to approximately 150 kW. When specifying high-voltage generators, the industry standard is to use the maximum tube current (mA) possible at 100 kVp for an exposure of 100 ms. That generally results in the maximum available power.

High voltage generator power (kW) is the maximum x-ray tube current (mA) at 100 kVp and 100 ms.

Power is the product of amperes multiplied by volts. This assumes constant current and voltage, which do not exist in single-phase x-ray imaging systems. However, the low-ripple power of three-phase and high-frequency circuits is so close to constant current that this power equation holds true.

Question: When a low-voltage ripple system is energized at 100 kVp and 100 ms, the maximum tube current possible is 800 mA. What is the power rating?

Answer: Power rating = Ampere × Volt
            = 800 mA × 100 kVp
            = 80,000 mA × kVp
            = 80,000 watt
            = 80 kW

Since the product of ampere × volt = watt, the product of milliampere × kilovolt = watt. However, power rating is expressed in kilowatt; therefore the defining equation for three-phase and high-frequency power is as follows:

$$\text{Power rating (kW)} = \frac{\text{mA} \times \text{kVp}}{1000}$$

Question: An interventional unit is capable of 1200 mA when operated in 100 kVp, 100 ms. What is the power rating?

Answer: $\text{Power rating (kW)} = \dfrac{1200 \text{ mA} \times 100 \text{ kVp}}{1000}$
            = 120 kW

Single-phase generators have 100% voltage ripple and are less efficient x-ray generators. Consequently, the single-phase expression of power rating is:

$$\text{Power rating (kW)} = (0.7)\frac{\text{mA} \times \text{kVp}}{1000}$$

Question: A single-phase radiographic unit installed in a private office has maximum capacity at 100 ms of 120 kVp and 500 mA. What is its power rating?

Answer: $\text{Power rating} = (0.7)\dfrac{(500 \text{ mA})(120 \text{ kVp})}{1000}$
            = 42 kW

X-RAY CIRCUIT

The three main sections of the x-ray imaging system—the x-ray tube, the operating console, and the high-voltage generator—are represented in Figure 9-30 by a simplified schematic. The location of all meters, controls, and components of importance are shown.

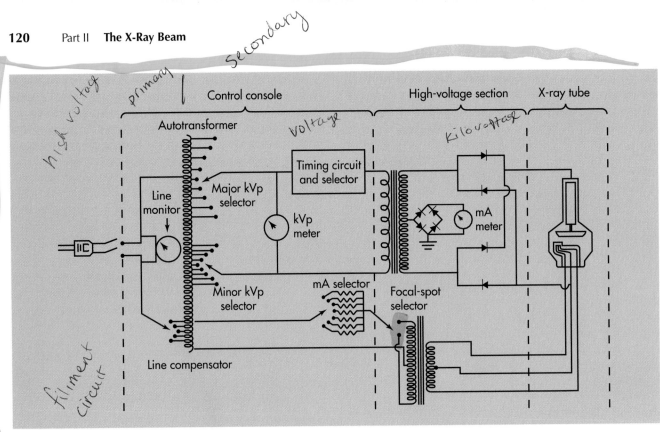

FIGURE 9-30 Schematic circuit of an x-ray imaging system.

SUMMARY

There are three principal sections of the x-ray imaging system: the x-ray tube, the operating console, and the high-voltage generator. The design and operation of the x-ray tube is discussed in Chapter 10.

The operating console consists of an on/off control, kVp selection, and mA and time (or mAs) selection. AECs are also located on the operating console.

The high-voltage generator provides power to the x-ray tube in three possible ways: single-phase power, three-phase power, and high-frequency power. The difference between single- and three-phase power involves the manner in which the high-voltage step-up transformer is electrically positioned. The waveforms for single-phase, three-phase, and three-phase fully rectified power were shown in Figure 9-21. With three-phase power, the voltage across the x-ray tube is nearly constant during exposure and never drops to zero, as does the voltage for single-phase power.

The components of an x-ray imaging system are sometimes identified by their power rating in kilowatt (kW). Maximum available power for high-voltage generators equal the maximum tube current (mA) at 100 kVp for an exposure of 100 ms.

CHALLENGE QUESTIONS

1. Define or otherwise identify:
   a. Automatic exposure control (AEC)
   b. Line compensation
   c. Capacitor
   d. mA meter location
   e. Diode
   f. Voltage ripple
   g. Autotransformer
   h. Rectification

2. Across 1200 windings of the primary coil of the autotransformer 220V is supplied. If 1650 windings are tapped, what voltage will be supplied to the primary coil of the high-voltage transformer?

3. A kVp meter reads 86 kVp, and the turns ratio of the high-voltage step-up transformer is 1200. What is the true voltage across the meter?

4. The supply voltage from the autotransformer to the filament transformer is 60 V. If the turns ratio of the filament transformer is 1/12, what is the filament voltage?

5. If the current in the primary of the filament transformer in Question 6 were 0.5 A, what would be the filament current?

6. The supply to a high-voltage step-up transformer with a turns ratio of 550 is 190 V. What is the voltage across the x-ray tube?

7. Locate the various meters and controls shown in Figure 9-30 on an x-ray imaging system you operate.

8. The radiographic table must be radiolucent. Define *radiolucent.*

9. When performing x-ray examinations in your clinical assignments, which examinations would not use the Bucky tray?

10. Describe the movements of a 90/20 table.

11. List three major controls on the operator's console.

12. What is the purpose of the autotransformer?

13. What is the relationship between the primary voltage and the secondary voltage in an autotransformer?

14. What does the prereading voltmeter allow?

15. Operating console controls are set at 200 mA with an exposure time of $\frac{1}{60}$ s. What is the mAs?

16. In an examination of a pediatric patient, the operating console controls are set at 600 mA and 30 ms. What is the mAs?

17. What is the difference between a high-voltage generator and a high-voltage transformer?

18. Why is rectification necessary in the x-ray circuit?

19. Match the power source with the voltage ripple.

POWER	VOLTAGE RIPPLE
Single-phase	1%
Three-phase, twelve-pulse	4%
Three-phase, six-pulse	14%
High frequency	100%

20. What is the only type of high-voltage generator that can be positioned in or on the x-ray tube housing?

The X-Ray Tube

OBJECTIVES

At the completion of this chapter, the student should be able to:

1. Describe the general design of an x-ray tube
2. List the external components that house and protect the x-ray tube
3. Identify the purpose of the glass or metal envelope
4. Discuss the cathode and filament current
5. Describe the parts of the anode and the induction motor
6. Define the line-focus principle and the heel effect
7. Identify the three causes of x-ray tube failure
8. Explain how to use x-ray tube rating charts to prevent tube failure

OUTLINE

Though x-ray tube is the part of the x-ray imaging system that is rarely seen by the radiologic technologist. The external structure of the x-ray tube consists of three parts: the support structure, the protective housing, and the glass or metal envelope. The internal structures include two electrodes called the *anode* and the *cathode*. This chapter discusses these external and internal structures as well as the causes and prevention of tube failure. With proper use, an x-ray tube should last many years.

EXTERNAL COMPONENTS
X-Ray Tube Support

The x-ray tube and housing assembly are quite heavy. Support mechanisms are required so that the radiologic technologist can move the weight of the tube to position it. Figure 10-1 illustrates the three main methods of x-ray tube support.

Ceiling support system. The ceiling support system is the most frequently used method of x-ray tube support (Figure 10-1, *A*). It consists of two sets of ceiling rails mounted directly over the radiographic table. The rails are mounted perpendicular to each other to allow for both longitudinal and transverse travel of the x-ray tube. A telescoping column attaches from the ceiling rails to the x-ray tube housing, and the column can change the distance to the radiographic table when the tube is manipulated by the radiographer. The distance for the tube to the x-ray cassette is called the **source-to-image receptor distance (SID).** When the tube is centered above the table at a standard SID, the tube is said to be in a detent, or locked, position. Other positions can be chosen and locked by the radiologic technologist.

Floor-to-ceiling support system. The floor-to-ceiling support system has a single column with rollers on each end, one attached to a ceiling-mounted rail and the other attached to a floor-mounted rail. The x-ray tube slides up and down the column as the column rotates. A variation of this type of support system is the floor-support system, which has a single col-

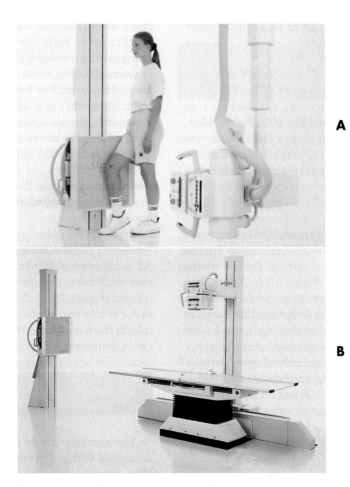

A

B

FIGURE 10-1 Three methods of supporting an x-ray tube. **A,** Ceiling support. **B,** Floor support. *(Courtesy Toshiba Corp.)*

Continued

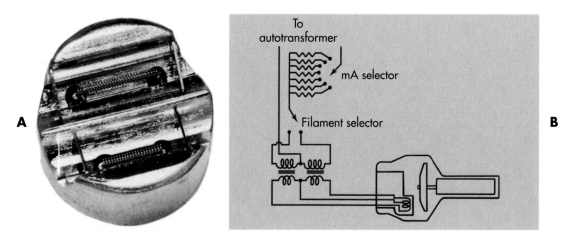

FIGURE 10-4 **A,** Dual-filament cathode designed to provide focal spots of 0.5 and 1.5 mm. **B,** Schematic for dual-filament cathode. (**A** *courtesy The Machlett Laboratories, Inc.*)

When this happens, arcing will occur and lead to tube failure. Such malfunction is usually abrupt.

Figure 10-4 shows a photograph of a dual-filament cathode and a schematic drawing of its electrical supply. The two filaments supply separate electron beams to produce two focal spots.

Focusing cup. The filament is embedded in a metal cup called the **focusing cup** (Figure 10-5). Since all the electrons accelerated from cathode to anode are electrically negative, the electron beam tends to spread out because of electrostatic repulsion. Some electrons even miss the anode completely.

The focusing cup is negatively charged so that it electrostatically confines the electron beam to a small area of the anode (Figure 10-6). The effectiveness of the focusing cup is determined by its size and shape, its charge, the filament size and shape, and the position of the filament within the focusing cup.

Certain types of x-ray tubes called **grid-controlled tubes** are designed to be turned on and off very rapidly. Grid-controlled tubes are used in portable capacitor-discharge imagers and in digital subtraction angiography, digital radiography, and cineradiography, all of which require multiple exposures at precise exposure times. The term *grid* is borrowed from vacuum tube electronics and refers to an element in the tube that acts as the switch. In a grid-controlled x-ray tube the focusing cup is the grid and therefore the exposure switch.

Filament current. When the x-ray imaging system is first turned on, a low current flows through the filament to warm it and prepare it for the thermal jolt necessary for x-ray production. At low filament current, no tube current flows because the filament does not get hot enough for thermionic emission. Once the filament current is high enough for thermionic emission, a small

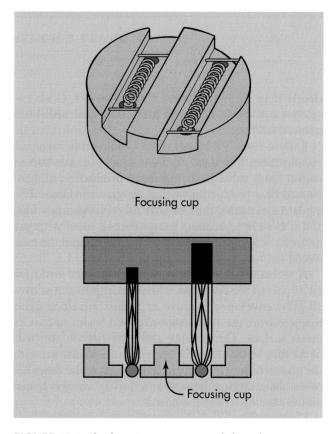

FIGURE 10-5 The focusing cup is a metal shroud surrounding the filament.

rise in filament current results in a large rise in tube current.

The x-ray tube current is adjusted by controlling the filament current. This relationship between filament current and tube current depends on the tube voltage (Figure 10-7). Fixed stations of 100, 200, and 300 mA and

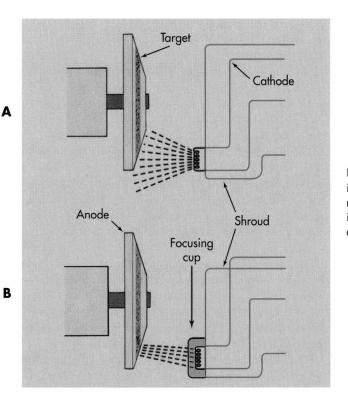

FIGURE 10-6   A, Without a focusing cup, the electron beam is spread beyond the anode because of mutual electrostatic repulsion among the electrons. **B,** With a focusing cup, which is negatively charged, the electron beam is condensed and directed to the target.

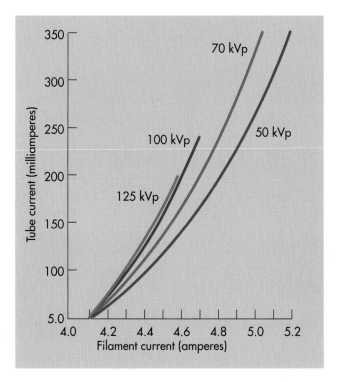

FIGURE 10-7 X-ray tube current is controlled by changing the filament current. Because of thermionic emission, a small change in filament current results in a large change in tube current.

no more can boil off

so on usually correspond to discrete connections on the filament transformer or to precision resistors.

When emitted from the filament, electrons momentarily remain in the vicinity of the filament before being accelerated to the anode. Since these electrons carry negative charges, they repel one another and tend to form a cloud around the filament. This cloud of electrons, called a **space charge,** makes it difficult for subsequent electrons to be emitted by the filament because of the electrostatic repulsion. This phenomenon is called the **space-charge effect.** X-ray tubes under certain conditions of low kVp and high mA are said to be space-charge limited. A major obstacle in producing x-ray tubes with currents exceeding 1000 mA is the design of adequate space-charge compensating devices.

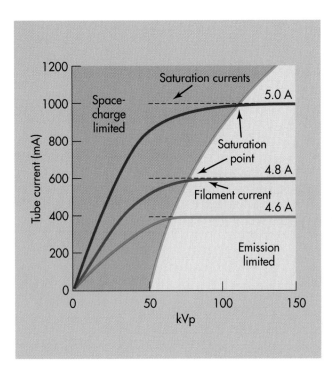

FIGURE 10-8 X-ray tube current reaches a maximum level called the *saturation current.*

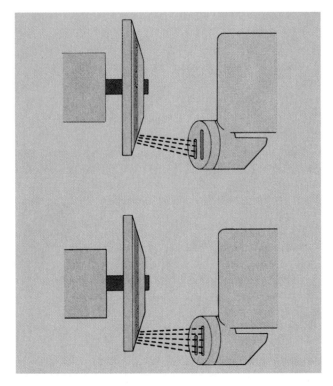

FIGURE 10-9 In a dual-focus x-ray tube, focal spot size is controlled by heating one of the two filaments.

At any given filament current, say 5.2 A (Figure 10-8), the x-ray tube current will rise with increasing kVp to a maximum value. A further increase in kVp will not result in a higher mA because all of the available electrons have been used. This is the **saturation current.** Saturation current is not reached at lower kVp because of space-charge limitation.

Dual-focus tube. Most diagnostic x-ray tubes are dual focus; that is, they have two focal spots, one large and the other small. The small focal spot is used when better spatial resolution is required. The large focal spot is used when large body parts are imaged and when other techniques that produce high heat are required.

The selection of one or the other focal spot is generally made with the mA station selector on the operating console. Normally, either filament can be used with the lower mA station, approximately 300 mA or less. At approximately 400 mA and up, only the larger focal spot is allowed because the heat capacity of the anode could be exceeded if the small focal spot were used.

Small focal spots range from 0.1 to 1.0 mm; large focal spots usually range from 0.4 to 2.0 mm. Each filament of a dual-filament cathode assembly is embedded in the focusing cup (Figure 10-9). The small focal spot size is associated with the small filament and the large focal spot size with the large filament. The electric current flows through the appropriate filament.

Anode

The anode is the positive side of the x-ray tube. There are two types of anodes: stationary and rotating (Figure 10-10). **Stationary anode** x-ray tubes are used in dental x-ray imaging systems, some portable imaging systems, and other special-purpose units in which high tube current and power are not required. General-purpose x-ray tubes use the **rotating anode** because they must be capable of producing high-intensity x-ray beams in a short time.

 The anode is the positive side of the tube; it conducts electricity, radiates heat, and contains the target.

The anode performs three functions in an x-ray tube.
1. The anode tube is an electrical conductor. It receives electrons emitted by the cathode and conducts them through the tube to the connecting cables and back to the high-voltage generator.
2. The anode provides mechanical support for the target.
3. The anode acts as a good thermal radiator.

When the projectile electrons from the cathode interact with the anode, approximately 99% of their kinetic energy is converted into heat. This heat must be conducted away quickly, before it can damage the anode. Adequate heat dissipation is the major engineering hurdle to higher-capacity x-ray tubes.

Target. The **target** is the area of the anode struck by the electrons from the cathode. In stationary anode tubes, the target consists of a tungsten alloy metal embedded in the copper anode (Figure 10-11, *A*). In rotating anode tubes, the entire rotating disc is the target (Figure 10-11, *B*). Alloying the tungsten (usually with rhenium) gives it added mechanical strength to withstand the stresses of high-speed rotation. High-capacity x-ray tubes have molybdenum, graphite or both, layered under the tungsten target as a thermal insulator (Figure 10-12). Both molybdenum and graphite have lower mass density than tungsten, making the anode easier to rotate.

Tungsten is the material of choice for the target in general radiography for the following reasons:
1. **Atomic number**—Tungsten's high atomic number, 74, results in high-efficiency x-ray production and in high-energy x-rays. The reason for this is discussed more fully in Chapter 11.
2. **Thermal conductivity**—Tungsten has a thermal conductivity nearly equal to that of copper. It is therefore an efficient metal for dissipating the heat produced.
3. **High melting point**—Any material, if heated sufficiently, melts and becomes liquid. Tungsten has a high melting point (3400° C compared with 1100° C for copper) and therefore can stand up under high tube current without pitting or bubbling.

Specialty x-ray tubes for mammography have molybdenum or rhodium targets principally because of their low atomic number and low K-characteristic x-ray energy. Table 10-1 summarizes the properties of these target materials, all of which have excellent heat dissapation.

A new generation of x-ray tubes have also been introduced that have very high heat capacity (6 to 8 MHU) that are predominantly used in CT imaging systems.

Rotating anode. Rotating anodes make higher tube currents and exposure times possible. The rotating anode x-ray tube allows the electron beam to interact with a much larger target area, and therefore the heating of the anode is not confined to one small spot as in a stationary anode tube. Figure 10-13 compares the target areas of typical stationary anode and rotating anode x-ray tubes with 1-mm focal spots. The actual target for the stationary tube is 1 mm × 4 mm = 4 mm². If the rotating anode diameter is 15 cm, then the radius of the target area is approximately 14 cm (140 mm). The total target area of the rotating anode is 2π(140) × 4 mm = 3519 mm².

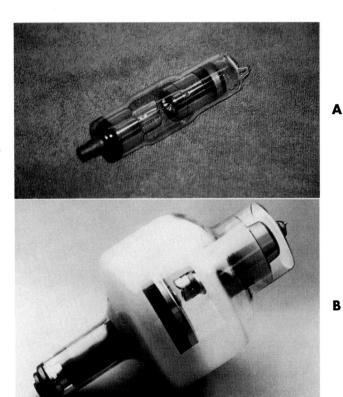

FIGURE 10-10 All diagnostic x-ray tubes can be classified according to their type of anode. **A,** Stationary anode. **B,** Rotating anode. *(Courtesy Philips Medical Systems.)*

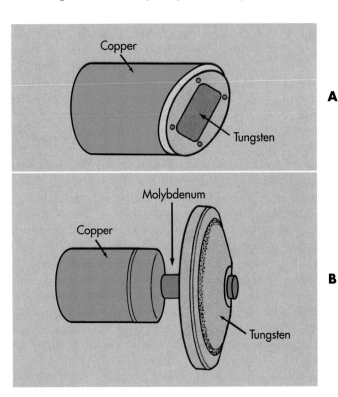

FIGURE 10-11 **A,** In a stationary anode tube the target is embedded in the anode. **B,** In a rotating anode tube the target is the rotating disc.

TABLE 10-1	Characteristics of X-Ray Targets			
Element	Chemical Symbol	Atomic Number	K X-Ray Energy (keV)	Melting Temperature (°C)
Tungsten	W	74	69	3400
Molybdenum	Mo	42	20	2600
Rhodium	Rh	45	23	3200

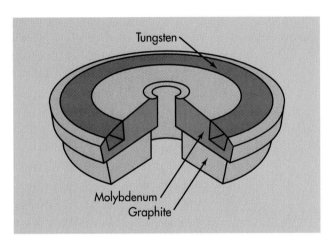

FIGURE 10-12 A layered anode consists of a target surface backed by one or more layers to increase capacity.

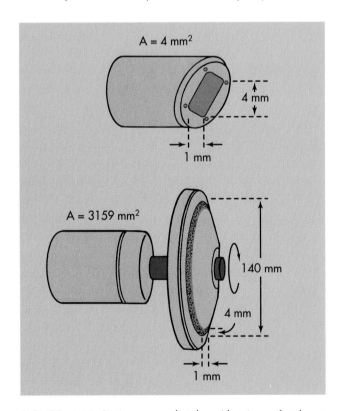

FIGURE 10-13 Stationary anode tube with a 1-mm focal spot may have a target area of 4 mm². A comparable 15-cm-diameter rotating anode tube can have a target area of approximately 3500 mm², which increases the heating capacity of the tube by a factor of nearly 1000.

Thus the rotating anode tube provides nearly 1000 times more area for the electron beam to interact than a stationary anode tube.

 Higher tube currents and shorter exposure times are possible with the rotating anode.

Heating capacity can be further improved by increasing the speed of rotation of the anode. Most rotating anodes revolve at 3400 revolutions per minute (rpm). The anodes of high-capacity tubes rotate at 10,000 rpm. The neck of the anode is the shaft between the anode and the rotor. This shaft is usually molybdenum because its poor heat conduction insulates the induction motor from anode heat.

Occasionally, the rotor mechanism of a rotating anode tube fails. When this happens, the anode becomes overheated and pits or cracks, causing tube failure (Figure 10-14).

Induction motor. How does the anode rotate inside a glass or metal envelope with no mechanical connection to anything outside the envelope? Most things that revolve are powerful by chains, axles, or gears. The rotating anode is driven by an electromagnetic induction motor. An induction motor consists of two principal parts separated from each other by the glass or metal envelope (Figure 10-15). The part outside the envelope, called the **stator,** consists of a series of electromagnets equally spaced around the neck of the tube. Inside the envelope is a shaft made of bars of copper and soft iron fabricated into one mass. This mechanism is called the **rotor.**

The induction motor works on electromagnetic induction similar to that for a transformer and on Lenz's law of induced currents. Current flowing in each stator winding induces a magnetic field that surrounds the rotor. The stator windings are energized sequentially so that the induced magnetic field rotates on the axis of the stator. This magnetic field interacts with the ferromagnetic rotor, causing it to rotate synchronously with the activated stator windings.

When the radiologic technologist pushes the exposure button of a radiographic imager, there is a small delay that allows the rotor to accelerate to its designed revolutions per minute. During this time, filament current is in-

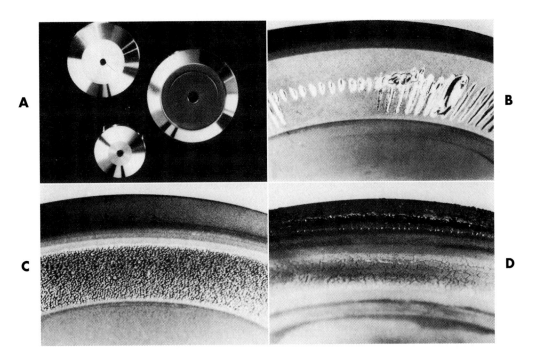

FIGURE 10-14 Comparison of smooth, shiny appearances of rotating anodes when new (**A**), and their appearance after failure (**B** to **D**). Examples of anode separation and surface melting shown were caused by slow rotation caused by bearing damage (**B**), repeated overload (**C**), and exceeding of maximum heat storage capacity (**D**). (*Courtesy Varian Medical Systems.*)

creased to provide the correct x-ray tube current. When a two-position exposure switch is used, it is important to push the switch to its final position in one motion. This maneuver minimizes the time that the filament is heated and prolongs tube life.

When the exposure is completed on imaging systems equipped with high-speed rotors, the rotor can be heard to slow down and stop within approximately 1 minute. The high-speed rotor slows down as quickly as it does because the induction motor is put into reverse. The rotor is a precisely balanced, low-friction device that if left alone might take many minutes to coast to rest after use. In a new x-ray tube, the **coast time,** or anode stop time, is about 60 s. With age, this is reduced because of wear of the rotor bearings. One design that allows the use of massive anodes employs spiral groove bearings and a direct oil-cooled anode (Figure 10-16). The main advantage is improved heat dissipation and higher-power capacity.

Line-focus principle. The focal spot is the area of the target from which x-rays are emitted. **Actual focal spot size** is the area on the anode target that is exposed to electrons from the tube current. Radiology requires small focal spots because the smaller the focal spot, the better the spatial resolution of the image. Unfortunately, as the size of the focal spot decreases, the heating of the target is concentrated onto a smaller area. This is the limiting factor to actual focal spot size.

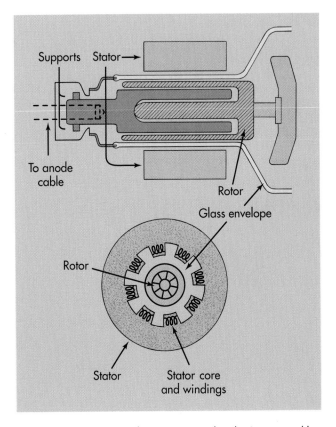

FIGURE 10-15 Target of a rotating anode tube is powered by an induction motor, the principal components of which are the stator and the rotor.

12° most common

Before the development of the rotating anode, another design was incorporated into x-ray tube targets to allow a large area for heating while maintaining a small focal spot. This design is known as the **line-focus principle.** Through angling of the target (Figure 10-17), the effective area of the target is made much smaller than the actual area of electron interaction. The effective target area, or **effective focal spot size,** is the area projected onto the patient and the image receptor. This is the value given when identifying large or small focal spots. When the target angle is made smaller, the effective focal spot

size is also made smaller. Diagnostic x-ray tubes have target angles varying from about 5 to 15 degrees. The advantage of the line-focus principle is that it simultaneously improves spatial resolution and heat capacity.

> The line-focus principle results in an effective focal spot size much smaller than the actual focal spot size.

Biangle targets are available that produce two focal spot sizes, designing two target angles on the anode (Figure 10-18). Combining biangular targets with different length filaments results in a very flexible combination.

A circular effective focal spot is preferred. Usually, however, it has a shape characterized as a double banana (Figure 10-19). These differences in x-ray intensity across the focal spot are controlled principally by the design of the filament and focusing cup and the voltage on the focusing cup. Round focal spots are particularly important for high-resolution magnification radiography.

The National Electrical Manufacturers Association (NEMA) has established standards and variances for focal-spot sizes. When a manufacturer states a focal-spot size, that is its nominal size. Table 10-2 shows the maximum measured size permitted to still be within the standard.

Heel effect. One unfortunate consequence of the line-focus principle is that the radiation intensity on the cathode side of the x-ray field is higher than that on the anode side. Electrons interact with target atoms at various depths into the target. The x-rays that constitute the useful beam are emitted from a depth in the target toward

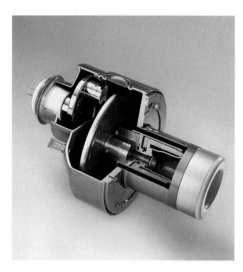

FIGURE 10-16 This very-high-capacity x-ray tube has spiral groove-liquid bearings and a direct oil-cooled anode. *(Courtesy Philips Medical Systems.)*

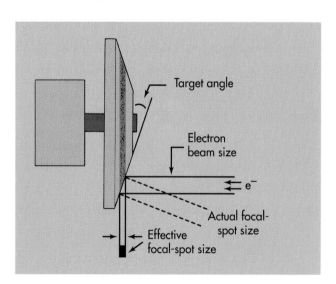

FIGURE 10-17 The line-focus principle allows high anode heating with small effective focal spots. As the target angle decreases, so does the effective focal spot size.

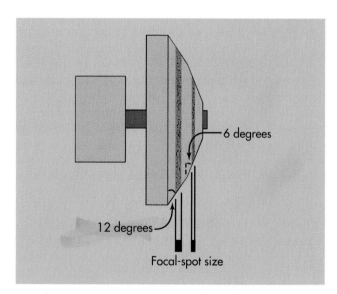

FIGURE 10-18 Some anodes have two angles to produce two focal spots.

the anode side and must traverse a greater thickness of target material than the x-rays emitted in the cathode direction (Figure 10-20). The intensity of x-rays that are emitted through the "heel" of the target is reduced because they have a longer path through the target and therefore increased absorption. This is the **heel effect.**

 The smaller the focal spot, the larger the heel effect.

The difference in radiation intensity across the useful beam of an x-ray field can vary as much as 45%. The **central ray** of the useful beam is the imaginary line generated by the centermost x-ray in the beam. If the radiation intensity along the central ray is designated as 100%, then the intensity on the cathode side may be as high as 120% and that on the anode side may be as low as 75%.

The heel effect is important when imaging anatomic structures that differ greatly in thickness or density. In general, positioning the cathode side of the x-ray tube over the thicker part of the anatomy provides more uniform optical density on the film. The cathode and anode directions are usually indicated on the protective housing, sometimes near the cable connectors.

In chest radiography, for example, the cathode should be down. The lower thorax in the region of the diaphragm is considerably thicker than the upper thorax and therefore requires higher radiation intensity if there is to be uniform exposure of the image receptor. Abdominal imaging, on the other hand, should be done so that the cathode is up. The upper abdomen is thicker than the lower abdomen and pelvis and requires a higher x-ray intensity for uniform optical density. Figure 10-21 shows two posterior-anterior (PA) chest images, one taken with the cathode down, the other with the cathode up. Can you tell the difference? Which do you think represents better radiographic quality? Resolve the difference before looking at the figure legend.

Another important consequence of the heel effect is changing focal-spot size. The effective focal spot is smaller on the anode side of the x-ray field than on the

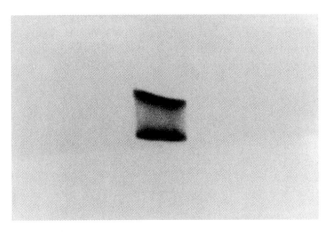

FIGURE 10-19   The usual shape of a focal spot is the double banana. *(Courtesy Donald Jacobson.)*

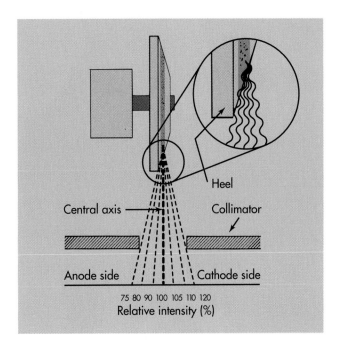

FIGURE 10-20   Heel effect results in reduced x-ray intensity on the anode side of the useful beam because of absorption in the "heel" of the target.

TABLE 10-2	Nominal Focal Spot Size Compared with that Permitted as Acceptable					
Nominal Focal Spot Size (mm)			**Acceptable Measured Focal Spot Size (mm)**			
Width	×	Length	Width	×	Length	
0.1	×	0.1	0.15	×	0.15	
0.2	×	0.2	0.3	×	0.3	
0.3	×	0.3	0.45	×	0.65	
0.4	×	0.4	0.6	×	0.85	
0.5	×	0.5	0.75	×	1.1	
1.0	×	1.0	1.4	×	2.0	
1.5	×	1.5	2.0	×	3.0	
2.0	×	2.0	2.6	×	3.7	

cathode side (Figure 10-22). Some manufacturers of mammography equipment take advantage of this property by angling the x-ray tube to produce the smaller focal spot along the chest wall.

> The heel effect results in smaller effective focal spot and less radiation intensity on the anode side of the x-ray beam.

Extrafocal radiation. X-ray tubes are designed so that projectile electrons from the cathode interact with the target only at the focal spot. However, some electrons bounce off the focal spot and land on other areas of the target, causing x-rays to be produced from outside of the focal spot (Figure 10-23). These x-rays are called **extrafocal radiation** or **off-focus radiation.** It is not unlike squirting a water pistol at a concrete pavement. Some of the water splashes off the pavement and lands in a larger area.

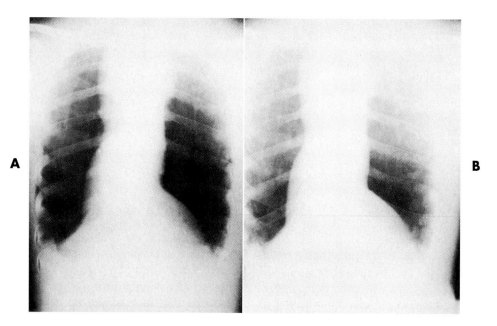

FIGURE 10-21 PA chest images demonstrating the heel effect. **A,** Images taken with the cathode up (superior). **B,** Image with cathode down (inferior). More uniform radiographic density is obtained with the cathode positioned to the thicker side of the anatomy, as in **B.** *(Courtesy Pat Duffy.)*

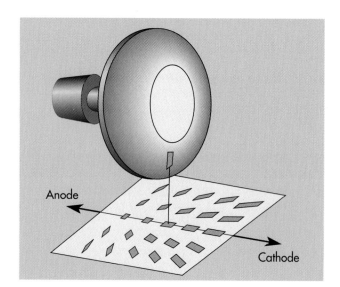

FIGURE 10-22 The effective focal spot changes size and shape across the projected x-ray field.

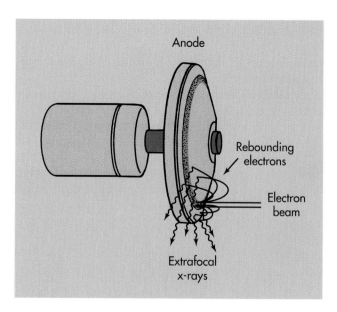

FIGURE 10-23 Extrafocal x-rays result from electrons interacting with the anode off of the focal spot, creating a larger-than-intended focal spot.

Extrafocal radiation is undesirable because it extends the size of the focal spot. The additional x-ray beam area increases skin dose modestly but unnecessarily. The extrafocal radiation can significantly reduce image contrast. Finally, extrafocal radiation can expose patient tissue that was not intended to be imaged. Examples of such undesirable images are the ears in a skull examination, soft tissue beyond the cervical spine, and lung beyond the borders of the thoracic spine.

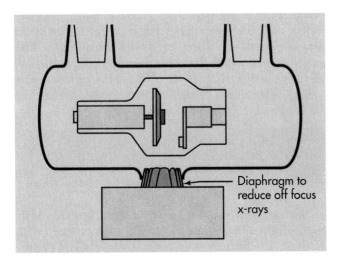

FIGURE 10-24   An additional diaphragm is positioned close to the focal spot to reduce extrafocal radiation.

Extrafocal radiation is reduced by designing a fixed diaphragm in the tube housing near the window of the x-ray tube (Figure 10-24). This is a geometric solution.

Another effective solution is the metal envelope x-ray tube. Electrons reflected from the focal spot are extracted by the metal envelope and conducted away. Therefore they are not available to be attracted to the target outside of the focal spot. The use of a grid does not reduce extrafocal radiation.

X-RAY TUBE FAILURE

With careful use, x-ray tubes can provide many years of service. With inconsiderate use, x-ray tube life may be shortened substantially, and the tube may even fail abruptly. The length of x-ray tube life is primarily under the control of the radiologic technologist. Basically, x-ray tube life is extended by using the minimum radiographic factors of mA, kVp, and exposure time that are appropriate for each examination. The use of faster image receptors has resulted in much longer tube life.

There are several causes of tube failure, all of which are related to the thermal characteristics of the x-ray tube. Enormous heat is generated in the anode of the x-ray tube during x-ray exposure. This heat must be dissipated for the x-ray tube to continue to function. This heat can be dissipated in three ways: radiation, conduction, and convection (Figure 10-25). Radiation is the transfer of heat by the emission of infrared radiation. Heat lamps emit not only visible light but also infrared

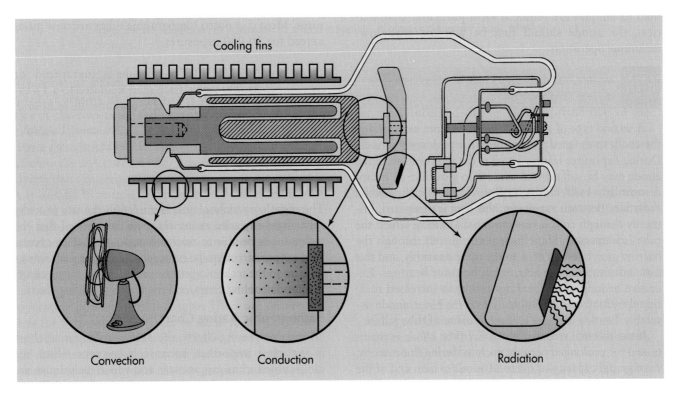

FIGURE 10-25   Heat from an anode is dissipated by radiation, conduction, and convection.

Answer: a. Unsafe b. Unsafe c. Safe d. Safe   e. Unsafe

Question: Radiographic examination of the abdomen with a tube that has a 0.6-mm focal spot and anode rotation of 10,000 rpm requires technique factors of 95 kVp and 150 mAs. What is the shortest possible exposure time for this examination?

Answer: Locate the proper radiographic rating chart (upper right in Figure 10-26) and the 95-kVp line (horizontal line near middle of chart). Beginning from the left (shorter exposure times), determine the mAs for the intersection of each mA curve with the 95 kVp level.

1. The first intersection is approximately 350 mA at 0.03 s = 10.5 mAs. Not enough.
2. The next intersection is approximately 300 mA at 0.2 s = 60 mAs. Not enough.
3. The next intersection is approximately 250 mA at 0.6 s = 150 mAs. This is sufficient.

Consequently, 0.6 s is the minimum possible exposure time.

Anode Cooling Chart

The anode has a limited capacity for storing heat. Although heat is dissipated to the oil bath and tube housing, it is possible through prolonged use or multiple exposures to exceed the heat storage capacity of the anode.

Thermal energy is conventionally measured in units of calories, British thermal units (BTU), or joules. In x-ray applications, thermal energy is measured in heat units (HU). The capacity of the anode and the housing to store heat is measured in heat units. A total of 1 HU is equal to the product of 1 kVp, 1 mA, and 1 s.

> Single-Phase
> HU = kVp × mA × s

Question: Radiographic examination of the lateral lumbar spine requires 98 kVp and 120 mAs. How many heat units are generated by this exposure?

Answer: Number of heat units = 98 kVp × 120 mAs
                          = 11,760 HU

Question: A fluoroscopic examination is performed at 76 kVp and 1.5 mA for 3½ minutes. How many heat units are generated?

Answer: Number of heat units = 76 kVp × 1.5 mA ×
                          3½ min × 60 s/min
                          = 23,940 HU

More heat is generated when three-phase and high-frequency equipment is used than when single-phase equipment is used. A modification factor is necessary for calculating three-phase or high frequency heat units.

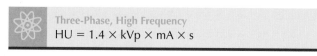

> Three-Phase, High Frequency
> HU = 1.4 × kVp × mA × s

Question: Six sequential skull films are exposed with a three-phase generator operated at 82 kVp and 120 mAs. What is the total heat generated?

Answer: Number of heat units/film = 1.4 × 82 kVp ×
                                     120 mAs
                          = 13,776 HU
                 Total HU = 6 × 13,776 HU
                          = 82,656 HU

The thermal capacity of an anode and its heat-dissipation characteristics are contained in a rating chart called an *anode cooling chart* (Figure 10-27). Unlike the radiographic rating chart, the anode cooling chart is not dependent on the filament size or the speed of rotation.

The tube represented in Figure 10-27 has a maximum anode heat capacity of 350,000 HU. The chart shows that if the maximum heat load were attained, it would take 15 minutes for the anode to completely cool. The rate of cooling is rapid at first and shows as the anode cools. In addition to determining the maximum heat capacity of the anode, the anode cooling chart is used to determine the length of time required for complete cooling after any level of heat input.

Question: A particular examination results in 50,000 HU being delivered to the anode in a matter of seconds. How long will it take the anode to cool completely?

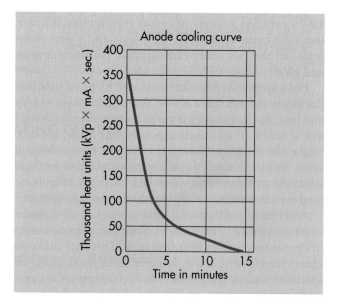

FIGURE 10-27 Anode cooling chart showing the time required for a heated anode to cool. *(Courtesy General Electric Medical Systems.)*

15 - time to cool to zero
if 4 min, 15 - 4 = 1 min

Answer: The 50,000-HU level intersects the anode cooling curve at approximately 6 minutes. From that point on the curve to complete cooling requires an additional 9 minutes (15 − 6 = 9). Therefore 9 minutes is required for complete cooling.

Although the heat generated in producing x-rays is expressed in heat units, joules are the equivalent. By definition:

> 1 watt = 1 volt × 1 amp
> = 1 KV × 1 mA

A total of 1 watt of electric power is also equal to 1 J/s.

> 1 watt = 1 volt × 1 amp
> = 1 J/C × 1 C/s
> = 1 J/s
> Therefore:
> 1 J/s = 1 kV × 1 mA
> and 1 J = 1 kV × 1 mA × 1 s
> Since HU = kVp × mA × s
> 1 HU = 1.4 J, 1 J = 0.7 HU

Question: How much heat energy (in joules) is produced during a single high-frequency mammographic exposure of 25 kVp and 200 mAs?

Answer: 25 kVp × 200 mAs = 5000 J
= 5 KJ

Housing Cooling Chart

The cooling chart for the housing of the x-ray tube has a shape similar to that of the anode cooling chart and is used in precisely the same way. Radiographic x-ray tube housings generally have maximum heat capacities in the range of several million HU. Complete cooling after maximum heat capacity requires from 1 to 2 hours. About twice that amount of time is required without auxiliary fan-powered air circulation.

SUMMARY

The primary support structure for the x-ray tube, which allows the greatest ease of movement and range of position, is the ceiling support system. The protective housing covers the x-ray tube and provides the following three functions: (1) it reduces leakage radiation to 100 mR/h at 1 m, (2) it provides mechanical support protecting the tube from damage, and (3) it serves as a way to conduct heat away from the x-ray tube target.

The glass or metal envelope surrounds the cathode (−) and anode (+), which are the electrodes of the vacuum tube. The cathode contains the tungsten filament, which is the source of electrons. The rotating anode is the tungsten-rhenium disk, which serves as a target for the electrons accelerated from the cathode. The line-focus principle results in an effective focal-spot size that is much smaller than the actual focal-spot size. The heel effect is defined as the variation in x-ray intensity across the x-ray beam because of absorption of x-rays in the heel of the target.

Safe operation of the x-ray tube is the responsibility of the radiographer. The causes of x-ray tube failure are threefold:

1. A single excessive exposure causes pitting or cracking of the anode.
2. Long exposure times cause excessive heating of the anode, resulting in damage to the bearings in the rotor assembly. Bearing damage causes warping and rotational friction of the anode.
3. Even with normal use, vaporization of the filament causes tungsten to coat the glass or metal envelope, which eventually causes arcing.

Tube rating charts printed by manufacturers of x-ray tubes aid the radiographer in using acceptable exposure levels to maintain x-ray tube life.

CHALLENGE QUESTIONS

1. Define or otherwise identify:
   a. Housing cooling chart
   b. Leakage radiation
   c. Heat unit (HU)
   d. Focusing cup
   e. Anode rotation speed
   f. Thoriated tungsten
   g. X-ray tube current
   h. Grid-controlled x-ray tube
   i. Convection
   j. Space charge
   k. Useful beam
2. List the main methods used to support the x-ray tube and briefly describe each.
3. Define *SID*.
4. What is the length and diameter of an x-ray tube?
5. What is done to ensure that the unsafe conditions shown on the radiographic rating chart are not exceeded?
6. Explain the phenomenon of thermionic emission.
7. Describe the principal cause of x-ray failure. What addition to the filament material prolongs tube life?
8. What is the reason for the filament to be embedded in focusing cup?
9. Why are x-ray tubes manufactured with two focal spots?
10. Is the anode or the cathode the negative side of the x-ray tube?

11. List and describe the two types of anodes.

12. What are the three functions the anode serves in an x-ray tube?

13. How does atomic number, thermal conductivity, and melting point affect the anode target material?

14. Draw diagrams of a stationary and a rotating anode.

15. How does the anode rotate inside a glass envelope with no mechanical connection to the outside?

16. Use a drawing to show the difference between the actual focal spot and the effective focal spot.

17. Define the heel effect and describe how it can be used advantageously. List the x-ray tube warm-up procedure.

18. List the three common anode materials. Explain the three causes of x-ray tube failure.

19. What happens when an x-ray tube is space charge limited?

X-Ray Production

OBJECTIVES

At the completion of this chapter, the student should be able to:

1. Discuss the interactions between projectile electrons and the x-ray tube target
2. Describe characteristic and bremsstrahlung x-ray production
3. Describe the x-ray emission spectrum
4. Explain how milliampere-second, peak kilovoltage, added filtration, target material, and voltage ripple affect the x-ray emission spectrum

OUTLINE

Chapter 10 discusses the internal components of the x-ray tube, the cathode and anode, within the evacuated glass or metal envelope. This chapter explains the interactions among the electrons accelerated from the cathode to the x-ray tube target. Those interactions produce two kinds of x-rays—characteristic and bremsstrahlung—which are described by the x-ray emission spectrum. Various conditions that affect the x-ray emission spectrum are also discussed.

ELECTRON TARGET INTERACTIONS

The primary function of the x-ray imaging system is to accelerate electrons from the cathode to the anode within the x-ray tube. The three principal parts of an x-ray imaging system—the operating console, the high-voltage generator, and the x-ray tube—are all designed to provide a large number of electrons focused to a small spot on the anode in such a manner that the electrons arriving at the anode have high kinetic energy.

 Kinetic energy is the energy of motion.

Kinetic energy is the energy of motion. Stationary objects have no kinetic energy; objects in motion have kinetic energy proportional to their mass and to the square of their velocity. The equation used to calculate kinetic energy follows:

> **Kinetic Energy**
> $KE = \frac{1}{2} mv^2$
> where
> KE = kinetic energy in joules
> m = mass in kilograms
> v = velocity in meters per second

For example, a 1000-kg automobile has four times the kinetic energy of a 250-kg motorcycle traveling at the same speed (Figure 11-1). If the motorcycle were to double its velocity, however, it would have the same kinetic energy as the automobile.

In determining the magnitude of the kinetic energy of a projectile, velocity is more important than mass. In an x-ray tube the projectile is the electron. All electrons have the same mass; therefore electron kinetic energy is increased by raising the peak kilovoltage (kVp). As electron kinetic energy is increased, both the intensity (quantity) and the energy (quality) of the x-ray beam are increased.

The modern x-ray imaging system is remarkable. It conveys to the x-ray tube target an enormous number of

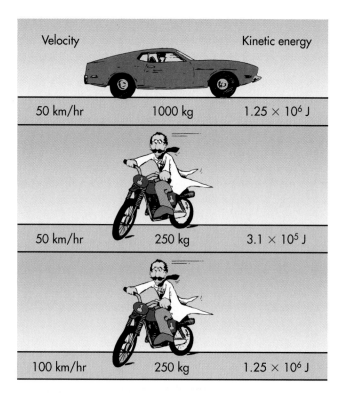

FIGURE 11-1 Kinetic energy is proportional to the product of mass and velocity squared.

electrons at a precisely controlled kinetic energy. At 100 mA, for example, 6×10^{17} electrons travel from the cathode to the anode every second. In an x-ray imaging system operating at 70 kVp, each electron arrives at the target with a maximum kinetic energy of 70 kiloelectron volts (keV). Since there are 1.6×10^{-16} J/keV, this energy is equivalent to the following:

> $(70 \text{ keV})(1.6 \times 10^{-16} \text{ J/keV}) = 1.12 \times 10^{-14} \text{ J}$

Inserting this energy into the expression for kinetic energy and solving for the velocity of the electrons, we find the following:

> $KE = \frac{1}{2} mv^2$
> $v^2 = \dfrac{2\ KE}{m}$
> $v^2 = \dfrac{(2)(1.12 \times 10^{-14} \text{ J})}{(9.1 \times 10^{-31} \text{ kg})}$
> $\quad = 0.25 \times 10^{17} \text{ m}^2/\text{s}^2$
> $v = 1.6 \times 10^8 \text{ m/s}$

Question: At what fraction of the velocity of light do 70-keV electrons travel?

Answer: $\dfrac{v}{c} = \dfrac{1.6 \times 10^8 \text{ m/s}}{3.0 \times 10^8 \text{ m/s}} = 0.53$

These calculations are not precisely correct; however, they do illustrate the point and demonstrate the use of this equation. According to the theory of relativity, an electron's mass increases as it approaches the speed of light; thus the actual value of v/c is 0.47 at 70 keV.

The distance between the filament and the x-ray tube target is only 1 to 3 cm. It is not difficult to imagine the intensity of the accelerating force required to raise the velocity of electrons from zero to half the speed of light in so short a distance.

The electrons traveling from cathode to anode constitute the x-ray tube current and are sometimes called *projectile electrons*. When these projectile electrons hit the heavy metal atoms of the x-ray tube target, they transfer their kinetic energy to the target atoms. These interactions occur within a very small depth of penetration into the target. As they occur, the projectile electrons slow and finally come nearly to rest, at which time they are conducted through the x-ray anode assembly and out into the associated electronic circuitry.

The projectile electron interacts with either the orbital electrons or the nuclear field of target atoms. These interactions result in the conversion of kinetic energy into thermal energy (heat) and electromagnetic energy in the form of infrared radiation (also heat) and x-rays.

Anode Heat

Most of the kinetic energy of projectile electrons is converted into heat (Figure 11-2). The projectile electrons interact with the outer-shell electrons of the target atoms but do not transfer sufficient energy to these electrons to ionize them. Rather, the outer-shell electrons are simply raised to an excited, or higher, energy level. The outer-shell electrons immediately drop back to their normal energy level with the emission of infrared radiation. The constant excitation and return of outer-shell electrons are responsible for most of the heat generated in the anodes of x-ray tubes.

 Approximately 99% of the kinetic energy of projectile electrons is converted to heat.

Only approximately 1% of the kinetic energy of projectile electrons is used for the production of x-radiation (99% is converted to heat). Therefore, sophisticated as it is, the x-ray tube is very inefficient.

The production of heat in the anode is directly proportional to an increase in x-ray tube current. Doubling the x-ray tube current doubles the quantity of heat produced. Heat production also increases directly with increasing kVp, at least in the diagnostic range. Although the relationship between varying kVp and varying heat production is approximate, it is sufficiently exact to allow the computation of heat units for use with anode cooling charts.

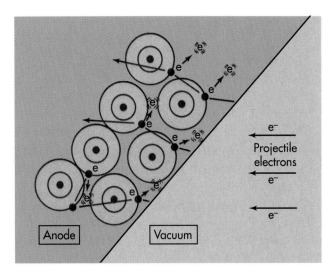

FIGURE 11-2 Most of the kinetic energy of projectile electrons is converted to heat by interactions with outer-shell electrons of target atoms. These interactions are primarily excitations rather than ionizations.

The efficiency of x-ray production is independent of the tube current. Consequently, regardless of what milliamperage (mA) station is selected, the efficiency of x-ray production remains constant.

The efficiency of x-ray production increases with increasing kVp. At 60 kVp, only 0.5% of the electron kinetic energy is converted to x-rays. At 100 kVp, approximately 1% is converted to x-rays, and at 20 MV, 70% is converted.

Characteristic Radiation

If the projectile electron interacts with an inner-shell electron of the target atom rather than with an outer-shell electron, **characteristic x-rays** can be produced. Characteristic x-rays result when the interaction is sufficiently violent to ionize the target atom by totally removing an inner-shell electron.

 Characteristic x-rays are emitted when an outer-shell electron fills an inner-shell void.

Figure 11-3 illustrates how characteristic x-rays are produced. When the projectile electron ionizes a target atom by removing a K-shell electron, a temporary electron void is produced in the K shell. This is a highly unnatural state for the target atom and is corrected by an outer-shell electron falling into the void in the K shell. The transition of an orbital electron from an outer to an inner shell is accompanied by the emission of an x-ray. The x-ray has energy equal to the difference in the binding energies of the orbital electrons involved.

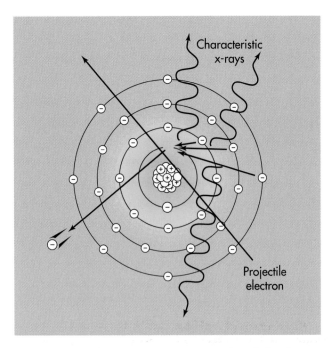

FIGURE 11-3 Characteristic x-rays are produced after the ionization of a K-shell electron. When an outer-shell electron fills the vacancy in the K shell, an x-ray is emitted.

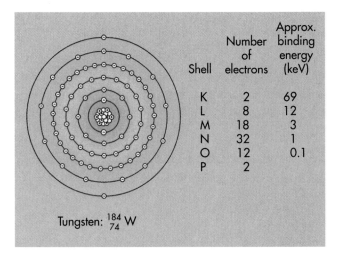

FIGURE 11-4 Atomic configuration and electron-binding energies for tungsten.

Question: A K-shell electron is removed from a tungsten atom and is replaced by an L-shell electron. What is the energy of the characteristic x-ray that is emitted?

Answer: Figure 11-4 shows that for tungsten, K-shell electrons have binding energies of 69 keV and L-shell electrons are bound by 12 keV. Therefore the characteristic x-ray emitted has energy of 69 − 12 = 57 keV

By the same procedure, the energy of x-rays resulting from M-to-K, N-to-K, O-to-K and P-to-K transitions can be calculated. Tungsten, for example, has electrons out to the P shell, and when a K-shell electron is ionized, its position can be filled with electrons from any of the outer-shells. All these x-rays are called *K x-rays* because they result from ionization of K-shell electrons.

Similar characteristic x-rays are produced when the target atom is ionized by the removal of electrons from shells other than K. Note that Figure 11-3 does not show the production of x-rays resulting from the ionization of an L-shell electron. Such a diagram would show the removal of an L-shell electron by the projectile electron. The vacancy in the L shell would be filled by an electron from any of the farther shells. X-rays resulting from electron transitions to the L shell are called *L x-rays* and are much less energetic than K x-rays, since the binding energy of an L-shell electron is much lower than that of a K-shell electron.

 Only the K-characteristic x-rays of tungsten are useful for making a diagnostic radiograph.

Similarly, M-characteristic x-rays, N-characteristic x-rays, and even O-characteristic x-rays can be produced in a tungsten target. Table 11-1 summarizes the production of characteristic x-rays in tungsten. Although many characteristic x-rays can be produced, it should be emphasized that they can be produced only at specific energies, equal to the differences in the electron binding energies for the various electron transitions. Except for K x-rays, all the characteristic x-rays have very low energy. The L x-rays with approximately 12 keV of energy penetrate only a few centimeters into soft tissue. Consequently, they are useless as diagnostic x-rays, as are all the other low-energy characteristic x-rays. The last column in Table 11-1 shows the effective energy for each characteristic x-ray of tungsten.

In summary, characteristic x-rays are produced by transitions of orbital electrons from outer to inner shells. Since the electron binding energy differs for every element, the energy of characteristic x-rays produced in the various elements also differs. This type of x-radiation is called *characteristic radiation* because it is characteristic of the target element. The effective energy of characteristic x-rays increases with increasing atomic number of the target element.

TABLE 11-1	Characteristic X-Rays of Tungsten and Their Effective Energies					
	ELECTRON TRANSITION FROM SHELL					**Effective Energy (keV)**
Characteristic X-Ray	**L**	**M**	**N**	**O**	**P**	
K	57.4	66.7	68.9	69.4	69.5	69
L		9.3	11.5	12.0	12.1	12
M			2.2	2.7	2.8	3
N				0.52	0.6	1
O					0.08	0.1

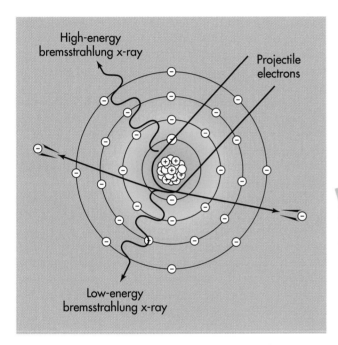

FIGURE 11-5 Bremsstrahlung x-rays result from an interaction between a projectile electron and a target nucleus. The electron is slowed, and its direction is changed.

Bremsstrahlung Radiation

The production of heat and characteristic x-rays involves interactions between the projectile electrons and the electrons of x-ray tube target atoms. A third type of interaction in which the projectile electron can lose its kinetic energy is an interaction with the nuclear field of a target atom. In this type of interaction, the kinetic energy of the projectile electron is also converted into electromagnetic energy.

A projectile electron that completely avoids the orbital electrons as it passes through a target atom may come sufficiently close to the nucleus of the atom to come under its influence (Figure 11-5). Since the electron is negatively charged and the nucleus is positively charged, there is an electrostatic force of attraction be-

tween them. The closer the projectile electron gets to the nucleus, the more it is influenced by the electric field of the nucleus. This field is very strong because the nucleus contains many protons and the distance between the nucleus and projectile electron is very small.

As the projectile electron passes by the nucleus, it is slowed, and it changes its course, leaving with reduced kinetic energy in a different direction. This loss in kinetic energy reappears as an x-ray. This interaction is somewhat analogous to a comet in its course around the sun.

 Bremsstrahlung x-rays are produced when a projectile electron is slowed by the electric field of a target atom nucleus.

These types of x-rays are called **bremsstrahlung x-rays**. *Bremsstrahlung* is a German word for "slowing down" or "braking." Bremsstrahlung radiation can be considered radiation resulting from the braking of projectile electrons by the nucleus.

A projectile electron can lose any amount of its kinetic energy in an interaction with the nucleus of a target atom, and the bremsstrahlung radiation associated with the loss can take on a corresponding range of values. For example, when an x-ray imaging system is operated at 70 kVp, projectile electrons have kinetic energies up to 70 keV. An electron with kinetic energy of 70 keV can lose all, none, or any intermediate level of that kinetic energy in a bremsstrahlung interaction. Therefore the bremsstrahlung x-ray produced can have any energy up to 70 keV.

This is different from the production of characteristic x-rays, which have very specific energies. Figure 11-5 illustrates the production of such a wide range of energies through the bremsstrahlung interaction. A low-energy bremsstrahlung x-ray results when the projectile electron is barely influenced by the nucleus. A maximum-energy x-ray occurs when the projectile electron loses all its kinetic energy and simply drifts away from the nucleus. Bremsstrahlung x-rays with energies between these two extremes occur more frequently.

In the diagnostic range, most x-rays are bremsstrahlung x-rays.

Bremsstrahlung x-rays can be produced at any projectile electron energy. K-characteristic x-rays require a tube potential of at least 70 kVp. At 65 kVp, for example, no useful characteristic x-rays are produced, and therefore the x-ray beam is all bremsstrahlung. At 100 kVp, approximately 15% of the x-ray beam is characteristic radiation, and the remaining percentage is bremsstrahlung.

X-RAY EMISSION SPECTRUM

Most people have seen or heard of pitching machines (the devices used by baseball teams for batting practice so that the pitchers do not get worn out). There are similar machines for automatically ejecting bowling balls, tennis balls, and even ping-pong balls.

Suppose there was a device that could eject all these types of balls at random at a rate of one per second. The most straightforward way to determine how often each type of ball was ejected on the average would be to catch each ball as it was ejected and then identify it and drop it into a basket; at the end of the observation period the total number of each type of ball could be counted.

Let us suppose that the results obtained for a 10-minute period are those shown in Figure 11-6. A total of 600 balls were ejected. Perhaps the easiest way to represent these results graphically would be to plot the total number of each type of ball emitted during the 10-minute period and represent each total by a bar (Figure 11-7).

Such a bar graph can be described as a discrete ball-ejection spectrum representative of the automatic pitching machine. It is a plot of the number of balls ejected per unit of time as a function of the type of ball. It is called *discrete* because only five distinct types of balls are involved. A discrete spectrum has only specific values of the variable considered.

Connecting the bars with a curve as shown would indicate a large number of different types of balls. Such a curve is called a *continuous ejection spectrum*. The word *spectrum* refers to the range of types of balls or values of any quantity such as x-rays. The total number of balls ejected is represented by the sum of the areas under the bars, in the case of the discrete spectrum and the area under the curve, in the case of the continuous spectrum. A continuous spectrum has all possible values of the variable considered.

Without regard to the absolute number of balls emitted, Figure 11-7 could also be identified as a *relative ball-ejection spectrum*, since at a glance you can tell the relative frequency with which each type of ball was ejected. Relatively speaking, baseballs are ejected most frequently and basketballs least frequently.

This type of relationship is fundamental to describing the output of an x-ray tube. If you could stand in the middle of the useful x-ray beam, catch each x-ray and measure its energy, you could describe what is known as the *x-ray emission spectrum* (Figure 11-8), in which the relative number of x-rays emitted is plotted as a function of the energy of each x-ray. X-ray energy is the variable considered.

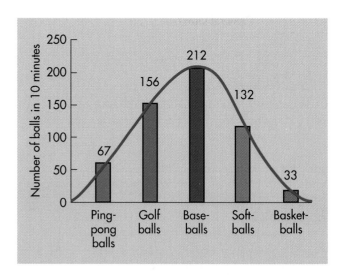

FIGURE 11-6 In a 10-minute period an automatic ball-throwing machine might eject 600 balls, distributed as shown.

FIGURE 11-7 Bar graph representing the results of the 10-minute observation of balls ejected by the automatic pitching machine in Figure 11-6. When the height of each bar is joined, a smooth emission spectrum is created.

Although we cannot catch and identify each individual x-ray, there are instruments that allow us to do essentially that. X-ray emission spectra have been measured for all types of x-ray imaging systems. Understanding x-ray emission spectra is a key to understanding how changes in kVp, mA, exposure time, and added filtration affect the optical density (OD) and contrast of an image.

Characteristic X-Ray Spectrum

The discrete energies of characteristic x-rays are characteristic of the differences between electron binding energies of a particular element. A characteristic x-ray from tungsten, for example, can have 1 of 15 different energies (Table 11-1) and no others. A plot of the frequency with which characteristic x-rays are emitted as a function of their energy would look like that shown for tungsten in Figure 11-9. Such a plot is called the *characteristic x-ray emission spectrum*. Five vertical lines represent K x-rays, and four vertical lines represent L x-rays. The other lower-energy lines represent characteristic emissions from the outer electron shells.

Characteristic x-rays have precisely fixed or discrete energies and form a discrete emission spectrum.

The relative intensity of the K x-rays is greater than that of the lower-energy characteristic x-rays because of the nature of the interaction process. K x-rays are the only characteristic x-rays of tungsten with sufficient energy to be of value in diagnostic radiology. Although there are five K x-rays, it is customary to represent them as one, as has been done with a single vertical line at 69 keV in Figure 11-8. Only this line will be shown in later graphs.

Bremsstrahlung X-Ray Spectrum

If it were possible to measure the energy contained in each bremsstrahlung photon emitted from an x-ray tube, you would find that these energies range from the peak electron energy all the way down to zero. In other words, when an x-ray tube is operated at 90 kVp, bremsstrahlung x-rays with energies up to 90 keV are emitted. A typical bremsstrahlung x-ray emission spectrum is shown in Figure 11-10.

Bremsstrahlung x-rays have a range of energies and form a continuous emission spectrum.

Question: At what kVp was the x-ray imaging system presented in Figure 11-10 operated?

Answer: Since the bremsstrahlung spectrum intersects the energy axis at approximately 90 keV, the imaging system must have been operated at approximately 90 kVp.

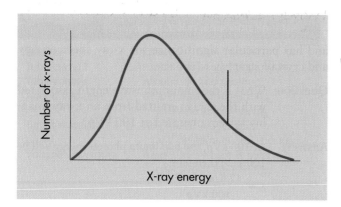

FIGURE 11-8 General form of an x-ray emission spectrum.

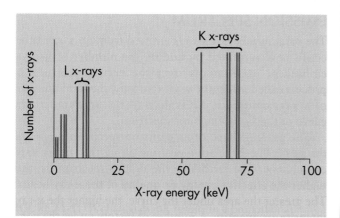

FIGURE 11-9 The characteristic x-ray emission spectrum for tungsten contains 15 x-ray energies.

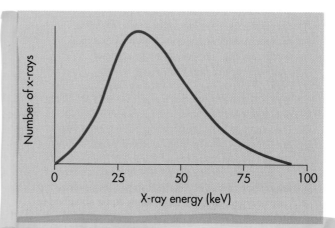

FIGURE 11-10 Bremsstrahlung x-ray emission spectrum extends from zero to maximum projectile electron energy, with the highest number of x-rays having approximately one third the maximum energy.

CHAPTER

12

X-Ray Emission

OBJECTIVES

At the completion of this chapter, the student should be able to:

1. Define *radiation quantity* and its relation to intensity
2. List and discuss the factors affecting the intensity of the x-ray beam
3. Explain x-ray quality and penetrability
4. List and discuss the factors affecting the quality of the x-ray beam

OUTLINE

The x-rays that are emitted through a window in the glass or metal envelope form a beam of varied energies. The x-ray beam is characterized by quantity (the number of x-rays in the beam) and quality (the penetrability of the beam). This chapter discusses the numerous factors that affect x-ray beam quantity and quality.

X-RAY QUANTITY
Output Intensity

The output intensity of an x-ray imaging system is measured in roentgen (R or mGy_a) or milliroentgen (mR) and is termed the **x-ray quantity,** the number of x-rays in the useful beam. Another term, **radiation exposure,** is often used instead of *x-ray intensity* or *x-ray quantity.* All have the same meaning and all are measured in roentgens.

The roentgen (mGy_a) is a measure of the number of ion pairs produced in air by a quantity of x-rays. Ionization of air increases as the number of x-rays in the beam increases. The relationship between the x-ray quantity as measured in roentgens and the number of x-rays in the beam is not always one to one. There are some small variations related to the effective x-ray energy.

Radiation Quantity
X-ray quantity is the number of x-rays in the useful beam.

These variations are unimportant over the x-ray energy range used in radiology, and we can therefore assume that the number of x-rays in the useful beam is the radiation quantity. Most general-purpose radiographic tubes, when operated at 70 kilovolt peak (kVp), produce x-ray intensities of approximately 5 mR/mAs (50 μGy_a) when the source-to-image receptor distance (SID) is 100 cm. Figure 12-1 is a nomogram for estimating x-ray intensity for a wide range of techniques. These curves apply only for single-phase, full-wave-rectified imaging systems.

Factors Affecting X-Ray Quantity

A number of factors affect x-ray quantity. Most are discussed briefly in Chapter 11, so this section is primarily a review. The factors affecting x-ray quantity are nearly the same as those controlling optical density (OD) on a radiograph. These relationships are summarized in Table 12-1.

mAs. X-ray quantity is directly proportional to the mAs. When mAs is doubled, the number of electrons striking the tube target is doubled, and therefore the number of x-rays emitted is doubled.

$$\frac{I_1}{I_2} = \frac{mAs_1}{mAs_2}$$

where I_1 and I_2 are the x-ray quantities at mAs_1 and mAs_2, respectively.

TABLE 12-1	Factors Affecting X-Ray Quantity and Radiographic OD	
Increase	**X-Ray Quantity**	**Radiographic OD**
mAs	Increases proportionately	Increases
kVp	Increases by $\left(\dfrac{kVp_2}{kVp_1}\right)^2$	Increases
Distance	Reduces by $\left(\dfrac{d_1}{d_2}\right)^2$	Reduces
Filtration	Reduces	Reduces

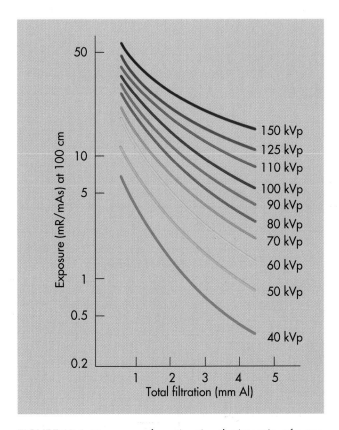

FIGURE 12-1 Nomogram for estimating the intensity of x-ray beams. From the position on the x-axis corresponding to the filtration of the machine, draw a vertical line until it intersects with the appropriate kVp. A horizontal line from that point will intersect the y-axis at the approximate x-ray intensity for the imaging system. *(Courtesy Edward McCullough.)*

Question: A lateral chest technique calls for 110 kVp and 10 mAs, which results in an x-ray intensity of 32 mR (0.32 mGy$_a$) at the position of the patient. If the mAs is increased to 20 mAs, what will the x-ray intensity be?

Answer:
$$\frac{x}{32 \text{ mR}} = \frac{20 \text{ mAs}}{10 \text{ mAs}}$$
$$x = \frac{(32 \text{ mAs})(20 \text{ mR})}{10 \text{ mAs}}$$
$$= 64 \text{ mR}$$

 X-ray quantity is proportional to mAs.

Question: The radiographic technique for a KUB (kidneys, ureters, and bladder) examination is 74 kVp and 60 mAs. The result is a patient exposure of 248 mR (2.5 mGy$_a$). What will the exposure be if the mAs can be reduced to 45 mAs?

Answer:
$$\frac{x}{248 \text{ mR}} = \frac{45 \text{ mAs}}{60 \text{ mAs}}$$
$$x = \frac{(248 \text{ mAs})(45 \text{ mR})}{60 \text{ mAs}}$$
$$= 186 \text{ mR}$$

Question: A radiograph is made at 74 kVp/100 mAs. How many electrons interact with the target?

Answer: 100 mAs = 100 mC
$$= 6.25 \times 10^{17} \text{ electrons}$$

mAs = mA × s
= mC/s × s
= mC, or the total number of electrons per exposure

Question: If the radiographic output intensity is 6.2 mR/mAs (62 μGy$_a$/mAs). How many electrons are required to produce 1.0 mR?

Answer: 6.2 mR/mAs = 6.2 mR/6.25 × 10^{15} electrons
Stated inversely: 6.25 × 10^{15} electrons/6.2 mR = 1 × 10^{15} electrons/mR

kVp. X-ray quantity varies rapidly with changes in kVp. The change in x-ray quantity is proportional to the square of the ratio of the kVp; in other words, if kVp is doubled, the x-ray intensity increases by a factor of four. Mathematically, this is expressed as follows:

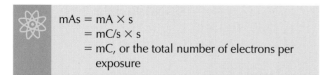

X-Ray Quantity and kVp
$$\frac{I_1}{I_2} = \left(\frac{kVp_1}{kVp_2}\right)^2$$
where I_1 and I_2 are the x-ray intensities at kVp$_1$ and kVp$_2$, respectively.

Question: A lateral chest technique calls for 110 kVp (kVp$_1$) and 10 mAs and results in an x-ray intensity of 32 mR (0.32 mGy$_a$) (I_1). What will the intensity (I_2) be if the kVp is increased to 125 (kVp$_2$) and the mAs remains fixed?

Answer:
$$\frac{32 \text{ mR}}{I_2} = \left(\frac{110 \text{ kVp}}{125 \text{ kVp}}\right)^2$$
$$I_2 = (32 \text{ mR})\left(\frac{125 \text{ kVp}}{110 \text{ kVp}}\right)^2$$
$$= (32 \text{ mR})(1.14)^2$$
$$= (32 \text{ mR})(1.29)$$
$$= 41.3 \text{ mR}$$

 X-ray quantity is proportional to kVp^2.

Question: An extremity is examined with a technique of 58 kVp and 8 mAs, resulting in an entrance skin exposure of 24 mR. If the technique is changed to 54 kVp and 8 mAs to improve contrast, what will the x-ray quantity be?

Answer:
$$\frac{I}{24 \text{ mR}} = \left(\frac{54 \text{ kVp}}{58 \text{ kVp}}\right)^2$$
$$I = 24 \text{ mR}\left(\frac{54 \text{ kVp}}{58 \text{ kVp}}\right)^2$$
$$= (24 \text{ mR})(0.93)^2$$
$$= (24 \text{ mR})(0.867)$$
$$= 20.8 \text{ mR}$$

In practice, a different situation prevails. Radiographic technique factors must be selected from a relatively narrow range of values: about 40 to 150 kVp. Theoretically, doubling the x-ray intensity by kVp manipulation alone would require an increase of 40% in kVp.

This relationship is not adopted clinically because as kVp is increased, the penetrability of the x-ray beam is increased and relatively fewer x-rays are absorbed in the patient. More x-rays go through the patient and interact with the image receptor. Consequently, maintaining a constant exposure of the image receptor and constant average OD would require an increase of 15% in kVp accompanied by a reduction of one-half in mAs.

Question: A radiographic technique calls for 80 kVp and 30 mAs and results in 135 mR (1.4 mGy$_a$). What is the expected entrance skin exposure if the kVp is increased to 92 kVp (+15%) and the mAs reduced by one-half to 15 mAs?

Answer:
$$\frac{I}{135 \text{ mR}} = \left(\frac{15 \text{ mAs}}{30 \text{ mAs}}\right)\left(\frac{92 \text{ kVp}}{80 \text{ kVp}}\right)^2$$
$$I = 135 \text{ mR}\left(\frac{15 \text{ mAs}}{30 \text{ mAs}}\right)\left(\frac{92 \text{ kVp}}{80 \text{ kVp}}\right)^2$$
$$= 135 \text{ mR}(0.5)(1.32)$$
$$= 89 \text{ mR}$$

Note that when the kVp is increased and the mAs is reduced, OD remains constant, and patient dose is significantly reduced. The disadvantage to such a technique adjustment is reduced image contrast.

Distance. X-ray quantity varies inversely with the square of the distance from the x-ray tube target. This relationship is known as the *inverse square law* (see Chapter 5).

X-Ray Quantity and Distance
$$\frac{I_1}{I_2} = \left(\frac{d_2}{d_1}\right)^2$$
where I_1 and I_2 are the x-ray quantities at distances d_1 and d_2, respectively.

Question: A portable radiograph is normally conducted at an SID of 100 cm (d_1) and results in an exposure of 12.5 mR (0.13 mGy$_a$) (I_1) at the image receptor. If 91 cm (d_2) is the maximum SID that can be obtained for a particular situation, what will be the image receptor exposure (I_2)?

Answer:
$$\frac{1.25 \text{ mR}}{I_2} = \left(\frac{91 \text{ cm}}{100 \text{ cm}}\right)^2$$
$$I_2 = (12.5 \text{ mR})\left(\frac{100 \text{ cm}}{91 \text{ cm}}\right)^2$$
$$= (12.5 \text{ mR})(1.1)^2$$
$$= (1.25 \text{ mR})(1.21)$$
$$= 15.1 \text{ mR}$$

X-ray quantity is inversely proportional to the square of the distance from the source.

Question: A posterior-anterior chest examination (120 kVp and 3 mAs) with a dedicated x-ray imaging system is taken at an SID of 300 cm (10 ft). The exposure at the image receptor is 12 mR (0.12 mGy$_a$). If the same technique is used at a SID of 100 cm, what will the x-ray quantity be?

Answer:
$$\frac{1}{12 \text{ mR}} = \left(\frac{300 \text{ cm}}{100 \text{ cm}}\right)^2$$
$$I = 12 \text{ mR}\left(\frac{300 \text{ cm}}{100 \text{ cm}}\right)^2$$
$$= (12 \text{ mR})(3)^2$$
$$= (12 \text{ mR})(9)$$
$$= 108 \text{ mR}$$

The Square Law
When the SID is increased, the mAs must be increased by SID^2 to maintain constant OD.

Compensating for a change in SID by changing the mAs by the factor SID^2 is known as the **square law**, a corollary to the inverse square law.

Question: What would the new mAs be in the previous question to reduce the x-ray quantity to 12 mR at 100 cm?

Answer:
$$\frac{x \text{ mAs}}{3 \text{ mAs}} = \frac{12 \text{ mR}}{108 \text{ mR}}$$
$$x \text{ mAs} = (3 \text{ mAs})\left(\frac{12 \text{ mR}}{108 \text{ mR}}\right)$$
$$= (3 \text{ mAs})(0.111)$$
$$= 0.3 \text{ mAs}$$

Filtration. X-ray imaging systems have metal filters, usually 1 to 3 mm of aluminum (Al), positioned in the useful beam. These filters reduce the number of low-energy x-rays that reach the patient. Low-energy x-rays contribute nothing useful to the image. They only increase patient dose unnecessarily because they are absorbed in superficial tissues and do not penetrate to reach the image receptor.

Adding filtration to the useful x-ray beam reduces patient dose.

When filtration is inserted in the x-ray beam, the patient dose is reduced because there are fewer low-energy x-rays in the useful beam. Calculation of the amount of reduction in exposure requires a knowledge of half-value layer (HVL), which is discussed in the following section.

An estimate of exposure reduction can be made from the nomogram in Figure 12-1, where it is shown that the reduction is not proportional to the thickness of added filter but is related in a complex way. The disadvantage to x-ray beam filtration is reduced image contrast resulting from beam hardening.

X-RAY QUALITY
Penetrability

As the energy of an x-ray beam is increased, the penetrability is also increased. **Penetrability** refers to the range of x-rays in tissue. High-energy x-rays are able to penetrate to deeper tissue than low-energy x-rays. The penetrability of an x-ray beam is called the **x-ray quality.** X-rays with high penetrability are of high quality and are termed **hard x-rays.** Those with low penetrability are of low quality and are called **soft x-rays.**

Penetrability
Penetrability is the ability of an x-ray to pass through tissue.

X-ray quality is identified numerically by the HVL. The HVL is affected by the kVp and the added filtration in the useful beam. Therefore x-ray quality is also influenced by kVp and filtration. Factors that affect beam quality also influence radiographic contrast. Distance and mAs do not affect radiation quality; they do affect radiation quantity.

Half-Value Layer

Attenuation is the reduction in x-ray intensity because of x-ray absorption and scattering. Although x-rays are attenuated exponentially, high-energy x-rays are more penetrating than low-energy x-rays. Whereas 100-keV x-rays are attenuated at only the rate of approximately 3% per centimeter of soft tissue, 10-keV x-rays are attenuated at approximately 15% per centimeter. X-rays of any given energy are more penetrating in material of low atomic number than in material of high atomic number.

Attenuation
Attenuation is the reduction in x-ray intensity resulting from absorption and scattering.

In radiography the quality of x-rays is measured by the HVL, which is the thickness of absorbing material necessary to reduce x-ray intensity by half. The HVL is therefore a characteristic of the useful x-ray beam. A diagnostic x-ray beam usually has an HVL in the range of 3 to 5 mm of Al or 3 to 6 cm of soft tissue.

Half-Value Layer
The HVL of an x-ray beam is the thickness of absorbing material necessary to reduce the x-ray intensity to half of its original value.

HVL is determined experimentally using a setup similar to that shown in Figure 12-2. There are three principal parts to this setup: the x-ray tube, a radiation detector, and graded thicknesses of filters, usually aluminum. First, a radiation measurement is made with no filter be-tween the x-ray tube and the detector. Then measurements of radiation intensity are made for successively thicker sections of filter. The thickness of filtration that reduces the x-ray intensity to half of its original value is the HVL.

A number of methods can be used to determine the HVL of an x-ray beam. Perhaps the most straightforward is to graph the results of x-ray intensity measurements made with an experimental setup like that in Figure 12-2. Figure 12-3 and Box 12-1 shows how this can be done when certain steps are completed. Sample numerical values are also shown in the figure.

BOX 12-1   Steps to Determine the HVL

1. Determine the x-ray quantity with no absorbing material in the beam and with known thicknesses of absorber.
2. Plot the ordered pairs of data (thickness of absorber, x-ray quantity).
3. Determine the x-ray quantity equal to half the original quantity and locate this value on the y-axis (vertical axis) of the graph (A).
4. Draw a horizontal line parallel with the x-axis from the point A in Step 3 until it intersects the curve (B).
5. From point B, drop a vertical line to the x-axis.
6. On the x-axis, read the thickness of absorber required to reduce the x-ray intensity to half of its original value point (C). This is the HVL.

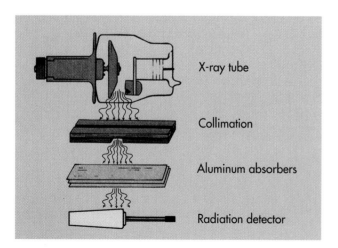

FIGURE 12-2 Typical experimental arrangement for the determination of the HVL.

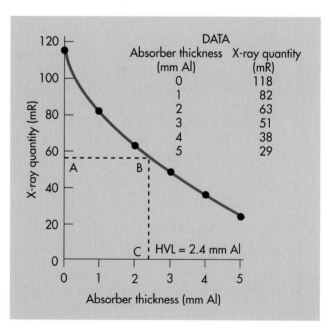

FIGURE 12-3 Data in the table are typical for HVL determination. The plot of these data shows an HVL of 2.4 mm of Al.

Question: The data from Figure 12-3 are obtained with the radiographic tube operated at 70 kVp while the detector is positioned 100 cm from the target with 1.0-mm Al filters inserted halfway between the target and the detector. Estimate the HVL from a simple observation of this data. Then plot the data to see how close you were.

Answer: Half of 118 is 59, and therefore the HVL must be between 2 and 3 mm of Al. A plot of the data shows the HVL to be 2.4 mm of Al.

 HVL is the most accurate method for specifying x-ray quality.

Question: The following graph was plotted from measurements designed to estimate HVL. What does this graph suggest the HVL to be?

Answer: At zero filtration, x-ray quantity appears to be 190 mR. Half of 190 mR is 95 mR. At the level of 95 mR, a horizontal line is drawn on the graph until it intersects the plotted curve. From that intersection a vertical line is dropped to the x-axis where it intersects at 2.8 mm of Al, the HVL.

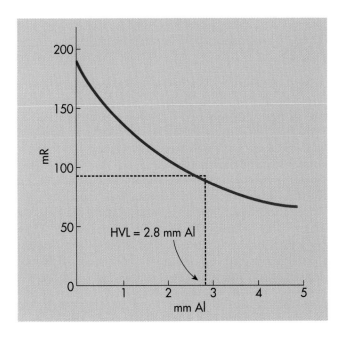

X-ray beam penetrability changes in a complex way with variations in kVp and filtration. Different combinations of added filtration and kVp can result in the same HVL for an x-ray beam. For example, measurements may show that a single x-ray imaging system has the same HVL when operated at 90 kVp with 2 mm of Al total filtration as when operated at 70 kVp with 5 mm of Al total filtration. In this case, x-ray penetrability remains constant, as does the HVL. X-ray beam quality can be identified by either kVp or filtration, but HVL is most accurate.

Factors Affecting X-Ray Quality

Many of the factors that affect x-ray quantity and radiographic OD have no effect on x-ray quality. These relationships are summarized in Table 12-2.

kVp. As the kVp is increased, so is x-ray beam quality and therefore the HVL. As discussed in Chapter 11, an increase in the kVp results in a shift of the x-ray emission spectrum toward the high-energy side, which increases the effective energy of the beam. The result is a more penetrating x-ray beam.

 Increasing the kVp increases the quality of an x-ray beam.

Table 12-3 shows the measured change in HVL as the kVp is increased from 50 to 150 kVp for a representative x-ray imaging system. The total filtration of the beam is 2.5 mm of Al.

Filtration. The primary purpose of adding filtration to an x-ray beam is to increase the quality of an x-ray beam by selectively removing low-energy x-rays that have no chance of getting to the image receptor. Figure 12-4 shows x-ray emission spectra with unfiltered and normally filtered x-ray beams.

The ideally filtered x-ray beam would be monoenergetic, or single energy. To reduce patient dose, it is desir-

TABLE 12-2	Factors Affecting X-Ray Quality and Quantity	
		EFFECT
Increase	**X-Ray Quality**	**X-Ray Quantity**
mAs	None	Increase
kVp	Increase	Increase
Distance	None	Reduce
Filtration	Increase	Reduce

TABLE 12-3	Relationship Between kVp and HVL
kVp	**HVL (mm Al)**
50	1.9
75	2.8
100	3.7
125	4.6
150	5.4

*For fixed radiographic imaging system having 2.5 mm of Al total filtration.

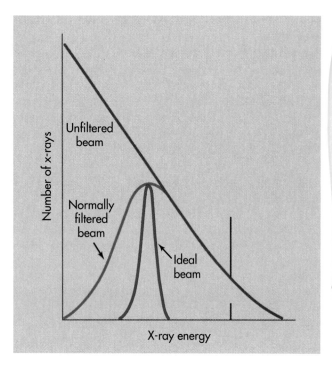

FIGURE 12-4 Filtration is used to selectively remove low-energy x-rays from the useful beam. Ideal filtration would remove all low-energy x-rays and create a more monoenergetic beam.

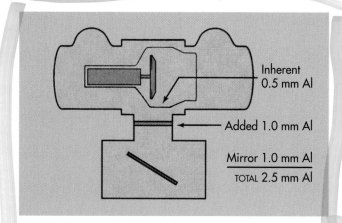

FIGURE 12-5 Total filtration consists of the inherent filtration of the x-ray tube, an added filter, and filtration by the mirror of the light-localizing collimator.

able to totally remove all x-rays below a certain energy determined by the type of x-ray examination. To improve image contrast, it is also desirable to remove x-rays with energies above a certain level. Unfortunately, such removal of regions of an x-ray beam is not normally possible.

Almost any material could serve as an x-ray filter. Aluminum (Z = 13) is chosen because it is efficient in removing low-energy x-rays through photoelectric effect and because it is readily available, inexpensive, and easily shaped. Copper (Z = 29), tin (Z = 50), gadolinium (Z = 64), and holmium (Z = 67) have been used sparingly in special situations. As filtration is increased, so is beam quality, but quantity is decreased.

 Increasing filtration increases the quality of an x-ray beam.

Filtration of diagnostic x-ray beams has two components: inherent and added. The glass or metal window of an x-ray tube filters the emitted x-ray beam. This type of filtration is called **inherent filtration** because it is an inherent, or already existing, kind of filtration. Inspection of an x-ray tube reveals that the part of the glass or metal envelope through which x-rays are emitted—the window—is very thin, and this provides for low inherent filtration.

The inherent filtration of a general-purpose x-ray tube is approximately 0.5 mm of Al equivalent. With age, in-

herent filtration tends to increase as some of the tungsten of both target and filament is vaporized and deposited on the inside of the window.

Special-purpose tubes, such as those used in mammography, have very thin x-ray tube windows. They are sometimes made of beryllium (Z = 4) rather than glass and have inherent filtration of approximately 0.1 mm of Al. Added filtration usually consists of a thin sheet of aluminum positioned between the protective x-ray tube housing and the x-ray beam collimator.

 Added filtration results in increased HVL.

The addition of a filter to an x-ray beam attenuates x-rays of all energies emitted, but it attenuates more low-energy than high-energy x-rays. This shifts the x-ray emission spectrum to the high-energy side, resulting in an x-ray beam with higher effective energy, greater penetrability, and higher quality. HVL increases, but the extent of increase in the HVL cannot be predicted even when the thickness of added filtration is known.

Because added filtration attenuates the x-ray beam, it affects x-ray quantity. This value can be predicted if the HVL of the beam is known. The addition of filtration equal to the beam HVL reduces the beam quantity to half its prefiltered value and results in a *harder* x-ray beam.

Question: A general-purpose x-ray imaging system has an HVL of 2.2 mm of Al. The exposure from this imager is 2 mR/mAs (20 μGy_a/mAs) at 100 cm SID. If 2.2 mm of Al is added to the beam, what will be the x-ray exposure?

Answer: This is an addition of one HVL; therefore the x-ray exposure will be 1 mR/mAs (10 μGy_a/mAs).

Added filtration usually has two sources and totals 2 and 3 mm of Al equivalent. First, 1- or 2-mm sheets of

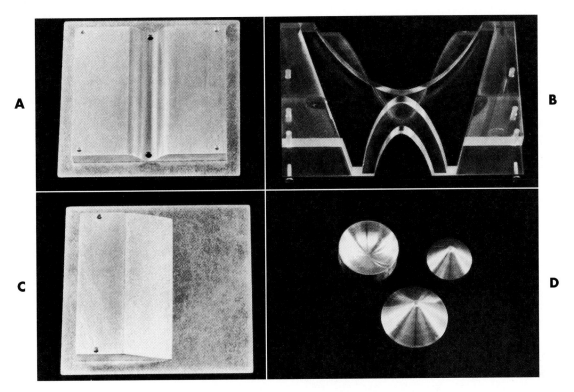

FIGURE 12-6 Compensating filters. **A,** Trough filter. **B,** "Bow-tie" filter for use in computed tomography. **C,** Wedge filter. **D,** Conic filters for use in digital fluoroscopy.

aluminum will be permanently installed in the port of the x-ray tube housing, between the housing and the collimator.

If the collimator is a conventional light-localizing, variable-aperture collimator, it will contribute an additional 1 mm of Al equivalent added filtration. This filtration results from the silver surface of the mirror in the collimator (Figure 12-5). One of the most difficult tasks facing the radiographic technologist is producing an image with a uniform OD when examining a body part that varies greatly in thickness or tissue composition.

When a filter is used in this fashion, it is called a *compensating filter* because it compensates for differences in subject radiopacity. Compensating filters can be fabricated for many procedures and therefore come in various sizes and shapes. They are nearly always constructed of aluminum, but plastic materials can also be used. Figure 12-6 shows some common compensating filters.

During posterior-anterior chest radiography, for instance, if the left chest is relatively radiopaque because of fluid, consolidation, or a mass, the image would appear with very low OD on the left side of the chest and very high OD on the right side. You could compensate for this variation by inserting a wedge filter so that the thin part of the wedge is positioned over the left side of the chest.

The wedge filter is used principally when radiographing a body part, such as the foot, that varies consider-

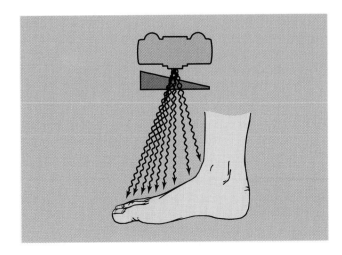

FIGURE 12-7 Use of a wedge filter for an examination of the foot.

ably in thickness (Figure 12-7). During an anterior-posterior projection of the foot, the wedge would be positioned with its thick portion shadowing the toes and the thin portion toward the heel.

A bilateral wedge filter, or trough filter, is sometimes used in chest radiography (Figure 12-8). The thin central region of the wedge is positioned over the mediastinum, and the lateral thick portions shadow the lung fields. The result is a radiograph with more uniform OD.

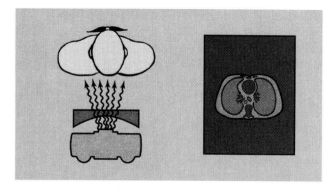

FIGURE 12-8 Use of a trough filter for examination of the chest.

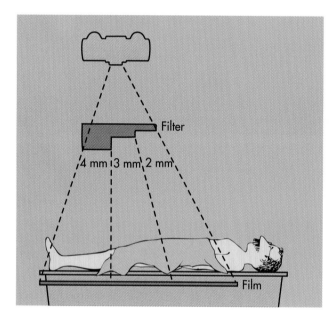

FIGURE 12-9 Arrangement of apparatus using an aluminum step-wedge for serial radiography of the abdomen and lower extremities.

Specialty compensating wedges of this type are generally utilized with dedicated apparatus, such as an x-ray imaging system used exclusively for chest radiography.

Special bow-tie–shaped filters are used with some computed tomographic units to compensate for the shape of the head or body. Conic filters, either concave or convex, find application in digital fluoroscopy, where the image receptor, the image intensifier tube, is round.

A step-wedge filter is an adaptation of the wedge filter (Figure 12-9). It is used in some special procedures, usually where long sections of the anatomy are imaged with two or three separate image receptors. A common application of this technique uses a three-step aluminum wedge and three 14 × 17 in (30 × 36 cm) films in a rapid change for translumbar and femoral arteriography and venography. These procedures call for careful selection of screens, grids, and radiographic technique.

Compensating filters are useful in maintaining image quality. They are not radiation protection devices.

SUMMARY

Radiation quantity is the number of x-rays in the useful beam. The factors affecting x-ray quantity are as follows:
1. mAs: X-ray quantity is directly proportional to mAs.
2. kVp: X-ray quantity is proportional to the square of the kVp.
3. Distance: X-ray quantity varies inversely with distance from the source.
4. Filtration: X-ray quantity is reduced by filtration.

Radiation quality is the penetrating power of the x-ray beam. The penetrability is quantified by the HVL, which is the thickness of additional filtration that reduces x-ray intensity to half its original value. The factors affecting beam penetrability or radiation quality follow:
1. kVp: X-ray penetrability is increased as kVp is increased.
2. Filtration: X-ray penetrability is increased when filtration is added to the beam.

The following are the three types of filtration: (1) inherent filtration of the glass or metal x-ray tube window, (2) added filtration in the form of aluminum sheets, and (3) compensating filters, which provide variation in intensity across the x-ray beam.

CHALLENGE QUESTIONS

1. Define or otherwise identify:
   a. Inherent filtration
   b. The unit of x-ray quantity
   c. A filtered x-ray spectrum
   d. A kVp change equal to twice the mAs
   e. Half-value layer
   f. Wedge filter
   g. The unit of x-ray quality
   h. The approximate HVL of your x-ray imaging system
   i. X-ray intensity

2. Describe the change in HVL with changing kVp (from 50 to 150 kVp) for an x-ray imaging system that has a total filtration of 2.5 mm of Al. Check your answer by plotting the data in Table 12-3.

3. An abdominal radiograph taken at 84 kVp and 150 mAs results in an exposure of 650 mR. The image is too light and is repeated at 84 kVp and 250 mAs. What is the exposure?

4. An image of the lateral skull taken at 68 kVp and 200 mAs has sufficient OD but too much contrast. If the kVp is increased to 78, what should be the new mAs?

5. A chest radiograph taken at an SID of 180 cm results in an exposure of 12 mR. What would the exposure be if the same radiographic factors were used at an SID of 100 cm?

6. The following data were obtained with a fluoroscopic x-ray tube operated at 80 kVp. The exposure levels were measured 50 cm above the tabletop with aluminum absorbers positioned on the surface. Estimate the HVL by visually inspecting the data; then plot the data and determine the precise value of the HVL.

Added Al (mm)	mR
0	65
1	48
3	30
5	21
7	16
9	13

7. When operated at 74 kVp and 100 mAs with 2.2 mm of Al added filtration and 0.6 mm of Al inherent filtration, the HVL of an x-ray imaging system is 3.2 mm of Al, and its output intensity at an SID of 100 cm is 350 mR. How much additional filtration is necessary to reduce the x-ray intensity to 175 mR?

8. The following technique produces good-quality radiographs of the cervical spine with an x-ray imaging system having 3 mm of Al total filtration. Refer to Figure 12-1 and estimate the x-ray intensity at an SID of 100 cm for each.
   a. 62 kVp, 70 mAs
   b. 70 kVp, 40 mAs
   c. 78 kVp, 27 mAs

9. A radiographic exposure is 80 kVp at 50 mAs. How many electrons will interact with the target?

10. An extremity is radiographed at 60 kVp and 10 mAs, resulting in an x-ray intensity of 28 mR. If the technique is changed to 55 kVp and 10 mAs, what is the resulting x-ray intensity?

11. State the inverse square law.

12. What is the primary purpose of x-ray beam filtration?

13. The kVp is reduced from 78 to 68 kVp. What, if anything, should be done with mAs?

14. What is the relationship between x-ray quantity and mAs?

15. What is the square law and how is it used?

16. List the two ways an x-ray beam can be shifted to a higher average energy.

17. Why is aluminum used for x-ray beam filtration?

18. Describe the use of a wedge filter when x-raying a foot.

19. Does adding filtration to the x-ray beam affect the quantity of x-rays reaching the film?

20. Fill in the following chart:

Increase	Effect on X-Ray Quality	Effect on OD
mAs		
kVp		
Distance		
Filtration		

X-Ray Interaction with Matter

OBJECTIVES

At the completion of this chapter, the student should be able to:

1. Describe each of the five x-ray interactions with matter
2. Define *differential absorption* and its effect on image contrast
3. Explain the effect of atomic number and mass density of tissue on differential absorption
4. Discuss why radiologic contrast agents are used to image some tissues and organs
5. Explain the difference between absorption and attenuation

OUTLINE

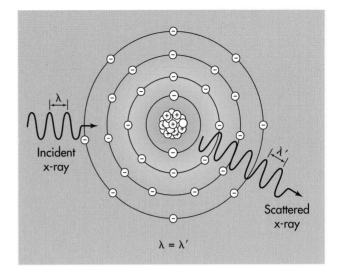

FIGURE 13-1 Coherent scattering is an interaction between low-energy x-rays and atoms. The x-ray loses no energy but changes direction slightly. The wavelength of the incident x-ray is equal to the wavelength of the scattered x-ray.

FIVE X-RAY INTERACTIONS WITH MATTER

In Chapter 5, the interaction between electromagnetic radiation and matter was described briefly. The interaction was said to have wavelike and particle-like properties. Basically, electromagnetic radiation interacts with structures similar in size to the wavelength of the radiation.

X-rays have very short wavelengths, no larger than approximately 10^{-8} to 10^{-9} m. The higher the energy of an x-ray, the shorter its wavelength. Consequently, low-energy x-rays tend to interact with whole atoms, which have diameters of approximately 10^{-9} to 10^{-10} m; moderate-energy x-rays generally interact with electrons, and high-energy x-rays generally interact with nuclei.

There are five mechanisms by which x-rays interact at these various structural levels: coherent scattering, Compton effect, photoelectric effect, pair production, and photodisintegration. Two of these—Compton effect and photoelectric effect—are of particular importance to diagnostic radiology and are discussed in some detail.

Coherent Scattering

X-rays with low energies (that is, those below approximately 10 keV) interact with matter by coherent scattering. Coherent scattering is also called *classical* or *Thomson scattering*, the latter after J.J. Thomson, the first person to describe the interaction between a low-energy x-ray and an electron.

Coherent scattering describes what happens when an incident x-ray interacts with a target atom (Figure 13-1). The target atom becomes excited and releases its excess energy as a scattered x-ray. The incident x-ray and the scattered x-ray have equal wavelength ($\lambda = \lambda'$) and therefore equal energy. However, the direction of the scattered x-ray is different from that of the incident x-ray.

Thus the result of coherent scattering is a change in the direction of the x-ray without a change in its energy. There is no energy transfer and therefore no ionization. Most coherently scattered x-rays are scattered in the forward direction.

Coherent scattering primarily involves low energy x-rays, which contribute little to the image. Therefore,

coherent scattering is generally of little importance to diagnostic imaging. Some coherent scattering, however, occurs within the diagnostic range. At 70 kVp, approximately 5% of x-rays undergo coherent scattering, which contributes slightly to **fog**, which is a general graying of a radiograph that reduces image contrast.

Compton Effect

Moderate-energy x-rays (that is, those throughout the diagnostic range) can undergo an interaction with outer-shell electrons that not only scatters the x-ray but also reduces its energy and ionizes the atom. This interaction is called the **Compton effect** or **Compton scattering** (Figure 13-2).

In the Compton effect, the incident x-ray interacts with an outer-shell electron and ejects it from the atom, ionizing the atom. The ejected electron is called a **Compton electron** or a **secondary electron**. The x-ray continues in a different direction with less energy. The energy of the Compton-scattered x-ray is equal to the difference between the energy of the incident x-ray and the energy of the ejected electron. The energy of the ejected electron is equal to its binding energy plus the kinetic energy with which it leaves the atom. Mathematically, this energy transfer is represented as follows:

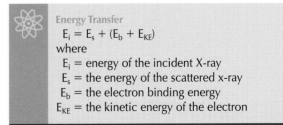

Energy Transfer
$$E_i = E_s + (E_b + E_{KE})$$
where
E_i = energy of the incident X-ray
E_s = the energy of the scattered x-ray
E_b = the electron binding energy
E_{KE} = the kinetic energy of the electron

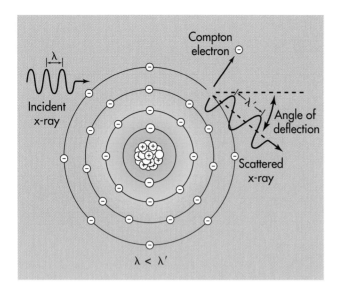

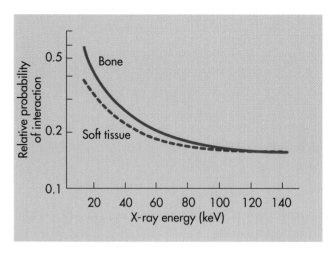

FIGURE 13-2 The Compton effect occurs between moderate-energy x-rays and outer-shell electrons. It results in ionization of the target atom, a change in x-ray direction, and a reduction of x-ray energy. The wavelength of the scattered x-ray is greater than that of the incident x-ray.

FIGURE 13-3 The probability that an x-ray will interact by the Compton effect is about the same for target atoms of soft tissue and bone. This probability decreases with increasing x-ray energy.

Question: A 30-keV x-ray ionizes an atom of barium by ejecting an O-shell electron with 12 keV of kinetic energy. What is the energy of the scattered x-ray?

Answer: Figure 4-9 shows that the binding energy of an O-shell electron of barium is 0.04 keV; therefore:

$$30 \text{ keV} = E_s + (0.04 \text{ keV} + 12 \text{ keV})$$
$$E_s = 30 \text{ keV} - (0.04 \text{ keV} + 12 \text{ keV})$$
$$= 30 \text{ keV} - (12.04 \text{ keV})$$
$$= 17.96 \text{ keV}$$

During a Compton interaction, most of the energy is divided between the scattered x-ray and the Compton electron, also called the *secondary electron.* Usually the scattered x-ray retains most of the energy. Both the scattered x-ray and the secondary electron may have sufficient energy to undergo more ionizing interactions before losing all their energy.

Ultimately, the scattered x-ray is absorbed photoelectrically. The secondary electron loses all its kinetic energy by ionization and excitation and drops into a vacancy in an electron shell previously created by some other ionizing event.

Compton-scattered x-rays can be deflected in any direction, including 180 degrees from the incident x-ray. At a deflection of zero, no energy is transferred. As the angle of deflection increases to 180 degrees, more energy is transferred to the secondary electron, but even at 180 degrees of deflection, the scattered x-ray retains at least two thirds of its original energy.

X-rays scattered back in the direction of the incident x-ray beam are called **backscatter radiation.** In diagnostic radiography, backscatter radiation is responsible for the cassette-hinge image sometimes seen on a radiograph even though the hinge was on the back side of the cassette. In such situations the radiation has backscattered from the wall or examination table, not the patient.

The probability that a given x-ray will undergo the Compton effect is a complex function of the energy of the incident x-ray. Generally the probability of Compton effect decreases as x-ray energy increases.

The probability of the Compton effect does not depend on the atomic number of the atom involved. Any given x-ray is just as likely to undergo the Compton effect with an atom of soft tissue as with an atom of bone (Figure 13-3). Table 13-1 summarizes Compton scattering.

 Compton scattering reduces contrast in an x-ray image.

Compton scattering can occur with all x-rays, and radiographs always appear duller and flatter because of Compton-scattered x-rays. Such x-rays produce no useful information on the radiograph. Rather, they produce fog: a uniform optical density on the radiograph that results in reduced image contrast. There are ways of reducing scattered radiation; they are discussed later, but none is totally effective.

The scattered x-rays from Compton interactions can create a serious radiation exposure hazard in radiography and particularly in fluoroscopy. A large amount of radiation can be scattered from the patient during fluoroscopy. Such radiation is the source of most of the occupational radiation exposure that radiologic technologists receive.

TABLE 13-1	Features of Compton Scattering
Most likely to occur	With outer-shell electrons
	With loosely bound electrons
As x-ray energy increases	Increased penetration through tissue without interaction
	Increased Compton scattering relative to photoelectric effect
	Reduced absolute Compton scattering
As atomic number of absorber increases	No effect on Compton scattering
As mass density of absorber increases	Proportional increase in Compton scattering

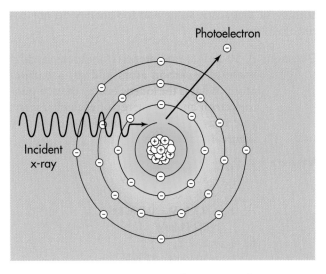

FIGURE 13-4 The photoelectric effect occurs when an incident x-ray is totally absorbed during the ionization of an inner-shell electron. The incident photon disappears, and the K-shell electron, now called a *photoelectron,* is ejected from the atom.

During radiography, the hazard is less severe because no one but the patient is normally in the examining room. Nevertheless, scattered radiation levels are sufficient to necessitate protective shielding of the x-ray examining room.

Photoelectric Effect

X-rays in the diagnostic range also undergo ionizing interactions with inner-shell electrons. The x-ray is not scattered, but it is totally absorbed. This process is called the **photoelectric effect** (Figure 13-4). The electron removed from the atom, called a **photoelectron,** escapes with kinetic energy equal to the difference between the energy of the incident x-ray and the binding energy of the electron. Mathematically, this is shown as follows:

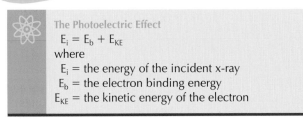

The Photoelectric Effect

$$E_i = E_b + E_{KE}$$

where

E_i = the energy of the incident x-ray

E_b = the electron binding energy

E_{KE} = the kinetic energy of the electron

The Photoelectric Effect
The photoelectric effect is an x-ray absorption interaction.

For low atomic number atoms, such as those found in soft tissue, the binding energy of even K-shell electrons is low (0.3 keV for carbon, for instance). Therefore the photoelectron is released with kinetic energy nearly equal to the energy of the incident x-ray. For target atoms of higher atomic number, the electron binding energies are higher (37 keV for barium K-shell electrons). Therefore the kinetic energy of the photoelectron from barium is proportionately lower. Table 13-2 shows the approximate K-shell binding energy for elements of radiologic importance.

TABLE 13-2	Atomic Number and K-Shell Electron Binding Energy of Radiologically Important Elements	
Element	Atomic Number	K-Shell Electron Binding Energy (keV)
Hydrogen	1	0.02
Carbon	6	0.3
Nitrogen	7	0.4
Oxygen	8	0.5
Aluminum	13	1.6
Calcium	20	4.1
Molybdenum	42	20
Rhenium	45	24
Iodine	53	33
Barium	56	37
Tungsten	74	69
Lead	82	88

Characteristic x-rays are produced after a photoelectric interaction in a manner similar to that described in Chapter 11. The ejection of a K-shell photoelectron by the incident x-ray results in a vacancy in the K shell. This unnatural state is immediately corrected when an outer-shell electron, usually from the L shell, drops into the vacancy.

This electron transition is accompanied by the emission of an x-ray whose energy is equal to the difference in the binding energies of the shells involved. These characteristic x-rays are **secondary radiation** and behave in the same manner as scattered radiation. They contribute

TABLE 13-4	Features of Photoelectric Effect
Most likely to occur	With inner-shell electrons
	With tightly bound electrons
	When x-ray energy is just higher than electron binding energy
As x-ray energy increases	Increased penetration through tissue without interaction
	Less photoelectric effect relative to Compton scattering
	Reduced absolute photoelectric effect
As atomic number of absorber increases	Increases proportionately with the cube of the atomic number (Z^3)
As mass density of absorber increases	Proportional increase in photoelectric effect

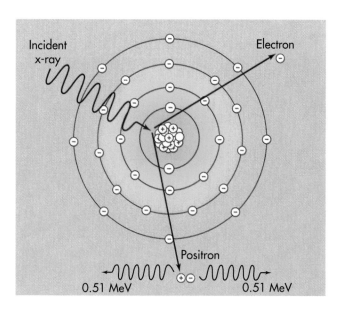

FIGURE 13-8 Pair production occurs with x-rays that have energies greater than 1.02 MeV. The x-ray interacts with the nuclear force field, and two electrons that have opposite electrostatic charges are created. The positron annihilates with an electron, creating two 0.51-MeV photons.

Pair Production

If an incident x-ray has sufficient energy, it may escape interaction with electrons and come close enough to the nucleus of the atom to be influenced by the strong electric field of the nucleus. The interaction between the x-ray and the nuclear electric field causes the x-ray to disappear, and in its place two electrons appear, one positively charged (positron) and one negatively charged. This process is called **pair production** (Figure 13-8).

 Pair production does not occur during x-ray imaging.

In Chapter 5, we calculated the energy equivalence of the mass of an electron to be 0.51 MeV. Since two electrons are formed in a pair-production interaction, the incident photon must have at least 1.02 MeV of energy. An x-ray with less than 1.02 MeV cannot undergo pair production. Any of the x-ray's energy in excess of 1.02 MeV is distributed equally between the two electrons as kinetic energy.

The electron produced by pair production eventually finds a vacancy in an atomic orbital shell. The positron unites with a free electron, and the mass of both particles is converted to energy in a process called *annihilation radiation.*

Because pair production involves only x-rays with energies greater than 1.02 MeV, it is unimportant in x-ray imaging but may influence radioisotope imaging in nuclear medicine.

Photodisintegration

Very-high-energy x-rays (that is, those with energy above approximately 10 MeV) can escape interaction

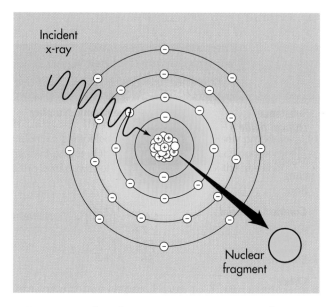

FIGURE 13-9 Photodisintegration is an interaction between very-high-energy x-rays and the nucleus. The x-ray is absorbed by the nucleus, and a nuclear fragment is emitted.

with electrons and the nuclear electric field and be absorbed directly by the nucleus. When this happens, the nucleus is raised to an excited state and instantaneously emits a nucleon or other nuclear fragment. This process is called **photodisintegration** (Figure 13-9). Because it involves only x-rays with energies greater than approximately 10 MeV, photodisintegration does not occur in diagnostic radiology.

DIFFERENTIAL ABSORPTION

Of the five ways an x-ray can interact with tissue, only two are important to radiology: the Compton effect and the photoelectric effect. More important than the x-ray interacting by these two effects, however, is the x-ray transmitted through the body without interaction. Figure 13-10 shows how each of these three types of x-ray contributes to an image.

The Compton-scattered x-ray contributes no useful information to the image. When a Compton-scattered x-ray interacts with the image receptor, the image receptor assumes that the x-ray came straight from the x-ray tube target (Figure 13-11). The image receptor does not recognize the scattered x-ray as representing an interaction off the straight line from the target.

These scattered x-rays result in **fog**, a generalized dulling of the image by optical densities not representing diagnostic information. To reduce this type of fog, we use techniques and apparatus to reduce the number of scattered x-rays that reach the image receptor.

X-rays that undergo photoelectric interaction produce diagnostic information on the image receptor. Since they do not reach the film, these x-rays are representative of anatomic structures with high x-ray absorption characteristics; such structures are radiopaque. The photoelectric absorption of x-rays results in the light areas of a radiograph (low optical density), such as those corresponding to bone.

Other x-rays penetrate the body and are transmitted to the image receptor with no interaction whatever. They result in the dark (high optical density) areas of a radiograph. The anatomic structures through which these x-rays pass are radiolucent.

Basically, an x-ray image results from the difference between the x-rays absorbed photoelectrically in the patient and those transmitted to the image receptor. This difference in x-ray interaction is called **differential absorption**. Differential absorption occurs because of Compton scattering, the photoelectric effect, and x-rays transmitted through the patient. Except at very low peak kilovoltage (kVp), most x-rays that interact do so by the Compton effect. This is one reason that radiographs are not as sharp and clear as photographs.

Generally less than 5% of the x-rays incident on a patient reach the film. Less than half of those that reach the film interact to form an image. Thus the radiographic image results from approximately 1% of the x-rays emitted by the x-ray tube target. Consequently, careful control and selection of the x-ray beam are necessary to produce high-quality radiographs.

 Differential absorption increases as the kVp is reduced.

Producing a high-quality radiograph requires the proper selection of kVp so that the effective x-ray en-

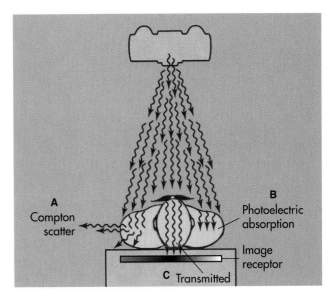

FIGURE 13-10 The three types of x-rays important to making a radiograph. **A,** Those scattered by Compton interaction. **B,** Those absorbed photoelectrically. **C,** Those transmitted through the patient without interaction.

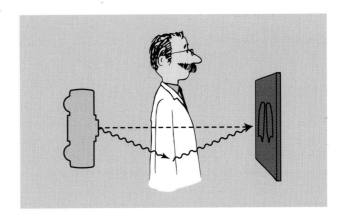

FIGURE 13-11 When an x-ray is Compton scattered, the image receptor thinks it came straight from the source.

ergy will result in maximum differential absorption. Unfortunately, reducing kVp to increase differential absorption and therefore image contrast results in increased patient dose. A compromise is necessary for each examination.

Dependence on Atomic Number

Consider the image of an extremity (Figure 13-12). An image of the bone is produced because many more x-rays are absorbed photoelectrically in bone than in soft tissue. Recall that the probability of an x-ray undergoing photoelectric absorption is proportional to the third power of the atomic number of the tissue. According to Table 13-3, bone has an atomic number of 13.8; soft tissue has an atomic number of 7.4. Consequently, the probability that an x-ray will undergo a photoelectric in-

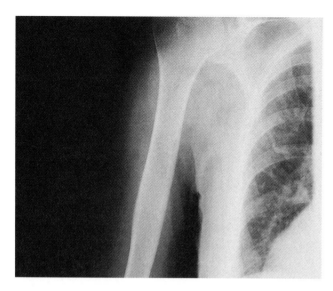

FIGURE 13-12 A radiograph of bony structures results from the differential absorption between bone and soft tissue. *(Courtesy John Lampignano.)*

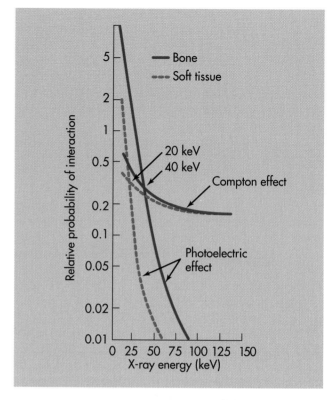

FIGURE 13-13 Graph showing probabilities of photoelectric and Compton interactions with soft tissue and bone. The interactions of these curves indicate the x-ray energies at which the probability of photoelectric absorption equals the chance for Compton scattering.

teraction is approximately seven times greater in bone than in soft tissue.

Question: How much more likely is an x-ray to interact with bone than muscle?

Answer: $\left(\dfrac{13.8}{7.4}\right)^3 = \dfrac{2628}{405} = 6.5$

These relative values of interaction are apparent in Figure 13-5 when particular attention is paid to the logarithmic scale of the vertical axis. Notice that the relative probability of interaction between bone and soft tissue (differential absorption) remains constant, whereas the absolute probability of each decreases with increasing energy. With higher x-ray energy, fewer interactions occur, so more x-rays are transmitted without interaction.

Question: What is the relative probability that a 20-keV x-ray will undergo photoelectric interaction in bone compared to fat?

Answer: $Z_{bone} = 13.8$, $Z_{fat} = 6.3$

$\left(\dfrac{13.8}{6.3}\right)^3 = 10.5$

Compton scattering of x-rays is independent of the atomic number of different tissue (Figure 13-3). The probability of Compton scattering for bone atoms and for soft tissue atoms is about equal and decreases with increasing x-ray energy. This decrease in scattering, however, is not as rapid as that occurring with photoelectric absorption. The probability of Compton scattering is inversely proportional to x-ray energy (1/E). The probability of photoelectric effect is inversely proportional to the third power of the x-ray energy $1/E^3$.

At low energies, the majority of x-ray interactions are photoelectric. At high energies, Compton scattering predominates. Of course, as x-ray energy is increased, the chance of any interaction at all decreases. As kVp is increased, more x-rays get to the image receptor, and therefore a lower x-ray quantity (lower milliampere-seconds [mAs]) is required.

Figure 13-13 combines all these factors into one graph. At 20 keV, the probability of photoelectric effect equals the probability of Compton scattering in soft tissue. Below this energy, most x-rays interact with soft tissue photoelectrically. Above this energy, the predominant interaction with soft tissue is Compton scattering. Low kVp resulting in increased differential absorption is the basis for mammography.

 To image small differences in soft tissue, use low kVp to get maximal differential absorption.

The relative frequency of the Compton interaction compared with the photoelectric interaction increases with increasing x-ray energy. The crossover point between photoelectric effect and Compton scattering for bone is about 40 keV. Therefore a high-kVp technique can be used for examining bony structures, resulting in much lower patient dose.

When a high-kVp technique is used in this manner, the amount of scattered radiation from surrounding soft tissue is less than the differential absorption in bone. When the amount of scattered radiation becomes too high, grids are used (see Chapter 18). Grids do not affect the magnitude of the differential absorption.

Differential absorption in bone and soft tissue results from photoelectric interactions, which greatly depends on the atomic number of tissue. The loss of contrast is due to fog caused by Compton scattering. Two other factors are also important in making an image: the x-ray emission spectrum and the mass density of patient tissue.

The crossover energies of 20 keV and 40 keV are a **monoenergetic** x-ray beam (that is, a beam containing x-rays that all have the same energy). In fact, as we saw in Chapter 11, clinical x-rays are **polyenergetic**. They are emitted over an entire spectrum of energies. Therefore the correct selection of kVp for optimal differential absorption depends on the other factors discussed in Chapter 11 that affect the x-ray emission spectrum. For instance, in anterior-posterior radiography of the lumbar spine at 110 kVp, more x-rays may be emitted with energy above the 40 keV crossover for bone than below it. Less filtration or a grid may then be necessary.

Dependence on Mass Density

Intuitively, we know that we could image bone even if differential absorption were not related to atomic number because bone has a higher mass density than soft tissue. Mass density is not to be confused with optical density. **Mass density** is the quantity of matter per unit volume, usually specified in units of kilograms per cubic meter (kg/m^3). Sometimes, mass density is reported in grams per cubic centimeter (gm/cm^3).

Question: How many grams per cubic centimeter are there in 1 kg/m^3?

Answer:
$$1\ kg/m^3 = \frac{1000\ gm}{(100\ cm)^3}$$
$$= \frac{10^3\ gm}{10^6\ cm^3}$$
$$= 10^{-3}\ gm/cm^3$$

Table 13-5 gives the mass densities of several radiologically important materials. Mass density is related to the mass of each atom and basically tells how tightly the atoms of a substance are packed. Water and ice are composed of precisely the same atoms, but ice occupies more volume. The mass density of ice is 917 kg/m^3 compared with 1000 kg/m^3 for water. Ice floats in water because of this difference in mass density. Ice is lighter than water.

 Regardless of the type of interaction, the interaction between x-rays and tissue is proportional to the mass density of the tissue.

TABLE 13-5	Mass Density of Various Materials Important to Diagnostic Radiology
Substance	**Mass Density (kg/m^3)**
Human tissue	
Lung	320
Fat	910
Muscle, soft tissue	1000
Bone	1850
Contrast material	
Air	1.3
Barium	3500
Iodine	4930
Other	
Calcium	1550
Concrete	2350
Molybdenum	10200
Rhenium	12500
Tungstate	19300
Lead	11350

The interaction between x-rays and the tissue being imaged is proportional to the mass density of the tissue. When mass density is doubled, the chance for x-ray interaction is doubled because twice as many electrons are available for interaction. Therefore even without the photoelectric effect related to atomic number, nearly twice as many x-rays would be absorbed and scattered in bone as in soft tissue. The bone would be imaged.

Question: What is the relative probability that 60-keV x-rays will undergo Compton scattering in bone compared to soft tissue?

Answer:
Mass density of bone = 1850 kg/m^3
Mass density of soft tissue = 1000 kg/m^3
$$\frac{1850}{1000} = 1.85$$

Lungs are imaged on a chest radiograph primarily because of differences in mass density. According to Table 13-5, the mass density of soft tissue is 770 times that of air (1000/1.3); for the same thickness, we can expect almost 770 times as many x-rays to interact with the soft tissue as with lung air.

The atomic numbers of air and soft tissue are about the same: 7.4 for soft tissue and 7.6 for air. Thus differential absorption in air-filled soft tissue cavities is due primarily to differences in mass density. Figure 13-14 demonstrates the differential absorption in air, soft tissue, and bone caused by differences in mass density. Table 13-6 summarizes the various relationships of differential absorption.

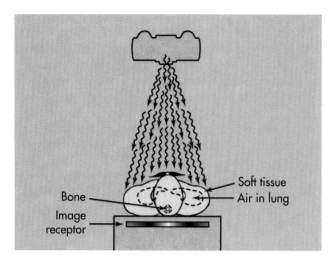

FIGURE 13-14 Even if x-ray interaction were not related to atomic number (Z), differential absorption would occur because of differences in mass density.

TABLE 13-6	Characteristics of Differential Absorption
As x-ray energy increases	Fewer Compton interactions
	Much fewer photoelectric interactions
	More transmission through tissue
As tissue atomic number increases	No change in Compton interactions
	Many more photoelectric interactions
	Less x-ray transmission
As tissue mass density increases	Proportional increase in Compton interactions
	Proportional increase in photoelectric interactions
	Proportional reduction in x-ray transmission

Question: Assume that all x-ray interactions during mammography are photoelectric. What is the differential absorption of x-rays in microcalcifications relative to fatty tissue?

Answer: Differential absorption as a result of atomic number =

$$\left(\frac{20}{6.3}\right)^3 = \frac{8000}{250} = 32{:}1$$

Differential absorption as a result of mass density

$$= \frac{1550}{910} = 1.7{:}1$$

Total differential absorption = (32)(1.7) = 54.4:1

CONTRAST EXAMINATION

Barium and iodine compounds are used as an aid for imaging internal organs with x-rays. The atomic number of barium is 56; that of iodine is 53. Each has a much higher atomic number and mass density that soft tissue. When used in this fashion, they are called **contrast agents.**

Question: What is the probability that an x-ray will interact with iodine rather than soft tissue?

Answer: Differential absorption as a result of atomic number $= \left(\frac{53}{7.4}\right)^3 = 367{:}1$

Differential absorption as a result of mass density $= \frac{4.93}{1.0} = 4.93{:}1$

Total differential absorption = 367 × 4.93 = 1809:1

When an iodinated compound fills the internal carotid artery or when barium fills the colon, these internal organs are readily visualized on a radiograph. A low-kVp technique (for example, below 80 kVp) produces excellent high-contrast radiographs of the organs of the gastrointestinal tract. A higher-kVp operation (for example, above 90 kVp) can often be used in these examinations not only to outline the organ under investigation but also to penetrate the contrast media to visualize the lumen of the organ more clearly.

Air was once used as a contrast medium in procedures such as pneumoencephalography and ventriculography. In these procedures, the normal body fluids filling these internal cavities were replaced by air. Such procedures have been discontinued, however, since the introduction of computed tomography and magnetic resonance imaging. Air, along with barium, is still used for contrast in some examinations of the colon; this type of study is called a **double-contrast examination.**

EXPONENTIAL ATTENUATION

When x-rays are incident on any type of tissue, they can interact with the atoms of that tissue via any of the five mechanisms discussed previously. The relative frequency of interaction of each mechanism depends primarily on the atomic number of the tissue atoms and the x-ray energy.

An interaction such as the photoelectric effect is called an *absorption process* because the x-ray disappears. Absorption is an all-or-nothing condition for x-ray interaction. Interactions in which the x-ray is only partially absorbed, such as the Compton effect, are scattering processes. Coherent scattering is also a scattering event because the x-ray emerging from the interaction travels in a direction different from that of the incident x-ray. Pair production and photodisintegration are absorption processes.

The total reduction in the number of x-rays remaining in an x-ray beam after penetration through a given thickness of tissue is called **attenuation.** When a broad beam of x-rays is incident on any tissue, some of the x-rays are absorbed, and some are scattered. The result is a reduced number of x-rays, a condition referred to as *x-ray attenuation.*

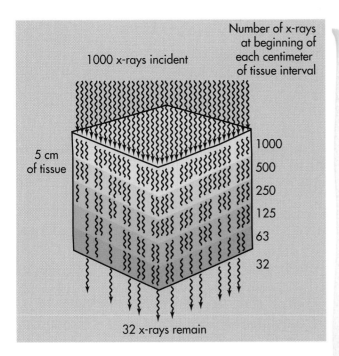

FIGURE 13-15 Interaction of x-rays by absorption and scatter is called *attenuation*. In this example the x-ray beam has been attenuated 97%; 3% of the x-rays have been transmitted.

 Attenuation is the product of absorption and scattering.

X-rays are attenuated exponentially, which means that they do not have a fixed range in tissue. They are reduced in number by a given percentage for each incremental thickness of tissue through which they go.

Consider the situation in Figure 13-15. A total of 1000 x-rays are incident on an abdomen 25 cm thick. The x-ray energy and the atomic number of the tissue are such that 50% of the x-rays are removed by the first 5 cm. Therefore in the first 5 cm, 500 x-rays are removed, leaving 500 available to continue penetration of the abdomen. By the end of the second 5 cm, 50% of the 500, or 250, x-rays have been removed, leaving 250 x-rays to continue. Similarly, entering the fourth 5-cm thickness are 125 x-rays, and entering the fifth and last 5-cm thickness are 63. Half of the 63 x-rays are attenuated in the next 5 cm of tissue, and therefore only 32 are transmitted to interact with the image receptor. The total effect of these interactions is 97% attenuation and 3% transmission of the x-ray beam.

A plot of this hypothetical x-ray beam attenuation, which closely resembles the actual situation, appears in Figure 13-16. Is it obvious that the assumed half-value layer in soft tissue was 5 cm? It should be clear that, theoretically at least, the number of x-rays emerging from any thickness of absorber will never reach zero. Each succeeding thickness can attenuate the x-ray beam only by a fractional amount and a fraction of any positive number is always greater than zero.

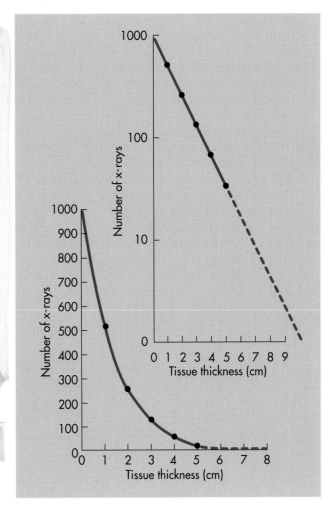

FIGURE 13-16 Linear and semilogarithmic plots of the exponential x-ray attenuation data in Figure 13-15.

This is not the way that alpha and beta particles interact with matter. Regardless of the energy of the particle and the type of tissue, these particulate radiations can penetrate only so far before they are absorbed. For example, beta particles with 2 MeV of energy have a range of about 1 cm in soft tissue. Substantially, no 2-MeV beta particles can penetrate beyond that thickness.

SUMMARY

The following are five fundamental interactions between x-rays and matter:

1. Coherent scattering is a change in the direction of an incident x-ray without a loss of energy.
2. The Compton effect occurs when incident x-rays ionize atoms and the x-ray then changes direction with a loss of energy.
3. The photoelectric effect occurs when the incident x-ray is absorbed in one of the inner electron shells and emits a photoelectron.
4. Pair production occurs when the incident x-ray interacts with the electric field of the nucleus. The

x-ray disappears and two electrons appear, one positively charged (positron) and one negatively charged.

5. Photodisintegration occurs when the incident x-ray is directly absorbed by the nucleus. The x-ray disappears, and nuclear fragments are released.

The interactions that are important to diagnostic x-ray imaging are the Compton effect and the photoelectric effect.

Differential absorption controls the contrast of an x-ray image. The x-ray image results from the difference between the x-rays absorbed by photoelectric interaction and those that pass through the body as image-forming radiation. Attenuation is the reduction of the x-ray beam intensity as it penetrates through tissue. Differential absorption and attenuation of the x-ray beam depend on the following factors:

1. The atomic number of the atoms in tissue
2. The mass density of the atoms in tissue
3. The x-ray energy

Radiologic contrast agents such as iodine and barium use the principles of differential absorption and attenuation to image soft tissue organs. Iodine is used in vascular, renal, and biliary imaging. Barium is used for gastrointestinal imaging. Both elements have high atomic numbers (iodine is 53, barium is 56) and mass densities much greater than soft tissue.

CHALLENGE QUESTIONS

1. Define or otherwise identify:
   a. Differential absorption
   b. Classical scattering
   c. Mass density
   d. 1.02 MeV
   e. Contrast agent
   f. Compton effect
   g. Attenuation
   h. Monoenergetic
   i. Secondary electron
   j. Photoelectric effect

2. What are the three primary factors important to differential absorption?

3. A 28-keV x-ray interacts photoelectrically with a K-shell electron of a calcium atom. What is the kinetic energy of the secondary electron? (See Table 4-3.)

4. Approximately what kVp is used to penetrate barium in a contrast examination?

5. Why are iodinated compounds such excellent agents for vascular contrast examinations?

6. Diagram the Compton interaction and identify the incident x-ray, positive ion, negative ion, secondary x-ray, and scattered x-ray.

7. Describe backscatter radiation.

8. Tungsten is sometimes alloyed into the beam-defining collimators of an x-ray imager. If a 63-keV x-ray undergoes a Compton interaction with an L-shell electron and ejects that electron with 12 keV of energy, what is the energy of the scattered x-ray? (See Figure 4-9.)

9. Of the five basic mechanisms of x-ray interaction with matter, three are not important to diagnostic radiology. Name them and explain why are they not important.

10. On average, 33.7 eV is required for each ionization in air. How many ion pairs would be a 22-keV x-ray probably produce in air and about how many ion pairs would be produced photoelectrically?

11. The energy of the Compton-scattered x-ray is equal to the difference of what two energies?

12. Does the probability of the Compton effect depend on the atomic number of the target atom?

13. When kVp is increased, is there an increase or a reduction of Compton scattering? Explain.

14. Describe the photoelectric effect.

15. When kVp is increased, what happens to the relative frequency of interaction of photoelectric effect vs. Compton scattering?

16. How much more likely is it that an x-ray will interact with bone than muscle?

17. What is the relationship between the atomic number of tissue and differential absorption?

18. What is the relationship between the mass density of tissue and differential absorption?

19. In a contrast radiographic examination using iodine, what is the relative probability that x-ray beam will interact with iodine rather than tissue?

PART III

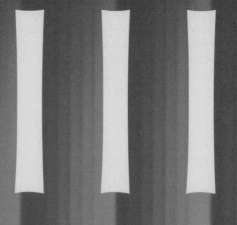

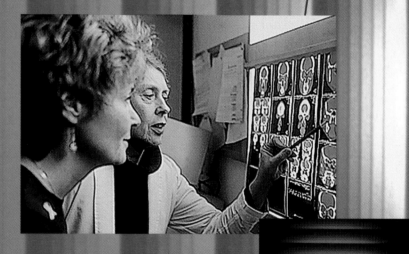

THE
RADIOGRAPHIC
IMAGE

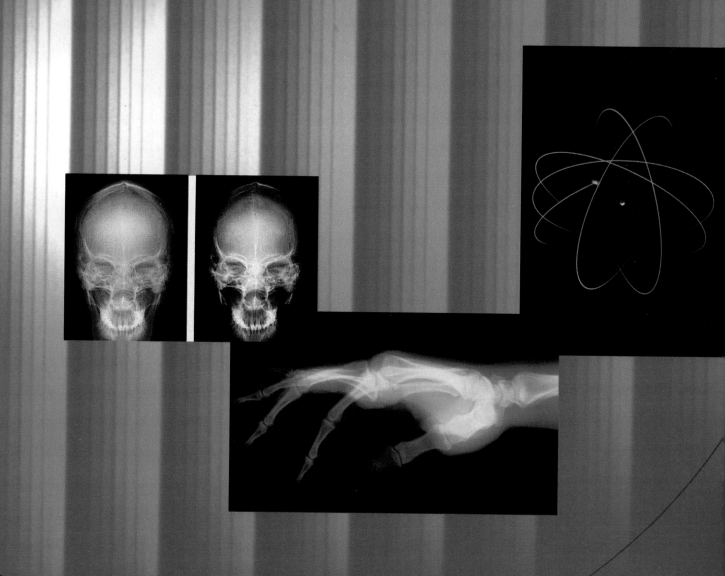

Radiographic Film

OBJECTIVES

At the completion of this chapter, the student should be able to:
1. Discuss the construction of radiographic film
2. Describe the formation of the latent image
3. List and define the characteristics of x-ray film
4. Identify the types of film used in diagnostic imaging departments
5. Explain proper storage and handling procedures for film

OUTLINE

During a diagnostic radiologic examination, image-forming x-rays exit the patient to expose radiographic intensifying screens placed in a protective radiographic cassette. These radiographic intensifying screens emit light, which exposes the radiographic film placed between the two screens.

This chapter discusses the construction of radiographic film and identifies the various types. This chapter also describes the formation of a latent image by x-ray exposure and presents tips for handling and storing radiographic film.

REMNANT RADIATION

The primary purpose of diagnostic radiologic apparatus and techniques is to transfer information with diagnostic value from an x-ray beam to the eye-brain complex of the radiologist. In other words, the x-ray beam must be transformed into something that can be seen and interpreted. The medium that transforms the x-ray beam into a visible image is called the **image receptor.** Radiographic film is still the most common type of image receptor.

The **useful beam** emerging from the x-ray tube contains x-rays nearly uniformly distributed in space. After interacting with the patient, however, the useful beam is no longer evenly distributed in space but rather varies in intensity according to the characteristics of the tissue through which it has passed (see Chapter 13). The beam is said to be **attenuated:** the intensity of radiation has been reduced as a result of absorption and scattering.

This beam of varied intensity is called the *remnant beam.* The **remnant beam** refers to the x-rays that remain after the useful beam exits the patient. It consists of x-rays scattered away from the image receptor and image-forming x-rays. **Image-forming x-rays** are the x-rays that interact with the image receptor to form a radiographic image. Image-forming x-rays are also known as *remnant radiation* or *exit radiation.* The American Registry of Radiologic Technologists uses the term *exit radiation.*

 Image-forming x-rays are the x-rays that exit the patient and interact with the image receptor.

Image-forming x-rays interact with the image receptor, which is usually film sandwiched between radiographic screens mounted in a protective cassette. The radiographic intensifying screens change x-ray energy into visible light. Visible light then exposes the film.

The construction and characteristics of radiographic film are similar to those of regular photographic film. Radiographic film is manufactured with high quality

control and has a spectral response different from that of photographic film; however, its mechanism of operation is much the same. The discussions in this chapter could be applied to photographic film with very few modifications.

FILM CONSTRUCTION

The manufacture of radiographic film is a precise, high-quality procedure. Manufacturing facilities are extremely clean, since the slightest bit of dirt or other contaminant limits the film's ability to reproduce the information of the x-ray beam. During the early 1960s, at the height of nuclear weapons testing, x-ray film manufacturers took extraordinary precautions to ensure that radioactive contamination from fallout did not invade their manufacturing environment.

Radiographic film basically has two parts: the **base** and the **emulsion** (Figure 14-1). Most x-ray film has the emulsion coated on both sides and therefore is called duplitized or **double-emulsion film.** Between the emulsion and the base is a thin coating of material called the **adhesive layer** to ensure uniform adhesion of the emulsion to the base. This adhesive layer allows the emulsion and base to maintain proper contact and integrity during use and processing.

The emulsion is enclosed by a protective covering of gelatin called the **overcoat** or **abrasion layer.** This overcoat protects the emulsion from scratches, pressure, and contamination during handling, processing, and storage and allows for relatively rough manipulation of x-ray film before exposure. Processed film may be handled with even less regard for damage. The thickness of radiographic film is approximately 150 to 300 μm.

Base

The base is the foundation for radiographic film. Its primary purpose is to provide a rigid structure onto which the emulsion can be coated. The base is flexible and fracture resistant to allow easy handling, but it is sufficiently rigid to be snapped into a viewbox. Conventional photographic film has a much thinner base than radio-

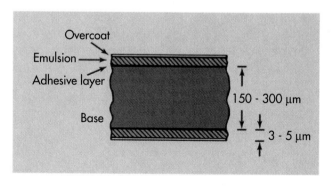

FIGURE 14-1 Cross-sectional view of radiographic film. The bulk of the film is the base. The emulsion contains the diagnostic information.

graphic film and therefore is not as rigid. Can you imagine attempting to snap a 14 × 17 inch photographic negative into a viewbox?

> The base of radiographic film is 150 to 300 μm thick, is semi-rigid, is lucent and is made of polyester.

The base of radiographic film maintains its size and shape during use and processing so that it does not contribute to image distortion. This property of the base is known as *dimensional stability*. The base is of uniform lucency, nearly transparent to light, so it causes no unwanted pattern of shading on the film.

During manufacturing, however, dye is added to the base of most radiographic film to slightly tint the film blue. Compared with untinted film, this coloring results in less eyestrain and fatigue for the radiologist and therefore is conducive to more efficient and accurate diagnoses.

The original radiographic film base was a glass plate; in fact, radiologists once referred to radiographs as *x-ray plates*. During World War I, the availability of high-quality glass became severely limited, and the medical applications of x-rays, particularly by the military, increased rapidly.

A substitute material, cellulose nitrate, soon became the standard base. Cellulose nitrate, however, had one serious deficiency: it was flammable. The improper storage and handling of some x-ray film files resulted in severe hospital fires during the 1920s and early 1930s.

By the mid 1920s, film using a "safety base," cellulose triacetate, was introduced. Cellulose triacetate has properties similar to those of cellulose nitrate but is not as flammable.

In the early 1960s a polyester base was introduced. Polyester has taken the place of cellulose triacetate as the film base of choice. Polyester is more resistant to warping from age and is stronger than cellulose triacetate, permitting easier transport through automatic processors. Its dimensional stability is superior. Polyester bases are also thinner than triacetate bases.

The polyester base is similar in composition to the polyester fibers in clothing. Principally, two chemicals, ethylene glycol and dimethyl terephthalate, are formed into a molten polymer (a very large molecule made from two or more smaller ones) by mixing at high temperature and low pressure. For clothing, the polyester is produced in thin strands like thread. For film, it is formed into thin sheets of appropriate size.

Emulsion

The emulsion is the heart of the x-ray film. It is the material with which x-rays or light photons from radiographic intensifying screens interact and transfer information. The emulsion consists of a homogeneous

mixture of gelatin and silver halide crystals. It is coated evenly with a 3- to 5-μm thick layer of this mixture.

The gelatin is similar to that used in salads and desserts but is of much higher quality. It is clear, so it transmits light, and is sufficiently porous for the processing chemicals to penetrate to the crystals of silver halide. Its principal function is to provide a support medium for the silver halide crystals by holding them uniformly dispersed in place.

The silver halide crystal is the active ingredient of the radiographic emulsion. In the typical emulsion, 98% of the silver halide is **silver bromide;** the remainder is usually **silver iodide.** These atoms have relatively high atomic numbers ($Z_I = 53$, $Z_{Br} = 35$, $Z_{Ag} = 47$) compared with the gelatin and base (for both, $Z \approx 7$). The interaction of x-rays and light photons with these atoms with high atomic numbers ultimately results in the formation of a latent image on the radiograph.

Silver halide crystals may be tabular, cubic, octahedral, polyhedral, or irregular in shape depending on the intended imaging application. Tabular grains are used in most radiographic films.

The tabular silver halide crystals are flat, typically 0.1 μm thick, with a triangular, hexagonal, or higher-order polygonal cross section, and are approximately 1 μm in diameter. The arrangement of atoms in the crystals is cubic, as shown in Figure 14-2. The crystals

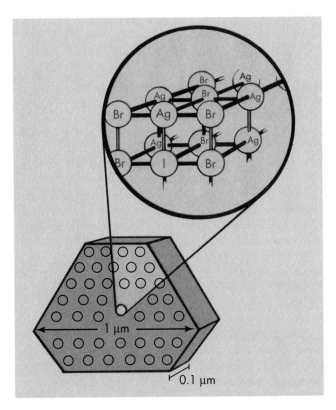

FIGURE 14-2 Example of a tabular silver halide crystal with a triangular cross section. The arrangement of atoms in the crystal is cubic.

are made by dissolving metallic silver (Ag) in nitric acid (HNO₃) to form silver nitrate (AgNO₃). The light-sensitive silver bromide (AgBr) crystals and potassium nitrate (KNO₃) are formed by mixing the silver nitrate with potassium bromide (KBr) in the following reaction:

Silver Halide Crystal Formation
$$AgNO_3 + KBr \rightarrow AgBr \downarrow + KNO_3$$
The arrow ↓ indicates that the silver bromide is precipitated while the potassium nitrate, which is soluble, is washed away.

The entire process takes place in the presence of gelatin, with the temperature, the pressure, and the rate at which ingredients are mixed being precisely controlled.

The shape and lattice structure of the silver halide crystals are not perfect, and some of the imperfections result in the imaging property of the crystals. The type of imperfection thought to be responsible is a chemical contaminant, usually silver-gold sulfide, which is introduced by chemical sensitization into the crystal lattice, usually at or near the surface. This contaminant has been given the name **sensitivity center.** During exposure, photoelectrons and silver ions are attracted to these sensitivity centers, where they combine to form a latent image center of metallic silver.

The differences in speed, contrast, and resolution among various radiographic films are determined by the process by which the silver halide crystals are manufactured and by the mixture of these crystals into the gelatin. The number of sensitivity centers per crystal, the concentration of crystals in the emulsion, and the size and distribution of the crystals also affect the performance characteristic of radiographic film.

Direct-exposure film, for example, contains a thicker emulsion with more silver halide crystals than screen-film. The size and concentration of silver halide crystals have a primary influence on speed. The composition of the radiographic emulsion is a proprietary secret closely guarded by each manufacturer.

The manufacture of radiographic film is conducted in total darkness. From the moment the emulsion ingredients are brought together until final packaging, no light is present.

FORMATION OF THE LATENT IMAGE

The image-forming x-rays exiting the patient and incident on the radiographic film deposit energy in the emulsion primarily by photoelectric interaction with the atoms of the silver halide crystal. This energy is deposited in a pattern representative of the object or anatomic part being radiographed. If you observe the film immediately after exposure, you would see no image. There is, however, an image present that cannot yet be seen; this image is called a **latent image.** With proper chemical processing, the latent image becomes a **manifest image.**

The latent image is the invisible change induced in the silver halide crystal.

The interaction between photons and silver halide crystals is fairly well understood, as is the processing of the latent image into the manifest image. However, the formation of the latent image, sometimes called the **photographic effect,** is not well understood and continues to be the subject of considerable research. The following discussion is an extraction of the Gurney-Mott theory, the accepted, although incomplete, explanation of latent image formation.

Silver Halide Crystal

The silver, bromine, and iodine atoms are fixed in the **crystal lattice** in ion form (Figure 14-3). Silver is a positive ion, and bromide and iodide are negative ions. When a silver halide crystal is formed, each silver atom releases an outer-shell electron, which becomes attached to a halide atom (either bromine or iodine). Now, the silver atom is missing an electron and therefore is a positively charged ion, identified as Ag^+. The bromine and iodine atoms each have one extra electron and therefore are negatively charged ions and identified as bromide and iodide (Br^- and I^-), respectively.

An ion is an atom that has either too many or too few electrons and therefore as a whole is electrically charged.

The silver halide crystal is not as rigid as some crystals such as diamond crystals. Under certain conditions, both atoms and electrons are free to migrate within the silver halide crystal. The halide ions, bromide and iodide, are

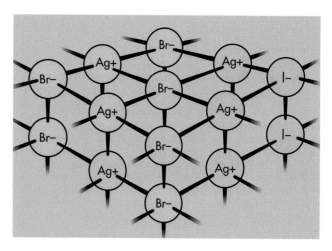

FIGURE 14-3 The crystal lattice of silver halide contains ions. Electrons from silver atoms have been "loaned" to bromine and iodine atoms.

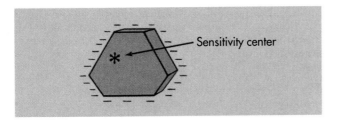

FIGURE 14-4 Model of a silver halide crystal emphasizing the sensitivity center and the concentration of negative ions on the surface.

generally in greatest concentration along the surface of the crystal. Therefore the crystal takes on a negative surface charge, which is matched by the positive charge of the **interstitial** silver ions, or the silver ions inside the crystal. An inherent defect in the structure of silver halide crystals, the Frankel defect, consists of interstitial silver ions and silver ion vacancies. A model of the silver halide crystal is shown in Figure 14-4.

Photon Interaction with the Silver Halide Crystal

When radiation interacts with film, the interaction with the silver and halide atoms (Ag, Br, I) responds to form the latent image. If the x-ray is totally absorbed, its interaction is photoelectric (Figure 14-5, A). If it is partially absorbed, its interaction is Compton. In both cases a secondary electron, either a photoelectron or Compton electron, is released with sufficient energy to travel a large distance in the crystal (Figure 14-5, B). While crossing the crystal, the secondary electron may have sufficient energy to dislodge additional electrons from the crystal lattice. Consequently, as a result of one x-ray interaction, a number of electrons are released and travel through the crystal lattice. The release of these secondary electrons is represented as follows:

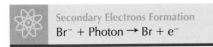

Secondary Electrons Formation
$$Br^- + Photon \rightarrow Br + e^-$$

Because light photons have lower energy, more are needed to produce an equal number of migrating secondary electrons as are produced by a single x-ray.

The result is the same if the interaction involves visible light from a radiographic intensifying screen or direct exposure by x-rays.

Secondary electrons liberated by the absorption event migrate to the sensitivity center and are trapped. Once a sensitivity center captures a photoelectron and becomes more negatively charged, it is attractive to mobile interstitial silver ions (Figure 14-5, C). The interstitial silver

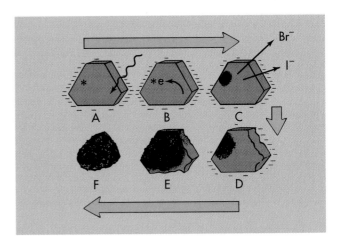

FIGURE 14-5 The production of the latent image and the conversion of the latent image into a manifest image follow several steps. **A,** The radiation interaction releases electrons. **B,** These electrons migrate to the sensitivity center. **C,** At the sensitivity center, atomic silver is formed by attracting an interstitial silver ion. **D,** This process is repeated many times, resulting in the buildup of silver atoms. **E,** The remaining silver halide is converted to silver during processing. **F,** The resulting silver grain.

ion combines with the electron trapped at the sensitivity center to form metallic silver atoms.

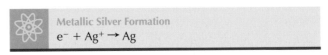

Metallic Silver Formation
$$e^- + Ag^+ \rightarrow Ag$$

Most of these electrons come from the bromide and iodide ions, since these negative ions have one extra electron. These negative ions therefore are converted to neutral atoms, and the loss of ionic charge results in disruption of the crystal lattice. The bromine and iodine atoms are now free to migrate, since they are no longer bound by ionic forces. They migrate out of the crystal into the gelatin portion of the emulsion. The deterioration of crystalline structure also makes it easier for remaining silver ions to migrate.

Latent Image

The concentration of electrons at the sensitivity center produces a region of negative electrification. As the halide atoms are removed from the crystal, the positive silver ions are electrostatically attracted to the sensitivity center. After migrating to the sensitivity center, the silver ions are neutralized by electrons and converted to atomic silver.

In an optimally exposed film, most developable silver halide crystals have collected 4 to 10 silver atoms at a sensitivity center (Figure 4-5, D). Consequently, this silver deposition is not observable, even microscopically. This group of silver atoms is called a **latent image center.** It is here that visible quantities of silver form during processing to create the radiographic image (Figure 14-5, *E*).

Crystals with silver deposited at the sensitivity center are developed into black grains (Figure 14-5, *F*). Crystals that have not been irradiated remain crystalline and inactive. The unobservable information contained in radiation-activated and inactivated silver halide crystals constitutes the latent image. **Processing** is the term applied to the chemical reactions that transform the latent image into a manifest image. Because of its importance, this subject is discussed separately in Chapter 15.

TYPES OF FILM

Medical imaging, especially radiologic imaging, is becoming extremely technical and sophisticated, and this is reflected in the number and variety of films used. Each major film manufacturer produces over 25 different films for medical imaging. When combined with the various film formats offered, over 500 selections are possible. Table 14-1 shows the standard film sizes in English and SI units. In most cases the sizes are not exactly equivalent, but they are usually interchangeable. By far the most commonly used film is that customarily referred to as screen-film. **Screen-film** is the kind of film used with radiographic intensifying screens.

The kind of film used without radiographic intensifying screens is **direct-exposure film,** sometimes called *nonscreen-film,* and special application films, such as those used in mammography, video recording, duplication, subtraction, cineradiography, and dental radiology. Each has particular characteristics that become more familiar to the technologist with use.

Screen-Film

Screen-film is the most widely used image receptor in radiology. There are several characteristics to be considered when selecting screen-film: contrast, speed, crossover, spectral matching, reprocity law, and safelights.

Contrast. Most manufacturers offer screen-film with multiple contrast levels. High-contrast film produces a very black-and-white image, whereas a low-contrast image is more gray. Contrast is discussed in more detail in Chapter 20.

The contrast of an image receptor is inversely proportional to its exposure **latitude** (that is, the range of exposure techniques that will produce an acceptable image). Consequently, screen-film is available in multiple latitudes. Usually, the manufacturer identifies these as medium-, high-, or higher-contrast films. The difference depends on the size and distribution of the silver halide crystal. A high-contrast emulsion contains smaller silver halide grains with a relatively uniform grain size. Lower-contrast films, on the other hand, contain larger grains having a wider range of sizes.

TABLE 14-1	Standard Film Sizes	
English Units (in)		SI Units (cm)
		18 × 43
8 × 10		20 × 25
		24 × 30
10 × 12		
		28 × 35
14 × 14		35 × 35
14 × 17		35 × 43

Speed. Screen-film is also available with different sensitivities or speeds. Usually, a manufacturer offers two or three different films with different speeds that result from different emulsions.

For direct-exposure film, speed is principally a function of the concentration and total content of silver halide crystals. For screen-film, silver halide grain size and shape are the principal determinates of film speed.

 Large-grain emulsions are more sensitive than small-grain emulsions.

To optimize speed, screen-films are almost always double emulsion; that is, an emulsion is layered on either side of the base. This is due primarily to the efficiency provided by using two radiographic intensifying screens to expose the film from both sides. This provides for twice the speed that could be obtained with single-emulsion film, even if the single emulsion is twice as thick.

There is a limit to film speed, however, because the light from the radiographic intensifying screen is absorbed very rapidly in the superficial layers of the emulsion. If the emulsion is too thick, the portion next to the film base remains largely unexposed. Compared to earlier technology, current emulsions contain less silver, yet produce the same optical density per unit exposure. This more efficient use of silver in the emulsion is termed the **covering power** of the emulsion.

The reported speed of a film is nearly always that for the image receptor: the film and two radiographic intensifying screens. When radiographic intensifying screens and film are properly matched, the reported speed will be accurate. Mismatch can result in significant error in exposure of the radiograph.

Crossover. Until recently, silver halide crystals were usually fat and three dimensional (Figure 14-6, *A*). Most emulsions now contain tabular grains (Figure 14-6, *B*), which are flat silver halide crystals, to provide a large surface area–to–volume ratio. The result is not only improved covering power but also significantly lower **crossover.**

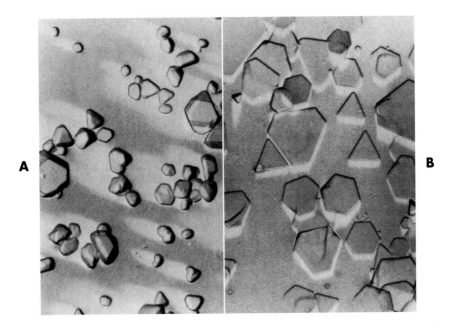

FIGURE 14-6 **A,** Conventional silver halide crystals are irregular in size. **B,** New technology produces flat, tabletlike grains. *(Courtesy Eastman Kodak Company.)*

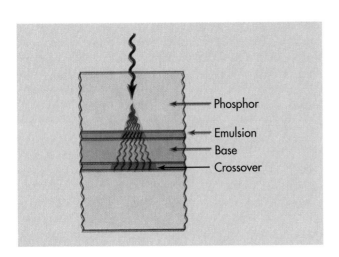

FIGURE 14-7 Crossover occurs when radiographic intensifying screen light crosses the base to expose the opposite emulsion.

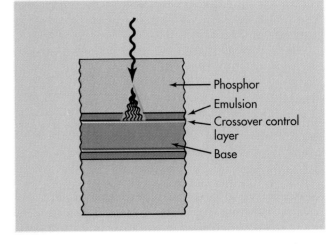

FIGURE 14-8 Crossover is reduced by adding a dye to the base; this dye is called a *crossover control layer.*

Crossover
Crossover is the exposure of an emulsion by light from the opposite-side radiographic intensifying screen.

When light is emitted by a radiographic intensifying screen, it not only exposes the adjacent emulsion but can also expose the emulsion on the other side of the base; this is crossover. When light crosses over the base, it causes increased blur on the image (Figure 14-7).

Crossover is reduced with the use of tabular-grain emulsions because the increased covering power, which relates to not only light absorption from the screen, which is increased, but also light transmitted through the emulsion to crossover. The addition of a light-absorbing dye in a crossover control layer reduces crossover to near zero (Figure 14-8). The crossover control layer has three critical characteristics: it absorbs most of the crossover light, it does not diffuse into the emulsion but remains as a separate layer, and it is completely removed during processing.

Crossover can also be reduced or eliminated by using radiographic intensifying screens, which emit short-wavelength light (blue or ultraviolet). Such light is more strongly absorbed by the silver halide crystals. Also, the polyester base is not transparent to ultraviolet light, so there is no crossover with ultraviolet-emitting screens.

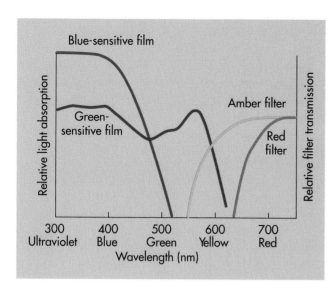

FIGURE 14-9 Radiographic films are either blue or green sensitive, and they require amber and red safelights, respectively.

TABLE 14-2	Approximate Reciprocity Law Failure	
Exposure Time	**Relative Speed (%)**	
1 ms	95	
10 ms	100	
100 ms	100	
1 s	90	
10 s	60	

nation of mA and exposure time as long as the product of mAs is equal. The reciprocity law is summarized as follows:

> **Reciprocity Law**
> Exposure = Intensity × Time
>   = Constant optical density

The reciprocity law is true for film exposed to x-rays. Industrial radiographers do not have to compensate for this effect. The reciprocity law fails when film is exposed to light from radiographic intensifying screens. Radiographers must be aware of this.

Reciprocity law failure is important when long exposure times are used, as in mammography, or short exposure times are used, as in angiography. The result for long or short exposures is reduced speed. An increase in technique may be required. Table 14-2 shows approximate speed loss as a function of exposure time.

Safelights. The use of radiographic film requires certain precautions in the darkroom. Most **safelights** are incandescent lamps with a color filter and provide sufficient illumination in the darkroom while ensuring that the film remains unexposed. Proper darkroom illumination depends not only on the color of the filter but also on the wattage of the bulb and the distance between the lamp and the work surface. A 15-watt bulb should be no closer than 5 feet from the work surface.

With blue-sensitive film, an amber filter is used. An **amber filter** transmits light with wavelengths longer than about 550 nm, which is above the spectral response of blue-sensitive film.

The use of an amber filter would fog green-sensitive film; therefore a **red filter,** which transmits only light above about 600 nm, must be used. A red filter is suitable with both green- and blue-sensitive film. Figure 14-9 shows the approximate transmission characteristics for an amber and a red safelight filter.

Direct-Exposure Film

The use of radiographic intensifying screens allows the radiologic technologist to reduce mAs and therefore lower patient dose, but intensifying screens have the disadvantage of producing a less sharp image than would

Spectral matching. Perhaps, the most important consideration in selecting modern screen-film is its spectral absorption characteristics. Since the introduction of rare earth screens in the early 1970s, radiologic technologists must be particularly careful to use a film whose sensitivity to various colors of light, its spectral response, is properly matched to the spectrum of light emitted by the screen. **Rare earth screens** use rare earth elements, so-called because they are relatively difficult and expensive to extract from the earth.

Calcium tungstate screens emit blue and blue-violet light. All silver halide films respond to violet and blue light but not to green, yellow, or red light unless they are spectrally sensitized with dyes. Many rare earth phosphors are now ultraviolet, blue, green, and red emitting. Although calcium tungstate screens may still be in limited use, they have largely been replaced by rare earth screens.

If green-emitting screens are used, they should be matched with a film that is sensitive not only to blue light but also to green light. Such film is **orthochromatic** and is called *green-sensitive film*. This is distinct from **panchromatic film,** which is used in photography and is sensitive to the entire visible light spectrum.

Figure 14-9 shows the spectral response of blue- and green-sensitive films. Blue-sensitive film should be used only with blue- or ultraviolet-emitting screens. Green-sensitive film is usually exposed with green-emitting screens. If films with sensitivity only in the ultraviolet and blue regions of the spectrum are used with green-emitting screens, the image receptor speed will be greatly reduced, and patient dose will increase. Proper **spectral matching** results in the correct screen-film combination.

Reciprocity law. The reciprocity law states that the density produced by a radiograph is equal for any combibe obtained without a screen. In the past, certain films were manufactured for use without screens, and they were used to image thin body parts, such as the hands and feet, that have high subject contrast and present low radiation risk. Most extremity examinations now use fine-grain, high-detail screens and double-emulsion film as the image receptor. Until the early 1970s, such film was also used for mammography; however, patient dose was much too high. This film typically requires 10 to 100 times more radiation than screen-film; today, such film is rarely used.

This type of film is identified as **direct-exposure film.** The emulsions of direct-exposure film are thicker than those of screen-film, and they contain higher concentrations of silver halide crystals to improve direct x-ray interaction. Direct-exposure film is less sensitive to light and therefore should not be used with screens. Direct-exposure film is usually used with a cardboard cassette, although some are available in individually packaged paper wrappings.

After processing, double-emulsion film is flat because the expansion and contraction characteristics of the two emulsion layers compensate for each other. With single-emulsion film, however, special attention must be paid to the swelling of the emulsion during processing and its shrinking during drying. The backside of the base of single-emulsion film is coated with clear gelatin, so during processing, the emulsion swells, and shrinkage is balanced, ensuring that the film does not curl.

Mammography Film

Mammography was originally performed with an industrial-grade, double-emulsion, direct-exposure film. The radiation doses associated with such a technique were much too high; consequently, specialty films were developed.

Mammography generally uses a single-emulsion film designed to be exposed with a single radiographic intensifying screen. All currently available mammography screen-film systems use green-emitting terbium-doped gadolinium oxysulfide screens with green-sensitive film. However, newer, improved systems are in development that will use different screens with different spectral emulsion characteristics. Digital mammography is also developing.

The surface of the base opposite the screen is coated with a special light-absorbing dye to reduce the reflection of screen light, which is transmitted through the emulsion and base. This effect is called **halation,** and the absorbing dye is an antihalation coating. Such antihalation coating is used on all single-emulsion screen-film, not just mammography film. It is removed during processing for better viewing.

Video Film

The use of video film is rapidly declining because of the increasing application of laser cameras. Video film and

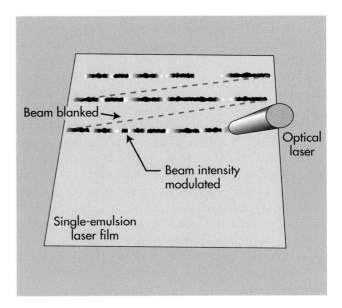

FIGURE 14-10 The laser beam writes in raster fashion.

laser film are used to record images from computed tomography (CT), digital radiography, ultrasound, and magnetic resonance imaging (MRI). In each of these systems, the image receptor is not film but rather some type of radiation detector. The image is formed by computer-assisted analysis of the detected radiation.

Laser Film

A laser printer uses the digital electronic signal from an imaging device. The intensity of the laser beam is varied in direct proportion to the strength of the image signal. This process is called laser-beam **modulation.** While being modulated, the laser beam writes in raster fashion over the entire film (Figure 14-10).

Laser printers provide exceptionally consistent image quality for multiple size films and multiple image formats per film. They can be electronically interfaced with multiple digital imaging modalities such as CT, MRI, and computed radiology. Dry processing of laser film at rates of two, 14″ × 17″ films per minute provides very high productivity (Figure 14-11).

Laser film is silver halide film sensitized to the red light emitted by the laser in much the same way that blue- and green-sensitive screen-film is sensitized. Different types of lasers are used in laser printers, and laser film is light sensitive; therefore laser film must be handled in total darkness.

Figure 14-12 illustrates in cross section a representative sample of single-emulsion film, such as that used for mammography, video imaging, and laser imaging.

Specialty Film

Occasionally, a radiographer is asked to perform a different type of task that requires a different type of film.

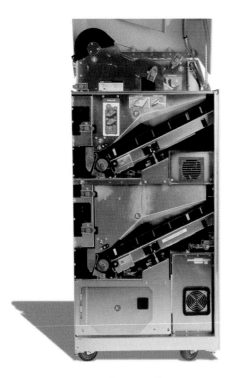

FIGURE 14-11 Cross-sectional view of laser image. (Courtesy Eastman Kodak.)

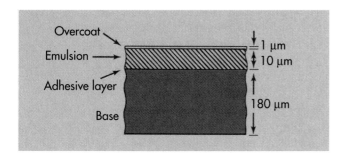

FIGURE 14-12 Cross section of single-emulsion mammography film.

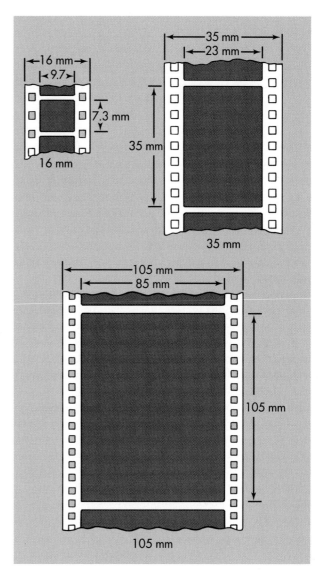

FIGURE 14-13 The format of 16- and 35-mm cine film and 105-mm spot film.

If you want to duplicate an existing radiograph, **duplicating film** is used. Duplicating film is designed for same-size use; that is, the size of duplicating film is equal to the size of the film being duplicated. Duplicating film is a single-emulsion film that is exposed to ultraviolet light or blue light through the existing radiograph to produce a copy.

Subtraction film is sometimes used in angiography, although with the increasing application of digital fluoroscopy, its use is declining. Subtraction film is single emulsion, and there are generally two types. One type is designed to prepare the subtraction mask, and the other accommodates the superimposed image of the original radiograph and subtraction mask. Subtraction film has a high contrast to enhance the existing subject contrast.

Cinefluorography is a special examination reserved al-most exclusively for the cardiac catheterization laboratory. The radiologic technologist who becomes involved in such procedures uses **cine film.** Cine film comes in two sizes, 16 mm and 35 mm, and is supplied in 100- and 500-foot rolls. Most cinefluorography uses 35-mm film, but some gastrointestinal studies can use 16-mm film to good advantage.

Spot Film

Roll films from 70 to 105 mm in width are used in many types of spot film cameras. These films are similar in composition to cine film but are called **spot films.** Spot film is larger than cine film and therefore can be viewed directly on a conventional viewbox without resorting to a projector. Figure 14-13 shows the format of the more popular sizes of cine and roll spot films.

The processing of cine film and spot film is critical to providing a quality image. Roll-type spot film can usually be adequately processed in the automatic processor used for conventional radiographs. Cine film, on the other hand, should be processed with specially designed movie film–processing equipment because when the image is magnified during projection, artifacts are likewise magnified.

HANDLING AND STORAGE OF FILM

Radiographic film is a sensitive radiation detector and must be handled accordingly. Improper handling and storage result in poor radiographs with artifacts that interfere with diagnosis. For this reason it is essential that when handling radiographic film, you take care not to bend, crease, or otherwise subject it to rough handling. Clean hands are a must, and hand lotion and creams should be avoided.

Improper handling or processing can cause **artifacts,** the marks or spurious images that sometimes appear on the processed radiograph. Artifacts can also be generated by the useful x-ray beam. Radiographic film is pressure sensitive, so rough handling or the imprint of any sharp object, such as a fingernail, is reproduced as an artifact on the processed radiograph.

Creasing the film before processing produces a line artifact. Dirt on the hands or on radiographic intensifying screens results in speckled artifacts. In a dry environment, static electricity can cause characteristic artifacts. During automatic processing, wear or dirt on the transport system can cause artifacts that are usually identifiable because they appear on radiograph after radiograph. Identifying artifacts and their causes is covered in Chapter 32.

Heat and Humidity

Radiographic film is sensitive to the effects of elevated temperature and humidity, especially for long periods of time. Heat reduces contrast and increases the fog of a radiograph. Consequently, radiographic film should not be stored at temperatures in excess of about 20° C (68° F). If storage temperatures exceed this, the longer the time of storage, the more severe the loss of contrast because of the increase in fog. Ideally, radiographic films should be refrigerated. Storage for a year or longer is acceptable if the film is maintained at 10° C (50° F). Film should never be stored near steam pipes or other sources of heat.

Humidity also affects film. Storage under conditions of elevated humidity (for example, over 60%) reduces contrast because of increased fog. Consequently, before use, radiographic film should be stored in a cool, dry place, ideally in a climate-controlled environment. However, conditions can be too dry. If the relative humidity dips below about 40%, static artifacts are possible.

Light

Radiographic film must be stored and handled in the dark. No white light can expose the emulsion before processing. If low-level, diffuse light exposes the film, fog will be increased. If bright light exposes or partially exposes the film, a gross, obvious artifact will be produced. Control of light is ensured by having a well-sealed darkroom and a light-proof storage bin for film that has been opened but not clinically exposed. The storage bin should have an electrical interlock to prevent its being opened while the door to the darkroom is ajar or open.

Radiation

Ionizing radiation, other than the useful beam, creates an image artifact by reducing contrast and increasing fog. Darkrooms are usually located next to x-ray rooms and are lead lined. However, this is not always necessary. It is usually acceptable to lead line only the storage shelf and film bin.

Radiographic film is far more sensitive to x-ray exposure than people, and therefore more lead is required to protect film than people. The fog level for unprocessed film is only 0.2 mR (2 μGy_a), and therefore the thickness of the lead barrier will be designed to keep the total exposure of unprocessed film below this level. This of course requires some assumptions about the storage time of the film. If the turnover of film is monthly, then the required lead shielding would be four times more than if it were weekly.

Care should be taken to ensure that the receiving area for radiographic film is not the same as that for the radioactive material used in nuclear medicine. Even though the packaging of radioactive material ensures the safety of those who handle it, the low-level radiation emitted can fog film if the radioactive material and film are stored together for even a short time.

Shelf Life

Most radiographic film is supplied in boxes of 100 sheets. Some film is packaged in an interleaved fashion with chemically treated protective paper between each sheet. Each box contains an expiration date, which indicates the maximum shelf life of the film. Under no circumstances should film be stored for longer periods. Film must be used before its expiration date, usually a year or so after purchase. Aging results in loss of speed and contrast and an increase in fog.

It is always wise to store boxes of film on edge rather than lying flat. When stored on edge, they are less likely to warp and in the case of noninterleaved packaging, less likely to stick to one another.

The storage of film should be sequenced so that the oldest film is used first. Rotation of the film, much like the rotation of perishables in a supermarket, is appropriate. Most hospitals receive film on a monthly basis and purchase enough for 5 weeks of use. The extra time is available in case of civil emergencies, when an unexpectedly large number of x-ray examinations might be necessary. Given a 5-week supply schedule and the first in–first out rule, 45 days is a reasonable maximum storage time for radiographic film.

SUMMARY

Image-forming x-radiation is the part of the x-ray beam that exits a patient and exposes the image receptor. The conventional radiographic image receptor is a cassette containing radiographic film sandwiched between two radiographic intensifying screens. Radiographic film is made of a polyester base covered on both sides with a film emulsion. The film emulsion contains light-sensitive silver bromide crystals, which are made from the mixture of silver nitrate and potassium bromide. During manufacturing, the emulsion is spread onto the base in darkness because the silver bromide molecule is light sensitive.

The unobservable latent image is formed in the film emulsion when light photons interact with the silver halide crystals. Processing converts the latent image into a manifest image.

The following are some important characteristics of radiographic film:

1. *Contrast.* High-contrast film produces black-and-white images. Low-contrast film produces images with shades of gray.
2. *Speed.* Speed is the sensitivity of the screen-film combination to x-rays and light. Fast screen-film combinations need fewer x-rays to produce a diagnostic image.
3. *Crossover.* When light is emitted from a radiographic intensifying screen, it exposes not only the adjacent film emulsion but also the emulsion on the other side of the base. The light crosses over the base and blurs the radiographic image.
4. *Spectral matching.* The x-ray beam does not directly expose the x-ray film. Radiographic intensifying screens emit light when exposed to x-rays and the light, which then exposes the radiographic film. The color of light emitted must match the response of the film.
5. **Reciprocity law.** When exposed to the light of radiographic intensify screens, radiographic film speed varies if a very short or a very long exposure time is used.

Film should be handled carefully and stored at specific temperatures and humidities to reduce artifacts. Artifacts on radiographic film can also be caused by rough handling.

CHALLENGE QUESTIONS

1. Define or otherwise identify the following:
   a. Polyester
   b. Sensitivity center
   c. Latent image
   d. Emulsion covering power
   e. Orthochromatic film
   f. Silver halide
   g. Spectral matching
   h. Artifact
   i. Radiation fog
   j. Shelf life
2. Diagram the cross-sectional view of a radiographic film designed for use with a pair of radiographic intensifying screens.
3. What does the term *dimensional stability* mean when applied to radiographic film? Which part of the film is responsible for this characteristic?
4. List the principal ingredients in the radiographic emulsion and their respective atomic numbers.
5. Silver bromide crystals are made from silver nitrate and potassium bromide. After exposure, some of the silver bromide is reduced to metallic silver. What are the chemical equations representing these interactions?
6. Desribe the process whereby a latent image is created in one crystal of the film emulsion.
7. What is the difference between panchromatic film and orthochromatic film?
8. What determines proper darkroom safelight selection?
9. What precautions are necessary when using films designed specifically for screen-film mammography?
10. What precautions are necessary when using and storing radiographic film?
11. Briefly discuss the history of the development of x-ray film.
12. Write the silver halide crystal reaction. What does the downward arrow represent?
13. What determines the speed of radiographic film?
14. What is the term for closely guarded information held by film manufacturers?
15. Explain the Gurney-Mott theory of the formation of a latent image.
16. What is the importance in spectral matching in choosing screen-film combinations?
17. Why do radiographers need to be aware of reciprocity law failure?
18. An amber filter on a safelight is used under what conditions? A red filter on a safelight is used under what conditions?
19. Discuss the difference between regular screen-film and mammography screen-film.
20. List the proper film storage conditions for (a) temperature, (b) humidity, and (c) shelf life.

Processing the Latent Image

OBJECTIVES

At the completion of this chapter, the student should be able to:

1. Discuss the historical development from manual processing to automatic processing
2. List the chemicals used in each processing step
3. Discuss the use of each chemical
4. Explain the systems of the automatic processor
5. Describe alternative processing methods

OUTLINE

Processing the invisible latent image creates the visible manifest image. Processing converts the light-exposed silver ions in the silver halide crystal to microscopic black grains of silver. The processing sequence has the following steps: (1) wetting, (2) developing, (3) fixing, (4) washing, and (5) drying.

These processing steps are completed in an automatic processor. The design of an automatic processor and its use are reviewed in this chapter. Alternative processing methods are also discussed.

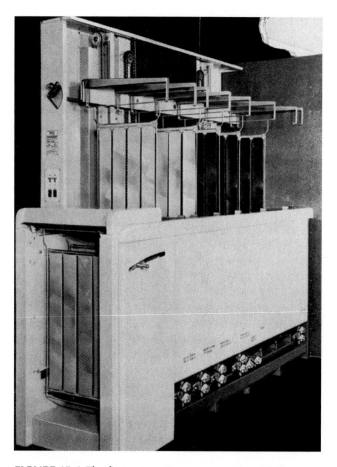

FIGURE 15-1 The first automatic processor, circa 1942. *(Courtesy Art Haus.)*

FILM PROCESSING

The latent image is invisible because only a few silver ions have been changed to metallic silver and deposited at the sensitivity center. Processing the film magnifies this action many millions of times until all the silver ions in an exposed crystal are converted to atomic silver, thus converting the latent image into a manifest radiographic image. The exposed crystal becomes a black grain that is visible microscopically. The silver contained in fine jewelry and tableware would also appear black except that it is highly polished, which smoothes the surface and makes it reflective.

Processing is as important as technique and positioning in making a quality radiograph. Further, a change from the vendor-recommended processing conditions always results in higher patient dose (see Chapter 40).

Manual Processing

Before the introduction of automatic film processing in radiography, x-ray films were processed manually. In manual processing, the exposed radiographic film was first immersed in a tank containing developer for approximately 5 minutes at 20° C (70° F). Films were then immersed in a stop bath, followed by a fixer solution. The film was washed in running water and hung to drip dry. It took approximately 1 hour to obtain a completely dry and ready-to-read radiograph.

Automatic Processing

The first phototype automatic x-ray film processor was introduced by Pako in 1942 (Figure 15-1). The first commercially available model could process 120 films/hr by using special film hangers. These film hangers were dunked from one tank to another. The total cycle time for processing one film was approximately 40 minutes.

A significant improvement in automatic x-ray film processing came in 1956 when the first roller transport system for processing medical radiographs was introduced by the Eastman Kodak Company. This processor accommodated all medical x-ray films that were de-

signed for exposure with radiographic intensifying screens. It was not necessary for hospitals to change film inventories, which obviated the complication of supplying different films to areas that did not have an automatic processor, such as the emergency room, surgery, and urology. The roller-transport automatic processor shown in Figure 15-2 was about 10 feet long, weighed nearly three quarters of a ton, and sold for approximately $225,000 in today's dollars.

Automatic processing revolutionized busy departments. Finished radiographs became available in 6 minutes, and the variability in results caused by the human element was eliminated from processing. It enabled radiologists and radiologic technologists to better standardize techniques so that fewer retakes were needed. Departmental efficiency, work flow, and radiographic quality all improved.

Another significant breakthrough in the production of radiographs was the introduction of 90-s rapid processing in 1965 by the Eastman Kodak Company. Rapid processing was possible because of the development of new chemistry, new emulsions, and the faster drying permitted by the polyester film base. This processor produces a radiograph in a dry-to-drop time of 90 s; 215 sheets of film/hr can be processed. This type of automatic film-processing system remains the standard.

In 1987, Konica introduced an automatic film processor that has a processing cycle of approximately 45 s. This processor, however, requires special films and chemicals. In the future, 20- to 45-s processing may become the standard.

Processing Sequence

A number of steps are involved in the processing of radiographic film, and these are summarized in Table 15-1.

All radiographic processing is done automatically today, and therefore the following discussion does not deal with manual processing. The chemicals involved in both are basically the same. In automatic processing the times for each step are shorter, and the chemical concentrations and temperature are higher.

The first step in the processing sequence is wetting. **Wetting** the film causes the emulsion to swell so that subsequent chemical baths can reach all parts of the emulsion uniformly. Actually, this step is often omitted, and the wetting agent is incorporated into the second step, **developing.**

Developing
Developing is the stage of processing during which the latent image is converted to a manifest image.

The developing stage of processing is very short and very critical. After development, the film is rinsed in an acid solution designed to stop the development process and remove excess developer chemicals from the emulsion. Photographers call this step *stop bath*, and in processing radiographs, the stop bath is included in the next step, **fixing.**

Fixing
Fixing is the stage of processing during which the silver halide that was not exposed to radiation is dissolved and removed from the emulsion.

The gelatin portion of the emulsion is hardened at the same time to make it structurally more sound. Fixing is followed by a vigorous washing of the film to remove any remaining chemicals from the previous processing steps.

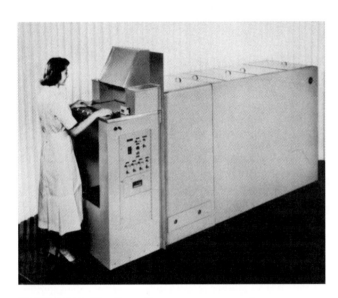

FIGURE 15-2 The first roller-transport automatic processor, circa 1956. *(Courtesy Eastman Kodak Company.)*

TABLE 15-1	Sequence of Events in Processing a Radiograph			
			APPROXIMATE TIME	
Event	**Purpose**		**Manual**	**Automatic**
Wetting	Swelling of the emulsion to permit subsequent chemical penetration		15 s	—
Developing	Production of a manifest image from the latent image		5 min	22 s
Stop bath	Termination of development and removal of excess chemical from the emulsion		30 s	—
Fixing	Removal of the remaining silver halide from the emulsion and hardening of the gelatin		15 min	22 s
Washing	Removal of excess chemicals		20 min	20 s
Drying	Removal of water and preparation of the radiograph for viewing		30 min	26 s

Washing
Washing is the stage of processing during which any remaining chemicals are removed from the film.

Finally, the film is dried to remove the water used to wash it and to make the film acceptable for handling and viewing.

Developing, fixing, and washing are important steps in the processing of radiographic film. The precise chemical reactions involved in these steps are not completely understood. A review of the general action, however, is in order because of the importance processing plays in producing a high-quality radiograph.

PROCESSING CHEMISTRY
Wetting

A **solvent** is a liquid into which various solids and powders can be dissolved. The universal solvent is water, which is the solvent for all the chemicals used in processing a radiograph. For these chemicals to penetrate through the emulsion, the radiograph must first be treated by a **wetting agent.** The wetting agent is water, and it penetrates through the gelatin of the emulsion, causing it to swell. In automatic processing the wetting agent is in the developer.

Developing

The principal action of developing is to change silver ions of the exposed crystals into metallic silver. The developer is the chemical that performs this task. The **developer** provides electrons to the sensitivity center of the crystal to change the silver ions to silver. In addition to the solvent, the developer contains a number of other ingredients. The composition of the developer and the function of each ingredient are outlined in Table 15-2.

For the ionic silver to be changed to metallic silver, an electron must be supplied to the silver ion. Chemically, the reaction is described as follows:

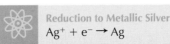

Reduction to Metallic Silver
$$Ag^+ + e^- \rightarrow Ag$$

When an electron is given up by a chemical, the **developing agent** in this case, to neutralize a positive ion, the process is called **reduction.** The silver ion is said to be reduced to metallic silver, and the chemical responsible for this is called a **reducing agent.**

The opposite of reduction is **oxidation,** a reaction that produces an electron. Oxidation and reduction occur simultaneously and are called **redox** reactions. To help recall the proper association, think of **EUR/OPE:** electrons are **u**sed in **r**eduction/**o**xidation **p**roduces **e**lectrons.

The precise chemical compositions of film developers are closely guarded as proprietary secrets. The principal component, however, is a compound called **hydroquinone.** Secondary constituents of the developing agent are **phenidone** and **metol.** Usually, hydroquinone and phenidone are combined for rapid processing. As reducing agents, each of these molecules has an abundance of electrons that can be easily released to neutralize positive silver ions.

Chapter 19 discusses certain aspects of film sensitometry.

The **optical density,** or degree of blackening on a radiograph, of a processed radiograph results from the synergistic action of hydroquinone and phenidone (Figure 15-3).

Synergism means that the action of two agents working together is greater than the sum of the action of each agent working independently.

The characteristic curve of a radiograph is shaped by the synergistic action of developing agents. Hydroquinone is rather slow acting but is responsible for the very blackest shades. Phenidone acts rapidly and influences the lighter shades of gray. Phenidone controls the

TABLE 15-2	Components of the Developer and Their Functions	
Component	**Chemical**	**Function**
Developing agent	Phenidone	Is a reducing agent, produces shades of gray rapidly
Developing agent	Hydroquinone	Is a reducing agent, produces black tones slowly
Buffering agent	Sodium carbonate	Helps swell gelatin, produces alkalinity, controls pH
Restrainer	Potassium bromide	Is an antifog agent, keeps unexposed crystals from being chemically attacked
Preservative	Sodium sulfite	Controls oxidation, maintains balance among developed components
Hardener	Glutaraldehyde	Controls emulsion swelling, aids archival quality
Sequestering agent	Chelates	Remove metallic impurities; stabilize developing agent
Solvent	Water	Dissolves chemicals for use

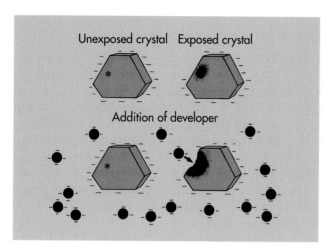

FIGURE 15-3 Development is the chemical process that amplifies the latent image. Only crystals that contain a latent image are reduced to metallic silver by the addition of developer.

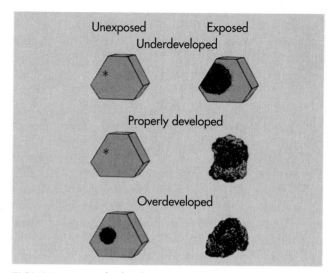

FIGURE 15-5 Underdevelopment results in a dull radiograph because the crystals that contain a latent image have not been completely reduced. Overdevelopment produces a similar radiograph because of the partial reduction of unexposed crystals. Proper development results in maximal contrast.

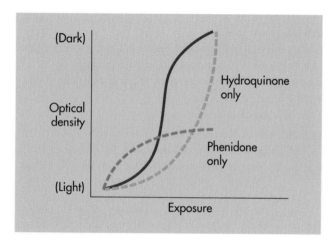

FIGURE 15-4 The shape of the characteristic curve is controlled by the developing agents. Phenidone controls the toe and hydroquinone the shoulder.

toe of the characteristic curve, and hydroquinone controls the shoulder (Figure 15-4).

An unexposed silver halide crystal has a negative electrostatic charge distributed over its entire surface. An exposed silver halide crystal, on the other hand, has a negative electrostatic charge distributed over its surface except in the region of the sensitivity center. The similar electrostatic charges on the developing agent and the silver halide crystal make it difficult for the developing agent to penetrate the crystal surface except in the region of the sensitivity center in an exposed crystal.

In an exposed crystal, the developing agent penetrates through the sensitivity center and reduces the remaining silver ions to atomic silver. The sensitivity center can be considered a metallic, conducting electrode through which electrons are transferred from the developing agent into the crystal. The difference between the development of exposed and unexposed crystals is illustrated in Figure 15-5.

Development occurs over a period of time and depends on factors such as crystal size, developer concentration, and temperature. If you could observe the process in action, you would see a slow buildup of metallic silver at the site of the sensitivity center. After complete development, exposed crystals are destroyed, and a grain of black metallic silver is all that remains. Unexposed crystals remain unaffected.

The reduction of a silver ion is accompanied by the liberation of a bromide ion. The bromide ion migrates through the remnant of the crystal into the gelatin portion of the emulsion. From there it is dissolved into the developer and removed from the film.

The developer contains alkali compounds such as **sodium carbonate** and **sodium hydroxide.** These **buffering agents** enhance the action of the developing agent by controlling the concentration of hydrogen ions: the pH. The pH measures the alkalinity needed by the developer solution. These alkali compounds are caustic; that is, they are very corrosive and can burn the skin. Sodium hydroxide is the strongest alkali and is commonly called **lye.** Be very cautious if you mix a developer solution containing sodium hydroxide. You should wear rubber gloves and, of course, never let it get near your mouth or eyes.

Potassium bromide and **potassium iodide** are added to the developer as restrainers. **Restrainers** restrict the action of the developing agent only to irradiated silver halide crystals. Without the restrainer, even crystals that had not been exposed would be reduced to metallic silver. This results in an increased fog that is termed **development fog.**

A **preservative** is also included in the developer to control the oxidation of the developing agent by air. Air is introduced into the chemistry when it is mixed, handled, and stored; when such oxidation occurs, it is called **aerial oxidation.** By controlling aerial oxidation, the preservative helps maintain the proper development rate.

Mixed chemistry lasts only a couple of weeks, so close-fitting floating lids on replenishment tanks are therefore essential for the control of aerial oxidation. Hydroquinone is particularly sensitive to aerial oxidation. It is easy to tell when the developing agent has been oxidized because it turns brownish. The addition of a preservative causes the developer to remain clear. **Sodium sulfite** is the usual preservative.

Developers used in automatic processors contain a **hardener,** usually glutaraldehyde. If the emulsion swells too much or becomes too soft, the film will not be transported properly through the system because of the very close tolerances of the transport system. The hardener controls the swelling and softening of the emulsion. When films that drop from the processor are damp, the cause is sometimes depletion of the hardener.

 Lack of a sufficient hardener such as glutaraldehyde may be the biggest cause of problems with automatic processing.

Metal impurities and soluble salts may exist in the developer. When these impurities are present, they can accelerate the oxidation of hydroquinone, rendering the developer unstable. **Chelates** are introduced as **sequestering agents** to form stable complexes with these metallic ions and salts.

Importance of Proper Development

Proper development implies that all exposed crystals containing a latent image are reduced to metallic silver, whereas unexposed crystals are unaffected. The development process, however, is not perfect; therefore some crystals containing a latent image remain undeveloped (unreduced), whereas other crystals that are unexposed may be developed. Both of these actions reduce the quality of the radiograph.

Film development is basically a chemical reaction. Like all chemical reactions, it is governed by three physical characteristics: time, temperature, and concentration (of the developer). A long development time leads to increased reduction of the silver in each grain and increased development of the total number of grains. A high developer temperature has the same effect. Similarly, silver reduction is controlled by the concentration of the developing chemicals. With increased developer concentration, the reducing agent becomes more powerful and can more readily penetrate both exposed and unexposed silver halide crystals.

Manufacturers of x-ray film and developing chemicals have very carefully determined the optimal conditions of time, temperature, and concentration for proper development. Optimal conditions of contrast, speed, and fog (see Figure 20-17) can be expected if the manufacturer's recommendations for development are followed. Deviation from the manufacturer's recommendations can result in loss of image quality. Figure 15-5 illustrates three degrees of development for exposed and unexposed crystals. The importance of proper development is obvious.

The image on a fogged film is gray and lacks proper contrast. There are many causes of fog, but perhaps the most important are those just mentioned: time, temperature, and developer concentration. A change in any of these factors above manufacturer recommendations results in increased development fog. Fog can also be produced by chemical contamination of the developer (**chemical fog**), by unintentional exposure to radiation (**radiation fog**), and by improper storage at elevated temperature and humidity. Chemical antifoggants, such as indozoles and triazoles are important ingredients in the developer.

Fixing

Once development is complete, the film must be treated so that the image will not fade but remain permanently. This stage of processing is termed **fixing.** The image is said to be fixed on the film, and this produces film of archival quality. **Archival quality** refers to the permanence of the radiograph: the image thus does not deteriorate with age but remains in its original state.

When the film is removed from the developer, some developer is trapped in the emulsion and continues its reducing action. If developing is not stopped, development fog will result. In manual processing, the step after developing is called *stop bath,* and its function is just that: to neutralize the residual developer in the emulsion and stop its action. The chemical used in the stop bath is **acetic acid.**

In automatic processing, a stop bath is not used because the rollers of the transport system squeeze the film clean. Furthermore, the fixer contains acetic acid that behaves as a stop bath. This acetic acid, however, is called an activator. An **activator** neutralizes the pH of the emulsion and stops developer action. Table 15-3 lists the chemical components of the fixer.

When referring to the fixing agent, you often hear the terms **clearing agent, hypo,** and **thiosulfate** used interchangeably. Fixing agents remove unexposed and undeveloped silver halide crystals from the emulsion. It is sodium thiosulfate that has been classically referred to as *hypo.* Ammonium thiosulfate, however, is the fixing agent used in most fixer chemistries.

TABLE 15-3	Components of the Fixer and Their Function	
Component	**Chemical**	**Function**
Activator	Acetic acid	Neutralizes the developer and stops its action
Fixing agent	Ammonium thiosulfate	Removes undeveloped silver bromine from emulsion
Hardener	Potassium alum	Stiffens and shrinks emulsion
Preservative	Sodium sulfite	Maintains chemical balance
Buffer	Acetate	Maintains proper pH
Sequestering agent	Boric acids/salts	Remove aluminum ions
Solvent	Water	Dissolves other components

Hypo retention is a term used to describe the undesirable retention of the fixer in the emulsion. Excess hypo slowly oxidizes and causes the image to discolor to brown over a long period of time. Fixing agents retained in the emulsion combine with silver to form silver sulfide, which appears yellow-brown.

 Silver sulfide stain is the most common cause of poor archival quality.

The fixer also contains a chemical called a **hardener.** As the developed and unreduced silver bromide is removed from the emulsion during fixation, the emulsion shrinks. The hardener accelerates this shrinking process and causes the emulsion to become more rigid or hardened. The purpose of hardeners is to ensure that the film is transported properly through the wash-and-dry section and to ensure rapid and complete drying. The chemicals commonly used as hardeners are **potassium alum, aluminum chloride,** and **chromium alum.** Normally, only one is used in a given formulation.

The fixer also contains a **preservative** that is of the same composition and that serves the same purpose as the preservative in the developer. The preservative is **sodium sulfite,** and it is necessary for maintaining the chemical balance because of the carryover of developer and fixer from one tank to another.

The alkalinity and acidity—the pH—of the fixer must remain constant. This is helped by adding a **buffer,** usually acetate, to the fixer.

In the same manner that metallic ions are sequestered in the developer, so must they be in the fixer. Aluminum ions are the principal impurity at this stage. Boric acids and boric salts are used for this purpose.

Finally the fixer contains drinking-quality water as the solvent. Other chemicals might be applicable as a solvent, but they would be thicker and more likely to gum up the transport mechanism of the automatic processor.

Washing

The next stage in processing is to wash away any residual chemicals in the emulsion, particularly hypo clinging to the surface of the film. Water is used as the wash agent. In automatic processing, the temperature of the wash wa-

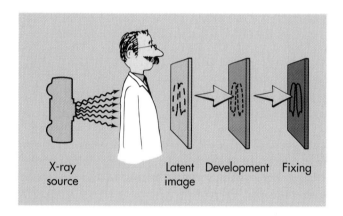

FIGURE 15-6 Converting the latent image to a manifest image is a three-step process.

ter should be maintained at approximately 3° C (5° F) below the developer temperature. In this way, the wash bath also serves to stabilize developer temperature. Inadequate washing leads to excess hypo retention and the production of an image that will fade, turn brown with time, and be of generally poor archival quality.

Drying

The final step in processing, drying the radiograph, is done by blowing warm, dry are over both surfaces of the film as it is transported through the drying chamber.

The total sequence of events involved in manual processing required over 1 hour. Most automatic processors are identified as 90-s processors and require a total time from start to finish—dry-to-drop time—of just that, 90 s.

The process of converting the latent image to a manifest image can be summarized as a three-step process in the emulsion (Figure 15-6). First, the latent image is formed by exposure of silver halide grains. Next, the exposed grains and only the exposed grains are made visible by development. Finally, fixing removes the unexposed grains from the emulsion and makes the image permanent.

SYSTEMS OF THE AUTOMATIC PROCESSOR

The principal components of an automatic processor are the transport system, the temperature-control sys-

TABLE 15-4	Principle Components of an Automatic Processor

System and Subsystem	Purpose
Transport	Transports film through various stages at precise time intervals
Roller	Moves film
Transport rack	Has rollers and guide shoes to move and change the direction of film
Drive	Provides power to turn rollers at a precise rate
Temperature control	Monitors and adjusts the temperature of each stage
Circulation	Agitates fluids
Developer	Continuously mixes, filters
Fixer	Continuously mixes
Wash	Provides water at a constant flow rate
Replenishment	Meters and replaces
Developer	Meters and replaces
Fixer	Removes moisture, vents exhaust
Dryer	Distributes fused power to above
Electrical	systems

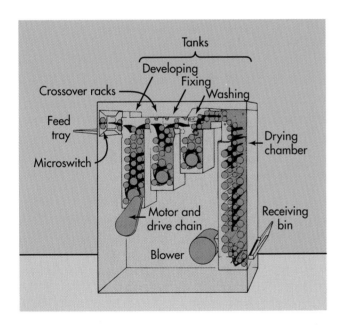

FIGURE 15-7 Cutaway view of an automatic processor with the major components identified.

tem, the circulation system, the replenishment system, the dryer system, and the electrical system (Table 15-4). Figure 15-7 is a cutaway view of an automatic processor.

Transport System

The transport system begins at the **feed tray**, where the film to be processed is inserted into the automatic

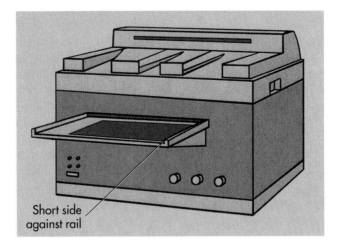

FIGURE 15-8 Place the short side of the film against the guide rail.

processor in the darkroom. There, **entrance rollers** grip the film to begin its trip through the processor. A microswitch is engaged while the film passes to control the replenishment rate of the processing chemicals. Always feed the film evenly using the side rails of the feed tray as a guide and alternate sides from film to film (Figure 15-8). This ensures even wear of the transport system components. From the entrance rollers, the film is transported by rollers and racks through the wet chemistry tanks and drying chamber and finally is deposited in the receiving bin.

 The shorter dimension of the film should always be against the side rail to maintain the proper replenishment rate.

The transport system not only transports the film but also controls processing by controlling the time the film is immersed in each wet chemistry. The sequence of times for each step in processing is accomplished by moving the film through each stage at a carefully controlled rate. The transport system consists of the following three principal subsystems: **rollers, transport racks,** and **drive motor.**

Roller subassembly. Three types of rollers are used in the transport system. **Transport rollers** are 1-inch-diameter rollers that convey the film along its path. They either are positioned opposite one another in pairs or are offset from one another (Figure 15-9). When the film makes a turn in the processor—most of the turns are designed to reverse the direction of the film—a 3-inch-diameter **master roller** or solar roller is used (Figure 15-10). The master roller usually has positioned around it a number of **planetary rollers** and metal or plastic guide shoes.

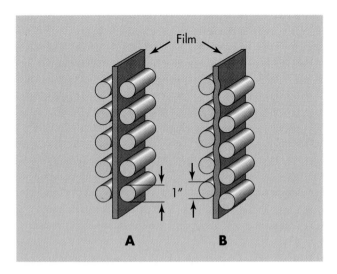

FIGURE 15-9 **A,** Transport rollers positioned opposite one another. **B,** Transport rollers positioned offset from one another.

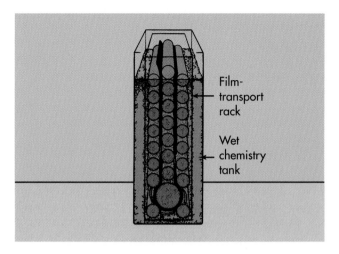

FIGURE 15-11 Transport rack subassembly.

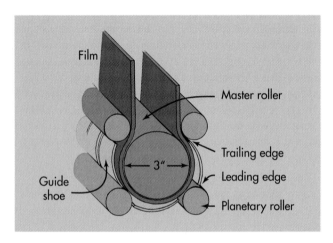

FIGURE 15-10 A master roller with planetary rollers and guide shoes is used to reverse the direction of film in a processor.

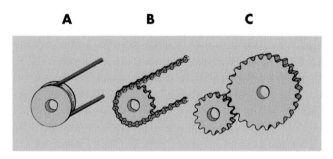

FIGURE 15-12 Three means by which the transfer of power to the transport rack can be accomplished. **A,** Belt and pulley. **B,** Chain and sprocket. **C,** Gears.

Transport-rack subassembly. Except for the entering rollers at the feed tray, most of the rollers in the transport system are positioned on a rack assembly (Figure 15-11). These racks are easily removable and provide for convenient maintenance and efficient cleaning of the processor.

When the film is transported in one direction along the rack assembly, only the 1-inch-diameter rollers are required to guide and propel it. At each bend, however, there is a curved metal lip with smooth grooves to guide the film around the bend. These are called **guide shoes.** For a 180-degree bend, the film is positioned for the turn by the leading guide shoe, is propelled around the curve by the master roller and its planetary rollers, and leaves the curve by entering the next straight run of rollers through the trailing guide shoe.

Such a system of a master roller, planetary rollers, and guide shoes is called a **turnaround assembly.** The turnaround assembly is located at the bottom of the transport rack assembly. Each wet chemistry cycle has a transport rack assembly positioned in the tank. When the film exits the top of the rack assembly, it is guided to the adjacent rack assembly through a **crossover rack.** The crossover rack is a smaller rack assembly composed of rollers and guide shoes.

Drive subsystem. Power for the transport system is provided by a fractional-horsepower drive motor. The shaft of the drive motor is usually reduced to 10 to 20 rpm through a gear-reduction assembly. A chain, pulley, or gear assembly transfers power to the transport rack and drives the rollers. Figure 15-12 illustrates the three principal mechanical devices: a belt and pulley, a chain and sprocket, and gears. These devices connect the mechanical energy of the drive motor to the drive motor mechanism of the rack assembly.

Film transport time should not vary by more than ±2% of the time specified by the manufacturer.

The speed of the transport system is controlled by both the speed of the motor and the gear reduction system used. The tolerance on this mechanical assembly is quite rigid.

Temperature-Control System

The developer, fixer, and wash require precise temperature control. The developer temperature is most critical, and it is usually maintained at 35° C (95° F). Wash water is 2.8° C (5° F) lower. Temperature is monitored at each stage by a thermocouple or thermistor. Control in each tank is provided by a thermostatically controlled heating element.

Circulation System

Anyone who has manually processed a radiograph knows how important it is to agitate the film during processing. Agitation is necessary to continually mix the processing chemistry, to maintain a constant temperature throughout the processing tank, and to aid in the exposure of the emulsion to the chemistry.

In automatic processing, a circulation system continuously pumps the developer and fixer, keeping each tank in constant agitation. This constant agitation keeps the chemicals mixed and keeps them from separating out. A filter that traps particles down to approximately 100 μm in size is required in the developer circulation system to trap flecks of gelatin that are dislodged from the emulsion. The particles thus have less chance of becoming attached to the rollers, where they can produce artifacts. These filters are not 100% efficient, and therefore sludge can build up on the rollers.

Cleaning the tanks and the transport system should be a part of the routine maintenance of any processor.

Filtration in the fixer circulation system is normally unnecessary, since the fixer hardens and shrinks the gelatin so that coating of the rollers does not occur. Furthermore, the fixer neutralizes the developer, and therefore the products of this reaction does not affect the final radiograph.

Circulation of water through the wash tank is necessary to remove all of the processing chemicals from the surface of the film before drying to ensure archival quality. Rather than use a closed circulation system, this is usually done with an open system. Fresh tap water is piped into the tank at the bottom and overflows out the top, where it is collected and discharged directly to the sewer system. The minimum flow rate for the wash tank in most processors is 12 l/min (3 gal/min).

Replenishment System

Each time a film makes its way through the processor, it uses some of the processing chemistry. Some developer is absorbed into the emulsion, and then it is neutralized during fixing. The fixer likewise is absorbed during that stage of processing, and some is carried over into the wash tank. If neither the developer nor the fixer is replenished, each will quickly lose chemical balance, the level of solution in each tank will drop, and short contact times of the film with the chemistry will result.

The replenishment system meters into each tank the proper amount of chemistry to maintain volume and chemical activity. Although the replenishment of the developer is more important, the fixer also has to be replenished. Wash water is not recirculated and therefore is continuously and completely replenished.

When a film is inserted into the feed tray with its widest dimension gripped by the leading rollers and its narrow side against the guide fence, a microswitch is activated and turns on the replenishment for as long as film travels through the microswitch. Replenishment rates are based on the amount of film processed: approximately 60 to 70 ml of developer and 100 to 110 ml of fixer for every 14 inches of film.

Exact film response to overreplenishment or underreplenishment depends on many emulsion variables, so accurate statements are difficult. Usually, if the replenishment rate is increased, a slightly increased radiographic contrast will result. If the rate is too low, a significant decrease in contrast will occur.

Dryer System

A finished radiograph that is wet or damp easily picks up dust particles in the air that could result in artifacts. Furthermore, a wet or damp film is difficult to handle in a viewbox. When stored, it can become sticky and be destroyed. The dryer system extracts all residual moisture from the processed radiograph and drops the dry radiograph into the receiving bin. It consists of a blower, ventilation ducts, drying tubes, and an exhaust system.

The blower is a fan that sucks in room air and blows it across heating coils through ductwork to the drying tubes. The room air therefore should be at low humidity and dust free. Sometimes as many as three heating coils of approximately 2500 watts are used. The temperature of the air entering the drying chamber is thermostatically regulated.

A finished radiograph that is wet or damp easily picks up dust particles in the air that could result in artifacts.

The drying tubes are long hollow cylinders with slit-like openings extending the length of the cylinder and facing the film. These ventilation ducts are positioned on both sides of the film as it is transported through the drying chamber. The hot, moist air is vented from the drying chamber to the outside, much like the air in a clothes dryer. Some fraction of the exhaust air may be recirculated in the dryer system.

When damp films drop into the receiving bin, the radiologic technologist should immediately suspect a malfunction of the dryer system. The developer and fixer replenishment should also be checked.

Electrical System

Electrical power must be provided to the thermal and mechanical components of each of these systems. This is done, of course, through proper wiring of the automatic processor. Normally, each major electrical component is fused. The fuse box is the only part of the electrical system of importance to the radiologic technologist.

ALTERNATIVE PROCESSING METHODS

We tend to think that most of the recent advances in medical x-ray imaging are associated with the imaging devices. This is certainly true. We forget, however, the excellent developments made by the radiographic film manufacturers that have improved image quality and the efficiency of radiology departments. Rapid processing and extended processing are attractive alternatives in many imaging facilities. Daylight processing is fast becoming standard in medical imaging.

Rapid Processing

No matter what the task, today we want to do it faster. Medical imaging is no exception, and the manufacturers of radiographic film have developed microprocessor-controlled equipment and specially formulated processing chemicals for this task. Processing as rapidly as 30 s is now available.

These rapid processors prove to be useful in angiography, special procedures, surgery, and emergency rooms, where time is most critical. In these situations, it is important to have radiographic images available for physicians as soon as possible. When used with proper chemistry, rapid processing produces images with sensitometric properties similar to those of 90-s processing.

For rapid processing, the chemicals are more concentrated, and developer and fixer temperatures are higher. Consequently, it is not possible to switch from standard to rapid processing between films.

Extended Processing

Extended processing finds particular application in mammography. Whereas the standard processing time is 90 s, extended processing may last as long as 3 minutes. Developer immersion time is nearly doubled, but it is not

necessary to alter developer temperature. Furthermore, standard chemicals may be used. The only significant disadvantage is the longer dry-to-drop time.

There are two principal advantages with extended processing: greater image contrast and lower patient dose. Contrast is increased approximately 15%. Image receptor sensitivity is increased by at least 30%. Thus patient radiation dose is reduced by at least 30%.

The improvements in contrast and patient dose with extended processing occur only with single-emulsion film. Extended processing is not recommended for double-emulsion films, since it does not significantly influence contrast or dose with such films.

Daylight Processing

Aside from the speed with which images are developed, there is a change quietly taking place in radiology department darkrooms. They are disappearing! Consequently, the position of darkroom technologist is also disappearing.

Daylight systems are being adopted. In a daylight system (Figure 15-13), the radiologic technologist need only position a cassette with an exposed film into the appropriate slot of the daylight system. The film is automatically extracted from the cassette and sent to the processor. The processor may be an integral part of the daylight system or a separate unit docked to the daylight system.

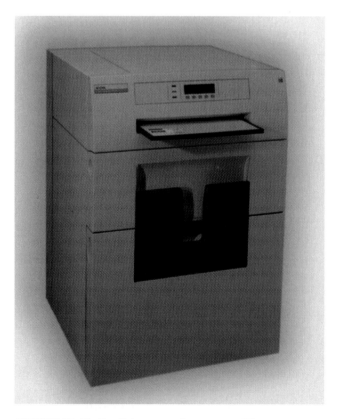

FIGURE 15-13 Daylight processing system. *(Courtesy Eastman Kodak).*

The cassette is reloaded with unexposed film of the proper size before it is released by the system for the next exposure.

Speed is the quality that makes the daylight system attractive. It takes only about 15 s for the radiologic technologist to insert the exposed cassette into the daylight loader and retrieve a fresh cassette. Loading, unloading, and processing time take about 2 minutes. Multiple film sizes are automatically accommodated.

Microprocessor technology makes daylight systems possible. The microprocessor monitors and controls the unloading and reloading of the cassette automatically by sensing the cassette size and film-consumption rate. Most systems can accommodate up to 1000 sheets of radiographic film of various sizes. Some units can also annotate data on the radiograph, including the date, time, and other examination characteristics. System status is continuously indicated with light-emitting diodes (LEDs) or liquid crystal displays (LCDs).

Some systems are designed for special specific applications, such as cardiovascular and interventional radiography. Most are rather small, having a footprint of no more than 1×1 m. Some models are on rollers for even greater flexibility.

SUMMARY

The process of converting the latent image to a manifest image is a three-step process. First, the latent image is formed when silver halide grains are exposed to light or x-rays. Next, only the grains so exposed are made visible by development. Finally, fixing removes the unexposed grains from the emulsion and makes the image permanent.

In 1965, the Eastman Kodak Company developed a 90-s radiographic film rapid processor, which is still the standard of the industry. The steps for manual and automatic processing are the same, but because manual processing takes up to an hour, it is no longer used. The sequence of processing steps are as follows: (1) wetting, (2) developing, (3) fixing, (4) washing, and (5) drying. Tables 15-2 and 15-3 list the chemicals and their functions in the developing and fixing processes.

The components of the automatic processor are (1) the transport system, (2) the temperature-control system, (3) the circulation system, (4) the replenishment system, (5) the dryer system, and (6) the electrical system. Diagnostic imaging departments may have alternative processing systems as well. Special chemicals and chemistry temperatures allow rapid 30-s processing. Extended processing is used to develop specialty films such as single-emulsion mammography screen-film. Daylight processing allows radiographers to maintain uninterrupted patient care; the daylight system commonly is used in critical care areas, such as the emergency department.

CHALLENGE QUESTIONS

1. Define or otherwise identify:
   a. Solvent
   b. Glutaraldehyde
   c. Reducing agent
   d. Synergism
   e. Archival quality
   f. Planetary roller
   g. Guide shoe
   h. Extended processing
   i. LED
   j. "Dry-to-drop"
2. Identify the steps involved in the automatic processing of a radiograph and the time of each step for a 90-s processor.
3. Describe the action of phenidone and hydroquinone in producing optical density on a radiograph.
4. By what other name is *fixer* known?
5. What are the characteristic features of daylight processing?
6. During the wash cycle, what restrictions are placed on temperature and flow rate?
7. What is a redox reaction?
8. When did automatic processing begin?
9. Which company invented the first roller-transport processing system?
10. What type of processors are used in the clinical sites you visit?
11. What is the universal wetting agent?
12. What is the principal action of development?
13. Give an example of a redox reaction.
14. Name the principal component in developer solutions.
15. Why should you wear gloves and goggles when mixing or handling developer solutions?
16. What happens over time if the preservative is not added to the developer?
17. If a film drops into the receiving bin damp or wet, what kind of problem does this probably indicate?
18. Why does the film need to go through the fixer tank?
19. If a radiographic film turns brown once it has been stored in the file room, what may be the problem?
20. How should each x-ray film be fed onto the feed tray of the automatic processor? Why is this important?

Radiographic Intensifying Screens

OBJECTIVES

At the completion of this chapter, the student should be able to:

1. Describe the component layers of a radiographic intensifying screen
2. Discuss luminescence and its relationship to phosphorescence and fluorescence
3. Define and use the term *intensification factor*
4. Identify how x-ray absorption efficiency and x-ray–to–light conversion efficiency affect screen speed
5. Define *image noise* and *image blur* and describe how to remedy them
6. Discuss the various screen-film combinations
7. Describe the handling and cleaning of radiographic intensifying screens

OUTLINE

Radiographic intensifying screens are part of the conventional image receptor. The image receptor includes the cassette, which is the protective holder; the radiographic intensifying screens; and the radiographic film.

Even though some x-rays reach the film emulsion, it is actually visible light from the radiographic intensifying screens that exposes the radiographic film. Visible light is emitted from the phosphor of the radiographic intensifying screens, which is activated by the image-forming x-rays exiting the patient.

This chapter discusses the components of radiographic intensifying screens and how these components contribute to a screen's performance characteristics. The properties of rare earth screens and the importance of spectral matching are also presented.

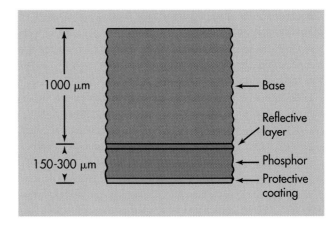

FIGURE 16-1 Cross-sectional view of an intensifying screen, showing its four principal layers.

SCREEN CONSTRUCTION

Using radiographic film to detect x-rays and image anatomic structures is inefficient. In fact, less than 1% of the x-rays incident on radiographic film interact with the film to contribute to the latent image. For increased efficiency, most radiographs are made with films placed in contact with radiographic intensifying screens. A **radiographic intensifying screen** is a device that converts the energy of the x-ray beam into visible light. This visible light then interacts with the radiographic film to form the latent image. Approximately 30% of the x-rays striking a radiographic intensifying screen interact with the screen. For each such interaction, a large number of visible light photons are emitted.

The radiographic intensifying screen acts as an amplifier of the remnant radiation reaching the screen-film cassette.

The use of a radiographic intensifying screen results in considerably lower patient dose but has the disadvantage of causing a slight blurring of the image. With modern screens, however, such image blur is not serious.

Radiographic intensifying screens resemble flexible sheets of plastic or cardboard. They come in sizes corresponding to film sizes. Usually, the radiographic film is sandwiched between two screens. The film used is called **double-emulsion film,** which has an emulsion coating on both sides of the base and a layer of supercoat over each emulsion. In most screens, there are four distinct layers: the protective coating, the phosphor, the reflective layers, and the base (Figure 16-1).

Protective Coating

The layer of the radiographic intensifying screen closest to the radiographic film is the **protective coating.** It is 10 to 20 μm thick and is applied to the face of the screen to make the screen resistant to abrasion and damage caused by handling. It also helps eliminate the buildup of static electricity and provides a surface for routine cleaning without disturbing the active phosphor. Naturally, the protective layer is transparent to light.

Phosphor

The active layer of the radiographic intensifying screen is the **phosphor.** The phosphor emits light during stimulation by x-rays. The active substance of most phosphors before about 1970 was crystalline calcium tungstate ($CaWO_4$) embedded in a polymer matrix. The **rare earth elements,** gadolinuim, lanthanum, and yttrium, are the phosphor material in newer, faster screens.

The term *rare earth* describes the elements of group III of the periodic table (see Figure 4-4) having atomic numbers of 57 to 71. These elements are transitional metals found in low abundance in nature. Those used in rare earth screens are principally gadolinium, lanthanum, and yttrium. The compositions of the four principal rare earth phosphors are terbium-activated gadolinium oxysulfide ($Gd_2O_2S{:}Tb$), terbium-activated lanthanum oxysulfide ($La_2O_2S{:}Tb$), terbium-activated yttrium oxysulfide ($Y_2O_2S{:}Tb$), and lanthanum oxybromide (LaOBr).

Phosphors convert the x-ray beam into light.

The action of the phosphor can be demonstrated by viewing an opened cassette in a darkened room through the protective barrier of the control booth. The radiographic intensifying screen glows brightly when exposed to x-rays. Many materials react in this way, but to be satisfactory for use in radiography, they must possess the characteristics given in Box 16-1. Calcium tungstate, zinc sulfide, barium lead sulfate, and the rare earth elements, gadolinium, lanthanum, and yttrium, exhibit these characteristics.

Roentgen accidently discovered x-rays when he observed the luminescence of barium platinocyanide, a phosphor that was never applied to diagnostic radiology with success. Within a year of Roentgen's discovery of x-rays, calcium tungstate was developed by the American inventor, Thomas A. Edison. Although Edison demonstrated the use of radiographic intensifying screens before the beginning of the twentieth century, screen-film combinations did not come into general use until about the time of World War I. The phosphor used at that time was calcium tungstate.

For a time, barium lead sulfate screens were used, particularly with techniques using high peak kilovoltage (kVp). Zinc sulfide was once used for low-kVp techniques but never gained wide acceptance. Calcium tungstate, because of improved manufacturing techniques and quality-control procedures, proved superior for nearly all radiographic techniques and until the 1970s was the phosphor used almost exclusively. Since then, **rare earth screens** have been used in diagnostic radiology. These screens are faster than those made of calcium tungstate, rendering them more useful for most types of radiographic imaging. The use of rare earth screens results in lower patient dose, less thermal stress on the x-ray tube, and a reduced shielding requirement for x-ray rooms.

Differences in screen-imaging characteristics are basically caused by differences in the composition of the phosphor. The thickness of the phosphor layer and the concentration and size of the phosphor crystals also influence the action of radiographic intensifying screens. The thickness of the phosphor layer ranges from approximately 150 to 300 μm, with individual phosphor crystals ranging from 5 to 15 μm.

Reflective Layer

Between the phosphor and the base is a **reflective layer** that is approximately 25 μm thick and made of a shiny substance, such as magnesium oxide or titanium dioxide (Figure 16-2). When x-rays interact with the phosphor, light is emitted isotropically. Less than half the light is emitted in the direction of the film. The reflective layer intercepts light headed in other directions and redirects it to the film. The reflective layer increases the efficiency of the radiographic intensifying screen, nearly doubling the number of light photons reaching the film.

Isotropic Emission
Isotropic emission of radiation means that radiation is emitted with equal intensity in all directions.

Some radiographic intensifying screens incorporate special dyes in the phosphor layer to selectively absorb the light photons emitted at a large angle to the film. These light photons increase image blur. Because they must travel a longer distance in the phosphor than those emitted perpendicular to the film, these photons are more easily absorbed by the dye. Unfortunately, this addition results in some reduction in screen speed.

Base

The layer farthest from the film is the **base**, which is about 1 mm thick and serves principally as a mechanical support for the active phosphor layer. It is made of high-grade cardboard or polyester. Polyester is the popular base material in the construction of radiographic inten-

---

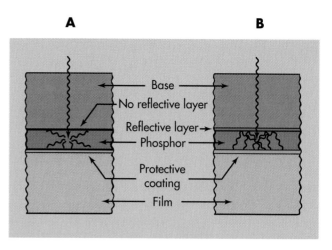

FIGURE 16-2 A, Screen without reflective layer. **B,** Screen with reflective layer. Screens without reflective layers are not as efficient as those with reflective layers because fewer light photons reach the film.

sifying screens just as it is for radiographic film. The requirements for a base material of high quality are given in Box 16-2.

LUMINESCENCE

Any material that emits light in response to some outside stimulation is called a *luminescent material* or a *phosphor*, and the visible light emitted is called **luminescence**. Materials can be caused to luminesce by a number of different stimuli, such as electric current (the fluorescent light), biochemical reactions (the lightning bug), visible light (a watch dial), and x-rays (a radiographic intensifying screen).

Luminescence is a process similar to characteristic x-ray emission. However, luminescence involves outer-shell electrons (Figure 16-3). In a radiographic intensifying screen, a single x-ray absorption causes thousands of light photons to be emitted.

When a luminescent material is stimulated, the outer-shell electrons far from the nucleus are raised to excited energy levels. This effectively creates a hole in the outer electron shell, which is an unstable condition for the atom. The hole is filled when the excited electron returns to its normal state, and this transition is accompanied by the emission of electromagnetic energy in the form of a visible light photon.

Energy is required to raise the outer-shell electron to an excited state, and this energy is released when the electron returns to its normal state. Only a narrow range of excited energy states for an outer-shell electron is possible, and these states depend on the structure of the luminescent material. The wavelength of the emitted light is determined by the level of excitation to which the electron was raised and is characteristic of a given luminescent material. Consequently, luminescent materials emit light of a characteristic color.

There are two types of luminescence. If visible light is emitted only while the phosphor is stimulated, the process is called **fluorescence**. If, on the other hand, the phosphor continues to emit light after stimulation, then the process is called **phosphorescence**. Some materials can phosphoresce for long periods after stimulation. For example, a light-stimulated watch dial fades slowly in a dark room. Radiographic intensifying screens fluoresce. Phosphorescence in an intensifying screen is called **screen lag** or **afterglow** and is objectionable.

There is a precise distinction between fluorescence and phosphorescence related to the motion of the excited electron around the nucleus. If the electron returns to its normal state with the emission of light within one revolution after stimulation, then fluorescence has occurred. If more than one revolution is required, then the process is phosphorescence. The time required for an electron to make one revolution about the nucleus is 10 ns (Table 16-1).

BOX 16-2   Favorable Properties of Radiographic Intensifying Screen Base

Is rugged and moisture resistant
Does not suffer radiation damage and discoloration with age
Is chemically inert and does not interact with the phosphor layer
Is flexible
Does not contain impurities that would be imaged by x-rays

TABLE 16-1	Luminescence	
Fluorescence		**Phosphorescence**
No lag		Afterglow
$<10^{-8}$ seconds		$>10^{-8}$ seconds

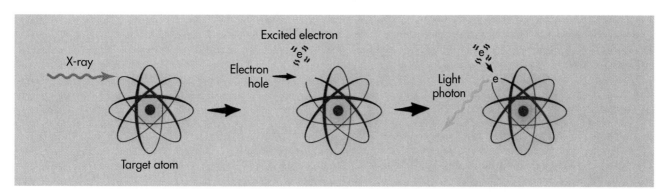

FIGURE 16-3 Luminescence occurs when an outer-shell electron is raised to an excited state and returns to its ground state with the emission of a light photon.

SCREEN CHARACTERISTICS

Three primary characteristics of radiographic intensifying screens are important to the radiologic technologist: screen speed, image noise, and spatial resolution.

Screen Speed

Screen speed is a relative number used to identify the efficiency of conversion of x-rays into usable light. There are many types of radiographic intensifying screens, and each manufacturer uses different names to identify them. Collectively, however, screens usually can be identified according to three broad categories: par speed, high speed, and fine detail. Par-speed calcium tungstate screens are assigned a value of 100 and are the basis for comparison of all other screens. Although calcium tungstate was the prominent phosphor used in radiographic intensifying screens for many years, today, rare earth phosphors have generally replaced it. High-speed rare earth screens have speeds up to 1200, and fine-detail screens have speeds of approximately 50 to 80. These and other characteristics are summarized in Table 16-2.

Since radiographic intensifying screens are used to reduce patient dose, it is important to know the magnitude of the dose reduction obtained. However, the speed of a radiographic intensifying screen conveys no information concerning dose reduction to the patient. This information is related by the **intensification factor (IF)**, which is the ratio of the exposures required to produce the same optical density with and without screens; as follows:

Intensification Factor

$$IF = \frac{\text{Exposure required without screen}}{\text{Exposure required with screens}}$$

The optical density chosen for comparing one radiographic intensifying screen with another is usually 1.0. The value of the intensification factor can be used to determine the dose reduction accompanying the use of a screen.

Question: A pelvic examination using a 100-speed radiographic intensifying screen is performed at 75 kVp and 50 mAs and results in an entrance skin exposure of 200 mR (2 mGy$_a$). A similar examination taken without screens would result in an entrance skin exposure of 6400 mR (64 mGy$_a$). What is the intensification factor of the screen-film combination?

Answer: $IF = \dfrac{6400}{200} = 32$

Several factors influence radiographic intensifying screen speed, some of which are under the control of the radiologic technologist. Ultimately, screen speed is determined by the relative number of x-rays interacting with the phosphor and the efficiency of conversion of x-ray energy into the visible light that interacts with the film.

The properties of radiographic intensifying screens that affect screen speed are given in Box 16-3 and cannot be controlled by the radiologic technologist. They are listed in their relative order of importance. Several conditions that affect radiographic intensifying screen speed are under the control of the radiologic technologist. They include radiation quality, image processing, and temperature.

Radiation quality. As x-ray tube potential is increased, the IF also increases (Figure 16-4). Although this may seem contrary to the discussion of x-ray absorption in Chapter 13, it is not.

In Chapter 13, x-ray absorption was shown to decrease with increasing kVp. Remember, however, that the IF is the ratio of x-ray absorption in a radiographic in-

TABLE 16-2	Some Characteristics of Typical Radiographic Intensifying Screens	
	TYPE OF SCREEN	
Type of Phosphor	**Calcium Tungstate**	**Oxysulfides or Oxybromides of Y, La, Gd**
Color of emission	Blue	Green or blue
Approximate speed	50-200	80-1200
Intensification factor	20-100	40-400
Resolution (lp/mm)	15	15

Y, yttrium; *La,* lanthanum; *Gd,* gadolinium; *lp,* line pairs.

BOX 16-3   Properties of Radiographic Intensifying Screen Speed that are Not Controlled by the Radiologic Technologist

Phosphor composition. Rare earth phosphors are very efficient at absorbing x-rays and converting them to visible light.
Phosphor thickness. The thicker the phosphor layer, the higher the relative number of x-rays converted into light. High-speed screens have thick phosphor layers; fine-detailed screens have thin phosphor layers.
Reflective layer. The presence of a reflective layer increases screen speed but also increases image blur.
Dye. Light-absorbing dyes are added to some phosphors to control the spread of light. These dyes improve spatial resolution but reduce speed.
Crystal size. Larger individual phosphor crystals produce more light emission per x-ray interaction. The phosphor crystals of high-speed screens are approximately 8 μm in size. The crystals of fine-detailed screens are approximately half that size.
Concentration of phosphor crystals. Higher crystal concentration results in higher screen speed.

tensifying screen to that in radiographic film alone. Screens have a higher effective atomic number than films, and therefore, although true absorption in the screen decreases with increasing kVp, the relative absorption compared with that in film increases. At 70 kVp, the IF for a typical par-speed screen is 60, whereas that for a rare earth screen is 150.

Image processing. Only the superficial layers of the emulsion are affected when radiographic film is exposed to light. However, the emulsion is affected uniformly throughout when the film is exposed to x-rays. Therefore excessive developing time for screen-film results in a lowering of the IF because the emulsion nearest the base contains no latent image, yet can be reduced to silver if the developer is allowed sufficient time to penetrate the emulsion to the depth. This too is relatively unimportant, since films manufactured for use with screens have thinner emulsion layers than those produced for direct exposure.

Temperature. Radiographic intensifying screens emit more light per x-ray interaction at low temperatures than at high temperatures. Consequently, the IF is less at higher temperature. This characteristic, although relatively unimportant in a clinic with a controlled environment, can be significant in field work in hot or cold climates.

Image Noise

Image noise appears on a radiograph as a speckled background. It occurs more often when fast screens and high-

kVp techniques are used. Noise reduces image contrast. Chapter 20 discusses noise more completely.

Rare earth radiographic intensifying screens have increased speed because of two important characteristics, both of which are higher compared to other types of screens. The percentage of x-rays that are absorbed by the screen is higher. This is called **detective quantum efficiency (DQE)**. The amount of light emitted for each x-ray absorbed is also higher. This is called **conversion efficiency (CE)**.

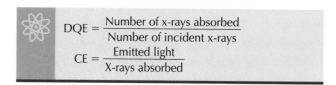

Figure 16-5 illustrates why an increase in the CE increases image noise but an increase in the DQE does not. In Figure 16-5, *A*, a calcium tungstate screen has a DQE of 20% and a CE of 5%. A radiographic technique of 10 mAs results in 1000 x-rays incident on the screen, 200 of which are absorbed, resulting in light photons equivalent to 10 x-rays. We could say that this system has a relative speed of 100.

Higher conversion efficiency results in increased noise.

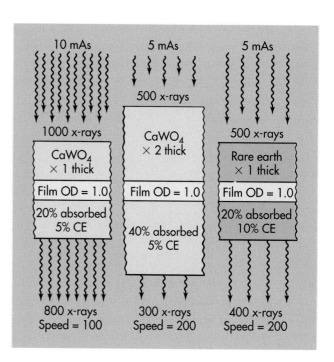

FIGURE 16-4 Approximate variation of the IF with kVp.

FIGURE 16-5 Image noise increases with higher CE but not with higher DQE.

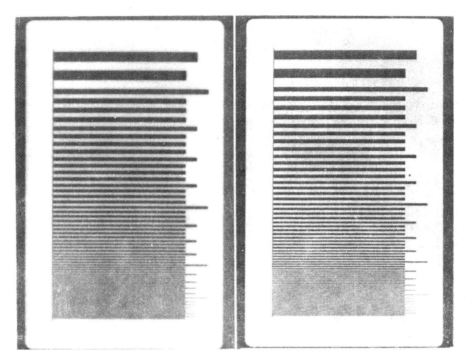

FIGURE 16-6 Radiographs of an x-ray test pattern made with direct-exposure film *(right)* and a par-speed screen-film combination *(left)*. The difference in image blur is obvious.

If the phosphor thickness is doubled as in Figure 16-5, *B*, the DQE increases to 40%, so the mAs can be reduced to 5. The speed is now 200, but there is no increase in noise because the same number of x-rays are used.

However, if the phosphor is changed to one that has a CE of 10%, the speed is doubled at the expense of increased noise (Figure 16-5, *C*). A 200-speed screen is attained because twice as much light is emitted per x-ray absorption. Only half as many x-rays are required, and this results in increased quantum mottle, a principal component of image noise. **Quantum mottle** is often a direct result of using very-fast-speed film-screen systems requiring very small amounts of exposure and resulting in a grainy, mottled, or splotchy image.

In practice, rare earth screens of the same spatial resolution are at least twice as fast as calcium tungstate screens with no significant increase in noise. Rare earth screens have higher DQE and CE, but the gain in speed is due principally to DQE.

Spatial Resolution

Unfortunately, when the remnant x-radiation is converted to visible light and the visible light in turn produces the latent image, some blurring of the image occurs. The **spatial resolution** of the screen is its ability to produce an accurate and clear image.

Radiographers often use the terms **image detail** or *visibility of detail* when describing image quality. These qualitative terms combine the quantitative measures of spatial resolution and contrast resolution. *Spatial resolution* refers to how small an object can be imaged. **Con-**trast resolution** refers to the ability to distinguish between and image similar tissues, such as the liver and pancreas or gray matter and white matter.

 Image detail is determined by spatial resolution and contrast resolution.

Although the use of radiographic intensifying screens adds one more step to the process of imaging the body with x-rays, such radiographs have the disadvantage of lower spatial resolution compared with direct-exposure radiographs.

Spatial resolution is measured in a number of ways and can be given a numerical value. Spatial resolution is influenced principally by effective focal spot size. Secondary factors affecting spatial resolution are geometry, crystal size of the radiographic intensifying screen phosphors, (screen blur), and crystal size of the film emulsion (film graininess) (see Chapter 20).

A photograph in focus shows good spatial resolution; one out of focus shows poor spatial resolution and therefore much image blur. Figure 16-6 shows the differences in spatial resolution between a direct-exposure film and a par-speed screen-film combination obtained when imaging an x-ray test pattern. Such a test pattern is called a *line pair test pattern*. It has lead grid lines separated by equal-size interspaces. As discussed more completely in Chapter 29, spatial resolution may be expressed by the number of line pairs per millimeter (lp/mm) that are imaged. The higher this number, the smaller the object that can be imaged and the better

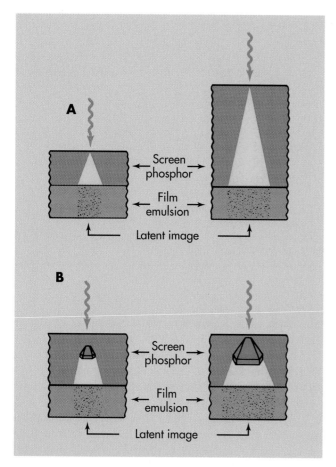

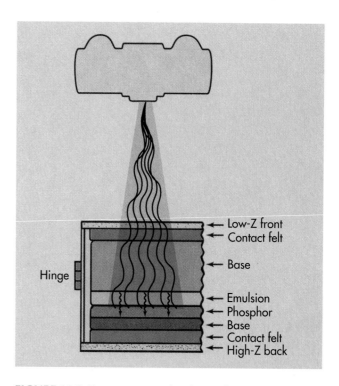

FIGURE 16-7 **A,** The reduction in spatial resolution is greater when phosphor layers are thick. **B,** The reduction is also greater when crystal size is large. These same conditions increase screen speed by producing more light photons per incident x-ray.

FIGURE 16-8 For mammography, the single screen is on the far side of the emulsion to reduce screen blur.

the spatial resolution. Very fast screens can resolve 7 lp/mm, and fine-detail screens can resolve 15 lp/mm (Table 16-2). Direct-exposure film can resolve 50 lp/mm. The unaided eye can resolve about 10 lp/mm.

When x-rays interact with the screen's phosphor, a larger area of the film emulsion is activated by the emitted light than would be with direct x-ray exposure. This results in reduced spatial resolution or more image blur.

 Generally, the conditions that increase the IF reduce spatial resolution.

High-speed screens have low spatial resolution, and fine-detail screens have high spatial resolution. Spatial resolution improves with smaller phosphor crystals and thinner phosphor layers. Figure 16-7 shows how these factors affect spatial resolution. Unfortunately, these factors are not under the control of the radiologic technologist.

In both parts of Figure 16-7 the x-ray is shown to interact with the phosphor soon after entering it. This re-

sults in screen blur. Screen blur is reduced in thinner screens. Figure 16-8 illustrates how spatial resolution is improved in mammography by placing the single-emulsion film on the tube side of the cassette. (See Chapter 23 for a more complete discussion.)

 In mammography, the screen is positioned in contact with the emulsion on the side of the film away from the x-ray source to reduce screen blur and improve spatial resolution.

SCREEN-FILM COMBINATIONS

Radiographic intensifying screens and films are manufactured for compatibility. The best results are obtained if screens and films are selected with this in mind. Radiographic intensifying screens are nearly always used in pairs. Figure 16-9 is a cross section of a properly loaded cassette containing front and back screens with a double-emulsion film. Production of the latent image is nearly evenly divided between front and back screens, with less than 1% being contributed directly by x-ray interaction. Each screen exposes the emulsion with which it is in contact.

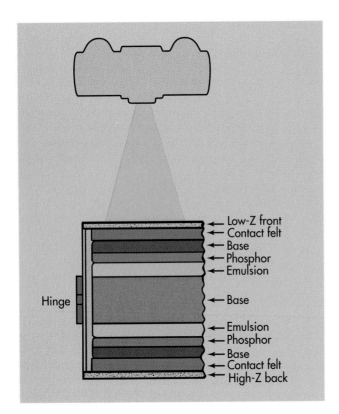

FIGURE 16-9 Cross-sectional view of a cassette containing front and back screens and double-emulsion film.

 Make sure that the film and screen are compatible. Use only the films for which the screens are designed.

In addition to reduced patient dose, the use of radiographic intensifying screens in an image receptor offers several advantages, which are summarized in Box 16-4. Proper selection, handling, and use of a screen-film combination are essential if all of these advantages are to be realized.

Cassettes

The **cassette** is the rigid holder that contains the film and radiographic intensifying screens. The front cover, the side facing the x-ray source, should be made of material with a low atomic number, such as plastic. It should be as thin as is practicable, yet sturdy. The front cover of the cassette is designed for minimal attenuation of the x-ray beam.

Attached to the inside of the front cover is the front screen, and attached to the back cover is the back screen. The radiographic film is sandwiched between the two screens.

Between each screen and the cassette cover is some sort of **compression device,** such as felt or rubber, which

maintains close screen-film contact when the cassette is closed and latched.

The back cover is usually made of heavy metal to minimize backscatter. The x-rays transmitted through the screen-film combination to the back cover are absorbed photoelectrically more readily in a material with a high atomic number than in a material with a low atomic number. X-rays could be transmitted through the entire cassette, and some might be scattered back to the film by the cassette-holding device or a nearby wall. This is called **backscatter radiation** and results in image blur. Sometimes the cassette hinges or hold-down clamps on the back cover are imaged. This is due to backscatter radiation and normally occurs only during high-kVp radiography when the x-ray beam is sufficiently penetrating.

One of the materials that the United States developed early in its space exploration program was carbon fiber. This material was developed for nose cone applications because of its excellent strength and heat resistance. It consists principally of graphite fibers ($Z_C = 6$) in a plastic matrix that can be formed to any shape or thickness.

This material is now widely used in radiology in devices designed to reduce patient exposure. A cassette with a front consisting of carbon fiber material absorbs only approximately half the x-rays absorbed in an aluminum or a cardboard cassette. Carbon fiber is also being used as pallet material for fluoroscopic examination tables and computed tomography couches. The use of carbon fiber not only reduces the patient exposure but may also result in longer x-ray tube life because of the lower radiographic techniques required.

Direct Film Exposure vs. Screen-Film Exposure

The principal advantage of the use of radiographic intensifying screens is that fewer x-rays are needed than in direct-exposure techniques. Table 16-3 shows the rela-

TABLE 16-3	Comparison of Relative Number of X-Rays and Light Photons for Direct and Screen-Film Exoposure*	
Stage	**TYPE OF EXPOSURE**	
	Direct	**Screen-Film**
Incident x-rays	1000	20
X-rays absorbed by film	10	<1
X-rays absorbed by screens	—	5
Light photons produced	—	5000
Light photons incident on film	—	3000
Light photons absorbed by film	—	1000
Latent images formed	10	10

*Intensification factor = 1000/20 = 50.

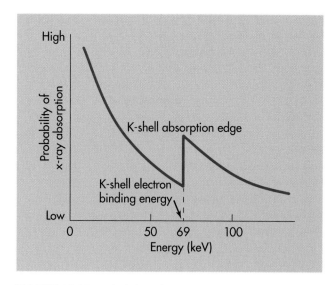

FIGURE 16-10 Probability of x-ray absorption in a calcium tungstate screen as a function of the incident x-ray energy.

TABLE 16-4	Composition and Emulsion of Radiographic Intensifying Screens	
Phosphor	**Activator**	**Emission**
Barium fluorochloride	Europium	Ultraviolet
Barium strontium sulfate	Europium	Ultraviolet
Barium sulfate	Lead	Ultraviolet
Zinc sulfide	Silver	Blue-ultraviolet
Calcium tungstate	Lead	Blue
Lanthanum oxybromide	Thulium	Blue
Yttrium oxysulfide	Terbium	Blue
Gadolinium oxysulfide	Terbium	Green
Lanthanum oxysulfide	Terbium	Green
Zinc cadmium sulfide	Silver	Yellow-green

tive number of x-rays and light photons at various stages for radiographs taken with direct exposure and with a par-speed screen-film combination. The major differences are caused by the interaction of x-rays with the screen phosphor and by the large number of visible light photons produced by each interaction. Unfortunately, the number of latent image centers formed is less than 1% of the number of light photons produced.

Rare Earth Screens

Table 16-4 lists the phosphors that are used in radiographic intensifying screens. Except for barium- and zinc-based phosphors and calcium tungstate, the other phosphors are rare earth elements, and therefore these screens have come to be known as *rare earth screens.*

Rare earth radiographic intensifying screens are manufactured to perform at several speed levels up to a relative level of 1200. This increase in speed is obtained without loss of resolution; however, with the fastest rare earth screens, the effects of quantum mottle (ra-

diographic noise) are noticeable and can become bothersome (see Chapter 21).

Since rare earth radiographic intensifying screens are faster, lower radiographic technique can be used, resulting in lower patient dose. Rare earth screens provide a general reduction in the radiation environment and when used exclusively, can influence the design of the radiographic facilities and reduce the need for protective lead shielding. The lower radiographic technique also results in a longer life for the x-ray tube.

Rare earth screens obtain their increased sensitivity through higher x-ray absorption (DQE) and more efficient conversion of x-ray energy into light (CE). The light emitted by these screens, however, differs from that of other screens, and therefore specially matched film is required when using rare earth screens. The **activators** identified in Table 16-4 are interstitial impurities of the phosphor crystal. The activators influence the intensity and wavelength of light emitted by the screen.

X-ray absorption. When diagnostic x-rays interact with a calcium tungstate screen, approximately 30% of the x-rays are absorbed. The mechanism of absorption is almost entirely the photoelectric effect. Recall that photoelectric absorption occurs readily with the inner-shell electrons of atoms of high atomic number. In a calcium tungstate screen, the tungstate atom determines its absorption properties. Tungsten has an atomic number of 74 and a K-shell electron binding energy of 69 keV. In the diagnostic range, x-ray absorption in tungsten follows the relationship shown in Figure 16-10.

At very low energies, photoelectric absorption is very high, but as the x-ray energy increases, the probability

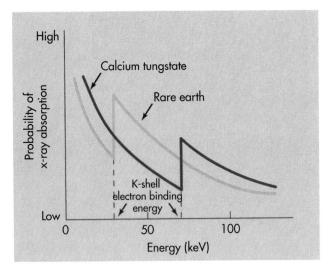

FIGURE 16-11 X-ray absorption probability in a rare earth screen compared with that for a calcium tungstate screen. In the energy interval between respective K-shell electron binding energies, absorption in a rare earth screen is higher.

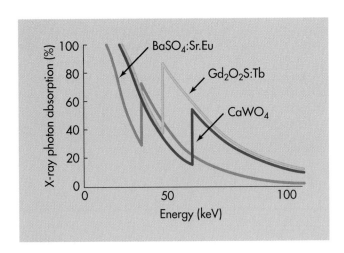

FIGURE 16-12 X-ray absorption for three intensifying screen phosphors.

TABLE 16-5	Atomic Number and K-Shell Electron Binding Energy of High-Atomic-Number Elements in Radiographic Intensifying Screen Phosphors		
Element	Chemical Symbol	Atomic Number	K-Shell Electron Binding Energy (keV)
Yttrium	Y	39	17
Barium	Ba	56	37
Lanthanum	La	57	39
Gadolinium	Gd	64	50
Tungsten	W	74	69

of absorption decreases rapidly until the x-ray energy is equal to the binding energy of the K-shell electrons. At x-ray energies below the K-shell electron binding energy, the incident x-ray does not have sufficient energy to ionize K-shell electrons.

When the x-ray energy equals the K-shell electron binding energy, the two K-shell electrons become available for photoelectric interaction. Consequently, at this energy, there is an abrupt increase in the probability of photoelectric absorption. This abrupt increase in absorption at this energy is called the *K-shell absorption edge,* and it is followed by another rapid reduction in photoelectric absorption with increasing x-ray energy.

The rare earth materials used for radiographic intensifying screens all have atomic numbers less than that for tungsten. Consequently, each has a lower K-shell, electron binding energy. Table 16-5 lists the important physical characteristics of the elements in radiographic intensifying screens.

Figure 16-11 shows that the probability for x-ray absorption in rare earth screens is lower than that for cal-cium tungstate screens at all x-ray energies except those between the respective K-shell electron binding energies. Below the K-shell absorption edge for the rare earth elements, x-ray absorption is higher in tungsten. At an x-ray energy equal to the K-shell electron binding energy of the rare earth elements, however, the probability of photoelectric absorption is considerably higher than that for tungsten.

The absorption probability of the rare earth elements decreases with increasing x-ray energy the same as tungsten. At x-ray energies above the K-shell absorption edge for tungsten, the rare earth elements again exhibit lower absorption than that for tungsten.

Each of the rare earth screens has an absorption curve characteristic of the phosphor that determines the speed of the screen and the way that it changes with kVp. Figure 16-12 shows the x-ray absorption in two phosphors relative to calcium tungstate ($CaWO_4$). For instance, barium strontium sulfate ($BaSO_4$) has a higher DQE at a lower keV than gadolinium oxysulfide ($Gd_2O_2S_2$).

The result of this complex interaction process is that in the x-ray energy range between the K-shell absorption edge for the rare earth elements and tungsten, the rare earth screen absorbs approximately five times more x-rays than calcium tungstate screens. Furthermore, for each x-ray absorbed, more light is emitted by the rare earth screens.

Rare earth radiographic intensifying screens exhibit better absorption properties than calcium tungstate screens only in the energy range between the respective K-shell absorption edges. This energy range extends from approximately 35 to 70 keV and corresponds to most of the useful x-rays emitted during routine x-ray examinations. Outside this energy range, calcium tungstate radiographic intensifying screens absorb more x-rays than rare earth screens.

Conversion efficiency. An additional property of the rare earth phosphors, the conversion efficiency (CE), the ratio of visible light energy emitted to the x-ray energy absorbed, contributes to their extraordinary speed.

When an x-ray interacts photoelectrically with a phosphor and is absorbed, its energy reappears as either heat or light through a rearrangement of electrons in the crystal lattice of the phosphor. If all the energy reappeared as heat, the phosphor would be worthless as an intensifying screen. In calcium tungstate, approximately 5% of the absorbed x-ray energy reappears as light. Rare earth phosphors exhibit a CE of 15% to 20%.

 The combination of improved CE and higher DQE results in the increased sensitivity or speed of rare earth radiographic intensifying screens.

Speed. Rare earth radiographic intensifying screens are available in many combinations with different films, resulting in varying relative speeds. When compared with par-speed calcium tungstate screens, rare earth screen-film combinations have relative speeds from 200 to 1200. Relative screen speeds of 200 to 800 provide image quality comparable to that of par-speed calcium tungstate screens.

When rare earth screen-film systems with relative speeds as high as 1200 are used, image quality may be degraded somewhat by increased quantum mottle, but this may be acceptable for some types of examinations, such as those of the chest and extremities, in view of the significantly reduced patient dose.

Spectrum matching. To be fully effective, rare earth screens must be used only in conjunction with film emulsions that have light absorption characteristics matched to the light emission of the screen. This is called **spectrum matching.** Calcium tungstate screens emit light in a

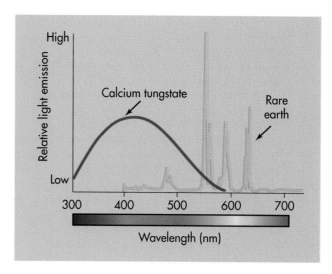

FIGURE 16-13 Calcium tungstate emits a broad spectrum of light centered in the blue region. Rare earth screens have discrete emissions centered near the green-yellow region.

rather broad, continuous spectrum centered in the violet-blue region with a maximum intensity at approximately 430 nm (Figure 16-13).

The spectral emission of rare earth phosphors is more discrete, as indicated by the many peaks in the spectrum (Figure 16-13). It is centered in the green region of the visible spectrum at approximately 540 mm. Terbium activation is responsible for the shape and intensity of this emission spectrum.

The emission spectrum can be altered somewhat by varying the concentration of terbium atoms in the phosphor, by adding activators, and by using light absorbing dyes. Phosphors are available that emit ultraviolet, blue, green, and red light.

Conventional x-ray film is sensitive to blue and blue-violet light and rather insensitive to light of longer wavelengths (Figure 6-14). Such blue-sensitive films were used with calcium tungstate screens because their absorption spectrum matches the calcium tungstate emission spectrum.

Specially designed green-sensitive film must be used with rare earth screens (Figure 16-15). If a green-emitting screen is used with blue-sensitive film, the strong emission in the green region will go undetected, and system speed will be sharply reduced. Obtaining maximal advantage and speed from rare earth screens requires that the film with which such screens are used must be sensitized for the emission of the screen.

Safelights. The use of a green-sensitive film creates problems in the darkroom. Safelight filters that are satisfactory for regular x-ray film fog film manufactured for use with rare earth screens. Safelights that are colored even more toward the red portion of the spectrum are required with rare earth screen-film.

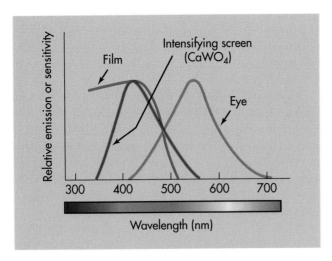

FIGURE 16-14 The importance of spectral matching is demonstrated by showing the relative emission spectrum for a calcium tungstate *(CaWO₄)* radiographic intensifying screen and the relative sensitivity of radiograph film to the light from that screen.

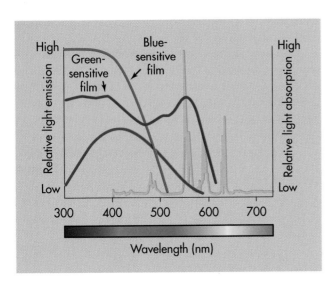

FIGURE 16-15 It is essential that blue-sensitive film be used with blue-emitting screens and green-sensitive film with green-emitting screens.

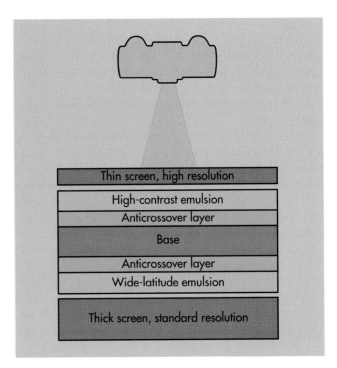

FIGURE 16-16 Asymmetric screens compensate for x-ray absorption in the front screen.

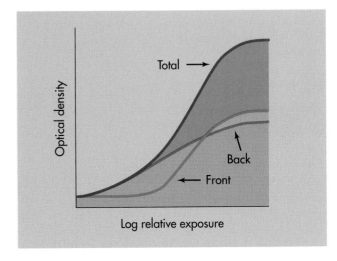

FIGURE 16-17 Characteristic curves from asymmetric screen emulsion image receptor.

Asymmetric screen-film. Consider the double-emulsion screen-film combination of Figure 16-16. If each screen has a DQE of 50%, the back screen will have only 50% of the x-rays transmitted with which to work. Therefore the back screen will absorb only 25% of the x-rays incident on the cassette, resulting in only half of the exposure of the back emulsion as the front emulsion.

This difference in exposure can be remedied by making the back radiographic intensifying screen thicker. It can also be remedied by using a different screen, exposing a different emulsion. Such screens and emulsions are

termed *asymmetric* and are used to great advantage in some applications, such as chest, pediatric, and portable radiography.

In chest radiography, for example, the front screen-emulsion is slower and has higher contrast. The back screen-emulsion is faster and has lower contrast (Figure 16-17). The result is a more balanced image of wide latitude and high contrast over both the lung fields and the mediastinum (Figure 16-18).

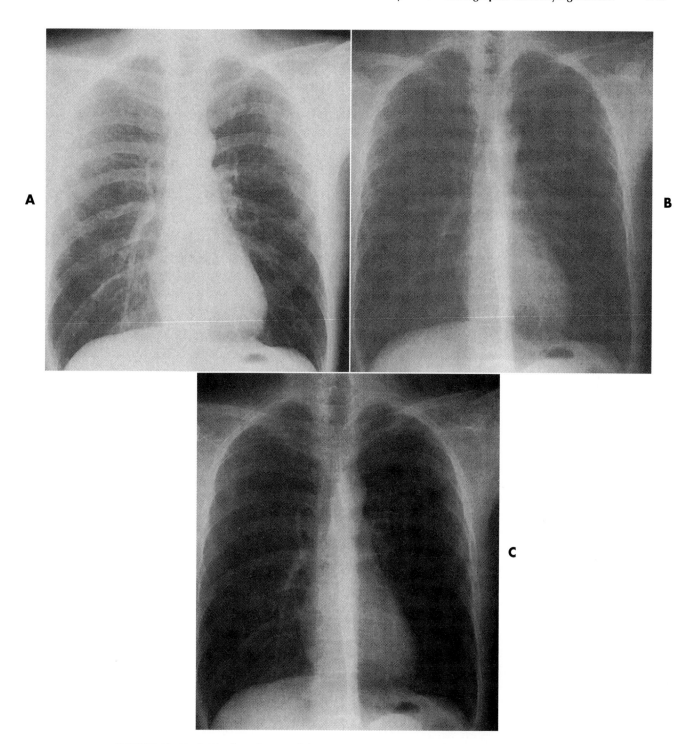

FIGURE 16-18 **A,** The front image of this asymmetric screen-emulsion image receptor shows high contrast. **B,** The back image shows wide latitude. **C,** The total image shows enhanced rendering of mediastinal and subdiaphragmatic tissue and pleural spaces.

CARE OF SCREENS

Radiographic intensifying screens must be properly cared for if high-quality radiographs are to be consistently produced. When handling screens, you should take the utmost care because even a small fingernail scratch can produce artifacts and degrade the radiographic image.

Screens should be handled only when they are new and being installed in cassettes and when they are being cleaned. When screens are mounted in a cassette, the manufacturer's instructions must be followed carefully.

When loading cassettes, do not slide the film in. A sharp corner or the edge can scratch the screen. Place the film in the cassette. Remove the film by rocking the cassette on the hinged edge and letting it fall to your fingers. Do not dig the film out of the cassette with your fingernails. Do not leave cassettes open because the screens can be damaged by falling objects, dust, and darkroom chemicals.

Periodically, radiographic intensifying screens must be cleaned. The required frequency of cleaning is determined primarily by two factors: the amount of use the screens receive and the degree to which the work environment is dust free. In a busy radiology department, it may be necessary to clean screens once a month or even more often. Under other circumstances, the cleaning frequency may safely be extended to 2 to 3 months.

When special screen-cleaning materials are used, the manufacturer's instructions should be followed carefully. One advantage of using these commercial preparations is that they often contain antistatic compounds, which can be quite helpful.

Radiographic intensifying screens can also be cleaned with mild soap and water. They should be carefully rinsed and thoroughly dried. If the screen is damp, the film emulsion layer may stick to it, possibly causing permanent damage.

An equally important requirement in caring for radiographic intensifying screens is maintaining good screen-film contact. Screen-film contact can be checked by radiographing a wire mesh (Figure 16-19). If there are any areas of blurring, as in Figure 16-20, then poor screen-film contact exists, and the problem should be corrected or the cassette replaced.

To test for screen-film contact, expose the cassette through the wire mesh at 50 kVp at 5 mAs and an SID of 100 cm. To view the result optimally, back away 2 to 3 m from the viewbox. Areas of poor screen-film contact appear blurred and cloudy, indicating that the cassette should be repaired or replaced.

When new radiographic intensifying screens are installed in a cassette, this examination for screen-film contact should be performed and the radiograph retained as a baseline evaluation. Additional wire-mesh radiographs for testing screen-film contact should be made and compared with the baseline film at least annually.

Box 16-5 summarizes the most common causes of poor screen-film contact. Nearly all the causes listed can result from rough handling of cassettes, which is the principal cause of loss of good screen-film contact. Although the cassettes appear sturdy, they are precision pieces of equipment and should be treated accordingly.

Properly maintained radiographic intensifying screens last indefinitely. X-ray interaction with the phosphor does not cause them to wear out. There is no such thing as radiation fatigue. The only way they become useless and need replacement is through improper handling and maintenance.

BOX 16-5   Common Causes of Poor Screen-Film Contact

Worn contact felt
Loose, bent, or broken hinges
Loose, bent, or broken latches
Warped screens resulting from excessive moisture
Warped cassette front
Sprung or cracked cassette frame
Foreign matter under the screen

FIGURE 16-19 Wire-mesh test tool used to check for screen-film contact. *(Courtesy Nuclear Associates.)*

FIGURE 16-20 A region of poor screen-film contact is seen on this radiograph of a wire-mesh test tool. *(Courtesy Barbara Smith Pruner.)*

SUMMARY

Radiographic intensifying screens are permanently placed within the radiographic cassette. The x-ray film used for each exposure is placed between them. The radiographic intensifying screens are so named because they change the energy of the image-forming x-ray beam exiting the patient into visible light, which exposes the radiographic film.

Radiographic intensifying screens are composed of the following four layers: (1) a protective coating, (2) the phosphor layer, (3) the reflective layer, and (4) the base. The phosphor layer has one purpose: to convert x-rays into visible light.

This process is called *luminescence.* Intensifying screens display a particular kind of luminescence called *fluorescence,* which means that the phosphor is stimulated to emit light only when struck by x-rays. Once the x-ray exposure is terminated, no lag or afterglow of light is present.

Radiographic intensifying screens display an x-ray absorption efficiency and an x-ray–to–light conversion efficiency. Intensification factor (IF) is a characteristic that compares nonscreen film exposure with screen-film exposure. The IF is defined as follows:

$$IF = \frac{Exposure\ required\ without\ screens}{Exposure\ required\ with\ screens}$$

Calcium tungstate phosphors were used almost exclusively until 1972, when rare earth phosphors were developed for medical x-ray use. Calcium tungstate par-speed intensifying screens are the standard for determining radiographic intensifying screen speed and have a value of 100. Table 16-2 summarizes optical density, resolution in line pairs per millimeter, image noise, and application of various intensifying screens.

Radiographic intensifying screens must be properly cared for if high-quality radiographs are to be consistently produced. Artifacts are avoided by careful handling of the screens and film. Spots show up on the radiograph if dust or other deposits are on the screen. Because of dust accumulation, screens need to be cleaned regularly.

CHALLENGE QUESTIONS

1. Define or otherwise identify:
   a. Afterglow
   b. Isotropic
   c. Spatial resolution
   d. Spectral matching
   e. Screen blur
   f. Image noise
   g. Phosphor
   h. Compression device
   i. Luminescence

2. Discuss the physical qualities that a material must possess to be used as a base for a radiographic intensifying screen.

3. Describe the composition of a typical radiographic intensifying screen.

4. Discuss the two types of luminescence and the ways that they are associated with radiographic intensifying screens and fluoroscopic screens.

5. What are the three main types of radiographic intensifying screens and the approximate speed of each?

6. The usual technique for an oblique radiograph of the foot uses direct-exposure film at 45 kVp and 180 mAs. If screens are used, the technique factors are changed to 45 kVp and 7.5 mAs to maintain the same average optical density. What is the approximate intensification factor for the screen-film combination?

7. Describe the technique for evaluating screen-film contact.

8. What characteristics of phosphor materials make them especially suited for radiographic intensifying screens?

9. Describe the construction of a film cassette, listing each layer from the tube side to the back cover.

10. List the most common cassette malfunctions.

11. What percentage of the x-ray beam exposing the image receptor contributes to the latent image?

12. Why are two intensifying screens placed in the radiographic cassette?

13. Why is afterglow objectionable as a characteristic of a radiographic intensifying screen?

14. Name five phosphors used in radiographic intensifying screens.

15. What is the difference between DQE and CE?

16. List some common causes of poor screen-film contact.

17. What is intensification factor? Write the formula for it.

18. Illustrate 20% x-ray absorption efficiency in the phosphor layer of a radiographic intensifying screen.

19. What is quantum mottle?

20. Why is it important to have radiographic film and radiographic intensifying screen phosphor spectrally matched?

21. Describe the factors involved in the care and handling of intensifying screens.

Beam-Restricting Devices

OBJECTIVES

At the completion of this chapter, the student should be able to:

1. Identify the x-rays that constitute image-forming radiation
2. List three factors that contribute to scatter radiation
3. Discuss three devices developed to minimize scatter radiation
4. Describe beam restriction and its effect on patient dose and image quality

OUTLINE

Three factors contribute to an increase in scatter radiation: increased kVp, increased x-ray field, size and increased patient or part thickness. Two principal devices are used to reduce scatter radiation: grids and beam restrictors. Grids are discussed in Chapter 18; this chapter focuses on beam-restricting devices. Beam-restricting devices are designed to control and minimize scatter radiation by limiting the x-ray field size to only the anatomic structure of interest. The three principal types of beam-restricting devices—aperture diaphragm, cones and cylinders, and collimators—are discussed in this chapter.

PRODUCTION OF SCATTER RADIATION

Two kinds of x-rays are responsible for the optical density, or the degree of blackening, on a radiograph: those that pass through the patient without interacting and those that are scattered in the patient through Compton interaction. X-rays that exit from the patient are remnant x-rays, and those that enter the image receptor are image-forming x-rays (Figure 17-1).

As scatter radiation increases, the radiograph loses contrast and appears gray and dull, and the imaged structures appear blurred. Three primary factors influence the relative intensity of scatter radiation reaching the image receptor: kilovolt peak (kVp), field size, and patient or part thickness.

Kilovolt Peak

As x-ray energy is increased, the relative number of x-rays that undergo Compton interaction increases also. The absolute number of the Compton interaction decreases with increasing x-ray energy, but the number of photoelectric interactions decreases much more rapidly (see Chapter 13).

Table 17-1 shows the percentage of x-rays incident on a 10-cm thickness of soft tissue that will undergo photoelectric interaction and Compton interaction at selected kVp levels from 50 to 120. Kilovoltage is one of the factors that affect the level of scatter radiation and can be controlled by the radiologic technologist.

It would be easy enough to say that all radiographs should be taken at the lowest reasonable kVp, since this technique would result in minimal scatter and thus higher image contrast. Unfortunately, it is not that simple. Table 17-1 shows that the percentage of x-rays interacting photoelectrically increases greatly as the kVp is lowered. This increase results in a considerable increase in patient dose. Also, fewer x-rays reach the image receptor at low kVp; this is usually compensated for by increasing the mAs. The result is still higher patient dose.

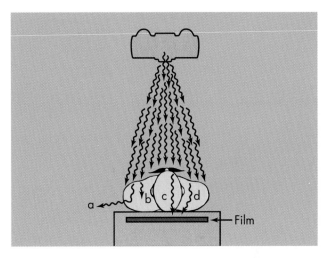

FIGURE 17-1 Some x-rays interact with the patient and are scattered away from the film *(a)*. Others interact with the patient and are absorbed *(b)*. X-rays that arrive at the image receptor are those transmitted through the patient without interacting *(c)*. Some x-rays are scattered in the patient and still reach the image receptor *(d)*. X-rays of type *c* and *d* are image-forming x-rays. X-rays of type *a, c,* and *d* are remnant radiation.

TABLE 17-1	Percent Interaction of X-Rays by Photoelectric and Compton Processes and Percent Transmission Through 10 cm of Soft Tissue			
	PERCENT INTERACTION			
kVp	**Photoelectric**	**Compton**	**Total**	**Percent Transmission**
50	79	21	>99	<1
60	70	30	>99	<1
70	60	40	>99	<1
80	46	52	98	2
90	38	59	97	3
100	31	63	94	6
110	23	70	93	7
120	18	73	91	9

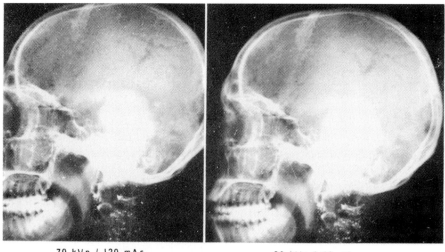

70 kVp / 120 mAs
665 mR

80 kVp / 60 mAs
545 mR

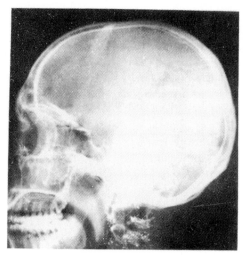

90 kVp / 30 mAs
230 mR

FIGURE 17-2   All these skull radiographs are of acceptable quality. The technique factors for each are shown, along with the resulting patient exposure.

On large patients, a high kVp must be used to ensure adequate penetration of the portion of the body being radiographed. If, for example, the normal technique factors for an anterior-posterior (AP) examination of the abdomen are insufficient to image the abdomen adequately, the technologist has a choice of increasing the mAs or the kVp.

Increasing the mAs usually generates enough x-rays to provide a satisfactory image but may result in an unacceptably high patient dose. On the other hand, a much smaller increase in kVp is usually sufficient to provide enough x-rays, and this can be done at a much lower patient dose. Unfortunately, when kVp is increased, the level of scatter radiation also increases, and therefore the radiographic contrast decreases.

Collimators and grids are used to reduce the level of scatter radiation. Figure 17-2 shows a series of radiographs of a skull phantom taken at 70, 80, and 90 kVp using appropriate collimation and grids with the mAs adjusted to produce radiographs of nearly equal optical density (OD). Most radiologists would accept any of these radiographs. Notice that the patient dose at 90 kVp is approximately one third that at 70 kVp. In general, because of this reduction in patient dose, a high-kVp technique is preferred to a low-kVp technique.

Field Size

Another factor that affects the level of scatter radiation and that is under the control of the radiologic technologist is x-ray beam field size. As field size is increased,

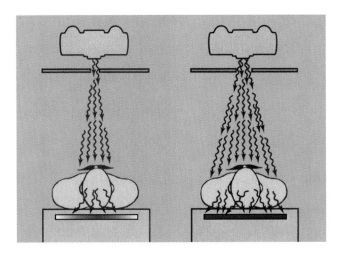

FIGURE 17-3 Collimation of the x-ray beam results in less scatter radiation, reduced dose, and improved contrast resolution.

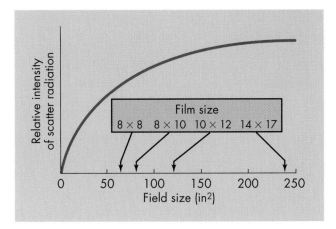

FIGURE 17-4 This graph is representative of operation at 70 kVp with a patient 20 cm thick. The relative intensity of scatter radiation increases with increasing field size.

scatter radiation also increases (Figure 17-3). The relative intensity of scatter radiation varies more when the x-ray field is small than when the field is large (Figure 17-4).

 Scatter radiation increases as the field size of the x-ray beam increases.

Figure 17-5 shows two radiographs of the abdomen and lumbar spine. Figure 17-5, *A*, was taken on a full frame, 14 × 17 in (35 × 43 cm) film, and Figure 17-5, *B*, has field size restricted to just the spinal column. There is a noticeable loss of contrast in the full-frame radiograph (Figure 17-5, *A*) because of the increased scatter radiation that accompanies a larger field size. The radiograph in Figure 17-5, *B*, demonstrates proper

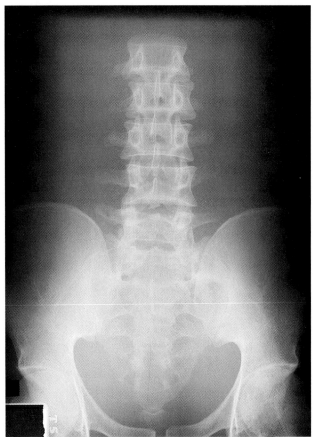

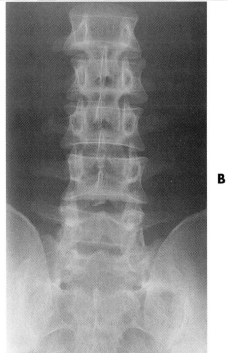

FIGURE 17-5 These images of the abdomen and lumbar spine show how the full-field technique results in reduced image contrast. **A,** Full-field technique: 75 kVp and 20 mAs. **B,** Preferred collimated technique: 75 kVp and 28 mAs. *(Courtesy Mike Enriquez.)*

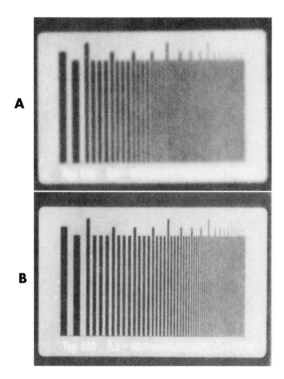

A

B

FIGURE 17-6 Spot films of a test pattern in the middle of 20 cm of tissue equivalent material taken with full-field exposure **(A)** and with the x-ray beam restricted to the area of the test pattern **(B).** The image in **B** is better because the smaller field size resulted in less scatter radiation.

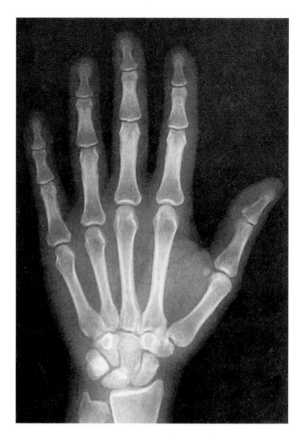

FIGURE 17-7 Extremity radiographs appear sharp because of less tissue; hence there is less scatter radiation. Posterior-anterior view of the hand. *(Courtesy Rees Stuteville.)*

collimation. When the x-ray beam is collimated, radiographic exposure factors may have to be increased. Reduced scatter radiation results in lower radiographic OD, which must be raised by increasing technique.

Restriction of field size to improve image quality is perhaps even more important during fluoroscopy. Figure 17-6 shows two spot films taken of a spatial-resolution bar phantom embedded in the middle of a tissue phantom 20 cm thick. The first image was taken with a full-field exposure, the second with the field size restricted to the area of the bar phantom. The difference in image contrast and spatial resolution is obvious.

Patient or Part Thickness

More scatter radiation results from imaging thick parts of the body than thin parts of the body such as the hand. A comparison of the bony structures in a radiograph of an extremity with the bony structures in a radiograph of the chest or pelvis demonstrates this. Even when the two are taken with the same screen-film combination, the extremity radiograph is much sharper because of the reduced amount of scatter radiation (Figure 17-7).

Figure 17-8 shows the relative intensity of scattered x-rays as a function of thickness of soft tissue for an 8 × 10 in (20 × 25 cm) field. Exposing a 3-cm-thick extremity at 70 kVp results in about 45% scatter radiation. Ex-

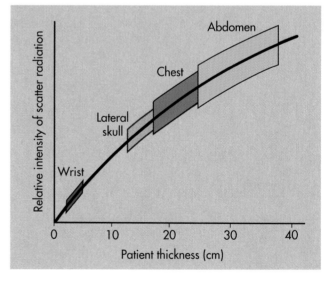

FIGURE 17-8 The relative intensity of scatter radiation increases with the increasing thickness of an anatomic part.

posing a 30-cm-thick abdomen results in nearly 100% of the x-rays exiting the patient as scattered x-rays. With increasing patient thickness, more x-rays undergo multiple scattering, so the average angle of scatter in the remnant beam is greater.

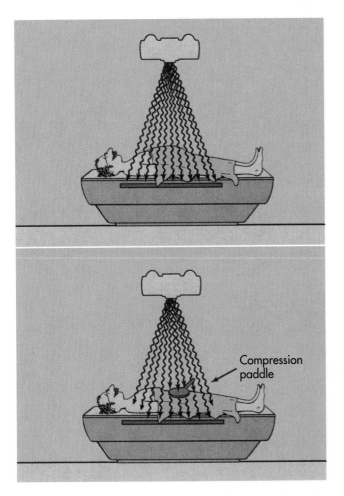

FIGURE 17-9 When tissue is compressed, scatter radiation is reduced, resulting in lower dose and improved contrast resolution.

Normally, tissue thickness cannot be controlled by the radiologic technologist. If you recognize that more x-rays are scattered with increasing tissue thickness, you can produce a high-quality radiograph by choosing the proper technique factors and by using devices such as a compression paddle to reduce the amount of scatter radiation reaching the image receptor (Figure 17-9).

> The compression of anatomic parts improves spatial and contrast resolution and lowers patient dose.

Compression devices improve spatial resolution by reducing patient thickness and bringing the object closer to the image receptor. Compression also reduces patient dose and improves contrast resolution. Compression is particularly important during mammography.

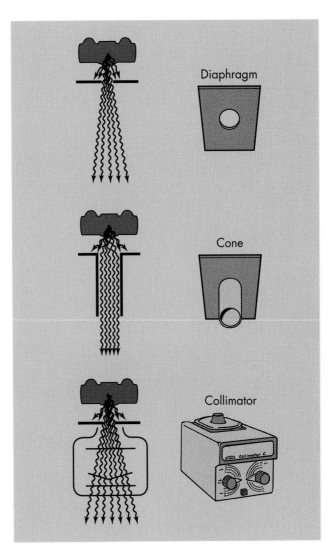

FIGURE 17-10 Three types of x-ray beam–restricting devices.

CONTROL OF SCATTER RADIATION

Beam restrictors limit the size of the x-ray field to only the anatomic structure of interest. There are two reasons to restrict any x-ray beam. Only the tissue being examined should be exposed. Larger x-ray fields result in unnecessary patient exposure. Large x-ray fields also result in more scatter radiation, which reduces image contrast.

Three types of beam-restricting devices are designed to reduce the amount of scatter radiation reaching the image receptor: the aperture diaphragm, cones or cylinders, and the variable-aperture collimator (Figure 17-10).

Aperture Diaphragm

An **aperture diaphragm** is the simplest of all beam-restricting devices. It is basically a lead or lead-lined metal diaphragm attached to the x-ray tube head. The opening in the diaphragm is usually designed to cover just less than the size of the image receptor used. Figure 17-11 shows the relationships among the x-ray tube, an

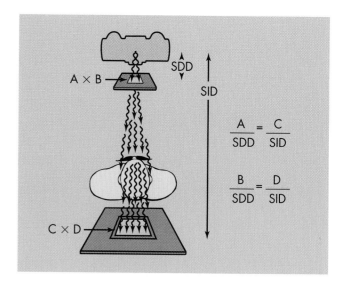

FIGURE 17-11 An aperture diaphragm is a fixed lead opening designed for a fixed image receptor size and constant source-to-image receptor distance *(SID)*. *SDD,* source-to-diaphragm distance.

$$\frac{A}{SDD} = \frac{C}{SID}$$

$$\frac{B}{SDD} = \frac{D}{SID}$$

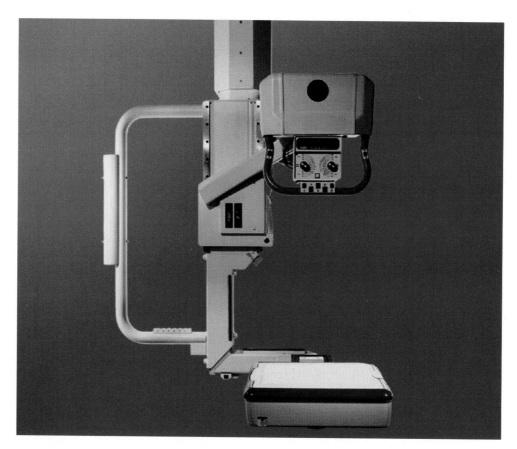

FIGURE 17-12 Digital trauma radiographic imager used for imaging the skull, spine, and extremities. Such imaging systems are flexible and adaptable for the examination of many body parts. *(Courtesy Fischer Imaging.)*

aperture diaphragm, and the image receptor. A properly designed aperture diaphragm projects onto the image receptor an image 1 cm smaller on all sides than the size of the image receptor. Therefore, when an aperture diaphragm is used, an unexposed border should be visible on each edge of the radiograph. Aperture diaphragms are sometimes used with a cone or cylinder.

Question: If a 20-cm² film is to be imaged at a 100-cm source-to-image receptor distance (SID) and the diaphragm is placed 10 cm from the target, what should be the dimension of one side of the diaphragm opening? NOTE: To leave an unexposed border of 1.0 cm on each side, reduce the beam size to 18 cm.

Answer:
$$\frac{A}{10 \text{ cm}} = \frac{18 \text{ cm}}{100 \text{ cm}}$$
$$A = \frac{(10 \text{ cm})(18 \text{ cm})}{100 \text{ cm}}$$
$$= 1.8 \text{ cm}$$

Trauma radiographic imaging systems present possibly the most familiar clinical example of the use of aperture diaphragms. The typical trauma system has a fixed SID and is equipped with diaphragms to accommodate film sizes of 5 × 7 in (13 × 18 cm), 8 × 10 in (20 × 25 cm), and 10 × 12 in (25 × 30 cm). Trauma radiographic imaging systems can be positioned to image all parts of the body (Figure 17-12).

When using an aperture diaphragm, the radiographer should take care that it is inserted into the x-ray tube head so that the long axis of the diaphragm is parallel to the long axis of the image receptor. If it is not, diaphragm cutoff can result, leaving large portions of the radiograph unexposed and causing unnecessary exposure to the patient because of possible repeat examinations.

X-ray imagers dedicated specifically for chest radiography are supplied with fixed aperture diaphragms. Usually, these diaphragms are securely fastened to the x-ray tube head and therefore are not easily removed. Such aperture diaphragms are designed for exposure of all but a 1-cm border of 14 × 17 in (35 × 45 cm) image receptors.

Dental radiography is another area in which aperture diaphragms are used. Dental radiographs are customarily obtained at a 20- or 40-cm SID. The diaphragm used in these techniques must provide a circular x-ray beam not exceeding 7 cm in diameter at the entrance skin of the patient. Typically, the diameter of an aperture diaphragm for a 20-cm SID is 18 mm and that for a 40-cm SID is 9 mm. Some dental apparatus is supplied with rectangular collimation, which requires precise alignment and positioning of the x-ray tube head, the patient, and the image receptor by the dental radiologic technologist.

Cones and Cylinders

Radiographic extension **cones and cylinders** are considered modifications of the aperture diaphragm. A typical extension cone and cylinder are diagrammed in Figure 17-13. In both, an extended metal structure restricts the useful beam to the required size. Unlike the beam produced by the aperture diaphragm, the useful beam produced by an extension cone or cylinder is usually circular. Both these beam restrictors are routinely called *cones*, even though the type used most commonly is actually a cylinder.

One difficulty with using cones is alignment. If the x-ray source, cone, and image receptor are not aligned on the same axis, one side of the radiograph may not be exposed because the edge of the cone may interfere with the x-ray beam. Such interference is called **cone cutting.**

The same limitations that apply to aperture diaphragms apply to cones and cylinders. Their openings are fixed so that they are appropriate for only specific types of examinations such as studies of the head and neck and dental radiography.

At one time, cones were used extensively in diagnostic radiology. Today, they are reserved primarily for examinations of the head and spine. Figure 17-14 shows the improvement in image contrast that results when a cone is used for examining the maxillary sinuses. In diagnostic radiography, the light-localizing variable-aperture collimator has replaced the cone in most examinations.

Beam-defining cones (more properly known as *position-indicating devices*) are used extensively in dental radiography. Figure 17-15 is a photograph of six typical dental cones. Dental cones are usually fabricated of plastic, and some are lead lined. The long, lead-lined dental cones result in slightly less exposure to the patient than the other types.

The 20-cm plastic pointer cones used on dental x-ray imagers result in unnecessarily high patient exposure

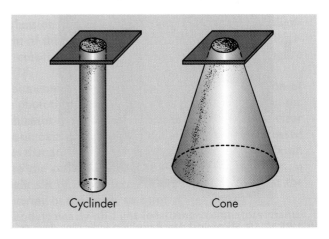

FIGURE 17-13 Radiographic cones and cylinders produce restricted useful x-ray beams of circular shape.

When a film-loaded cassette is inserted in the Bucky tray and clamped into place, sensing devices in the tray identify the size and alignment of the cassette. An electric signal is transmitted to the collimator housing and actuates the synchronous motors that drive the collimator leaves to a precalibrated position so that the x-ray beam is restricted to the image receptor size in use.

When properly adjusted, the automatic collimator provides an unexposed border on all sides of the finished radiograph. Even with PBL, the radiologic technologist should manually collimate more tightly to reduce patient dose and improve image quality.

 Under no circumstances should the x-ray beam exceed the size of the image receptor.

Depending on the tube potential, additional collimator filtration may be necessary to produce high-quality radiographs with minimal patient exposure. Some collimator housings are designed to allow easy changing of the added filtration. Most commonly, filtration stations of zero and 1, 2, and 3 mm of Al are provided.

Even in the zero position, however, the added filtration to the x-ray tube is not zero because collimator structures intercept the beam. The exit port, usually plastic, and the reflecting mirror provide filtration in addition to the inherent filtration of the tube. The added filtration of the collimator assembly is usually equivalent to approximately 1 mm of Al.

SUMMARY

Two types of image-forming x-rays exit the patient: (1) x-rays that pass through tissue without interacting and (2) x-rays that are scattered in tissue by Compton interaction and therefore contribute only noise to the image. The three factors that contribute to an increase in scatter radiation and ultimately to image noise are increasing kVp, increasing x-ray field size, and increasing anatomic part thickness.

Although an increase in kVp does increase scatter radiation, there is a trade-off with reduced patient exposure. The increase in scatter can be controlled and minimized by using beam-restricting devices such as the aperture diaphragm, extension cones and cylinders, and the variable-aperture collimator. The variable-aperture collimator is the most commonly used beam-restricting device in diagnostic imaging.

CHALLENGE QUESTIONS

1. Define or otherwise identify:
   a. Three factors affecting scatter radiation
   b. Approximate equivalent collimator filtration
   c. Aperture diaphragm
   d. Cone cutting
   e. Automatic collimation
   f. Off-focus radiation
   g. PBL
   h. Two reasons to collimate
   i. Image-forming x-rays
   j. Compression

2. Why should a radiograph of the lumbar vertebrae be well collimated?

3. A chest x-ray imager is designed for only 14 × 17 in (35 × 43 cm) radiographs. If the SID is 180 cm and the source-to-diaphragm distance is 10 cm, what should the diaphragm opening be to allow an unexposed border of 1 cm around the film?

4. An acceptable intravenous pyelogram can be obtained with technique factors of 74 kVp and 120 mAs or 82 kVp and 80 mAs. Discuss possible reasons for selecting one technique over the other.

5. One mode for skull radiography uses a 10 × 12 in (25 × 30 cm) film format. What should be the size of the diaphragm located 12 cm from the target if the SID is 80 cm?

6. What happens to image contrast and patient dose as more filtration is added to the beam?

7. What is the difference between remnant radiation and image-forming radiation?

8. At the 80-kVp level, what percentage of the x-ray beam is scattered through Compton interaction?

9. Name the types of devices used to reduce the level of scatter radiation.

10. Name the three types of beam-restricting devices.

11. Compression of tissue is particularly important during what examination?

12. List the two reasons for restricting the x-ray beam.

13. Describe the design of the aperture diaphragm.

14. Why show an unexposed 1-cm border on the edge of the radiograph?

15. Explain a difficulty that can occur when using extension cones.

16. What is viewed in the light field of a variable-aperture light-localizing collimator?

17. Where do the two crossed lines used to mark central ray location on the tissue to be radiographed originate?

18. If the light field and the radiation field do not coincide, what needs to be adjusted?

19. When should the x-ray field exceed the size of the image receptor?

CHAPTER

18

The Grid

OBJECTIVES

At the completion of this chapter, the student should be able to:

1. Recognize the relationship between scatter radiation and image contrast
2. Describe grid construction
3. Calculate grid ratio, grid frequency, contrast improvement factor, Bucky factor, and selectivity
4. Describe eight types of grids
5. Discuss the four common errors when using grids
6. Evaluate the circumstances for proper grid selection
7. Describe advantages and disadvantages of the use of grids in relation to patient dose

OUTLINE

ontrast is one of the most important characteristics of image quality. Contrast is the light, dark, and shades of gray on the x-ray image. These variations make up the radiographic image. Contrast resolution is the ability to image adjacent similar tissues.

Scatter radiation produced by Compton scattering results in noise, reducing contrast and contrast resolution and making the manifest image less visible. Two types of devices used to reduce scatter radiation are beam-restricting devices, which are discussed in Chapter 17, and grids, which are discussed in this chapter. By removing scattered x-rays from the remnant beam, the grid removes a major source of noise and thus improves contrast.

CONTROL OF SCATTER RADIATION

The relative intensity of scatter radiation was previously shown to be a complex function of many factors, primarily kilovolt peak (kVp), field size, and patient or part thickness. The amount of scatter radiation is reduced as the kVp is lowered because of enhanced differential absorption. There are, however, a number of disadvantages to low-kVp radiography, principally increased patient dose.

The beam-restricting devices discussed in the previous chapter are very efficient in reducing the scatter radiation, but their effect is not enough. Even under the most favorable conditions, most of the remnant x-rays have

been scattered. Figure 18-1 illustrates that scattered x-rays are emitted in all directions from the patient.

SCATTER RADIATION AND IMAGE CONTRAST

Chapter 20 discusses in detail many characteristics that affect the quality of a radiograph. One of the most important characteristics of film quality is **contrast,** the degree of difference between the light and dark areas of a radiograph. **Contrast resolution** is the ability to image and distinguish various soft tissues.

If you could radiograph a long bone in cross section using only transmitted unattenuated x-rays, the image would be very high contrast (Figure 18-2, *A*). The change in optical density (OD) from light to dark, corresponding to the bone–soft tissue interface, would be very abrupt.

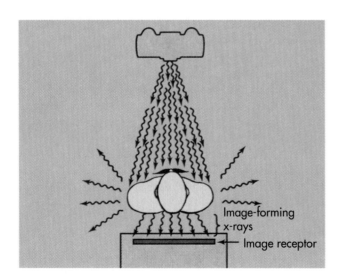

FIGURE 18-1 When primary x-rays interact with the patient, x-rays are scattered from the patient in all directions.

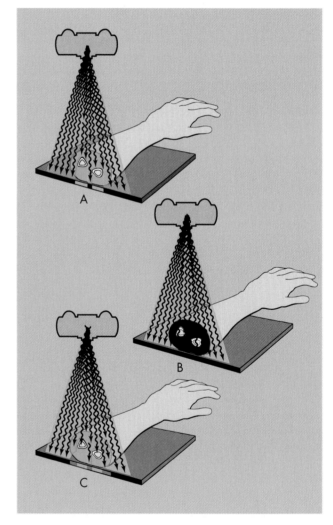

FIGURE 18-2 Radiographs of a long bone. **A,** High contrast would result from using only transmitted unattenuated x-rays. **B,** No contrast would result from using only scattered x-rays. **C,** Moderate contrast results from using both transmitted and scattered x-rays.

Reduced image contrast results from scattered x-rays.

On the other hand, if the radiograph were taken with only scatter radiation and no transmitted, unattenuated x-rays reached the image receptor, the image would be dull gray (Figure 18-2, *B*). The radiographic contrast would be very low. In the normal situation, however, the x-rays arriving at the image receptor consist of both transmitted and scattered x-rays. If the radiograph were properly exposed, the image in cross-sectional view would appear as in Figure 18-2, *C*. The image would have moderate contrast. The loss of contrast results from the presence of scattered x-rays. The more scattered x-rays, the lower the contrast.

The scattered x-rays that reach the image receptor are part of image-forming x-rays and indeed those that are scattered forward to contribute to the image. Most that are scattered at a large angle are removed by the grid and are part of the remnant x-rays, not the image-forming x-rays.

GRIDS

An extremely effective device for reducing the level of scatter radiation is the **grid,** a carefully fabricated series of sections of radiopaque material (**grid lines**) alternating with sections of radiolucent material (**interspace material**). In 1913, Gustave Bucky first demonstrated this technique for reducing the amount of scatter radiation reaching the image receptor. Over the years, Bucky's grid has been improved by more precise manufacturing, but the basic principle has not changed.

The grid is designed to transmit only the x-rays whose direction is on a straight line from the source to the image receptor. Scattered x-rays are absorbed in the grid material. Figure 18-3 is a schematic of how a grid "cleans up" scatter radiation.

X-rays exiting the patient that strike the radiopaque grid material are absorbed and do not reach the image receptor. For instance, a typical grid may have grid strips approximately 50 μm thick separated by interspace material approximately 350 μm thick. Consequently, up to 12.5% of all photons striking the grid interact with radiopaque grid material and are absorbed.

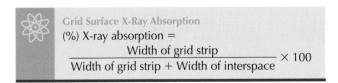

Grid Surface X-Ray Absorption

$$\text{(\%) X-ray absorption} = \frac{\text{Width of grid strip}}{\text{Width of grid strip} + \text{Width of interspace}} \times 100$$

Question: A grid is constructed with 50-μm strips and a 350-μm interspace. What percentage of x-rays incident on the grid will be absorbed by its entrance surface?

Answer: $\dfrac{50\ \mu m}{50\ \mu m + 350\ \mu m} = 0.125$

$= 12.5\%$

Primary beam x-rays striking the interspace material are transmitted through to the image receptor. Scattered x-rays striking interspace material may or may not be absorbed, depending on their angle of incidence and the physical characteristics of the grid. If the angle of a scattered x-ray is great enough to cause it to intersect the grid material, it will be absorbed. If the angle is slight, the scattered x-ray will be transmitted like a primary x-ray. Laboratory measurements show that high-quality grids can attenuate 80% to 90% of the scatter radiation. Such a grid is said to exhibit good cleanup.

Grid Construction

Many types of grids are available, and to make an informed judgment about which grid is best for a certain procedure, the radiographer needs to understand the three aspects of grid construction: grid ratio, grid frequency, and grid material.

Grid ratio. There are three important dimensions on a grid: the width of the grid strip *(T)*, the width of the interspace material *(D)*, and the height of the grid *(h)*. The **grid ratio** is the height of the grid strip divided by the interspace width (distance between the grid strips), as follows:

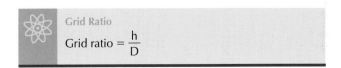

Grid Ratio

$$\text{Grid ratio} = \frac{h}{D}$$

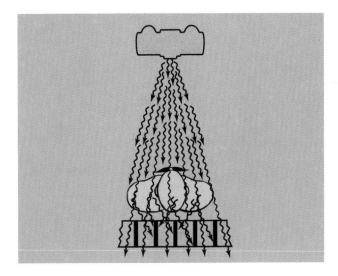

FIGURE 18-3 The only x-rays transmitted through a grid are those traveling in the direction of the interspace. X-rays scattered obliquely through the interspace are absorbed.

Grid ratio can best be understood by reference to Figure 18-4.

High-ratio grids are more effective in cleaning up scatter radiation than low-ratio grids because the angle of scatter allowed by high-ratio grids is less than that permitted by low-ratio grids (Figure 18-5).

Unfortunately, grids with high ratios are more difficult to manufacture than grids with low ratios. High-ratio grids are fabricated by reducing the width of the interspace, increasing the height of the grid material, or combining both techniques. The higher the grid ratio, the higher the exposure necessary to get a sufficient number of x-rays through the grid to the image receptor and the higher the patient dose.

 High-ratio grids increase patient radiation dose.

Generally, grid ratios range from 5:1 to 16:1, with the higher-ratio grids most often used in high-kVp radiography. An 8:1 to 10:1 grid is frequently used with general-purpose x-ray imaging systems. A 5:1 grid cleans up approximately 85% of the scatter radiation, whereas a 16:1 grid may clean up as much as 97%

Question: A certain grid is fabricated of 30-μm grid strips sandwiched between interspace material 300 μm thick. The height of the grid is 2.4 mm. What is the grid ratio?

Answer:
$$\text{Grid ratio} = \frac{h}{D}$$
$$= \frac{2400 \ \mu m}{300 \ \mu m}$$
$$= 8:1$$

Grid frequency. The number of grid strips or grid lines per inch or per centimeter is called the **grid frequency.** Grids with high frequencies show less distinct grid lines on a radiograph than grids with low frequencies. The higher the frequency of a grid, the thinner its strips of innerspace material and the higher the grid ratio.

 The use of high-frequency grids requires high radiographic technique and results in a higher patient radiation dose.

As grid frequency increases, there is relatively more grid material to absorb x-rays, and therefore patient dose is high because higher radiographic technique is required. The disadvantage of the increased patient dose associated with high-frequency grids can be overcome by reducing the width of the grid strips, but this effectively reduces the grid ratio and therefore the cleanup.

Most grids have frequencies in the range of 25 to 45 lines/cm (60 to 110 lines/in). Grid frequency can be calculated if the widths of the grid strip and the interspace are known. Grid frequency is computed by dividing the width of one line pair (T + D, where *T* is the width of the grid strip and *D* is the width of the interspace material) and is expressed in micrometers into 1 cm:

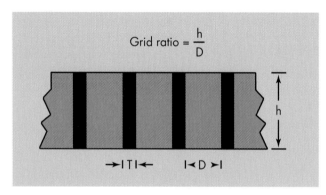

FIGURE 18-4 *Grid ratio* is defined as the height of the grid strip *(h)* divided by the width of the interspace material *(D)*. *T,* Width of grid strip.

> **Grid Frequency**
> $$\text{Grid frequency} = \frac{10,000 \ \mu m/cm}{(T + D) \ \mu m/\text{line pair}}$$

Question: What is the grid frequency of a grid having a grid strip width of 30 μm and an interspace width of 300 μm?

Answer: If 1 line pair = 300 μm + 30 μm = 330 μm, how many line pairs are in 10,000 μm (10,000 μm = 1 cm)?
$$\frac{10,000 \ \mu m/cm}{330 \ \mu m/\text{line pair}} = 30.3 \ \text{lines/cm}$$
30.3 lines/cm × 2.54 cm/in = 77 lines/in

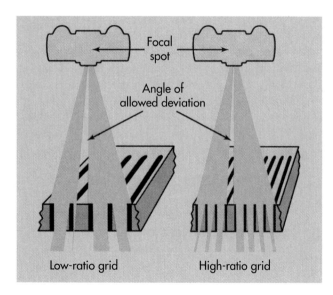

FIGURE 18-5 High-ratio grids are more effective than low-ratio grids because the angle of deviation is smaller.

Specially designed grids are used for mammography. Usually a 4:1 or a 5:1 grid is used. These low-ratio grids have grid frequencies of approximately 80 lines/cm (200 lines/in).

Grid material. Theoretically the grid strip should be infinitely thin and have high absorption properties. There are several possible materials out of which to form these strips. **Lead** is the most widely used because it is easy to shape and is relatively inexpensive. Its high atomic number and high mass density make lead the material of choice in the manufacture of grids. Tungsten, platinum, gold, and uranium have all been tried, but none has the overall desirable characteristics of lead.

The purpose of the interspace material is to maintain a precise separation between the delicate lead strips of the grid. The interspace material of most grids is either aluminum or plastic fiber; there are conflicting reports as to which is better. Aluminum has a higher atomic number than plastic and therefore may provide some selective filtration of scattered x-rays not absorbed in the grid material. Aluminum also has the advantage of producing less visible grid lines on the radiograph.

On the other hand, the use of aluminum as interspace material increases the absorption of primary x-rays in the interspace, especially at low kVp. The result is higher mAs and higher patient dose. Above 100 kVp, this property is unimportant, but at low kVp, the patient dose may be increased by 20% or more. For this reason, plastic fiber interspace grids are usually preferred to aluminum interspace grids.

Still, aluminum has two additional advantages over fiber. It is nonhygroscopic; that is, it does not absorb moisture as plastic fiber does. Fiber interspace grids can become warped if they absorb moisture. Also, aluminum interspace grids are easier to manufacture with high quality because aluminum is easier to form and roll into sheets of precise thickness.

Regardless of its composition, the grid is encased completely by a thin cover of aluminum. The aluminum casing provides rigidity and helps seal out moisture. Table 18-1 is a summary of the characteristics of the most popular commercially available grids. The types of grids shown in the table are discussed on pp. 237-240.

Grid Performance

Contrast improvement factor. The characteristics of grid construction previously described, especially the grid ratio, are usually specified when identifying a grid. Grid ratio, however, does not relate the ability of the grid to improve radiographic contrast. This property of the grid is specified by the **contrast improvement factor (k)**.

The principal function of a grid is to improve image contrast.

The contrast improvement factor of a grid is the ratio of the contrast of a radiograph made with the grid to the contrast of a radiograph made without the grid. A contrast improvement factor of 1 indicates no improvement whatsoever. Most grids have contrast improvement factors between 1.5 and 2.5. In other words, the radiographic contrast is approximately doubled when grids are used. Mathematically, the contrast improvement factor *(k)* is expressed as follows:

Contrast Improvement Factor
$$k = \frac{\text{Radiographic contrast with grid}}{\text{Radiographic contrast without grid}}$$

Question: After an aluminum step wedge is placed on a tissue phantom 20 cm thick, a radiograph is made. Without a grid, analysis of the radiograph shows an average gradient (a measure of contrast) of 1.1. With a 12:1 grid, radiographic contrast is 2.8. What is the contrast improvement factor of this grid?

TABLE 18-1	Construction Characteristics of Some Popular Grids		
Type	**Interspace**	**Grid Frequency (lines/in)**	**Grid Ratio**
Focused	Aluminum	145	14:1, 12:1, 10:1, 8:1
Focused	Aluminum	103	12:1, 10:1, 8:1, 6:1
Parallel	Aluminum	103	6:1
Focused	Aluminum	85	12:1, 10:1, 8:1, 6:1, 5:1
Parallel	Aluminum	85	6:1, 5:1
Parallel	Aluminum	196	3.5:1, 2:1
Crossed focused	Aluminum	85	6:1, 5:1
Crossed focused	Aluminum	85	6:1, 5:1
Focused	Fiber	80	12:1, 8:1, 5:1
Crossed focused	Fiber	80	8:1, 5:1
Focused	Fiber	60	6:1
Parallel	Fiber	60	6:1

Answer: $k = \dfrac{2.8}{1.1}$

$= 2.55$

The contrast improvement factor is usually measured at 100 kVp, but it should be realized that the contrast improvement factor is a complex function of the x-ray emission spectrum, patient or part thickness, and the area irradiated. Other factors, such as lead content, also influence this measure of grid performance. The contrast improvement factor is higher for high-ratio grids.

Bucky factor. Although the use of a grid improves contrast, a penalty is paid in the form of patient dose. The amount of image-forming radiation transmitted through a grid is much less than the image-forming radiation incident on the grid. Therefore, when a grid is used, the radiographic technique must be increased to produce the same OD. The amount of such increase is given by the **Bucky factor (B)**, as follows:

Bucky Factor

$$B = \frac{\text{Incident image-forming radiation}}{\text{Transmitted image-forming radiation}} = \frac{\text{Patient dose with grid}}{\text{Patient dose without grid}}$$

The Bucky factor, sometimes called the *grid factor,* is named for Gustave Bucky, the inventor of the grid. It is an attempt to measure the penetration of both primary and scatter radiation through the grid. Table 18-2 gives representative values of the Bucky factor for several popular grids.

Two generalizations can be made from the data presented in Table 18-2:

1. The higher the grid ratio, the higher the Bucky factor. The penetration of primary radiation through a grid is rather independent of grid ratio. The penetration of scatter radiation through a grid becomes less likely with increasing grid ratio, and therefore the Bucky factor increases.
2. The Bucky factor increases with increasing kVp. At high kVp, more scatter radiation is produced. This scatter radiation has a more difficult time penetrating the grid, and thus the Bucky factor increases.

TABLE 18-2	Approximate Bucky Factor Values for Popular Grids.			
	BUCKY FACTOR			
Grid ratio	70 kVp	90 kVp	120 kVp	Average
No grid	1	1	1	1
5:1	2	2.5	3	2
8:1	3	3.5	4	4
12:1	3.5	4	5	5
16:1	4	5	6	6

As the Bucky factor increases, radiographic technique and patient dose increase proportionately.

Whereas the contrast improvement factor measures an improvement in image quality when using grids, the Bucky factor measures how much of an increase in technique will be required compared with nongrid exposure. The Bucky factor also indicates how much of an increase in patient dose accompanies the use of a particular grid.

Selectivity. The ideal grid would be constructed so that all primary x-rays would be transmitted and all scattered x-rays would be absorbed. The ratio of transmitted primary radiation to transmitted scatter radiation is called the **selectivity** of the grid and is usually identified by the Greek letter sigma (Σ):

Selectivity

$$\Sigma = \frac{\text{Primary radiation transmitted through the grid}}{\text{Scatter radiation transmitted through the grid}}$$

Selectivity is primarily a function of the construction characteristics of the grid rather than the characteristics of the x-ray beam. This is not the case for the contrast improvement factor.

Selectivity is related to grid ratio, but the total lead content in the grid has the primary influence on selectivity. Figure 18-6 shows how two grids can have the same grid ratio, yet greatly different lead content. This is usually accomplished with a small loss in grid frequency.

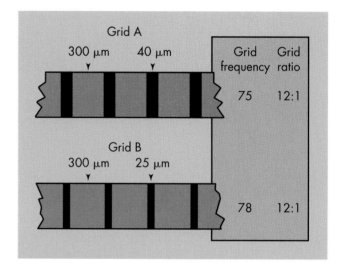

FIGURE 18-6 Because grids *A* and *B* have the same height and interspace thickness, they have the same grid ratio. Grid *A* has 60% more lead but a slightly lower frequency. Grid *A* has higher selectivity and therefore a higher contrast improvement factor.

The heavier a grid is, the more lead it contains, the higher its selectivity, and the more efficient it is in cleaning up scatter radiation. Of course, the lead must be properly arranged. A flat sheet of lead with high mass would make a very poor grid.

The radiologic technologist normally selects a grid based on its ratio. The radiologic engineer or medical physicist takes into account grid ratio, grid frequency, contrast improvement factor, and selectivity in setting up the apparatus for a particular radiologic suite or procedure. The relationships among these grid characteristics are complicated; however, a few general rules regarding them follow:

> **Grid Characteristics**
> 1. High-ratio grids have high contrast improvement factors.
> 2. High-frequency grids have low contrast improvement factors.
> 3. Heavy grids have high selectivity and high contrast improvement factors.

Grid Types

Parallel grids. The simplest type of grid is the **parallel grid,** which is diagrammed in cross section in Figure 18-7. In the parallel grid, all lead grid strips are parallel. This type of grid is the easiest to manufacture, but it has some properties that are clinically undesirable, namely **grid cutoff,** the undesirable absorption of primary x-rays by the grid.

Nearly all grids are large enough to cover a 35 × 43 cm (14 × 17 in) image receptor. As Figure 18-7 illustrates, the attenuation of primary x-rays becomes greater as the x-rays approach the edge of the image receptor. The lead strips in 35 × 43 cm grids are 43 cm long. Across the 35-cm dimension a variation in OD may be observed because of the primary x-ray attenuation. The OD reaches a maximum along the center line of the image receptor and decreases toward the sides.

Grid cutoff can be partial or complete and can result in reduced OD or total absence of film exposure, respectively. The term is derived from the fact that the primary x-rays are "cut off" from getting to the image receptor. Grid cutoff can occur with any type of grid if the grid is improperly positioned, but it is most common with parallel grids.

Parallel grid cutoff is most pronounced when the grid is used at a short source-to-image receptor distance (SID) or with an image receptor with a large area. Figure 18-8 demonstrates the geometric relationship for attenuation of primary x-rays by a parallel grid. The distance from the central ray at which complete cutoff will occur is given by the following:

> **Grid Cutoff**
> $$\text{Distance to cutoff} = \frac{\text{SID}}{\text{Grid ratio}}$$

For instance, theoretically a 10:1 grid when used at 100-cm SID should completely absorb all primary x-rays farther than 10 cm from the central axis. When this grid is used with a 35 × 43 cm image receptor, OD should be apparent only over a 20 × 43 cm area of the image re-

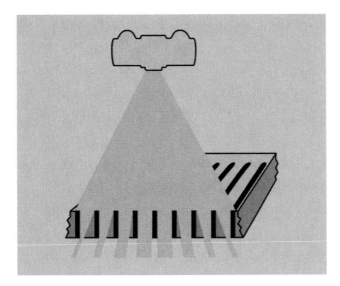

FIGURE 18-7   A linear grid is constructed with parallel grid strips. At a short source-to-image receptor distance, some grid cutoff may occur.

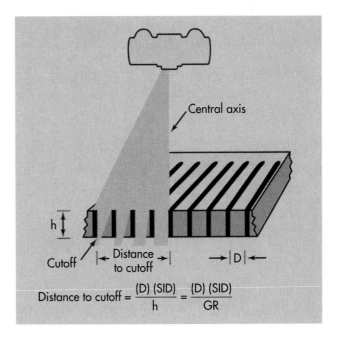

FIGURE 18-8   With a linear grid, OD decreases toward the edge of the image receptor. The distance to grid cutoff is the SID divided by the grid ratio.

ceptor. The radiographs in Figure 18-9 were taken with a 6:1 parallel grid at 76 and 61 cm SID (*A* and *B*, respectively). They demonstrate increasing degrees of grid cutoff with decreasing SID.

Question: A 16:1 parallel grid is positioned for chest radiography at 180-cm SID. What is the distance from the central axis to complete grid cutoff? Will the image satisfactorily cover a 35 × 43 cm image receptor?

Answer: Distance to cutoff = $\dfrac{180}{16}$ = 11.3 cm

Distance to edge of image receptor = 35 ÷ 2
= 17.5 cm

No! Grid cutoff will occur on the lateral 6.2 cm (17.5 − 11.3) of the image receptor.

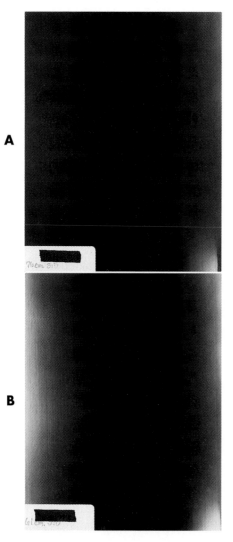

FIGURE 18-9 A, Radiograph taken with a 6:1 parallel grid at an SID of 76 cm. **B,** Radiograph taken with a 6:1 parallel grid at an SID of 61 cm. OD decreases from the center to the edge and complete cutoff. *(Courtesy Dawn Sturk.)*

Crossed grids. Parallel grids clean up scatter radiation in only one direction: along the axis of the grid. Crossed grids are made to overcome this deficiency. **Crossed grids** have lead grid strips running parallel to both the long and short axes of the grid (Figure 18-10). They are usually made by sandwiching two linear grids together with their grid strips perpendicular to one another. They are not too difficult to manufacture and therefore are not excessively expensive. They have, however, found restricted application in clinical radiology. (Interestingly, Bucky's original grid was crossed.)

Crossed grids are much more efficient than linear grids in cleaning up scatter radiation. In fact, a crossed grid has a higher contrast improvement factor than a linear grid of twice the grid ratio. A 6:1 crossed grid cleans up more scatter radiation than a 12:1 linear grid. This advantage increases as the kVp of operation is increased. A crossed grid identified as having a grid ratio of 6:1 is constructed with two 6:1 linear grids.

 The main disadvantage of linear and crossed grids is grid cutoff.

There are two serious disadvantages to using crossed grids. First, positioning the grid is critical; the central ray of the x-ray beam must coincide with the center of the grid. Second, tilt table techniques are possible only if the tube and table are properly aligned. If the table is horizontal and the tube is angled, grid cutoff will occur.

Focused grids. The focused grid is designed to minimize grid cutoff. The lead grid strips of a **focused grid** lie on the imaginary radius lines of a circle centered at the focal

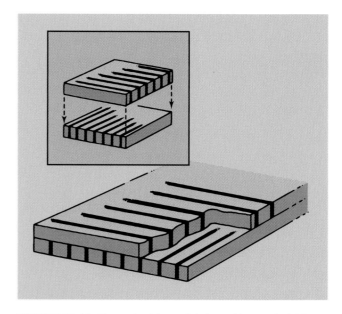

FIGURE 18-10 Crossed grids are fabricated by sandwiching two linear grids together so that their grid strips are perpendicular.

spot so that they coincide with the divergence of the x-ray beam. The x-ray tube target should be placed at the center of this imaginary circle (Figure 18-11).

Focused grids are more difficult to manufacture than linear grids. They are characterized by all the properties of linear grids, except that when properly positioned, they have no grid cutoff. The radiologic technologist must take care when positioning focused grids because of their geometric limitations.

 High-ratio grids have less positioning latitude than low-ratio grids.

Every focused grid is marked with its intended focal distance and the side of the grid that should face the x-ray tube. If radiographs are made at distances other than those intended, grid cutoff will occur. All grids have focusing ranges. A focused grid intended for use at 100-cm SID usually has sufficient latitude to produce acceptable radiographs when used at an SID between 90 and 100 cm. The use of a 100-cm SID, 16:1 focused grid at 180 cm produces severe grid cutoff.

Moving grid. An obvious and annoying shortcoming of the grids previously discussed is that they produce grid lines on the radiograph. **Grid lines** are the images made when primary x-rays are absorbed in the grid strips. Even though the grid strips are very small, their image is still observable. The presence of grid lines can be demonstrated simply by radiographing a grid. Generally, high-frequency grids present less obvious grid lines than low-frequency grids. This is not always the case, since the visibility of grid lines is related directly to the width of the grid strips.

A major improvement in grid development occurred in 1920. Hollis E. Potter hit on a very simple idea: move the grid while the x-ray exposure is being made. The grid lines disappear at little cost of increased radiographic technique. The device that does this is now called a **moving grid,** although the terms *Potter-Bucky diaphragm, Bucky diaphragm,* and *Bucky grid* are still widely used (Figure 18-12).

Focused grids are usually used as moving grids. They are placed in a holding mechanism that is moved at the time of x-ray exposure. There are two basic types of moving grid mechanisms in use today: reciprocating and oscillating.

A reciprocating grid is motor driven back and forth several times during x-ray exposure. The total distance of drive is approximately 2 cm.

An oscillating grid is positioned in a frame with 2 to 3 cm of tolerance on all sides between the frame and grid. Delicate springlike devices located in the four corners hold the grid centered in the frame. A powerful electromagnet pulls the grid to one side and releases it at the beginning of the exposure. Thereafter, the grid oscillates in a circular fashion around the grid frame, coming to rest after 20 to 30 s.

The main difference between reciprocating and oscillating grids is their pattern of motion. The motion of a reciprocating grid is to and fro, whereas that of an oscillating grid is circular. There are disadvantages of moving grids. Moving grids require a bulky mechanism that is subject to failure. The distance between the patient and the image receptor is increased with moving grids because of this mechanism; that extra distance may create an unwanted increase in magnification and image blur. Moving grids can introduce motion into the cassette-holding device, which can result in additional image blur.

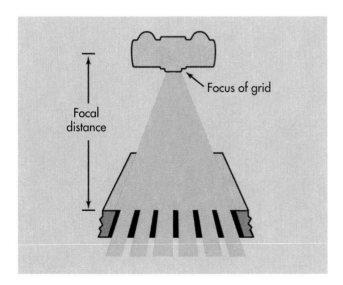

FIGURE 18-11 A focused grid is fabricated so that the grid strips are parallel to the primary x-ray path across the entire image receptor.

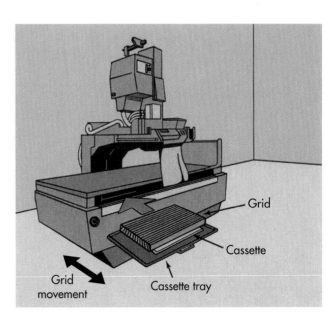

FIGURE 18-12 Proper installation of a moving grid.

If not properly designed, moving grids can produce a stroboscopic effect when used with half- or full-wave-rectified x-ray generators because of synchronization between x-ray pulsation and grid movement. This effect results in the presence of pronounced grid lines. Also, the minimum exposure time is longer with moving grids than with stationary grids.

Fortunately, the advantages of moving grids far outweigh the disadvantages. The types of motion blur discussed are for descriptive purposes only. The motion blur generated by properly functioning moving grids is undetectable. Only malfunctioning moving grid systems create problems, and these problems occur very infrequently. The moving grids are usually the technique of choice and therefore are rather universally used.

Grid Problems

Most grids in diagnostic imaging are the moving type. They are permanently mounted in the moving mechanism just below the tabletop or just behind the vertical chest board. To be effective, of course, the grid must move from side to side. If the grid is installed incorrectly and moves in the same direction as the grid strips, grid lines will appear on the radiograph (Figure 18-13). Stationary grids are either fastened to the front surface of a cassette or built into specially designed cassettes.

The most frequent error in the use of grids is improper positioning. For the grid to function correctly, it must be precisely positioned relative to the x-ray tube target and to the central ray of the x-ray beam. Four situations characteristic of focused grids must be avoided

(Table 18-3). Only an off-level grid is a problem with parallel and crossed grids.

Off-level grid. A properly functioning grid must lie in a plane perpendicular to the central ray of the x-ray beam (Figure 18-14). The **central ray of the x-ray beam** is the x-ray traveling along the center of the useful x-ray beam.

Despite its name, an **off-level grid** is usually produced by having an improperly positioned radiographic tube and not an improperly positioned grid. However, this can occur when the grid tilts during horizontal beam radiography or during mobile radiography when the image receptor sinks into the patient's bed. If the central ray is incident on the grid at an angle, then all incident x-rays will be angled and grid cutoff will occur across the entire radiograph, resulting in lower OD.

The condition can be prevented by paying careful attention to the installation of grids and the positioning of the x-ray tube. Grid cutoff caused by off-level grids can

TABLE 18-3	Types of Grid Errors
Type of Grid Misalignment	**Result**
Off level	Grid cutoff across image; underexposed, light image
Off center	Grid cutoff across image; underexposed, light image
Off focus	Grid cutoff toward edge of image
Upside down	Severe grid cutoff toward edge of image
Combined off-center and off-focus	Image that is dark on one side and light on the other

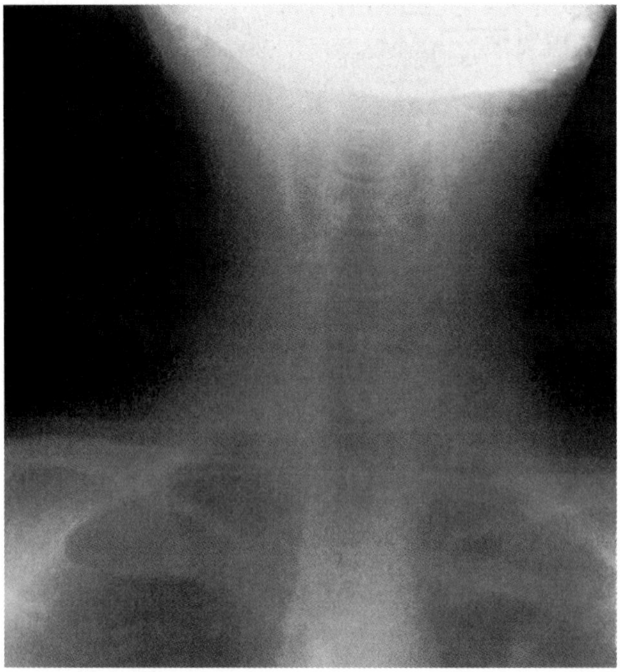

FIGURE 18-13 If the focused grid is tilted or the central ray is angled toward the grid strips, overall density decreases, and grid lines appear across the radiograph.

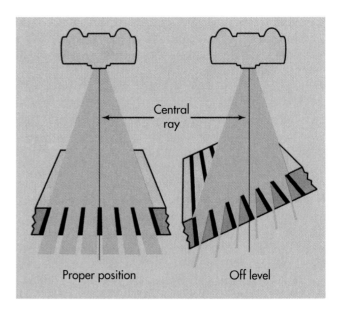

FIGURE 18-14 If a grid is off level so that the central ray is not perpendicular to the grid, partial cutoff will occur over the entire image receptor.

occur with all types of grids. It is the only positioning problem that occurs with parallel and crossed grids.

Off-center grid. A grid can be perpendicular to the central ray of the x-ray beam and still produce grid cutoff if it is shifted laterally. This is a problem with focused grids, as shown in Figure 18-15, in which an off-center grid is shown with a properly positioned grid.

The center of a focused grid must be positioned directly under the x-ray tube target so that the central ray of the x-ray beam passes through the centermost interspace of the grid. Any lateral shift results in grid cutoff across the entire radiograph, resulting in a lower OD. This error in positioning is called **lateral decentering.**

As with an off-level grid, an off-center grid is more a matter of positioning the tube than the grid. In practice, it means that the radiologic technologist must carefully line up the center of the light-localized field with the center of the cassette. Marks on both the light field and the cassette and sometimes on the table, are provided so that this can be done quickly and easily.

Off-focus grid. A major problem with using a focused grid arises when radiographs are taken at SIDs unspecified for that grid. Figure 18-16 illustrates what happens when a focused grid is not used at the proper focal distance. The farther the grid from the specified focal distance, the more severe the grid cutoff. In Figure 18-16, the grid cutoff is not uniform across the image receptor but is more severe to the periphery.

This condition is not normally a problem if all chest radiographs are taken at 180 cm SID and all table radiographs at 100 cm SID. Occasionally, table radiographs are taken at an SID other than 100 cm and with a grid

having a 100 cm focal distance. Positioning the grid at the proper focal distance is more important with high-ratio grids. More positioning latitude is possible with low-ratio grids.

Upside-down grid. The explanation of an upside-down grid is obvious. If it occurs it will be noticed immediately. A radiographic image taken with an upside-down focused grid shows sever grid cutoff on either side of the central ray (Figure 18-17). Every focused grid has a clear

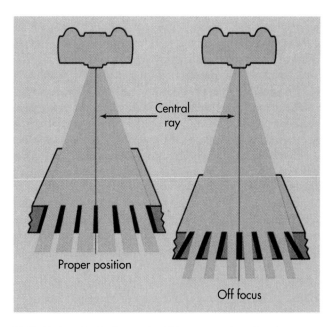

FIGURE 18-16 If a focused grid is not positioned at the specified focal distance, grid cutoff will occur, and OD will decrease with distance from the central ray.

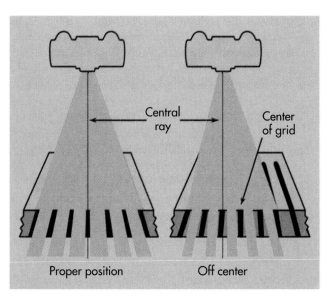

FIGURE 18-15 When a focused grid is positioned off center, partial grid cutoff occurs over the entire image receptor.

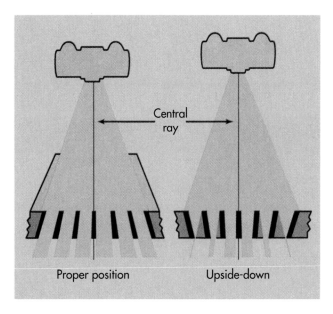

FIGURE 18-17 A focused grid positioned upside down should be detected on the first radiograph. Complete grid cutoff occurs except in the region of the central ray.

label on one side and sometimes on both. Labels indicate the tube side, the image receptor side, or both, and the prescribed focal distance. With even moderate attention, upside-down grid errors will not occur.

Combined off-center, off-focus grid. Perhaps the most common improper grid position occurs if the grid is both off-center and off-focus. Without proper attention, this can easily occur during mobile radiography. It is an easily recognized grid-positioning artifact because the result is uneven exposure. The resulting radiograph appears dark on one side and light on the other.

Grid Selection

Modern grids are sufficiently well manufactured that many radiologists do not find the grid lines of stationary grids objectionable, especially for portable radiography and horizontal views of an upright patient. Stationary grids are also cheaper than moving grids. Moving grid mechanisms, however, rarely fail, and image degradation rarely occurs. Therefore in most situations, it is appropriate to design radiographic procedures around moving grids. When moving grids are used, parallel grids can be used, but focused grids are more common.

Focused grids are generally far superior to parallel grids, but they require care and attention in use. When focused grids are used, the indicators on the x-ray apparatus must be in good adjustment and properly calibrated. The SID indicator, the source-to-tabletop distance (STD) indicator, and the light-localizing collimator must all be properly adjusted.

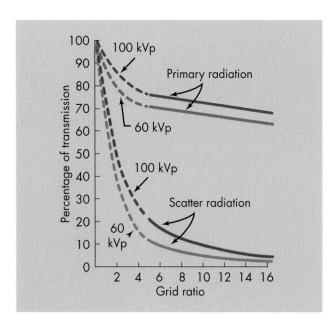

FIGURE 18-18 As grid ratio increases, the transmission of scatter radiation decreases faster than the transmission of primary radiation. Therefore cleanup of scatter radiation increases.

Selection of a grid with the proper ratio depends on an understanding of three interrelated factors: kVp, degree of cleanup, and patient dose. When a high kVp is used, high-ratio grids should be too. Of course, the choice of grid is also influenced by the size and shape of the anatomic part being radiographed.

As grid ratio increases, the amount of cleanup also increases. Figure 18-18 shows the approximate percentage of scatter radiation and primary radiation transmitted as a function of grid ratio. Note that the difference between the grid ratios of 12:1 and 16:1 is small. The difference in patient dose is large, however, and therefore, 16:1 grids are not often used. Many general-purpose x-ray examination facilities find that an 8:1 grid is a good compromise between the desired levels of scatter radiation cleanup and patient dose.

 Generally, grid ratios up to 8:1 are satisfactory at tube potentials below 90 kVp. Grid ratios above 8:1 are used when the kVp exceeds 90.

The use of one grid also reduces the likelihood of grid cutoff because improper grid positioning can easily accompany frequent changes of grids. In facilities where a high-kVp technique for chest radiography is used, 16:1 grids can be used.

Patient dose. One major disadvantage that accompanies the use of x-ray grids is increased patient dose. For any examination, using a grid may require several times more radiation to the patient than not using one. The use of a moving grid instead of a stationary grid with similar physical characteristics requires approximately 15% more radiation to the patient. Table 18-4 is a summary of approximate patient doses for various grid techniques with a 200-speed image receptor.

Low-ratio grids are used during mammography. All dedicated mammographic equipment is equipped with a 4:1 or a 5:1 moving grid. Even at the low kVp used for mammography, considerable scatter radiation occurs.

TABLE 18-4	Approximate Entrance Skin Exposure for Examining the Adult Pelvis with a 200-Speed Image Receptor		
	ENTRANCE EXPOSURE (mR)		
Type of Grid	70 kVp	90 kVp	120 kVp
No grid	85	70	50
5:1	270	215	145
8:1	325	285	205
12:1	425	395	290
16:1	520	475	365
5:1 crossed	535	405	295
8:1 crossed	585	530	405

The use of such grids greatly improves image contrast, with no loss of spatial resolution. The only disadvantage is the increased patient dose, which can be as much as twice that without a grid. However, with dedicated equipment and grid, patient dose still is very low.

The concern about exposure to the patient is important. Grid selection, however, should not be compromised so far that the loss of contrast enhancement interferes with diagnostic interpretation.

Three factors must be kept in mind when choosing a grid: (1) the patient dose increases with increasing grid ratio, (2) high-ratio grids are usually used for high-kVp examination, and (3) the patient dose at high kVp when

x-rays are transmitted through tissue is less than that at low kVp when x-rays are absorbed in tissue.

Grid-Selection Factors
1. Patient dose increases with increasing grid ratio.
2. High-ratio grids are usually used for high-kVp examinations.
3. Patient dose at high kVp is less than that at low kVp.

In general, compared with the use of low kVp and low-ratio grids, the use of high kVp and high-ratio grids will result in lower patient dose and radiographs of equal quality.

One additional disadvantage of using grids is the increased radiographic technique required. When a grid is used, the technique factors must be increased over what they were for nongrid examinations; either the mAs or the kVp must be increased. Table 18-5 presents approximate changes in technique factors required by standard grids. Usually, the mAs is increased rather than the kVp. (One exception is chest radiography.) Increased time can result in motion blur. Table 18-6 summarizes the clinical factors that should be considered in the selection of various types of grids.

TABLE 18-5 Approximate Change in Radiographic Technique for Standard Grids

Grid Ratio	mAs Increase	kVp Increase
No grid	1×	—
5:1	2×	+8 to 10
8:1	4×	+13 to 15
12:1	5×	+20 to 25
16:1	6×	+30 to 40

TABLE 18-6 Clinical Considerations in Grid Selection

Type of Grid	Degree of Scatter Removal	Positioning Latitude Off Center	Off Focus	Recommended Technique	Remarks
5:1, linear	+	Very wide	Very wide	Up to 80 kVp	It is the least expensive. It is the easiest to use.
6:1, linear	+	Very wide	Very wide	Up to 80 kVp	It is the least expensive. It's ideally suited for bedside radiography.
8:1, linear	++	Wide	Wide	Up to 100 kVp	It is used for general stationary grids.
10:1, linear	+++	Wide	Wide	Up to 100 kVp	Reasonable care is required for proper alignment.
5:1, crisscross	+++	Narrow	Very wide	Up to 100 kVp	Tube tilt is limited to 5 degrees.
12:1, linear	++++	Narrow	Narrow	Over 110 kVp	Extra care is required for proper alignment. It is usually used in fixed mount.
6:1, crisscross	++++	Narrow	Very wide	Up to 110 kVp	It is not suited for tilted-tube techniques.
16:1, linear	+++++	Narrow	Narrow	Over 100 kVp	Extra care is required for proper alignment. It is usually used in fixed mount.
8:1, crisscross	+++++	Narrow	Wide	Up to 120 kVp	It is not suited for tilted-tube techniques.

Adapted from *Characteristics and applications of x-ray grids*, c. 1980, Liebel-Florsheim, Cincinnati.

Radiographic Exposure

OBJECTIVES

At the completion of this chapter, the student should be able to:

1. List the four prime exposure factors
2. Discuss milliampere-second and kilovolt peak in relation to x-ray beam quantity and quality
3. Describe characteristics of the imaging system that affect x-ray beam quantity and quality

OUTLINE

Exposure factors are a few of the tools that radiographers use to create high-quality radiographs. Radiographic quality is discussed in Chapter 20. This chapter introduces the student radiographer to the prime exposure factors that are under the radiographer's control: kilovolt peak (kVp), mA, exposure time, and source-to-image receptor distance (SID).

Properties of the x-ray imaging system that influence the selection of exposure factors are reviewed, including focal spot size, total x-ray beam filtration, and the source of high voltage.

EXPOSURE FACTORS

Proper exposure of a patient to x-radiation is necessary to produce a diagnostic radiograph. The factors that influence and determine the quantity and quality of x-radiation to which the patient is exposed are called **exposure factors** (Table 19-1). Recall from Chapter 12 that *radiation quantity* refers to radiation intensity (measured in mR or mR/mAs) and *radiation quality* refers to x-ray beam penetrability (best measured by half-value layer [HVL]).

All of these factors are under the control of the radiologic technologist, except those fixed by the design of the x-ray imaging system. For example, focal-spot size is limited to two selections. Sometimes the added x-ray beam filtration is fixed. The high-voltage generator provides characteristic voltage ripple that cannot be changed.

The four prime exposure factors are kVp, mA, exposure time, and SID. mA and exposure time(s) are usually combined (mAs). Of these, the most important are kVp and mAs, the factors principally responsible for x-ray quality and quantity. Focal-spot size, distance, and filtration are secondary factors that may require manipulation for particular studies.

TABLE 19-1	Exposure Factors Influencing X-Ray Quantity and Quality	
Factor Increased	**Resulting Change in Quantity**	**Resulting Change in Qualtiy**
Kilovolt peak	Increase	Increase
Milliampere	Increase	No change
Exposure time	Increase	No change
Milliampere-second	Increase	No change
Distance	Decrease	No change
Voltage ripple	Decrease	Decrease
Filtration	Decrease	Increase

kVp

The effects of kVp on the x-ray beam are described in previous chapters. To understand kVp as an exposure technique factor, assume that the kVp is the primary control of beam quality and therefore **beam penetrability,** the ability of the x-ray beam to penetrate tissue. A higher-quality x-ray beam is one with higher energy and thus is more likely to penetrate the anatomic part of interest.

 The kVp controls radiographic contrast.

The kVp has more effect than any other factor on image-receptor exposure because it affects beam quality and to a lesser degree influences beam quantity. With increasing kVp, more x-rays are emitted that have higher energy and greater penetrability. Unfortunately, because they have higher energy, they also interact more by the Compton effect and produce more scatter radiation, which results in increased image noise.

The kVp selected greatly determines the number of x-rays in the image-forming beam and therefore the resulting average optical density (OD). Finally, and perhaps most important, the kVp controls the scale of contrast on the finished radiograph because of the increased image noise produced. Therefore a high kVp results in reduced image contrast.

mA

The mA station selected for patient exposure determines the number of x-rays produced and therefore the radiation quantity. Recall that the unit of electric current is the ampere (A). One ampere is equal to one coulomb (C) of electrostatic charge flowing each second in a conductor, as follows:

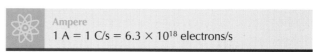 **Ampere**
$$1\ A = 1\ C/s = 6.3 \times 10^{18}\ electrons/s$$

Therefore when the 100-mA station on the operating console is selected, 6.3×10^{17} electrons flow through the x-ray tube each second.

Question: What is the electron flow from cathode to anode when the 500-mA station is selected?

Answer: 500 mA = 0.5 A
$$= (0.5\ A)\ (6.3 \times 10^{18}\ electrons/s/A)$$
$$= 3.15 \times 10^{18}\ electrons/s$$

As more electrons flow through the x-ray tube, more x-rays are produced. Assuming a constant exposure time, this relationship is directly proportional. When the 200-mA station is changed to the 300-mA station, the number of electrons flowing through the x-ray tube is increased by 50%. The number of x-rays produced increases by 50% and therefore so does patient dose. A change from 200 to 400 mA would be a 100% increase or a doubling of the x-ray tube current and patient dose if exposure time remains constant.

 With a constant exposure time, mA controls x-ray quantity and therefore patient dose.

Question: At 200 mA the entrance skin exposure (ESE) is 752 mR (7.5 mGy$_a$). What will be the ESE at 500 mA if no change is made in exposure time?

Answer:
$$ESE = 752 \text{ mR} \left(\frac{500 \text{ mA}}{200 \text{ mA}} \right)$$
$$= 1880 \text{ mR}$$

A change in the mA does not change the kinetic energy of electrons flowing from cathode to anode. It simply changes the number of electrons. Consequently, the energy of the x-rays produced is not changed; only the number is changed.

 X-ray quality remains fixed with a change in the mA.

Often, x-ray imaging systems are identified by the maximum x-ray tube current (mA) possible. Inexpensive radiographic imaging systems designed for private physicians' offices normally have a maximum capacity of 600 mA. The available mA stations may be 50, 100, 200, 300, 400, and 600. High-powered special-procedure equipment may have a capacity of 1200 mA. The available mA stations are those previously listed plus 800, 1000, and 1200.

Exposure Time

Radiographic exposure times are usually kept as short as possible. The purpose is not to minimize patient radiation dose but rather to minimize motion blur that can occur because of patient motion.

 Short exposure time reduces motion blur.

Producing a diagnostic radiograph requires that a patient be exposed to a certain amount of radiation. Therefore, when exposure time is reduced, the mA must be increased proportionately to provide the required x-ray intensity. On older x-ray imagers, exposure time is expressed in fractional seconds, whereas current x-ray imaging systems identify exposure time in milliseconds (ms). Table 19-2 shows how the different units of time are related.

An easy way to identify an x-ray imaging system as either single phase, three phase, or high frequency is to

TABLE 19-2	Relationships Among Different Units of Exposure Time	
Fractional (s)	**Seconds (s)**	**Milliseconds (ms)**
1.0	1.0	1000
4/5	0.8	800
3/4	0.75	750
2/3	0.67	667
3/5	0.6	600
1/2	0.5	500
2/5	0.4	400
1/3	0.33	333
1/4	0.25	250
1/5	0.2	200
1/10	0.1	100
1/20	0.05	50
1/60	0.017	17
1/120	0.008	8

note the shortest exposure time possible. Single-phase imaging systems cannot produce an exposure time less than ½ cycle or its equivalent 8 ms. Three-phase and high-frequency generators can normally provide exposure times as short as 1 ms.

mAs

mA and exposure time (in seconds) are usually combined and used as one factor—mAs—in radiographic technique selection.

 mAs
mAs = Milliampere (mA) × Exposure Time (s)

Although the radiologic technologist may be required to select an exposure time, it is always selected with consideration of the mA station. The important parameter is the product of the exposure time and tube current.

 mAs controls radiation quantity, optical density, and patient dose.

The mAs determines the number of x-rays in the primary beam, and therefore the mAs principally controls radiation quantity in the same way that mA and exposure time do; it does not influence radiation quality. The mAs is the key factor in the control of OD on the radiograph.

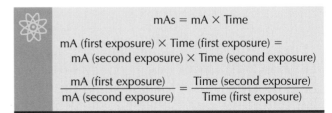
mAs = mA × Time
mA (first exposure) × Time (first exposure) = mA (second exposure) × Time (second exposure)
$$\frac{\text{mA (first exposure)}}{\text{mA (second exposure)}} = \frac{\text{Time (second exposure)}}{\text{Time (first exposure)}}$$

Question: A radiographic technique calls for 600 mA at 200 ms. What is the mAs?

Answer: 600 mA × 200 ms = 600 mA × 0.2 s
= 120 mAs

Time and mA can be used to compensate for each other in an indirect fashion. This is described by the following:

Question: A radiograph of the abdomen requires 300 mA and 500 ms. The patient is unable to hold his breath, which results in motion blur. A second exposure is made with an exposure time of 200 ms. Calculate the new mA that is required.

Answer:
$$\frac{x}{300\ mA} = \frac{500\ ms}{200\ ms}$$
(200 ms)x = (500 ms) (300 mA)
(0.2 s)x = (0.5 s)(300 ms)
(0.2 s)x = 150 mAs
$$x = \frac{150\ mAs}{0.2\ s}$$
x = 750 mA
or
$$New\ mA = \frac{Original\ mAs}{New\ time}$$
$$new\ mA = \frac{0.5\ s \times 300\ mA}{0.2\ s}$$
New mA = 750 mA

If the high-voltage generator is properly calibrated, the same mAs and therefore the same OD can be produced with various combinations of mA and time (Table 19-3). This is according to the reciprocity law, which states that OD will be constant for any combination of mA and exposure time that results in constant mAs.

mAs is the product of x-ray tube current and exposure time. Since x-ray tube current is electron flow per unit time, mAs is therefore simply a measure of the total number of electrons conducted through the x-ray tube for a particular exposure.

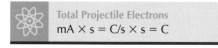
Total Projectile Electrons
mA × s = C/s × s = C

Question: How many electrons are involved in x-ray production at 100 mAs?

Answer: 100 mAs = 0.1 As = 0.1 C/s × s = 0.1 C
1 C = 6.3 × 10^18 electrons
Therefore 100 mAs = 6.3 × 10^17 electrons

mAs is one measure of electrostatic charge.

TABLE 19-3	Product of mA and Time (ms) for 10 mAs				
mA		ms		mAs	
100	×	100	=	10	
200	×	50	=	10	
300	×	33	=	10	
400	×	25	=	10	
600	×	17	=	10	
800	×	12	=	10	
1000	×	10	=	10	

On an x-ray imaging system in which only mAs can be selected, the exposure factors are automatically adjusted to the highest mA at the shortest exposure time allowed by the high-voltage generator. Such a design is called a **falling-load generator.**

Question: A radiologic technologist selects a technique of 200 mAs. The operating console is automatically adjusted to the maximum mA station: 1000 mA. What will be the exposure time?

Answer: $\frac{200\ mAs}{1000\ mA} = 0.2\ s = 200\ ms$
The actual exposure time will be somewhat longer than 200 ms because the tube current falls as the anode heats up.

Varying the mAs changes only the number of electrons conducted during an exposure, not the energy of those electrons. The relationship is directly proportional; a doubling of the mAs doubles the x-ray quantity.

Only the x-ray quantity is affected by changes in the mAs.

Question: A cervical spine examination calls for 68 kVp and 30 mAs and results in an entrance skin exposure (ESE) of 114 mR (1.14 mGy_a). The next patient is examined at 68 kVp and 25 mAs. What will be the ESE?

Answer: $ESE = 114\ mR \left(\frac{25\ mAs}{30\ mAs}\right) = 95\ mR$

Distance

Distance affects exposure of the image receptor according to the inverse square law, which was discussed in Chapter 5. The SID largely determines the intensity of the x-ray beam at the image receptor and has no effect on radiation quality.

Distance has no effect on radiation quality.

The following relationship, termed the **square law** by some, is derived from the inverse square law. It allows a radiologic technologist to calculate the required change in mAs after a change in SID to maintain constant OD.

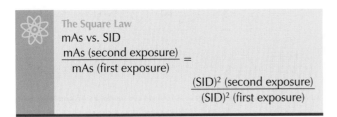

The Square Law
mAs vs. SID

$$\frac{\text{mAs (second exposure)}}{\text{mAs (first exposure)}} = \frac{(SID)^2 \text{ (second exposure)}}{(SID)^2 \text{ (first exposure)}}$$

Note that both the original mAs and the original SID are in the denominator rather than reversed as in the inverse square law.

Question: An examination requires 100 mAs at 180-cm SID. If the distance is changed to 90-cm SID, what should be the new mAs?

Answer:

$$\frac{x}{100} = \frac{90^2}{180^2}$$

$$x = 100\left(\frac{90}{180}\right)^2$$

$$= 100\left(\frac{1}{2}\right)^2$$

$$= 100\left(\frac{1}{4}\right)$$

$$= 25 \text{ mAs}$$

 Distance (SID) affects OD.

When preparing to make a radiographic exposure, the radiologic technologist selects specific settings for each of the factors described: kVp, mAs, and SID. The control panel selections are based on an evaluation of the patient, the thickness of the anatomic part, and the type of accessories used.

Standard SIDs have been in use for many years now. For tabletop radiography, 100 cm is common, whereas dedicated chest examination is usually conducted at 180 cm. With advances in generator design and image receptors, even larger SIDs are anticipated. Tabletop radiography at 120 cm and chest radiography at 300 cm are now in use. The use of a longer SID results in less magnification, less focal-spot blur, and improved spatial resolution. However, more mAs must be used because of the effects of the square law.

IMAGING SYSTEM CHARACTERISTICS
Focal-Spot Size

Most x-ray tubes are equipped with two possible focal-spot sizes. On the operating console, they are usually identified as small and large. Conventional tubes have two fo-

cal spots of normal size: 0.6 mm/1.2 mm, 0.5 mm/1.0 mm, or 1.0 mm/2.0 mm available. X-ray tubes used in special procedures or magnification radiography have 0.3 mm/1.0 mm focal spots. Most mammography tubes have 0.1 mm/0.3 mm focal spots. These are called **microfocus tubes** and are designed specifically for imaging very small microcalcifications at relatively short SIDs.

For normal imaging, the large focal spot is used. This ensures that a sufficient mAs can be used to image thick or dense body parts. The large focal spot also provides for a shorter exposure time, which minimizes motion blur.

One difference between the large and small focal spots is the capacity to produce x-rays. Many more x-rays can be produced with the large focal spot because anode heat capacity is higher. With the small focal spot, electron interaction occurs over a much smaller area of the anode, and the resulting heat limits the capacity of x-ray production.

 Changing the focal spot for a given kVp/mAs does not change x-ray quantity or quality.

A small focal spot is reserved for fine-detail radiography, in which the quantity of x-rays is relatively low. Small focal spots are always used for magnification radiography. They are normally used during extremity radiography and during the examination of other thin body parts in which higher x-ray quantity is not necessary. Changing the focal spot for a given kVp/mAs does not change x-ray quantity or quality.

Filtration

Inherent filtration. All x-ray beams are affected by the inherent filtration properties of the glass or metal envelope of the x-ray tube. For general-purpose tubes, the value of inherent filtration is approximately 0.5 mm of aluminum (Al) equivalent. The variable-aperture light-localizing collimator usually provides an additional 1.0 mm of Al equivalent. Most of this is due to the reflective surface of the mirror of the collimator. To meet the required total filtration of 2.5 mm of Al, the manufacturer inserts an additional filter of 1.0 mm of Al between the x-ray tube housing and the collimator. The radiologic technologist has no control over these sources of filtration.

Added filtration. Some x-ray imagers have selectable added filtration as shown in Figure 19-1. Usually the equipment is placed into service with the lowest allowable added filtration. Radiographic technique charts usually are formulated at the lowest filtration position. If a higher filter position is used, a radiographic technique chart usually must be developed at that position.

Under normal conditions, it is unnecessary to change the filtration. Some facilities may be set for higher filtration during examinations of tissue with high subject con-

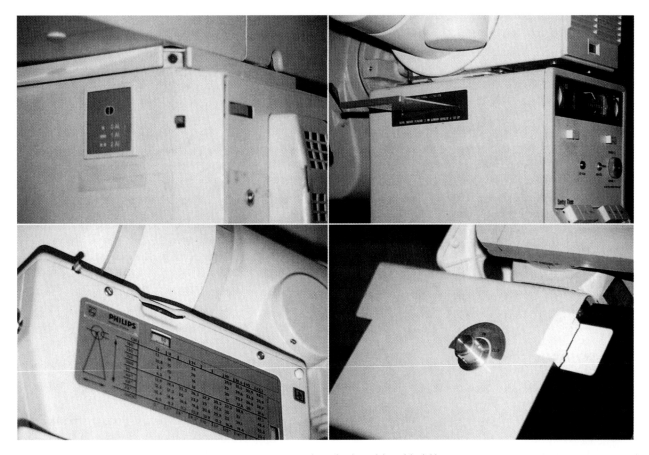

FIGURE 19-1 Four examples of selectable added filtration.

TABLE 19-4	Characteristics of the Various Types of High-Voltage Generators				
				EQUIVALENT TECHNIQUE (kVp/mAs)	
Generator Type	Ripple (%)	Relative Quantity		Chest	Abdomen
Half-wave	100	100		120/20*	74/40*
Full-wave	100	200		120/20	74/40
Three phase, 6 pulse	14	260		115/6	72/34
Three phase, 12 pulse	4	280		115/4	72/30
High frequency	<1	300		112/3	70/24
*The mAs equal that for full-wave rectification; the exposure time is doubled.					

trast, such as studies of the extremities, joints, and chest. When properly used, higher filtration for these examinations results in lower patient dose. *When filtration is changed, be sure to return it to its normal position before the next examination.*

As added filtration is increased, the result is increased x-ray beam quality and penetrability. The result on the image is the same as that for increased kVp: more scatter radiation, increased image noise, and reduced image contrast.

High-Voltage Generation

The radiologic technologist *cannot* select the type of high-voltage generator to be used for a given examination. This

is fixed by the type of x-ray imaging system. Still, it is important to understand how the various high-voltage generators affect radiographic technique and patient dose.

Three basic types of high-voltage generators are available: single phase, three phase, and high frequency. The radiation quantity and quality produced in the x-ray tube are influenced by the type of high-voltage generator. Review Figure 9-25 for the shape of the voltage waveform associated with a high-voltage generator. Table 19-4 lists the percentage of ripple of various types of high-voltage generators, the variation in their output, and the change in the radiographic technique for two common examinations associated with each generator.

Half-wave rectification. A half-wave-rectified generator has 100% voltage ripple. During exposure with such a generator, x-rays are produced and emitted only half the time. Half-wave rectification results in the same radiation quality as that for full-wave rectification, but the radiation quantity is halved. During each negative half-cycle, no x-rays are emitted.

Half-wave rectification is rarely used. Some mobile x-ray imagers and most dental x-ray imagers are half wave rectified. No general-purpose x-ray imagers have this type of high-voltage generator.

Full-wave rectification. The voltage waveform for full-wave rectification is identical to that of half-wave rectification, except there is no dead time. During exposure, x-rays are continually emitted in pulses. The radiation quality does not change when going from half-wave to full-wave rectification; however, the radiation quantity doubles. Consequently, the required exposure time for full-wave rectification is only half that for half-wave rectification.

Three-phase power. Three-phase power comes in two principal forms: 6 pulse or 12 pulse. The difference is determined by the manner in which the high-voltage step-up transformer is engineered. The difference between the two forms is minor but does cause a detectable change in x-ray quantity and quality. Three-phase power is more efficient than single-phase power. More x-rays are produced per mAs, and the average energy of those x-rays is higher, so three-phase power results in higher x-ray quantity and quality. The x-radiation emitted is nearly constant rather than pulsed.

High-frequency generation. High-frequency generators were developed in the 1980s and are increasingly used, especially with low-power x-ray systems. The voltage waveform is nearly constant with less than 1% ripple. High frequency generation results in even higher x-ray quantity and quality.

At present, high-frequency generators are being increasingly used with dedicated mammography systems and mobile x-ray imagers. It is likely that most high-voltage generators of the future will be of the high-frequency type, regardless of the required power levels.

SUMMARY

Radiographic exposure factors (mAs, kVp, and distance) are manipulated by radiologic technologists to produce high-quality radiographs. The exposure factors influence quantity (number of x-rays) and quality (penetrability of the x-rays). Proper selection of these exposure factors optimizes both the spatial resolution and contrast resolution of the image. Table 19-4 summarizes the effects of primary and secondary factors on the quantity and quality of the beam.

CHALLENGE QUESTIONS

1. Define or otherwise identify:
   a. Kilovolt peak (kVp)
   b. Milliampere-second (mAs)
   c. Beam penetrability
   d. Microfocus tubes
   e. Source-to-image receptor distance (SID)
   f. Falling-load generator
   g. Square law
2. Discuss how an increase in kVp changes x-ray quantity, x-ray quality, and contrast scale.
3. What mA stations are typically available on an operating console?
4. What is normally the shortest radiographic exposure time on single-phase, three-phase, and high-frequency equipment?
5. Describe how a change in SID from 100 to 180 cm should be accompanied by a change in kVp, mA, and exposure time.
6. Why does an x-ray tube have two focal-spot sizes?
7. Discuss how an increase in mAs changes x-ray quantity, x-ray quality, and contrast scale.
8. Why are short radiographic exposure times necessary?
9. A radiographic technique calls for 800 mA at 50 ms. What is the mAs?
10. The normal lateral chest technique is 120 kVp, 100 mA, and 15 ms. To reduce motion blur, the radiologic technologist shortens the exposure time to 5 ms. What is the new mA?
11. Explain the following statement: the mA does not change the kinetic energy of electrons flowing across the x-ray tube.
12. Why is it important to keep exposure time as short as possible?
13. Write three mA and exposure times that equal 100 mAs. Explain the advantages of each choice.
14. An examination requires 78 kVp/150 mAs at 100-cm SID. If the distance is changed to 180 cm, what is the new mAs?
15. What are the two types of focal spots available in x-ray tubes? Explain how each is typically used.
16. List the three types of high-voltage generators.
17. Explain how high-voltage generation influences x-ray beam quantity and quality.
18. What are the sources of x-ray beam filtration?
19. What is the principal advantage of exposure with a large focal spot compared with a small focal spot?
20. Identify each control and meter on an x-ray imager that you operate.

CHAPTER

20

Radiographic Quality

OBJECTIVES

At the completion of this chapter, the student should be able to:

1. Define *radiographic quality, resolution, noise,* and *speed*
2. Interpret the shape of the characteristic curve
3. Identify the toe, shoulder, and straight-line portion of the characteristic curve
4. Distinguish the geometric factors affecting radiographic quality
5. Analyze the subject factors affecting radiographic quality
6. Examine the tools and techniques available to create high-quality images

OUTLINE

Definitions
   Radiographic Quality
   Resolution
   Noise
   Speed
Film Factors
   Characteristic Curve
   Optical Density
   Film Processing
Geometric Factors
   Magnification
   Distortion
   Focal-Spot Blur
   Heel Effect

Subject Factors
   Subject Contrast
   Motion Blur
Tools for Improved Radiographic Quality
   Patient Positioning
   Image Receptors
   Selection of Technique Factors

*R*adiographic quality is defined as the exactness of representation of the patient's anatomic part on the radiograph. High-quality radiographs are required so that radiologists can make accurate diagnoses. To produce quality images, radiographers apply knowledge of the three major interrelated categories of radiographic quality: film factors, geometric factors, and subject factors. Each of these factors influences the quality of a radiographic image and is under the partial control of the radiologic technologist. The selection of radiographic technique factors is discussed in this chapter.

DEFINITIONS
Radiographic Quality

The term *radiographic quality* refers to the fidelity with which the anatomic structure being examined is imaged on the radiograph. A radiograph that faithfully reproduces structure and tissues is identified as a high-quality radiograph. The radiologist needs high-quality radiographs to make accurate diagnoses. Poor-quality radiographs contain images that are difficult for the human eye to interpret. They can lead to reexamination or sometimes, missed diagnoses.

The quality of a radiograph is not easy to define, and it cannot be measured precisely. A number of factors affect radiographic quality, but there are no precise, universally accepted measures by which to judge it. Perhaps, the most important characteristics of radiographic quality are spatial resolution, contrast resolution, noise, and artifacts. Artifacts are discussed in Chapter 32. Resolution and noise are discussed next.

Resolution

Resolution is the ability to image two separate objects and visually detect one from the other. **Spatial resolution** refers to the ability to image small objects that have high subject contrast, such as a bone–soft tissue interface, a breast microcalcification, or a calcified lung nodule. Conventional radiography has excellent spatial resolution. The measure of spatial resolution is discussed more completely in Chapter 29.

Contrast resolution is the ability to distinguish anatomic structures of similar subject contrast such as liver-spleen and gray matter–white matter. The actual size of objects that can be imaged is always smaller under conditions of high contrast than under conditions of low contrast. Computed tomography (CT) has excellent contrast resolution, and that of magnetic resonance imaging (MRI) is even better.

The less precise terms, **detail** or **recorded detail,** are sometimes used instead of *spatial* and *contrast resolution.* These items refer to the degree of sharpness of structural lines on a radiograph. *Visibility of detail* refers to the ability to visualize recorded detail when image contrast and optical density (OD), the degree of blackening on a radiograph, are optimized (see later discussion on OD in this chapter and in Chapter 21).

Noise

Noise is a term borrowed from electrical engineering. The flutter, hum, and whistle heard from a stereo system is audio noise that is inherent in the design of the system. The "snow" on television screens, especially in areas receiving weak signals, is video noise, and it too is inherent in the system.

Radiographic noise also is inherent in the imaging system. **Radiographic noise** is the undesirable fluctuation in the OD of the image. A number of factors contribute to radiographic noise, including some that are under the control of the radiologic technologist. Lower noise results in a better radiographic image because it improves contrast resolution.

Radiographic Noise
Radiographic noise is the undesirable fluctuation in the OD of the image.

Radiographic noise has four components: film graininess, structure mottle, quantum mottle, and scatter radiation. We discuss the principal source of radiographic noise—scatter radiation—in Chapters 18 and 19.

Film graininess refers to the distribution in size and space of the silver halide grains in the emulsion. **Structure mottle** is similar to film graininess but refers to the phosphor of the radiographic intensifying screen. Film graininess and structure mottle are inherent in the image receptor. They are not under the control of the radiologic technologist, and they contribute very little to radiographic noise, with the exception of mammography.

Quantum mottle is somewhat under the control of the radiologic technologist, and it is a principal contributor to radiographic noise in many radiographic imaging procedures. *Quantum mottle* refers to the random nature in which x-rays interact with the image receptor. If an image is produced with just a few x-rays, the quantum mottle will be higher than if the image is formed from a large number of x-rays (Figure 20-1). Figure 20-2 demonstrates this property with the exposure of a contrast-detail test object. The use of very fast intensifying screens results in increased quantum mottle.

The use of high mAs, low kVp, and slower image receptors reduces quantum mottle.

Quantum mottle is like sowing grass seed. If very little seed is cast, the resulting grass will be thin, with only a few blades. Likewise, when fewer x-rays are "cast" at the radiographic intensifying screen, the resulting image appears mottled or blotchy. On the other hand, if a lot of

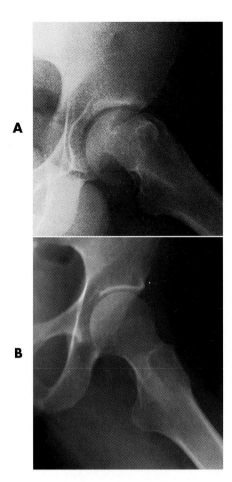

FIGURE 20-1 **A,** This hip radiograph demonstrates the mottled, grainy appearance associated with quantum mottle resulting from a low number of x-rays being used to produce the image. **B,** In comparison, an optimal hip image shows greater recorded detail.

seed is cast, the resulting grass will be thick and smooth. In the same way, when more x-rays interact with the radiographic intensifying screen, the image appears smooth like a lush lawn.

Speed

Two of the characteristics of radiographic quality—resolution and noise—are intimately connected with a third characteristic—speed. Although the speed of the image receptor is not apparent on the radiographic image, it very much influences resolution and noise. In fact, a variation in any one of these characteristics alters the other two. As a general rule, the following apply:

Radiographic Quality Rules
1. Fast image receptors have high noise and low spatial and contrast resolution.
2. High spatial and contrast resolution require low noise and slow image receptors.
3. Low noise accompanies slow image receptors with high spatial and contrast resolution.

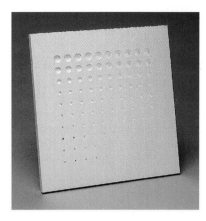

FIGURE 20-2 Contrast-detail test object consisting of various hole sizes (detail) drilled to various depths (contrast) in an aluminum block. *(Courtesy Gammex RMI.)*

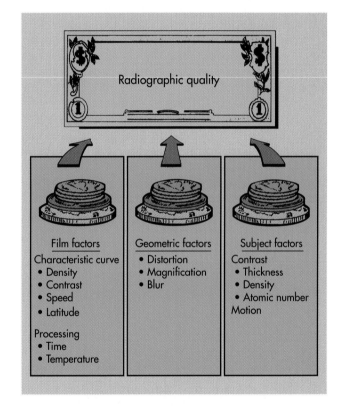

FIGURE 20-3 Organizational chart of principal factors affecting radiographic quality.

The radiologic technologist is provided with all the physical tools required to produce quality radiographs. The skillful radiologic technologist properly manipulates these tools according to each clinical situation. Generally, the quality of a radiograph is directly related to an understanding of the basic principles of x-ray physics and the factors affecting radiographic quality. Figure 20-3 is an organizational chart of the principal factors affecting radiographic quality, most of which are under the control of the radiologic technologist. Each is considered in detail in this chapter.

FILM FACTORS

Unexposed x-ray film that has been processed appears quite lucent, like frosted window glass. It easily transmits light but not images. On the other hand, exposed, processed x-ray film can be quite opaque. Properly exposed film appears with various shades of gray, and heavily exposed film appears black.

The study of the relationship between the intensity of exposure of the film and the blackness after processing is called **sensitometry.** The radiologic technologist may be involved in sensitometric measurements during quality-control activities. Therefore knowledge of sensitometric aspects of radiographic film is essential for maintaining adequate quality control.

Characteristic Curve

The two principal measurements involved in sensitometry are the exposure to the film and the percentage of light transmitted through the processed film. Such measurements are used to describe the relationship among OD, the degree of blackness of the film, and radiation exposure. This relationship is called a **characteristic curve** or sometimes the *H & D curve* after Hurter and Driffield, who first described this relationship.

A typical characteristic curve is shown in Figure 20-4. At low and high exposure levels, large variations in exposure result in only a small change in OD. These portions of the characteristic curve are called the **toe** and **shoulder,** respectively. At intermediate exposure levels, small changes in exposure result in large changes in OD. This intermediate region, called the **straight-line portion,** is the region in which a properly exposed radiograph appears.

Two pieces of apparatus are needed to construct a characteristic curve: an optical step wedge, sometimes called a **sensitometer,** and a **densitometer,** a device that measures OD. The steps involved are outlined in Figure 20-5, where an aluminum step wedge, or penetrameter, is shown as an alternative to the sensitometer.

First the image receptor under investigation is exposed—flashed—through the sensitometer. When processed, the film has areas of increasing OD corresponding to optical wedge steps. The sensitometer is fabricated so that the relative intensity of light exposure to the film under each step can be determined.

The processed film is analyzed in the densitometer, a device that has a light source focused through a pinhole. A light-sensing device is positioned on the opposite side of the film. The radiographic film is positioned between the pinhole and the light sensor, and the amount of light transmitted through each step of the radiographic image is measured. These data are recorded, analyzed, and when plotted, result in a characteristic curve.

Radiographic film is sensitive over a wide range of exposures. Film-screen, for example, responds to radiation intensities from under 1 to over 1000 mR (0.01 to 10 mGy$_a$). Consequently, the exposure values for a characteristic curve are presented in logarithmic fashion. Furthermore, it is not the absolute exposure that is of interest but rather the change in OD over each exposure interval. Therefore **log relative exposure (LRE)** is used as the scale along the x-axis.

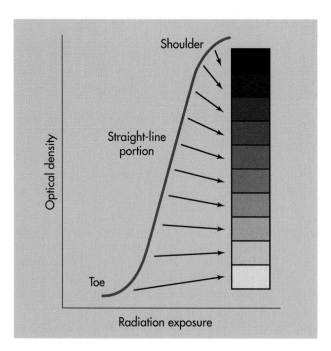

FIGURE 20-4 Characteristic curve of radiographic film is the graphic relationship between OD and radiation exposure.

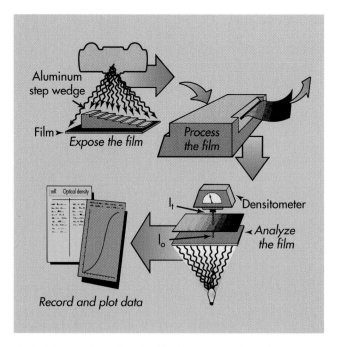

FIGURE 20-5 Steps involved in the construction of a characteristic curve.

Figure 20-6 shows the exposure in mR, the LRE, and the relative mAs for a representative film-screen combination. The LRE scale is usually presented in increments of 0.3 because the log of 2, doubling the exposure, is 0.3. Doubling the exposure can be achieved by doubling the mAs, as the x-axis scale in Figure 20-7 shows.

An increase of 0.3 in the LRE results from doubling the radiation exposure.

Optical Density

It is not enough to say that OD is the degree of blackening of a radiograph or that a clear area of the radiograph represents low OD and a black area represents high OD. OD has a precise numerical value that can be calculated if the level of light incident on a processed film (I_o) and the level of light transmitted through the film (I_t) can be measured. The OD is defined as follows:

Optical Density
$$OD = \log_{10} \frac{I_o}{I_t}$$

Question: The lung field of a chest radiograph transmits only 0.15% of incident light as determined with a densitometer. What is the OD?

Answer: 0.15% = 0.0015
$$OD = \log_{10} \frac{1}{0.0015}$$
$$= 2.8$$

OD is a logarithmic function. Logarithms allow a wide range of values to be expressed by small numbers. Radiographic film contains ODs ranging from near zero to 4. These ODs correspond to clear and black, respectively. An OD of 4 actually means that only 1 in 10,000 light photons (10^4) is capable of penetrating the x-ray film. Table 20-1 shows the range of light transmission corresponding to various levels of OD.

Question: The OD of a region of a lung field is 2.5. What percentage of visible light is transmitted through that region of the image?

Answer: Reference to Table 20-1 shows that an OD of 2.5 is equal to 2 of every 625 light photons being transmitted, or 0.32%.

High-quality glass has an OD of zero, which means that all light incident on such glass is transmitted. Unexposed radiographic film allows no more than about 80% of incident light photons to be transmitted. Most unexposed and processed radiographic film has an OD in the

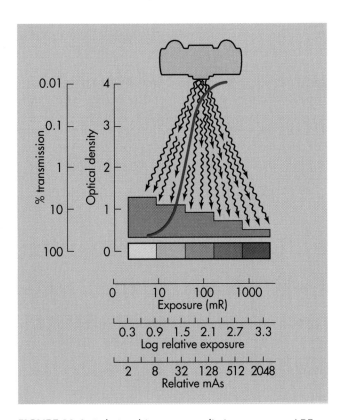

FIGURE 20-6 Relationship among radiation exposure, LRE, and relative mAs for typical film-screen combination. The relationship between the percent transmission and OD is shown along the y-axis.

TABLE 20-1	Relationship of OD of Radiographic Film to Light Transmission Through the Film.	
LIGHT TRANSMITTED		
Percentage ($I_t/I_o \times 100$)	Fraction (I_t/I_o)	OD ($\log_{10} I_o/I_t$)
100	1	0
50	1/2	0.3
32	8/25	0.5
25	1/4	0.6
12.5	1/8	0.9
10	1/10	1
5	1/20	1.3
3.2	4/25	1.5
2.5	1/30	1.6
1.25	1/80	1.9
1	1/100	2
0.5	1/200	2.3
0.32	2/625	2.5
0.125	1/800	2.9
0.1	1/1000	3
0.05	1/2000	3.3
0.032	1/3125	3.5
0.01	1/10,000	4

range of 0.1 to 0.3, corresponding to 79% and 50% transmission, respectively.

These ODs in unexposed film are due to **base density,** the OD inherent in the base of the film, and **fog density,** the development of silver grain that contains no useful information (Figure 20-7). Base density is due to the composition of the base and the tint added to the base to make the radiograph more pleasing to the eye. Base density has a value of approximately 0.1. Fog density results from inadvertent exposure of film during storage, undesirable chemical contamination, improper processing, and a number of other influences. Fog density on a processed radiograph should not exceed 0.2 because a higher fog density reduces radiograph contrast.

 Higher fog density levels reduce the contrast of the radiograph.

Question: The light incident on the radiograph of a long bone has a relative value of 1500. If the light transmitted through the radiopaque bony structures has an intensity of 480 (relatively white) and the light transmitted through the radiolucent soft tissue has an intensity of 2 (relatively black), what are the approximate respective ODs? Refer to Table 20-1 if necessary.

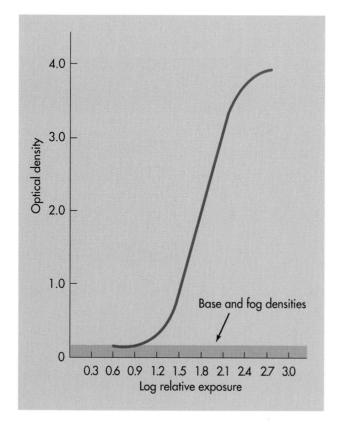

FIGURE 20-7 Base and fog densities reduce radiographic contrast and should be as low as possible.

Answer: $OD = \log_{10} \frac{I_o}{I_t}$

  a. For bone:
  $$OD = \log_{10} \frac{1500}{480}$$
  $$= 0.5$$
  b. For soft tissue:
  $$OD = \log_{10} \frac{1500}{2}$$
  $$= 2.9$$

The useful range of OD is approximately 0.25 to 2.5. Most radiographs, however, show image patterns in the range of 0.5 to 1.25 OD. Attention to this part of the characteristic curve is essential. However, very low OD may be too light to contain an image pattern, whereas very high OD requires a hot light to view the imager.

 Base plus fog OD has a range of approximately 0.1 to 0.3.

The most useful range of OD is highly dependent on viewbox illumination, viewing conditions, and the shape of the characteristic curve. For example, with image receptors for high-contrast mammography and high-luminance viewboxes and good viewing conditions, the most useful OD range is approximately 0.25 to 2.5 with gross features and as high as 3.5 with fine features such as skin lines.

Reciprocity law. You might think that the OD on a radiograph would be strictly dependent on the total exposure, mAs, and would be independent of the time of exposure. This, in fact, is the **reciprocity law,** which states that whether a radiograph is exposed over a very short period of time (for example, 1 ms) or over hours or even days, the OD will be the same if the total energy imparted to the radiograph, and therefore the mAs, is constant.

 Reciprocity Law
The reciprocity law states that the OD on a radiograph is proportional only to the total energy imparted to the radiographic film.

The reciprocity law holds for direct exposure with x-rays but it does not hold for exposure of film by the visible light from radiographic intensifying screens. Consequently, *the reciprocity law fails for screen-film exposures* at exposure times less than approximately 10 ms or longer than approximately 5 s.

OD is somewhat less at such short or long exposure times than exposure times within that range, even though the radiation exposure is the same. The reciprocity law is important in some special procedures that require very short or very long exposure times, such as cardiovascular and interventional radiography and mammography, respectively. For these situations, increasing the mAs may be required if the automatic exposure control (AEC) does not compensate for reciprocity law failure.

Contrast. When a high-quality radiograph is placed on an illuminator, the differences in OD are obvious in the image. Such OD variations are called **radiographic contrast** (see Chapter 21 for further explanation of contrast.) A radiograph that has marked differences in OD is a high-contrast radiograph. On the other hand, if the OD differences are less distinct, the radiograph is of low contrast. Figure 20-8 illustrates the difference between high and low contrast with a photograph.

Radiographic contrast is the product of two separate factors:

1. **Image receptor contrast** (historically referred to as *film contrast*) is inherent in the film and is influenced somewhat by processing of the film.

2. **Subject contrast** is determined by the size, shape, and x-ray attenuating characteristics of the subject being examined and the energy (kVp) of the x-ray beam.

 Radiographic contrast is the combined result of image receptor contrast and subject contrast.

Radiographic contrast can be greatly affected by changes in either image receptor contrast or subject contrast. In the clinical setting, it is usually best to standardize the image receptor contrast and alter the subject contrast according to the needs of the examination. Subject contrast is dealt with in greater detail later.

Image receptor contrast is inherent in the type of film and radiographic intensifying screen being used. It can however, be influenced by two other factors: the range of ODs and the film-processing technique. Film selection is generally limited and determined somewhat by the intensifying screen used. Film-screen images always have higher contrast than direct-exposure images.

The best control the radiologic technologist can exercise is exposing the image receptor properly so that the ODs lie within the diagnostically useful range, 0.25 to 2.5 (a bit higher in mammography). When the exposure of the image receptor results in an OD outside this range, contrast is lost because the image is in either the toe or the shoulder of the characteristic curve (Figure 20-9).

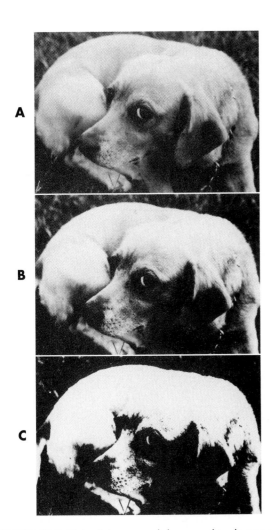

FIGURE 20-8 This vicious guard dog posed to demonstrate differences in contrast. **A,** Low contrast. **B,** Moderate contrast. **C,** High contrast.

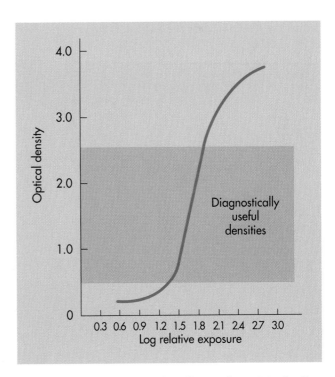

FIGURE 20-9   If exposure of the film results in ODs that lie in the toe or shoulder regions, where the slope of the curve is less, contrast is reduced.

Standardized film-processing techniques are absolutely necessary for consistent film contrast and good radiographic quality. Deviation from the manufacturer's recommendations results in reduced contrast.

 Radiographic contrast is equal to the slope of the straight-line portion of the characteristic curve.

The characteristic curve of an image receptor allows the radiologic technologist to judge at a glance the relative degree of contrast. If the slope or steepness of the straight-line portion of the characteristic curve had a value of 1, then it would be angled at 45 degrees. An increase of 1 unit along the LRE axis would result in an increase of 1 unit along the OD axis. The contrast would be 1.

An image receptor that has a contrast of 1 has very low contrast. Image receptors with a contrast higher than 1 amplify the subject contrast during x-ray examination. An image receptor with a contrast of 3, for instance, would show large OD differences over a small range of x-ray exposure.

Generally, it is not necessary for the radiologic technologist to have a precise knowledge of image receptor contrast, but from the appearance of the characteristic curve, the technologist should be able to distinguish high-contrast image receptors from low-contrast image receptors. Figure 20-10 shows the characteristic curves for two different image receptors. Image receptor A has higher contrast than image receptor B, as shown by the fact that the slope of the straight-line portion of the characteristic curve is steeper for A than for B.

Several methods are used to numerically specify image receptor contrast. The one most often used is **average gradient.** The average gradient is the slope of a straight line drawn between the two points on the characteristic curve at ODs 0.25 and 2.0 above base and fog densities, which is the approximate useful range of OD on most radiographs.

Image Receptor Contrast

$$\text{Average gradient} = \frac{OD_2 - OD_1}{LRE_2 - LRE_1}$$

where:
OD_2 = the OD of 2.0 plus base and fog densities
OD_1 = the OD of 0.25 plus base and fog densities
LRE_2 and LRE_1 = the LREs associated with OD_2 and OD_1, respectively

This method is diagrammed in Figure 20-11 for a film having a combined base and fog density of 0.1.

Most radiographic image receptors have an average gradient in the range of 2.5 to 3.5. Because of this, the image receptor acts as an amplifier of subject contrast. The range of the number of x-rays producing the latent image is effectively expanded, and the subject contrast is enhanced.

Question: A radiographic film has a base density of 0.06 and a fog density of 0.11. At what ODs should you evaluate the characteristic curve to determine the film contrast?

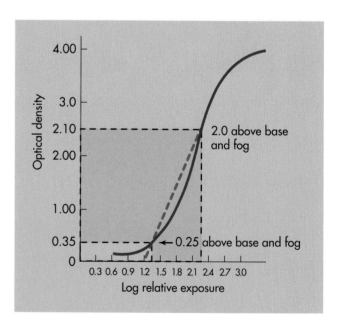

FIGURE 20-10 Slope of the straight-line portion of the characteristic curve is greater for image receptor A than for image receptor B. Image receptor A has higher contrast.

FIGURE 20-11 The average gradient is the slope of the line drawn between the points on the characteristic curve that correspond to the OD levels 0.25 and 2.0 above base and fog densities.

Answer: The curve should be evaluated at ODs 0.25 and 2.0 above base plus fog densities. Therefore at ODs of:
$$OD_1 = 0.06 + 0.11 + 0.25 = 0.42$$
and
$$OD_2 = 0.06 + 0.11 + 2.0 = 2.17$$

Image receptor contrast may also be identified by **gradient**. The gradient is the slope of the tangent *at any point* on the characteristic curve (Figure 20-12). Toe gradient is probably more important than average gradient for general radiography, since many clinical ODs appear in the toe region of the characteristic curve. Midgradient or shoulder gradient is more important for mammography.

Question: If the ODs of 0.42 and 2.17 on the characteristic curve in the preceding example correspond to LREs of 0.95 and 1.75, what is the average gradient?

Answer:
$$\text{Average gradient} = \frac{OD_2 - OD_1}{LRE_2 - LRE_1}$$
$$= \frac{2.17 - 0.42}{1.75 - 0.95}$$
$$= \frac{1.75}{0.8}$$
$$= 2.19$$

Note that the numerator in the expression for average gradient always equal 1.75.

Another way to evaluate image receptor contrast is to replot the data of a characteristic curve (an H & D curve) into an H & H contrast curve as done in Figure 20-13. The H & H curve is named for Art Haus and Ed Hendrick, the medical physicists who first demonstrated this technique.

Speed. The ability of an image receptor to respond to a low x-ray exposure is a measure of its sensitivity or more commonly, its speed. An exposure of less than 1 mR can be detected with a film-screen combination, whereas an exposure of several mR are necessary to produce a measurable exposure with direct-exposure film.

The characteristic curve of an image receptor is also useful in identifying speed. Figure 20-14 shows the characteristic curves of two different image receptors. Since image receptor *A* requires less exposure than image receptor *B* to produce any OD, *A* is faster than *B*.

The characteristic curve of a fast image receptor is positioned to the left—closer to the y-axis—of that of a slow image receptor. Radiographic image receptors are identified as either *fast* or *slow* according to their sensitivity to x-ray exposure. Usually the identification of a given image receptor as so many times faster than another is sufficient for the radiologic technologist. If *A* were twice as fast as *B*, image receptor *A* would require only half the mAs required by *B* to produce a given OD. Moreover, the image on image receptor *A* might be of poor quality because of increased radiographic noise.

When numbers are used to express speed, all are relative to 100, termed *per speed*. Numbers higher than 100 refer to fast or high-speed image receptors. Numbers less than 100 refer to "detail" image receptors. Do not be deceived into thinking that slower image recep-

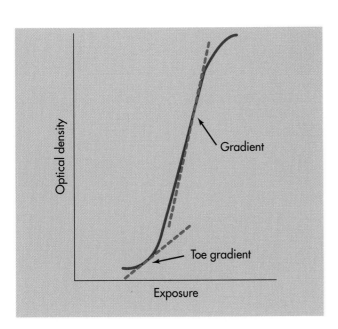

FIGURE 20-12 Gradient is the slope of the tangent at any point on the characteristic curve. Toe gradient is more important clinically than average gradient.

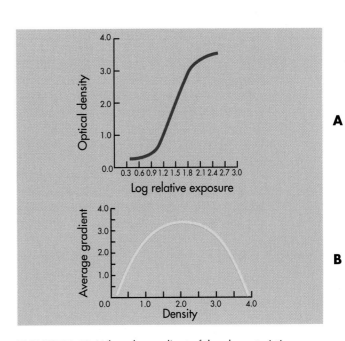

FIGURE 20-13 When the gradient of the characteristic curve **(A)** is plotted as a function of optical density, a contrast curve, **(B)** results.

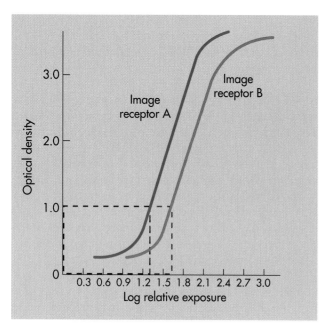

FIGURE 20-14 The speed of an image receptor is the reciprocal of the exposure, in roentgens, needed to produce an OD of 1.0. Image receptor *A* is faster than image receptor *B*.

tors are better because they have less noise. Slower image receptors also require more patient radiation dose. A balance is required.

In sensitometry, the OD specified for determining image receptor speed is 1.0 above base plus fog density, and the speed is measured in **reciprocal roentgens (1/R),** as follows:

Image Receptor Speed

$$Speed = \frac{1}{\text{Exposure in roentgens to produce an OD of 1.0 plus base + fog}}$$

Question: The characteristic curve of a given screen-film shows that 10 mR is needed to produce an OD of 1.0 above base plus fog density on that image receptor. What is the image receptor speed?

Answer: $Speed = \dfrac{1}{10 \text{ mR}} = \dfrac{1}{0.01 \text{ R}} = 100 \text{ R}^{-1}$

Question: How much exposure is required to produce an OD of 1.0 above base plus fog density on a 600-speed image receptor?

Answer: $Speed = \dfrac{1}{\text{exposure}}$

Therefore:

$Exposure = \dfrac{1}{\text{speed}}$

$= \dfrac{1}{600}$

$= 0.00167 \text{ R}$

$= 1.7 \text{ mR}$

When imaged receptors are replaced, a change in the mAs may be necessary to maintain the same OD. For example, if image receptor speed is doubled, the mAs must be halved. No change is required in kVp. This relationship is expressed as follows:

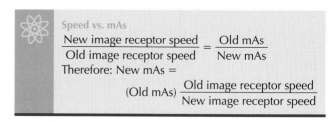

Speed vs. mAs

$$\frac{\text{New image receptor speed}}{\text{Old image receptor speed}} = \frac{\text{Old mAs}}{\text{New mAs}}$$

Therefore: New mAs =

$(\text{Old mAs}) \dfrac{\text{Old image receptor speed}}{\text{New image receptor speed}}$

Question: A posterior-anterior (PA) chest film requires 120 kVp and 8 mAs with a 250-speed image receptor. What radiographic technique should be used with a 400-speed image receptor?

Answer: New mAs = $(8 \text{ mAs}) \dfrac{250}{400}$

$= 5 \text{ mAs}$

Therefore the new technique is 120 kVp and 5 mAs.

Latitude. An additional image receptor feature easily obtained from the characteristic curve is the latitude. **Latitude** refers to the range of exposures over which the image receptor responds with ODs in the diagnostically useful range. It can also be thought of as the margin of error in technical factors. With wider latitude, the mAs can vary more and still result in a diagnostic image. Figure 20-15 shows two image receptors with different latitudes. Image receptor *B* responds to a much wider range of exposures than image receptor *A* and is said to have a wider latitude than *A*.

 Latitude and contrast are inversely proportional.

Image receptors with wide latitude are said to have *long gray scale,* and those with narrow latitude have *short gray scale.* (See Chapter 21 for an explanation of gray scale.) When slopes of the curves in Figure 20-16 are compared, it should be clear that a high-contrast image receptor has narrow latitude and a low-contrast image receptor has wide latitude.

Film Processing

Proper film processing is required for optimal image receptor contrast because the degree of development has a pronounced effect on the level of fog density and on the ODs resulting from a given exposure at a given image receptor speed. The important factors affecting the degree of development are listed in Box 20-1.

Development time. As development time is varied, the characteristic curve for any film changes in shape and

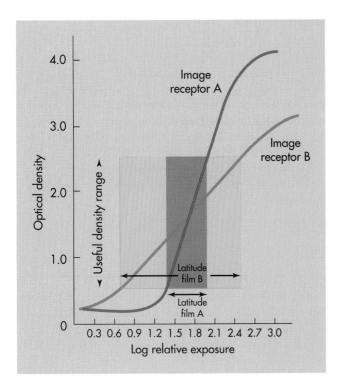

FIGURE 20-15 The latitude of an image receptor is the exposure range over which it responds with diagnostically useful OD.

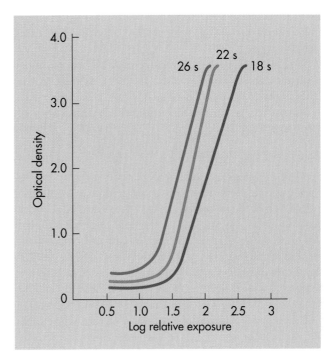

FIGURE 20-16 As development time increases, changes occur in the shape and relative position of the characteristic curve.

BOX 20-1   Factors Affecting the Finished Radiograph

Concentration of processing chemicals
Degree of chemistry agitation during development
Development time
Development temperature

---

position along the LRE axis (Figure 20-16). If the characteristic curves were analyzed for contrast, speed, and fog level, each would be shown to vary as in Figure 20-17. Speed and fog increase with longer development time.

The development time recommended by the manufacturer is the time that will result in maximal contrast at relatively high speed and with low levels of fog. When development time extends far beyond the recommended period, the image receptor contrast decreases, the relative speed increases, and the fog level increases.

Development temperature. The relationships just described for variations in development time apply equally well to variations in development temperature. When the average gradient, speed, and fog level for the characteristic curves representative of various temperatures are plotted as a function of development temperature, the results appear also as in Figure 20-17. As with develop-

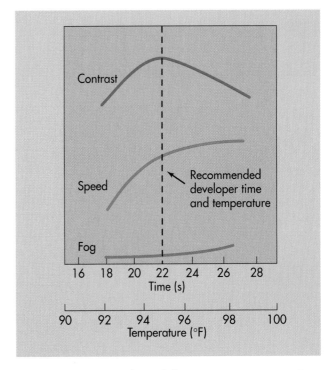

FIGURE 20-17 An analysis of characteristic curves at various development times and temperatures yields these relationships for contrast, speed, and fog for 90-s automatically processed film.

ment time, maximal contrast is obtained at the recommended development temperature. The fog level increases with increasing temperature, as does the image receptor speed.

Within a small range, a change in either time or temperature can be compensated for by a change in the other. However, a small change in either alone can result in a large change in the sensitometric characteristics of the image receptor.

GEOMETRIC FACTORS

Making a radiograph is similar in many ways to taking a photograph. Proper exposure time and intensity are required for both processes. Images are recorded in both because the x-rays and the visible light photons travel in straight lines. In that regard, an x-ray image may be considered analogous to a shadowgraph. Figure 20-18 shows the familiar shadowgraph that can be made to appear on a wall if light is shone on a properly contorted hand. The sharpness of the shadow image on the wall is a function of a number of geometric factors. For example, the closer the hand to the wall, the sharper the shadow image. Similarly, the farther the hand from the light source, the sharper the shadow.

These geometric conditions also apply to the production of high-quality radiographs. Three principal geometric factors affect radiographic quality: magnification, distortion, and focal-spot blur.

 Magnification, distortion, and focal-spot blur are the three principal geometric factors that affect radiographic quality.

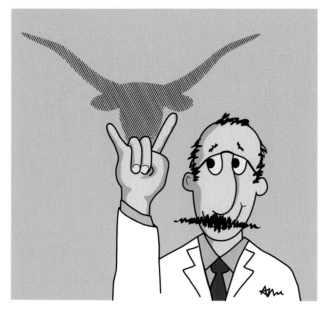

FIGURE 20-18 A shadowgraph is analogous to a radiograph. *(Dedicated to Xie Nan Zhu, Guangzhou, People's Republic of China.)*

Magnification

All images on the radiograph are larger than the object they represent, a condition called **magnification.** For most clinical examinations, the smallest magnification possible should be maintained. During some situations, however, magnification is desirable and is carefully planned into the radiographic examination. This type of examination is called magnification radiography. It is discussed in Chapter 22.

Quantitatively, magnification is measured and expressed by the magnification factor (MF), which is defined as follows:

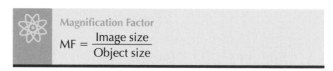

Magnification Factor
$$MF = \frac{\text{Image size}}{\text{Object size}}$$

The MF is dependent on the geometric conditions of the examination. For most radiographs taken at a source-to-image receptor (SID) of 100 cm, the MF is approximately 1.1. For radiographs taken at 180-cm SID, the MF is approximately 1.05.

Question: If a heart measures 12.5 cm from side to side at its widest point and its image on a chest radiograph measures 14.7 cm, what is the MF?

Answer: $MF = \dfrac{14.7 \text{ cm}}{12.5 \text{ cm}} = 1.176$

In the usual radiographic examination, it is not possible to determine the object size. The image size may be measured directly from the radiograph. In such situations the MF can be determined from the ratio of the SID to the source-to-object distance (SOD):

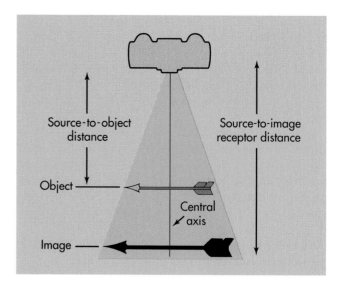

FIGURE 20-19 Magnification is the ratio of image size to object size, or SID to SOD.

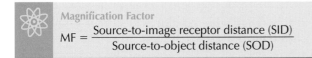

Magnification Factor

$$MF = \frac{\text{Source-to-image receptor distance (SID)}}{\text{Source-to-object distance (SOD)}}$$

Minimizing Magnification
Large SID: Use as large an SID as possible.
Small OID: Place the object as close to the image receptor as possible.

Figure 20-19 shows that this method of calculating the MF results from the basic geometric relationship between similar triangles. If two right triangles have a common hypotenuse, the ratio of the height of one to its base will be the same as the ratio of the height of the other to its base.

This is the situation that generally is encountered in radiology. The SID is known and can be measured directly. The SOD can be estimated relatively accurately by a radiologic technologist who has a good foundation in human anatomy. The image size can be measured accurately; therefore the object size can be calculated as follows:

Magnification Factor

$$MF = \frac{\text{Image size}}{\text{Object size}} = \frac{\text{SID}}{\text{SOD}}$$

$$\text{Object size} = \text{Image size}\left(\frac{\text{SOD}}{\text{SID}}\right)$$

Question: A renal calculus measures 1.2 cm on the radiograph. The SID is 100 cm, and the SOD is estimated at 92 cm. What is the size of the calculus?

Answer: $\text{Object size} = 1.2\left(\frac{92}{100}\right)$
$= 1.1 \text{ cm}$

Question: A lateral film of the lumbar spine taken at 100-cm SID results in the image of a vertebral body with maximum and minimum dimensions of 6.4 cm and 4.2 cm, respectively. What is the object size if the vertebral body is 25 cm from the image receptor?

Answer: $MF = \frac{100}{100-25} = \frac{100}{75} = 1.33$
Therefore the object size is as follows:
$\frac{6.4}{1.33} \times \frac{4.2}{1.33} = 4.81 \text{ cm} \times 3.16 \text{ cm}$

You might ask if these relationships hold for objects off the central axis (Figure 20-20). The MF will be the same for objects positioned off the central axis as for those lying on the central axis if the object-to-image receptor distance (OID) is the same and if the object is essentially flat.

In summary, there are two factors that affect image magnification: SID and OID.

The SID is standard in most radiology departments at 180 cm for chest imaging, 100 cm for routine examinations, and 90 cm for some special studies such as mobile radiography and skull radiography.

There are three familiar clinical situations in which magnification is routinely minimized. Most chest radiographs are taken at 180-cm SID from the PA projection. This projection results in a smaller heart-to-image receptor distance than at 100-cm SID. Magnification is reduced because of the large SID.

Dedicating mammography imaging systems are designed for a 50- to 70-cm SID. This is a relatively short SID, but it is necessary, considering the low kVp and low radiation intensity of mammography imaging systems. Such systems have a device for vigorous compression of the breast to reduce magnification by reducing OID.

Distortion

The previous discussion assumed that the object being magnified was very simple (for example, an arrow lying perpendicular to the central x-ray beam at a fixed OID). If any one of these conditions is changed, as they all are in most clinical examinations, the magnification will not be the same over the entire object. Unequal magnification of different portions of the same object is called **distortion.**

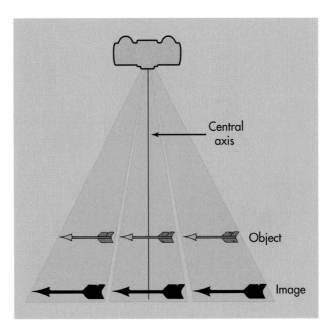

FIGURE 20-20 The magnification of an object positioned off the central x-ray axis is the same as that for an object on the central axis if the objects are in the same plane.

Distortion can interfere with diagnosis. The following conditions contribute to image distortion: object thickness, object position, and object shape.

 Distortion depends on the thickness, position, and shape of the object.

Object thickness. With a thick object, the OID changes measurably across the object. Consider, for instance, two rectangular structures of different thicknesses (Figure 20-21). Because of the change in OID across the thicker structure, the image of that structure is more distorted than the image of the thinner structure.

 Thick objects are more distorted than thin objects.

Consider the images produced by a disc and a sphere of the same diameter (Figure 20-22). When positioned on the central axis, the images of both objects appear as circles. The image of the sphere appears less distinct because of its varying thickness, but it does appear circular. When these objects are positioned laterally to the central axis, the disc still appears circular. The sphere appears not only less distinct but also elliptical because of its thickness. This distortion resulting from object thickness is shown more dramatically in Figure 20-23 by the image of an irregular object.

These statements about discs and spheres are clinically insignificant because lateral distances off the central axis are too small. Only irregular objects, such as those shown in Figure 20-23 or the human body, show significant distortion.

Object position. If the object plane and the image plane are parallel, the image will not be distorted. However, distortion is possible in every radiographic examination if proper patient positioning is not maintained.

 If the object plane and image plane are not parallel, image distortion will occur.

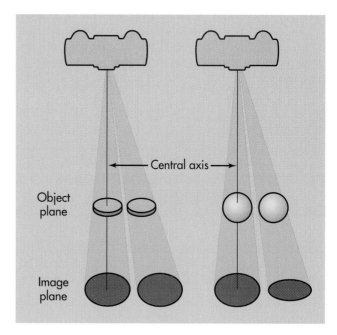

FIGURE 20-22 Object thickness influences distortion. Radiographs of a disc or sphere appear as circles if the object is on the central axis. When lateral to the central axis, the disc appears as a circle and the sphere as an ellipse.

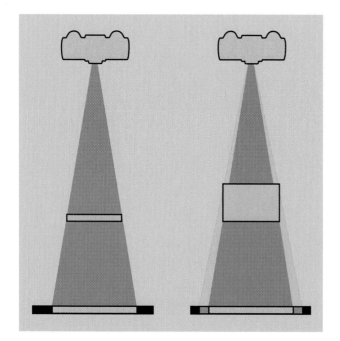

FIGURE 20-21 Thick objects result in unequal magnification and therefore more distortion than thin objects.

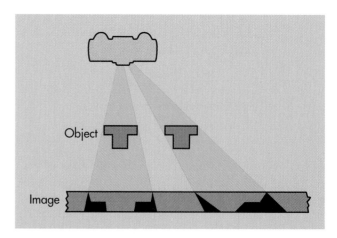

FIGURE 20-23 Irregular objects such as anatomic structures or these items can cause considerable distortion when radiographed off the central axis.

With multiple objects positioned at various OIDs, spatial distortion can occur. **Spatial distortion** is the misrepresentation in the image of the actual spatial relationships among objects. Figure 20-24 demonstrates this condition for two arrows of the same size, one of which lies on top of the other. Because of the position of the arrows, only one image should be seen, representing the superimposition of the arrows.

Unequal magnification, however, of the two objects causes arrow *A* to appear larger than arrow *B* and to be positioned more laterally. This distortion is minimal for objects lying along the central x-ray beam. As object position is shifted laterally from the central axis, spatial distortion can become more significant.

This illustrates the projection nature of x-ray images; a single image is not enough to define the three-dimensional configuration of a complex object. Therefore most x-ray examinations are made with two or more projections.

Object shape. Figure 20-25 is an example of gross distortion and shows that the image of an inclined object can be smaller than the object itself, a condition called **foreshortening.** The amount of foreshortening, the amount of reduction in image size, increases as the angle of inclination increases.

If an inclined object is not located on the central x-ray beam, the degree of distortion will be affected by the object's angle of inclination and its lateral position from the central axis. Figure 20-26 illustrates this situation and shows that the image of an inclined object can be severely foreshortened or made to appear longer than it really is, a condition call **elongation.** Collectively, these conditions of foreshortening and elongation are sometimes called **shape distortion.**

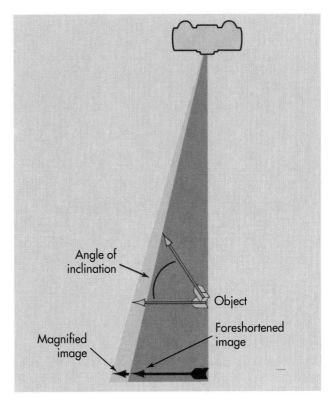

FIGURE 20-25 Inclination of an object results in a foreshortened image.

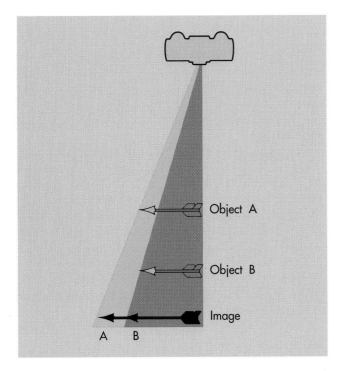

FIGURE 20-24 When objects of the same size are positioned at different distances from the image receptor, spatial distortion occurs.

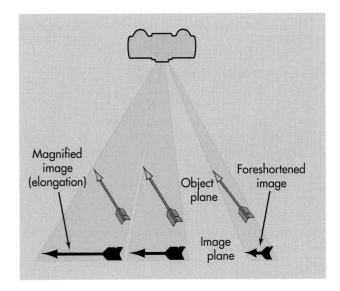

FIGURE 20-26 An inclined object positioned lateral to the central axis beam may be severely distorted by elongation or foreshortening.

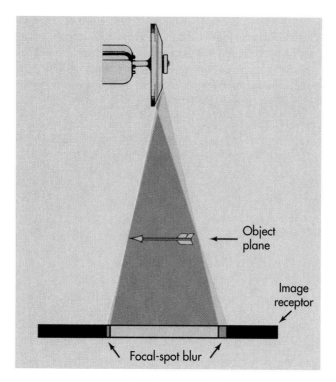

FIGURE 20-27   Focal-spot blur is caused by the effective size of the focal spot, which is larger to the cathode side of the image.

Focal-Spot Blur

So far, our discussion of the geometric factors affecting radiographic quality has assumed that x-rays are emitted from a point source. In actual practice, there is not a point source of x-radiation but rather a roughly rectangular source varying in size from approximately 0.1 to 1.5 mm on a side, depending on the type of x-ray tube in use.

Figure 20-27 illustrates the result of using x-ray tubes with measurable effective focal spots as imaging devices. (Recall that effective focal spot is the area of the focal spot projected to the image receptor.) The point of the object arrow in Figure 20-27 does not appear as a point in the image plane because the x-rays used to image that point originate throughout the rectangular source.

A blurred region on the radiograph over which the radiologic technologist has little control will result because the effective focal spot has size. This phenomenon is called **focal spot blur,** and as illustrated, it is greater on the cathode side of the image. Focal-spot blur occurs because the focal spot is not a point. Focal spot blur is undesirable and is the most important factor in determining spatial resolution. Focal-spot blur is caused by a large effective focal spot, a short SID, and a long OID.

Focal-spot blur is the most important factor in determining spatial resolution.

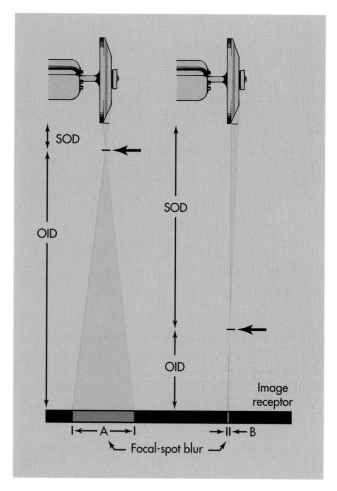

FIGURE 20-28   The focal-spot blur is small when the OID is small.

The geometric relationships governing magnification also influence focal-spot blur. As the geometry of the source, object, and image are altered to produce greater magnification, they also produce increased focal-spot blur. Consequently, these conditions should be avoided when possible.

The region of focal-spot blur can be calculated using similar triangles. If an arrowhead were positioned near the x-ray tube target, the size of the focal-spot blur would be larger than that of the effective focal spot (Figure 20-28, *A*). Generally, the object is much closer to the image receptor, and therefore the focal-spot blur is much smaller than the effective focal spot (Figure 20-28, *B*).

From these drawings, you can see that two similar triangles are described. Therefore the ratio of SOD to the OID is the same as the ratio of the sizes of the effective focal spot and the focal-spot blur.

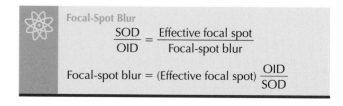

Focal-Spot Blur

$$\frac{SOD}{OID} = \frac{Effective\ focal\ spot}{Focal\text{-}spot\ blur}$$

$$Focal\text{-}spot\ blur = (Effective\ focal\ spot)\frac{OID}{SOD}$$

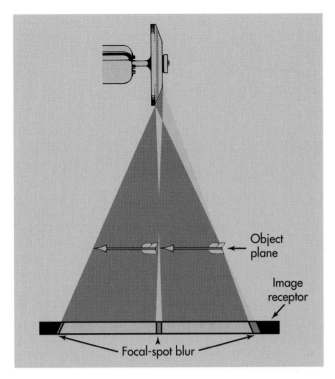

FIGURE 20-29 The effective focal-spot size is largest on the cathode side, and therefore the focal-spot blur is greatest on the cathode side.

TABLE 20-2	Patient Positioning for Examinations That Can Take Advantage of the Heel Effect	
Examination	**Toward the Cathode**	**Toward the Anode**
PA chest	Abdomen	Neck
Abdomen	Abdomen	Pelvis
Femur	Hip	Knee
Humerus	Shoulder	Elbow
AP thoracic spine	Abdomen	Neck
AP lumbar spine	Abdomen	Pelvis

AP, Anterior-posterior.

BOX 20-2	Subject Factors

Subject contrast
Patient or part thickness
Tissue mass density
Effective atomic number
Object shape
kVp

Question: An x-ray tube target having a 0.6-mm effective focal spot is used to image an object in a chest cavity estimated to be 8 cm from the anterior chest wall. If the radiograph is taken PA at 180-cm SID with a tabletop film separation of 5 cm, what will be the size of the focal-spot blur?

Answer:
$$\text{Focal spot blur} = (0.6 \text{ mm}) \frac{8+5}{180-(8+5)}$$
$$= (0.6 \text{ mm}) \frac{13}{167}$$
$$= (0.6 \text{ mm})(0.078)$$
$$= 0.047 \text{ mm}$$

To minimize focal-spot blur, you should use small focal spots and position the patient so that the part of the body under examination is close to the image receptor. The SID is usually fixed but should be as large as possible. High-contrast objects smaller than the focal-spot blur cannot normally be imaged.

The terms *penumbra* and *geometric unsharpness* have been used to describe focal-spot blur. These terms were borrowed from the scientific disciplines of astronomy and mathematics, and their use in medical imaging should be discouraged because imaging scientists have adopted *blur* as a term specific to medical imaging.

Heel Effect

The heel effect, introduced in Chapter 10, is described as a varying intensity across the x-ray field caused by the attenuation of x-rays in the heel of the anode. Another characteristic of the heel effect is unrelated to x-ray intensity but affects focal-spot blur.

The size of the effective focal spot is not constant across the radiograph. A tube said to have a 1-mm focal spot has a smaller effective focal spot on the anode side and a larger effective focal spot on the cathode side (Figure 20-29).

 Focal-spot blur is small on the anode side and large on the cathode side.

This variation in focal-spot size results in a variation in focal-spot blur. Consequently, images toward the cathode side of a radiograph have higher blur and poorer spatial resolution than those to the anode side. This is clinically significant when x-ray tubes with small target angles are used at short SIDs. Table 20-2 lists radiographic examinations that should be performed with regard for the varying radiation intensity of the heel effect.

SUBJECT FACTORS

The third general group of factors affecting radiographic quality concerns the patient (Box 20-2). These factors are associated not so much with the positioning of the patient as with the selection of a radiographic technique that properly compensates for the patient's size, shape, and tissue composition. Patient positioning is basically a requirement associated with the geometric factors affecting radiographic quality.

Subject Contrast

The contrast of a radiograph viewed on an illuminator is called *radiographic contrast*. As indicated previously, radiographic contrast is a function of image receptor contrast and subject contrast. In fact, the radiographic contrast is simply the product of image receptor contrast and subject contrast.

> **Radiographic Contrast**
> Radiographic contrast =
>   Image receptor contrast × Subject contrast

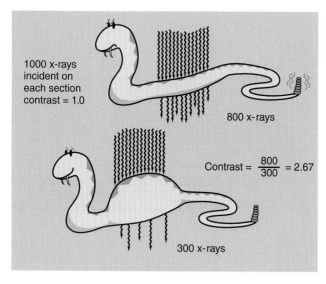

FIGURE 20-30 The different thicknesses of anatomic parts contribute to subject contrast.

Question: Screen-film with an average gradient of 3.1 is used to radiograph a long bone having a subject contrast of 4.5. What is the radiographic contrast?

Answer:
$$\text{Radiographic contrast} = (3.1)(4.5)$$
$$= 13.95$$

Several of these subject factors are discussed in Chapter 13 in relation to the effective attenuation of an x-ray beam. The effect of each on subject contrast is a direct result of differences in attenuation in body tissues.

Patient thickness. Given a standard composition, a thick body section attenuates more x-rays than a thin body section (Figure 20-30). The same number of x-rays is incident on each section, and therefore the contrast of the incident x-ray beam is zero; there is no contrast.

If the same number of x-rays left each section, the subject contrast would be 1.0. Since more x-rays are transmitted through thin body sections than through thick ones, however, subject contrast is greater than 1. The degree of subject contrast is directly proportional to the relative number of x-rays leaving those sections of the body.

Tissue mass density. Different sections of the body may have equal thicknesses, yet different mass densities. Tissue mass density is an important factor affecting subject contrast. Consider, for example, the radiograph of several tissuelike items in water (Figure 20-31). The items have approximately the same thickness and chemical composition. However, they have a slightly different

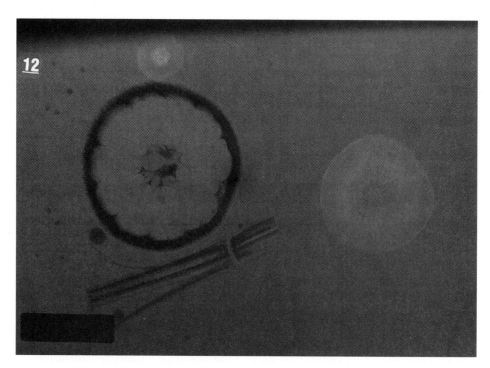

FIGURE 20-31 A radiograph of an orange, a kiwi, a piece of celery, and a chunk of carrot shows the subtle differences on mass density. *(Courtesy Marcy Barnes.)*

mass density from water and therefore will be imaged. The effect of mass density on subject contrast is demonstrated in Figure 20-32.

Effective atomic number. Another important factor affecting subject contrast is the effective atomic number of the tissue being examined. In Chapter 13, it is shown that Compton interactions are independent of atomic number but photoelectric interactions vary in proportion to the cube of the atomic number. The effective atomic numbers of tissues of interest are reported in Table 13-3. In the diagnostic range of x-ray energies, the photoelectric effect is very important; therefore the subject contrast is greatly influenced by the effective atomic number of the tissue being radiographed. When the effective atomic number of adjacent tissues is very much different, subject contrast is very high.

Subject contrast can be greatly enhanced by the use of contrast media. The high atomic number of iodine (Z = 53) and barium (Z = 56) result in extremely high subject contrast. Contrast media are effective because they accentuate subject contrast through increased photoelectric absorption.

Object shape. The shape of the anatomic structure under investigation influences the radiographic quality not only through its geometry but also through its contribution to subject contrast. Obviously, a structure having a form that coincides with the x-ray beam has maximal subject contrast (Figure 20-33, *A*). All other anatomic shapes have reduced subject contrast because of the change in thickness that they present across the x-ray beam. Figure 20-33, *B* and *C,* show examples of two shapes that result in reduced subject contrast.

This characteristic of the subject affecting subject contrast is sometimes termed **absorption blur.** It reduces both spatial resolution and contrast resolution of any anatomic structure, but is most troublesome during angiographic procedures, in which vessels with small diameters are being examined.

kVp. The radiologic technologist has no control over the four previous factors influencing subject contrast. The absolute magnitude of subject contrast, however, is greatly controlled by the kVp of operation. kVp also influences film contrast but not to the extent that it controls subject contrast.

Figure 20-34 shows a composite of a series of radiographs of an aluminum step wedge taken at kVps ranging from 40 to 100. A low kVp results in high subject contrast, sometimes called *short gray-scale contrast,* since the radiographic image appears either black or white with few shades of gray. On the other hand, a high kVp results in low subject contrast, or *long gray-scale contrast.* (See Chapter 21 for an explanation of gray-scale contrast.)

It would be easy to jump to the conclusion that low-kVp techniques are always more desirable than high-kVp techniques. However, low-kVp radiography has two major disadvantages. As the kVp is lowered for any radiographic examination, the x-ray beam becomes less penetrating, requiring a higher mAs to produce an acceptable range of ODs. The result is higher patient dose. A method to estimate the amount of increased patient dose is given in Chapter 40. A radiographic technique that produces low subject contrast allows for wide latitude in exposure factors. Optimization of radiographic technique by mAs selection is not so critical when using high kVp.

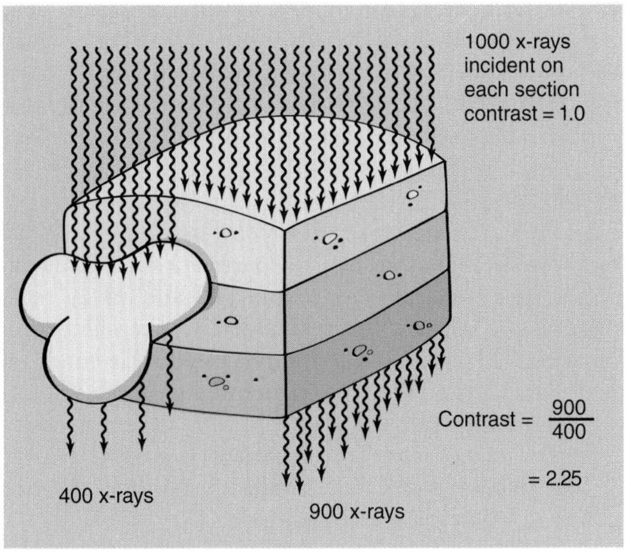

FIGURE 20-32 The variation in tissue mass density contributes to subject contrast.

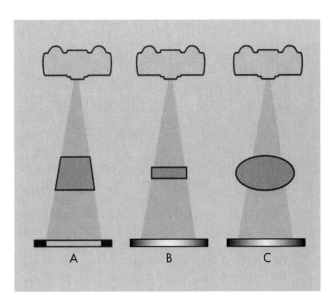

FIGURE 20-33 The shape of the structure under investigation contributes to absorption blur.

FIGURE 20-34 Radiographs of an aluminum step wedge demonstrating change in contrast with varying kVp. *(Courtesy Eastman Kodak Co.)*

Motion Blur

Movement of either the patient or the x-ray tube during exposure results in a blurring of the radiographic image. This loss of radiographic quality, called **motion blur,** may result in repeated radiographs and therefore should be avoided.

Normally, motion of the x-ray tube is not a problem. In tomography (see Chapter 22), the x-ray tube is deliberately moved during exposure to blur the images of structures on either side of the plane of interest. Sometimes the table or a restraining device is moved by auxiliary equipment, such as a moving grid mechanism.

 Patient motion is usually the cause of motion blur.

The radiographer can reduce motion blur by carefully giving instructions to the patient, as follows: "Take a deep breath and hold it. Don't move."

Motion blur is primarily affected by four factors. By observing the guidelines listed in Box 20-3, the radiologic technologist can reduce motion blur. Note that the last two items in this list have the same relation to mo-

tion blur as to focal-spot blur. With the use of low-ripple power and high-speed image receptors, motion has been virtually eliminated as a common clinical problem.

TOOLS FOR IMPROVED RADIOGRAPHIC QUALITY

The radiologic technologist normally has the tools available to produce high-quality radiographs. Proper patient preparation, the selection of proper imaging devices, and proper radiographic technique are complex, related concepts. For any given radiographic examination, a proper interpretation and application of each of these factors must be made. A small change in one may require a compensating change in another.

Patient Positioning

The importance of patient positioning should now be clear. Proper patient positioning requires that the anatomic structure under investigation be placed as close to the image receptor as is practical and that the axis of this structure lie in a plane parallel to the plane of the image receptor. The central axis x-ray beam should be incident on the center of the structure. Finally the patient must be effectively restrained to minimize motion blur.

To be able to position patients properly, the radiologic technologist must have a good knowledge of human anatomy. If multiple structures are being radiographed and are to be imaged with uniform magnification, they must be the same distance from the film. The various techniques applied to radiographic positioning are designed to produce radiographs with minimal image distortion and maximal image resolution.

Image Receptors

Usually, a standard type of screen-film combination is used throughout a radiology department for a given examination. Generally, extremity and soft tissue radiographs are taken with the fine-detail screen-film combinations. Most other radiographs use double-emulsion film with screens. The new, structured-grain x-ray films used with high-resolution intensifying screens produce exquisite images with limited patient dose.

The following principles should be considered when planning a particular examination:

1. The use of intensifying screens decreases patient dose by a factor of at least 20.

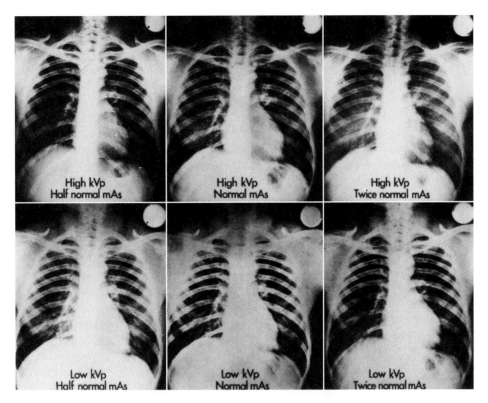

FIGURE 20-35 Chest radiographs demonstrating two advantages of a high-kVp technique: greater latitude and wider margin for error. *(Courtesy Eastman Kodak Co.)*

2. As the speed of the image receptor increases, radiographic noise increases, and contrast resolution decreases.
3. Low-contrast imaging procedures have a wider latitude, and larger margin of error, in producing an acceptable radiograph.

Selection of Technique Factors

Before each examination, the radiologic technologist must select the optimal radiographic technique factors: kVp, mA, and exposure time. Many considerations determine the value of each of these factors, and they are complexly interrelated. Few generalizations are possible.

One generalization that can be made for all radiographic exposures is that the time of exposure should be as short as possible. Image quality is improved with short exposure times as a result of reduced motion blur. One of the reasons three-phase and high-frequency generators are better than single-phase generators is that shorter exposure times are possible with the former.

 Keep exposure time as short as possible.

Similar simple statements cannot be made about the selection of kVp or mA. Since time is to remain at a minimum, the selection of kVp, mA, and the resulting mAs should be carefully considered. The radiographer should strive for optimal radiographic contrast and ODs by exposing the patient to the proper quantity and quality of x-radiation.

 The primary control of radiographic contrast as kVp.

As kVp is increased, both the quantity and quality of x-radiation increase; more x-rays are transmitted through the patient, so a higher portion of the primary beam reaches the image receptor. Thus the kVp also affects the OD. Of the x-rays that interact with the patient, the relative number of Compton interactions increases with increasing kVp, resulting in less differential absorption and reduced subject contrast. Furthermore, with increased kVp the scatter radiation reaching the film is higher, and therefore radiographic noise is higher. The result of increased kVp is loss of contrast. When radiographic contrast is low, latitude is high, and there is greater margin for error.

The principal advantages of using high kVp are the great reduction in patient dose and the wide latitude of exposures allowed in the production of a diagnostic radiograph. Figure 20-35 shows a series of chest radiographs that demonstrates the increased latitude resulting from a high-kVp technique; the relative technique factors are indicated on each radiograph. To some extent, the use of grids can compensate for the loss of contrast accompanying a high-kVp technique.

 The primary control of OD is mAs.

As mAs is increased, the radiation quantity increases, and therefore the number of x-rays arriving at the image receptor increases, resulting in a higher OD and lower radiographic noise.

In a secondary way the mAs also influences contrast. Recall that maximal contrast is obtained only when the film is exposed over a range that results in an OD along the straight-line portion of the characteristic curve. Too low an mAs results in a low OD and reduced radiographic contrast. Too much mAs results in a high OD and a loss of radiographic contrast.

A number of other factors influence OD, radiographic contrast, and therefore radiographic quality. For example, adding filtration to the x-ray tube reduces the x-ray beam intensity but increases the quality, and a change in SID results in a change in OD because x-ray intensity varies with distance. Table 20-3 summarizes the principal factors that influence the making of a radiograph.

The continuing trend in radiographic technique is to use high kVp with a compensating reduction in mAs to produce a radiograph of satisfactory quality while reducing patient exposure and the likelihood of reexamination because of an error in technique. Such considerations are discussed in detail in Chapter 21.

SUMMARY

Radiographic quality is the exactness of representation of the anatomic structure on the radiograph. Characteristics that make up radiographic quality are as follows:
1. Spatial resolution or the ability to image small, high-contrast structures
2. Low noise and elimination of ODs that do not reflect anatomic structures
3. Proper speed of the screen-film combination, which limits patient dose but produces a quality radiograph

These characteristics and three others—film factors, geometric factors, and subject factors—combine to determine radiographic quality. Film factors involve quality control in film processing and characteristics of film. The graph on semilogarithmic paper resulting from sensitometry and densitometry data of film OD is the characteristic curve. The characteristic curve shows film contrast (slope of the straight-line portion), speed, and latitude (range of exposures in diagnostically useful range of the characteristic curve).

Geometric factors of radiographic quality involve preventing magnification and distortion as well as using object thickness, position, focal-spot blur, and the heel effect advantageously. Subject factors that affect radiographic quality depend on the patient. A radiographer must prevent motion blur by encouraging patient cooperation. Also, by measuring patient or part thickness, recognizing tissue mass density, examining anatomic shape, and evaluating optimal kVp levels, a radiographer can create a high-quality radiograph.

TABLE 20-3	Principal Factors Affecting the Making of a Radiograph*						
	Patient Dose	Magnification	Focal-Spot Blur	Motion Blur	Absorption Blur	OD	Radiographic Contrast
Film speed	−	0	0	−	0	+	0
Screen speed	−	0	0	−	0	+	+
Grid ratio	+	0	0	0	0	−	+
Processing time/temperature	0	0	0	0	0	+	−
Patient or part thickness	+	+	+	+	+	−	−
Field size	+	0	0	0	0	+	−
Use of contrast media	0	0	0	0	0	+	−
Focal-spot size	0	0	+	0	0	0	0
SID	−	−	−	−	0	−	0
OID	0	+	+	+	0	0	+
Screen-film contact	0	0	0	0	0	0	−
mAs	+	0	0	0	0	+	+ or −
Time	+	0	0	+	0	+	+ or −
kVp	+	0	0	0	0	+	−
Voltage ripple	+	0	0	−	0	−	−
Total filtration	−	0	0	0	0	−	−

*As the factors in the left-hand column are increased, *while all other factors remain fixed*, cross-referenced conditions are affected as shown: +, increase; −, decrease; 0, no change.

CHALLENGE QUESTIONS

1. Define or otherwise identify the following:
   a. Average gradient
   b. Foreshortening
   c. Focal-spot blur
   d. Densitometer
   e. Motion blur
   f. Distortion
   g. Quantum mottle
   h. Latitude
   i. Contrast resolution

2. What principally determines radiographic spatial resolution?

3. Describe the equipment used in sensitometry.

4. How does proper film processing affect image contrast and optical density.

5. Have the manufacturer's representative help construct a characteristic curve from the data obtained from the sensitometry and densitometry data of a screen-film combination used in your department.

6. The intensity of light emitted by a viewbox is 1000. The intensity of the light transmitted through the film is 1. What is the OD of the film? Will it be light, gray, or black?

7. Base and fog densities on a given radiograph are 0.35. At densities 0.25 and 2 above base and fog densities, the characteristic curve shows LREs of 1.3 and 2. What is the average gradient?

8. List the factors affecting the finished radiograph in relation to film processing.

9. X-ray image receptors A and B require 15 mR and 45 mR, respectively, to produce an OD of 1.0. Which is faster and what is the speed of each?

10. What are the three principal geometric factors that affect radiographic quality?

11. What are standard SIDs?

12. List and explain the five factors that affect subject contrast.

13. What is the difference between foreshortening and elongation?

14. Describe the H & D contrast curve.

15. Discuss the factors that influence radiographic OD and contrast.

16. Construct a characteristic curve for a typical screen-film combination and carefully label the axes.

17. An x-ray examination of the heart taken at 100-cm SID shows a cardiac silhouette measuring 13 cm in width. If the OID distance is estimated at 15 cm, what is the actual width of the heart?

18. The subject contrast of a thorax is 5.3, and the image receptor contrast is 3.2. What is the radiographic contrast?

19. State the reciprocity law and describe its influence on radiography.

20. Does the use of a radiographic intensifying screen increase contrast compared to direct exposure?

Radiographic Technique

OBJECTIVES

At the completion of this chapter, the student should be able to:

1. List the four patient factors and explain their effect on radiographic technique
2. Identify four image quality factors and how they influence the characteristics of a radiograph
3. Discuss the four types of radiographic-technique charts
4. Explain the three types of automatic-exposure control

OUTLINE

Radiographic technique is the combination of settings selected on the control panel of the x-ray imaging system to produce a quality image on the radiograph. The geometry and position of the x-ray tube, the patient, and the image receptor are included in this description.

Radiographic technique may be described by identifying three groups of factors. The first group includes patient factors such as anatomic thickness and body composition. The second group consists of image-quality factors such as optical density (OD), contrast, detail, and distortion. The final group includes exposure-technique factors such as kilovolt peak (kVp), milliampere (mA), exposure time, and source-to-image receptor distance (SID); these factors determine the basic characteristics of radiation exposure of the image receptor and patient dose and are discussed in previous chapters.

These factors also provide the radiologic technologist with a specific and orderly means of producing, evaluating, and comparing radiographs. Understanding them is essential for the production of quality images.

PATIENT FACTORS

Perhaps, the most difficult task for the radiologic technologist is evaluation of the patient. The patient's size, shape, and physical condit ion greatly influence the required radiographic technique.

The general size and shape of a patient is called the **body habitus,** and there are four such states (Figure 21-1). The **sthenic** patient—meaning "strong, active"— is the average patient. The **hyposthenic** patient is thin but healthy appearing. Such a patient requires less radiographic technique. The **hypersthenic** patient is big in frame and usually overweight. The **asthenic** patient is small, frail, sometimes emaciated, and often elderly. Radiographic technique charts are based on the sthenic patient.

Recognition of body habitus is essential to the selection of radiographic technique. Once this is established, the thickness and composition of the anatomic part being examined must be determined.

Thickness of Part

The thicker the patient, the more x-radiation required to penetrate through the patient to the image receptor. For this reason, the radiologic technologist must use **calipers,** an instrument with two bent or curved legs used for measuring the thickness of a solid, to measure the thickness of the anatomic part being irradiated. Never guess at patient or part thickness.

Depending on the type of radiographic technique being practiced, either the mAs or the kVp will be altered as a function of the thickness of the part. Table 21-1 shows an example of how the mAs changes when imaging the abdomen if a fixed-kVp technique is used. Table 21-2 reports the change in radiographic-technique factors as a function of thickness of part when a variable-kVp technique is used.

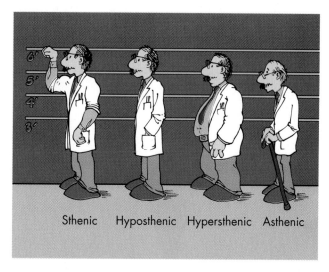

FIGURE 21-1 The four general states of body habitus.

TABLE 21-1	Fixed-kVp Technique for an Anterior-Posterior Abdominal Examination							
kVp	80	80	80	80	80	80	80	80
Patient thickness (cm)	16	18	20	22	24	26	28	30
mAs	12	15	22	30	45	60	90	120

TABLE 21-2	Variable-kVp Technique for an Anterior-Posterior Pelvic Examination							
mAs	100	100	100	100	100	100	100	100
Patient thickness (cm)	15	16	17	18	19	20	21	22
kVp	56	58	60	62	64	66	68	70

Body Composition

The thickness of the anatomic part is not the only factor that must be selected to ensure good radiographic quality. The thorax and the abdomen may have the same thickness, but the radiographic technique used for each will be considerably different from that used with the other. The radiologic technologist must estimate the mass density of the anatomic part and the range of mass densities involved.

Generally speaking, when only soft tissue is being imaged, low kVp and high mAs are used. With an extremity, however, which has both soft tissue and bone, low kVp is used because the body part is thin.

When imaging the chest, the radiologic technologist takes advantage of the high subject contrast. Lung tissue has very low mass density, the bony structures have high mass density, and the mediastinal structures have inter-mediate mass density. Consequently, high kVp and low mAs can be used to good advantage. This results in an image with satisfactory contrast and low patient radiation exposure.

 The chest has high subject contrast; the abdomen has low subject contrast.

These various tissues are often described by their degree of **radiolucency** or **radiopacity** (Figure 21-2). Radiolucent tissue attenuates few x-rays and appears black on the radiograph. Radiopaque tissue absorbs x-rays and appears white on the radiograph. Table 21-3 shows the relative degree of radiolucency for various body habitus and tissues.

Pathology

The type of pathology, its size, and its composition influence radiographic technique. In these cases, the patient examination request form and previous images may be of some help. The radiologic technologist should not hesitate to seek more information from the referring physician, the radiologist, or the patient regarding the suspected pathology.

 Pathologies can appear with increased radiolucency or radiopacity.

Some pathologies are destructive, causing the tissue to be more radiolucent. Others can constructively increase mass density or composition, causing the tissue to be more radiopaque. Practice and experience will guide your clinical judgment. Box 21-1 lists some radiolucent and radiopaque conditions.

IMAGE-QUALITY FACTORS

The phrase image-quality factors refers to the characteristics of the radiographic image; these include OD, con-

TABLE 21-3	Relative Degrees of Radiolucency		
		Body Habitus	**Tissue Type**
Radiolucent	Black		
		Asthenic	Lung
		Hyposthenic	Fat
		Sthenic	Muscle
		Hypersthenic	Bone
Radiopaque	White		

Radiopaque
OD = 2.5

Radiolucent
OD = 2.5

FIGURE 21-2 Relative radiolucency and OD are shown on this radiograph. *(Courtesy Bette Shans.)*

BOX 21-1 Classifying Pathology	
Radiolucent (Destructive)	**Radiopaque (Constructive)**
Active tuberculosis	Aortic aneurysm
Atrophy	Ascites
Bowel obstruction	Atelectasis
Cancer	Cirrhosis
Degenerative arthritis	Hypertrophy
Emphysema	Metastases
Osteoporosis	Pleural effusion
Pneumothorax	Pneumonia
	Sclerosis

trast, image detail, and distortion. These factors provide a means for the radiologic technologist to produce, review, and evaluate radiographs. Image-quality factors are considered the "language" of radiography, and often it is difficult to separate one factor from another.

Optical Density

As you recall from Chapter 20, optical density (OD), sometimes called *radiographic density,* can be thought of as the degree of blackening of the finished radiograph. OD is actually the logarithm to the base of 10 of the ratio of light incident on a film to the light transmitted through the film (Figure 21-3). A completely black image represents an OD of 4 or greater; a clear image has an OD of less than 0.2.

In medical radiography, a poor-quality radiographic image can be described as "too dark" or "too light." If a radiograph is too dark, it has a high OD: too much x-radiation reached the image receptor, and the film is **overexposed.**

If a radiograph is too light, it has a low OD: too little x-radiation reached the image receptor, and the film is **underexposed.** Both overexposure and underexposure may require that the radiographic examination be repeated. Figure 21-4 shows clinical examples of two extremes of exposure.

OD can be controlled in radiography by two major factors: mAs and SID. A significant number of problems would arise if the SID were continually changed. Therefore it is usually fixed at 90 cm for mobile examinations, 100 cm for table studies, and 180 cm for upright chest examinations. Figure 21-5 illustrates the change in OD at these SIDs when other exposure-technique factors remain constant.

When distance is fixed, however, as is usually the case, the mAs becomes the primary variable technique

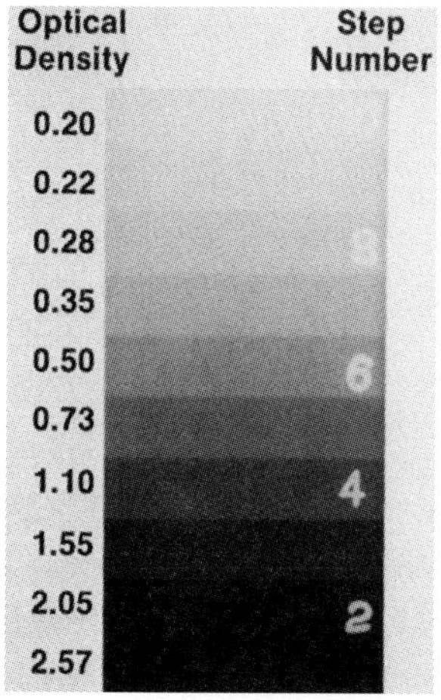

Optical Density	Step Number
0.20	
0.22	
0.28	8
0.35	
0.50	6
0.73	
1.10	4
1.55	
2.05	2
2.57	

FIGURE 21-3 Amount of light transmitted through a radiograph is determined by the OD of a film. The step-wedge radiograph shows a representative range of ODs.

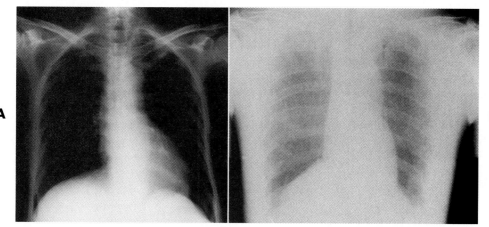

FIGURE 21-4 **A,** This overexposed radiograph of the chest is too black to be diagnostic. **B,** Likewise, this underexposed chest radiograph is unacceptable because there is no detail in the lung fields.

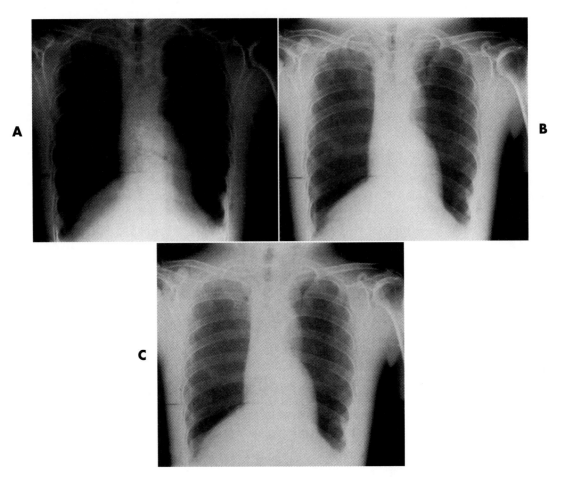

FIGURE 21-5 Normal chest radiograph taken at 100-cm SID **(B).** If the exposure-technique factors are not changed, a similar radiograph at 90-cm SID **(A)** will be overexposed and at 180-cm SID **(C),** underexposed.

factor used to control OD. OD increases directly with mAs, which means that if the OD is to be increased on a radiograph, the mAs needs to be increased accordingly.

OD can be affected by other factors, but mAs becomes the factor of choice for its control (Figure 21-6). A change in mAs of approximately 30% is required to produce a visible change in OD. As a general rule, when only the mAs is changed, it should be halved or doubled (Figure 21-7). If such a change is not required, another exposure is probably not required.

 The mAs must be changed by approximately 30% to produce a perceptible change in OD.
The kVp must be changed by approximately 4% to produce a perceptible change in OD.

Since an increase in OD on the finished radiograph is accomplished with a proportionate increase in mAs, is the same true with kVp? Yes, there is an increase in kVp, but it is not proportionate. As kVp is increased, the qual-

ity of the x-ray beam is increased, and more x-rays penetrate the anatomic part of interest. This results in more remnant radiation exposing the image receptor. As discussed in Chapter 12, x-ray intensity at the patient is proportional to kVp^2 and at the image receptor to kVp^5.

Other qualitative factors are affected when the kVp is changed to adjust the OD. This makes it much more difficult to optimize the OD with kVp. It takes the eye of an experienced radiologic technologist to determine whether OD is the only factor to be changed or if contrast should also be changed to optimize the radiographic image.

Technique changes involving kVp become complicated. A change in the kVp affects penetration, scatter radiation, patient dose, and especially contrast. Generally, if the OD on the radiograph is to be increased using kVp, an increase in kVp by 15% is equivalent to doubling the mAs. This is known as the **fifteen-percent rule.** Figure 21-8 illustrates the OD change when this rule is applied. If only OD is to be changed, the fifteen-percent rule should not be used because such a large change in kVp will change image contrast.

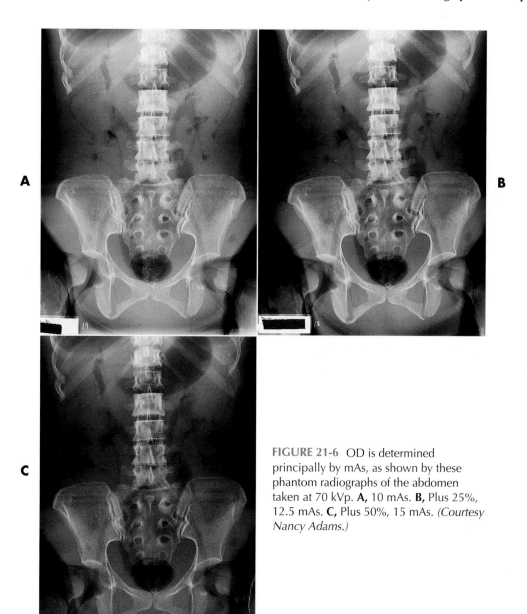

FIGURE 21-6 OD is determined principally by mAs, as shown by these phantom radiographs of the abdomen taken at 70 kVp. **A,** 10 mAs. **B,** Plus 25%, 12.5 mAs. **C,** Plus 50%, 15 mAs. *(Courtesy Nancy Adams.)*

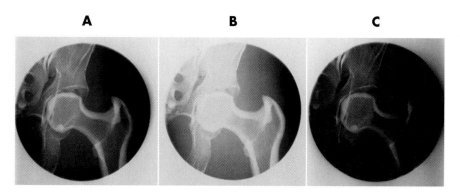

FIGURE 21-7 Changes in the mAs have a direct effect on OD. **A** is the original image. **B** shows the decrease in OD when the mAs is decreased by half. **C** shows the increase in OD when the mAs is doubled.

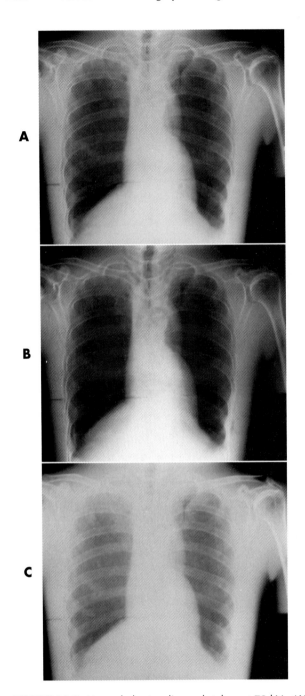

FIGURE 21-8 Normal chest radiograph taken at 70 kVp (**A**). If the kilovoltage is increased 15% to 80 kVp, overexposure occurs (**B**). Similarly, at 15% less, or 60 kVp, the radiograph is underexposed (**C**).

 A 15% increase in kVp accompanied by a half reduction in mAs will result in the same OD.

The simplest method for increasing or decreasing the OD on a radiograph is to increase or decrease the mAs. This reduces other possible factors that could affect the finished image. The various factors that affect OD are listed in Table 21-4.

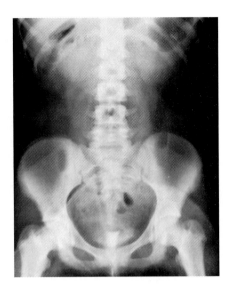

FIGURE 21-9 Radiograph of the abdomen showing the vertebral column with its high subject contrast. The kidneys, pelvis, and psoas muscle are low-contrast tissues that are better visualized with low kVp.

TABLE 21-4	Technique Factors Affecting OD	
Factor Increased	**Effect on OD**
mAs	Increase
kVp	Increase
SID	Decrease
Thickness of part	Decrease
Mass density	Decrease
Development time	Increase
Image receptor speed	Increase
Collimation	Decrease
Grid ratio	Decrease

Contrast

Contrast is an important factor in the evaluation of radiographic image quality because the purpose of contrast is to make anatomic parts visible for diagnosis. **Contrast** is thus defined as the difference in OD between adjacent anatomic structures or as the variation in OD on the radiograph.

Contrast is the result of differences in attenuation of the x-ray beam as it penetrates various tissues of the body. It is the relative penetrability of the beam through different tissues that determines image contrast.

Figure 21-9 shows an image of a spinal column and pelvis, illustrating the difference in OD between adjacent structures. High contrast is visible at the bone–soft tissue interface along the spinal column. The soft tissues of the psoas muscle and kidneys exhibit much less contrast, although details of these structures are readily visible. The contrast resolution of the soft tissues can be enhanced with reduced kVp but at the expense of higher patient dose.

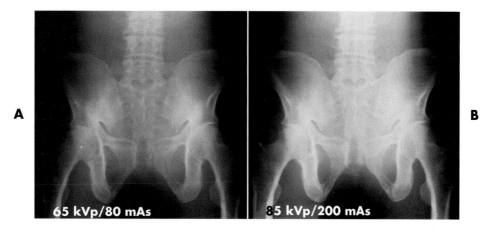

FIGURE 21-10 Radiographs of a pelvis phantom demonstrate a short scale of contrast (**A**) and a long scale of contrast (**B**).

 kVp is the major factor for controlling radiographic contrast.

The penetrability of the primary x-ray beam is controlled by kVp. Obtaining adequate contrast requires that the anatomic part be adequately penetrated; therefore penetration becomes the key to understanding radiographic contrast. Compare the radiographs shown in Figure 21-10. Figure 21-10, *A*, shows high contrast, or "short gray scale," whereas Figure 21-10, *B*, shows low contrast, or "long gray scale."

Gray scale of contrast means the range of ODs from the whitest to the blackest part of the radiograph. For example, think of using scissors to cut a small patch representing each OD on the radiograph and then arranging the patches in order from the lightest to darkest. The resulting OD range would be the gray scale of contrast.

High-contrast radiographs produce **short gray scale.** They exhibit black to white in just a few apparent steps. Low-contrast radiographs produce **long gray scale** and have the appearance of many shades of gray. Figure 21-11 presents two radiographs of a step wedge, which demonstrates scale of contrast. The one taken at 50 kVp shows that only five steps are visible. At 90 kVp, all thirteen steps are visible because of the long scale of contrast.

Often the radiologic technologist is required to increase or decrease contrast because of an unacceptable image. For increased contrast, the range of ODs must be made more black and white with a greater difference in the OD of adjacent structures. In other words, a radiograph with a shorter contrast scale must be produced. Accomplishing this requires a reduction in the kVp.

To reduce contrast, the radiographer must produce a radiograph with a longer contrast scale and therefore with more grays. This is done by increasing the

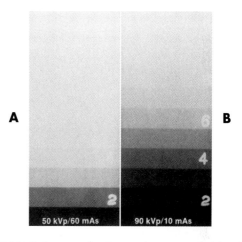

FIGURE 21-11 Images of a step wedge exposed at low kVp (**A**) and high kVp (**B**) illustrate the meaning of short scale and long scale of contrast, respectively.

kVp. Normally, a change of approximately 4 kVp is required to visually affect the scale of contrast in the 50- to 90-kVp range (Figure 21-12). At a lower kVp, a 2-kVp change may be sufficient, whereas at a higher kVp, a 10-kVp change may be required.

The phrases *high contrast, high degree of contrast,* and *a lot of contrast* all define a short scale of contrast and are obtained by the use of low-kVp exposure techniques. *Low contrast* and *low degree of contrast* are the same as a long scale of contrast and result from high-kVp exposure techniques. These relationships in radiographic contrast are summarized in Table 21-5.

In addition to kilovoltage, many other factors influence radiographic contrast. Although mAs affects only x-ray quantity, not quality, it still influences contrast. If the mAs is too high or two low, the predominant OD will fall on the shoulder or toe of the characteristic curve, respectively. Radiographic contrast is low on the shoulder and toe regions because the gradient of the characteristic curve is low in these regions. Structures look the same despite differences in subject contrast.

The use of intensifying screens results in shorter contrast scale when compared with nonscreen exposures. Collimation removes some scatter radiation from the radiograph, producing a radiograph of shorter contrast scale. Grids also help reduce the amount of scatter that reaches the film, thus producing radiographs of shorter contrast scale. Grids with high ratios increase the contrast. The exposure-technique factors that affect contrast are summarized in Table 21-6.

A typical clinical problem faced by the radiologic technologist is the adjustment of image contrast. An image is made, but the contrast scale is either too long—too many grays—or too short—too much black and white. Usually, it is the latter, so a longer scale of contrast is required. To solve such a problem, apply the fifteen-percent rule. Increase the kVp by 15% while reducing the mAs by half.

Question: A patient's knee measures 14 cm, and an exposure is made at 62 kVp and 12 mAs. The resulting contrast scale is too short. What should the second technique be?

Answer: Increase the kVp by 15%:
$$62 \text{ kVp} \times 0.15 = 9.3 \text{ kVp}$$
Therefore the new kVp = 62 + 9 = 71 kVp
Reduce the mAs to half:
$$12 \text{ mAs} \times 0.5 = 6 \text{ mAs}$$
Second technique = 71 kVp and 6 mAs

A smaller technique compensation for a change in contrast scale may be required. An increase of 5% in kVp may be accompanied by a 30% reduction in mAs to produce the same OD at a slightly reduced contrast scale. This is known as the **five-percent rule.** The proper technique compensation by the radiologic technologist is a judgment call. The anatomic part, body habitus, suspected pathology, and x-ray image receptor characteristics must all be considered by the skillful radiologic technologist. With practice and experience this becomes routine.

Question: A modest reduction in image contrast is required for a knee exposed at 62 kVp and 12 mAs. What technique should be tried?

TABLE 21-5	Relationship Between kVp and Scale of Contrast
High kVp	**Low kVp**
Long scale	Short scale
Low contrast	High contrast
Less contrast	More contrast

TABLE 21-6	Exposure Technique Factors that Affect Radiographic Contrast*	
Factor Increased	**Change in Contrast**	
kVp	Decrease	
Grid ratio	Increase	
Beam restriction	Increase	
Image receptor used	Variable	
Development time	Decrease	
mAs	Decrease (toe, shoulder)	
*In approximate order		

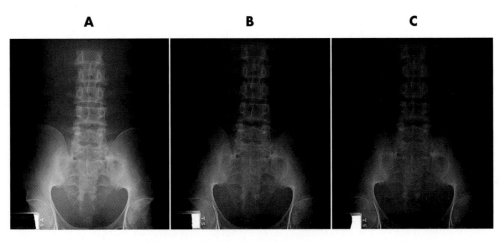

A   **B**   **C**

FIGURE 21-12 These radiographs of the pelvis and abdomen show that a 4-kVp increase results in a perceptible change in contrast. **A,** 75 kVp and 28 mAs. **B,** 79 kVp and 28 mAs. **C,** 81 kVp and 28 mAs. *(Courtesy Mike Enriquez.)*

Answer: Apply the five-percent rule:

$$62 \text{ kVp} \times 0.05 = 3.1 \text{ kVp}$$
$$62 + 3 = 65 \text{ kVp}$$
$$12 \text{ mAs} \times 0.30 = 3.6 \text{ mAs}$$
$$12 - 4 = 8 \text{ mAs}$$
$$\text{Second technique} = 65 \text{ kVp and 8 mAs}$$

Image Detail

Image detail describes the sharpness of small structures on the radiograph. With adequate detail, even the smallest parts of anatomy are visible and the radiologist can more readily detect tissue abnormalities. Image detail must be evaluated by two means: sharpness of image detail and visibility of image detail.

Sharpness of image detail refers to the structural lines or borders of tissues in the image and the amount of clarity or blur of the image. The factors that generally control the sharpness of detail are the geometric factors discussed in Chapter 20: focal-spot size, source-to-image receptor distance (SID), and object-to-image receptor distance (OID). Sharpness of image detail is also influenced by the type of intensifying screens used and the presence of motion.

 Sharpness of image detail is best measured by spatial resolution.

To produce the sharpest image detail, the radiologic technologist should use the smallest appropriate focal spot and the longest SID and place the anatomic part as close to the image receptor as possible—in other words, minimize OID. Figure 21-13 shows two radiographs of a foot phantom. One was taken under optimal conditions and the other with poor technique. The difference in sharpness of image detail is obvious.

Visibility of image detail describes the ability to see the detail on the radiograph and is best measured by contrast resolution. *Loss of visibility* refers to any factor that causes the deterioration or obscuring of the image detail. For example, fog reduces the ability to see structural lines on the image. An attempt to produce the best defined image can be accomplished by using all the correct factors, but if the film is fogged by light or radiation, the detail present will not be fully visible (Figure 21-14). You might conclude that good detail is still present but that its visibility is poor. Because kVp and mAs influence image contrast, these factors must be chosen with care for each examination.

 The visibility of image detail is best measured by contrast resolution.

The assumption is that any factor affecting OD and contrast also affects the visibility of image detail. Key factors that provide the best visibility of image detail are collimation, use of grids, and all other methods that prevent scatter radiation from reaching the image receptor.

Distortion

The fourth image quality factor is distortion, the misrepresentation of object size and shape on the finished radiograph. Because of the position of the x-ray tube, the

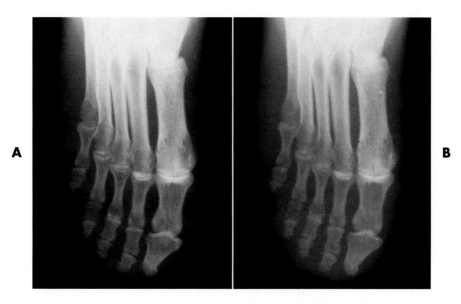

FIGURE 21-13 Radiograph taken with a 1.0-mm focal spot **(A)** that exhibits far greater detail than radiograph that was taken with a 2.0-mm focal spot x-ray tube **(B)**.

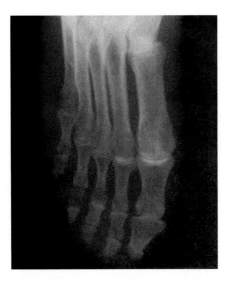

FIGURE 21-14 Same radiograph as shown in Figure 21-13, **A,** except the visibility of image detail is reduced because of safelight fog.

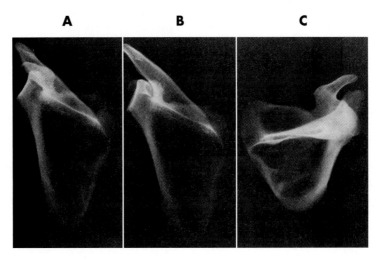

FIGURE 21-15 **A,** Normal projection of the scapula. **B,** Elongation of the scapula. **C,** Foreshortening of the scapula.

anatomic part of interest, and the image receptor, the final image may misrepresent the object.

Poor alignment of the image receptor or the x-ray tube can result in elongation of the image. *Elongation* means the object or part of interest appears larger than normal. Poor alignment of the anatomic part may also result in foreshortening of the image. *Foreshortening* means that the anatomic part appears smaller than normal. Figure 21-15 provides examples of elongation and foreshortening. Many body parts are naturally foreshortened as a result of shape (for example, ribs and facial bones).

Distortion can be minimized by proper alignment of the tube, the anatomic part of interest, and the image re-

ceptor. This alignment is fundamentally important for patient positioning.

 Distortion is reduced by positioning the anatomic part of interest in a plane parallel to that of the image receptor.

Distortion can also be used to advantage. The Towne's view of the skull is such an example.

Table 21-7 summarizes the principal radiographic image quality factors. The primary controlling technique factor for each image quality factor is given, as well as secondary technique factors that influence each image quality factor.

Factor	Controlled by	Influenced by
OD	mAs	kVp
		Distance
		Thickness of part
		Mass density
		Development time and temperature
		Image receptor speed
		Collimation
		Grid ratio
Contrast	kVp	mAs (toe, shoulder)
		Development time and temperature
		Image receptor used
		Collimation
		Grid ratio
Detail	Focal-spot size	SID
		OID
		Motion
		All factors related to density and contrast
Distortion	Patient positioning	Alignment of tube, anatomic part, and image receptor

TABLE 21-7   Principal Radiographic Image Quality Factors

EXPOSURE-TECHNIQUE FACTORS

kVp, mA, exposure time, and SID are the principal exposure technique factors. It is important for the radiologic technologist to know how to manipulate these exposure technique factors to produce the desired OD, radiographic contrast, image detail, and distortion on the finished radiograph.

For each radiographic imaging system a guide or chart should be available that describes standard methods for consistently producing high-quality images. Such an aid is called a **radiographic-technique chart.** Radiographic-technique charts are written tables that provide a means for determining the specific technical factors to be used for a given radiographic examination.

For a radiographic-technique chart to meet with success, the radiologic technologist must understand its purpose, how it was constructed, and how it is to be used. Most important, the technologist must know how to make adjustments for body habitus and pathologic processes. When used properly, the radiographic-technique chart allows for consistently good diagnostic images. The scale of contrast and OD are more predictable than if no standard chart is used.

Radiographic technique charts can be prepared to accommodate all types of facilities. The four principal types of charts are based on variable kVp, fixed kVp, high kVp, and automatic exposure. Each chart provides a guide for the selection of exposure factors for all patients and all examinations.

Most facilities select a particular type of imaging system for use and then prepare similar charts for each radiographic examination room. The type of chart selected usually depends on the technical director of radiology,

the type of imaging systems available, the screen-film combination, and the accessories available.

Radiographic-technique charts and their use have become an important issue in patient protection. Radiologic technologists are required to use their skills in producing the best possible image with a single exposure. Repeated examinations only increase the radiation dose to the patient. The preparation of these charts becomes an important and challenging task, and once in use, the charts must constantly be evaluated and changed when necessary.

The preparation of a chart does not require that it be created completely from scratch. Many authors have guides that can be used in the preparation of specific charts. Each radiographic imager is unique in its radiation characteristics. Therefore a specific chart should be prepared and tested for each examination room.

 Radiographic-technique charts from books, pamphlets, and manufacturers should not be used as printed.

Before the preparation of the radiographic-technique chart begins, the x-ray equipment must be calibrated by a medical physicist, and the processing system must be thoroughly evaluated. The total filtration should also be determined. Although 2.5 mm of Al is the prescribed standard, one may find 3 mm of Al total filtration or more available on the collimator housing. This significantly alters contrast and makes a considerable difference in any technique chart.

The type of grid to be used should be known and the collimator or beam restrictor checked for accurate light field and x-ray beam coincidence. This is most important so that all variables are reduced to a minimum. When a radiographic technique chart is found to be inadequate, these factors should be checked first.

Variable-kVp Technique Chart

The variable-kVp radiographic technique chart uses a fixed mAs and a kVp that varies according to the thickness of the anatomic part. The basic characteristic of the variable kVp chart is an inherently short scale of contrast. Generally, exposures made with this method provide radiographs of shorter contrast scale because of the use of a lower kVp.

 kVp varies with the thickness of the anatomic part by 2 kVp/cm.

Exposure directed by the variable-kVp chart usually results in higher patient dose and less exposure latitude. For success, the radiologic technologist must be accurate in measuring the anatomic part before selecting the exposure factors from the chart. Without such care and attention, the anatomic part may not be fully penetrated as a result of the lower kVp.

There are approximate procedures for establishing a kVp to begin formulating a variable-kVp technique chart. The beginning kVp depends on the voltage ripple as follows:

Variable kVp
Beginning kVp (single phase) =
$\qquad$ 2 × Thickness of anatomic part (cm) + 30

To begin preparation of a variable-kVp radiographic technique chart, select the body part for examination. For example, if the knee is chosen, use a knee phantom for all test exposures.

First, measure the thickness of the knee phantom accurately, using a caliper designed for that purpose. Multiply the part thickness by 2 and add 30; this indicates a kVp with which to begin if the high-voltage generator is single phase. If the high-voltage generator is three phase or high frequency, 25 or 23, respectively, are the additive factors.

Question: A phantom knee measures 14 cm thick. What single-phase kVp should be used to begin construction of a variable-kVp technique chart?

Answer: $14 \text{ cm} \times 2 = 28 + 30$
$\qquad = 58 \text{ kVp}$

The kVp setting for examination of the knee will be 58 kVp. The next task is to select the optimal mAs at this kVp. This depends on the image receptor characteristics and effectiveness of scatter radiation control. For example, when using a 200-speed image receptor with an 8:1 grid, make test exposures at 58 kVp with 9 mAs, 12 mAs, and 20 mAs (Figure 21-16). Select the radiograph that produces the best OD or make additional exposures at other mAs values if necessary.

The result of this exercise is the first line of the variable kVp technique chart. The kVp and mAs to be used when radiographing a knee measuring 14 cm have been established at 58 kVp and 12 mAs, as shown in Table 21-8.

At this point, the chart can be expanded to include knees with other thicknesses. The same procedure is used to prepare a variable-kVp radiographic technique chart for other anatomic parts. Because radiologists prefer similar contrast scales for examination of the same atomic parts, the variable-kVp technique chart has been replaced largely by the fixed-kVp technique chart.

Fixed-kVp Technique Chart

The fixed-kVp radiographic technique chart is the one used most often. Developed by Arthur Fuchs, it is a

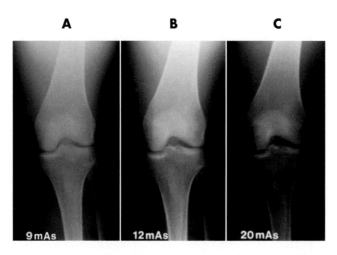

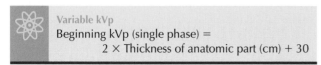

FIGURE 21-16 Radiographs of a knee phantom taken at 58 kVp. That obtained at 12 mAs (**B**) was selected to begin the variable-kVp chart.

method for selecting exposures that produce radiographs with a longer scale of contrast. The kVp is selected as the optimum required for penetration of the anatomic part. This usually results in somewhat higher kVp values for most examinations than with the variable-kVp technique.

 For each anatomic part there is an optimum kVp.

Once selected, the kVp is fixed at that level for each type of examination and not varied according to different thicknesses of the anatomic part. The mAs, however, is changed according to the thickness of the anatomic part to provide the proper OD. For example, all examinations of the knee might require 60 kVp with the mAs adjusted to accommodate for differences in thickness.

Since the fixed-kVp technique generally requires a higher kVp, one benefit is lower patient dose. There is greater latitude and more consistency with exposures of the same anatomic part.

Measurement of the part is not as critical because part size is grouped as small, medium, or large. For most x-ray examinations of the spine and trunk, the optimum kVp is approximately 80. Approximately 70 kVp is appropriate for the soft tissue of the abdomen. For most extremities, the optimum would be approximately 60 kVp.

To prepare a fixed-kVp radiographic technique chart, separate the anatomic part thickness into the three groups by identifying the range of thickness that is to be included in each group. Using the abdomen as an example, small might be 14 to 20 cm; medium 21 to 25 cm; and large, 26 to 32 cm.

For test exposures, use a medium-sized phantom and begin with 80 kVp. Produce radiographs at mAs increments of 40, 60, 80, and so on until the proper OD is obtained (Figure 21-17). Again, the OD selected depends on the type of image receptor and available scatter radiation–control devices.

Once the proper OD has been established, the chart can then be expanded to include small and large anatomic parts. For small anatomic parts, reduce the mAs by 30%. For large anatomic parts, increase the mAs by 30%. For a part that is swollen as a result of trauma, a 50% increase may be required. Table 21-9 presents the results of a representative procedure.

Fixed-kVp charts can also be calculated with specific mAs values for every 2-cm thickness. This approach is more accurate than the subjective small, medium, and large labels.

High-kVp Technique Chart

The kVp selected for high-kVp technique charts is generally greater than 100. For example, overhead radiographs for procedures using a barium contrast medium would use 120 kVp for each exposure. High-kVp exposure techniques are ideal for barium work to ensure adequate penetration of the barium.

This type of exposure technique could also be used for routine chest radiography to provide improved visualization of the various tissue mass densities present in the lung fields and mediastinum. Lower or more conventional kVp settings provide increased subject contrast between bone and soft tissue. When 120 kVp is selected for chest radiography, however, all skeletal tissue will be penetrated and exhibit increased visualization of the different soft tissue mass densities present.

To prepare a high-kVp technique chart, use the same basic procedure as for the fixed-kVp technique chart. All exposures for a particular anatomic part would use the same kVp. Obviously, the mAs would be much less.

Test exposures are made using a phantom to determine the appropriate mAs for adequate ODs. Figure 21-18 shows a chest radiograph made at 120 kVp. Note the improved visualization of the tissue markings of the bronchial tree and the mediastinal structures, compared with the low-kVp radiographs in Figure 21-8. An additional advantage to the high-kVp exposure technique is reduced patient dose.

TABLE 21-8	Variable kVp Chart for Examination of the Knee	
Knee*	**Part Thickness (cm)**	**kVp**
mAs: 12	8	50
SID: 100 cm	9	52
Grid: 12:1	10	54
Collimation: to part	11	56
Image receptor speed:		
200	**12**	**58**
	13	60
	14	62
	15	64
	16	66

*Anterior-posterior/lateral.

TABLE 21-9	Fixed-kVp Chart for Examination of the Abdomen		
Abdomen*	**Part Thickness (cm)**		**Required mAs**
kVp: 80	Small:	14-20	56
SID: 100 cm	Medium:	21-25	80
Grid: 12:1	Large:	26-32	104
Collimation: to part			
Image receptor speed: 200			

*Anterior-posterior.

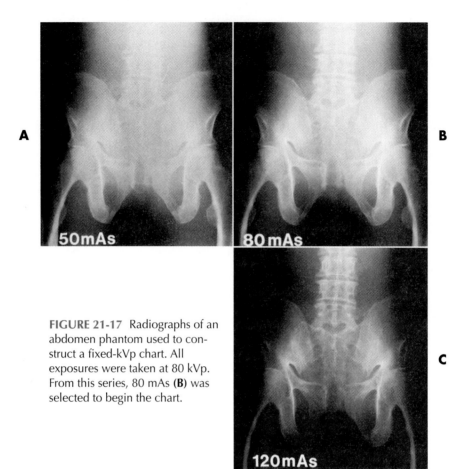

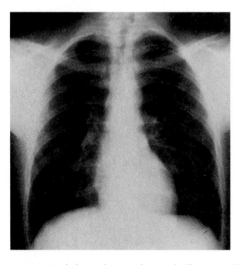

FIGURE 21-17 Radiographs of an abdomen phantom used to construct a fixed-kVp chart. All exposures were taken at 80 kVp. From this series, 80 mAs (**B**) was selected to begin the chart.

FIGURE 21-18 High-kVp chest radiograph illustrates the improved visualization of mediastinal structures.

AUTOMATIC-EXPOSURE TECHNIQUES

The appearance of the operating consoles of x-ray imaging systems is changing in response to the ability to incorporate computer-assisted technology. Several automated-exposure techniques are now available, but none relieves the radiologic technologist of the respon-sibility of identifying certain characteristics of the patient and the anatomic part to be imaged.

Computer-assisted automatic-exposure systems use an electronic exposure timer, such as those described in Chapter 9. The radiation intensity is measured by either a photocell or an ionization chamber and terminates the exposure when the proper OD on the image receptor has been reached. The principles associated with automatic-exposure systems have already been described, but the importance of using radiographic exposure charts with these systems has not.

Automatic control x-ray systems are not completely automatic. It is incorrect to assume that because the radiologic technologist does not have to select a kVp, an mA, and a time for each examination, a less qualified or less skilled operator can use the system.

Generally, the radiologic technologist must use a guide for the selection of the kVp and OD settings. Sometimes, only OD as a function of patient size must be selected. The kVp selection is similar to that of the fixed-kVp method. OD selections are numerically scaled to allow for different thicknesses of the anatomic part.

Patient positioning must be absolutely accurate because the specific body part must be placed over the phototiming device to ensure proper exposure. In addition to the accuracy in positioning, it is recommended that

TABLE 21-10	Factors to Consider When Constructing an Exposure Chart for Automatic Systems
Factor for Selection	**Rationale**
kVp	To select for each anatomic part
Density control	To adjust according to the thickness of a part
Collimation	To reduce patient dose and ensure proper response of an automatic-exposure control
Accessory selection	To optimize the radiation dose image quality ratio

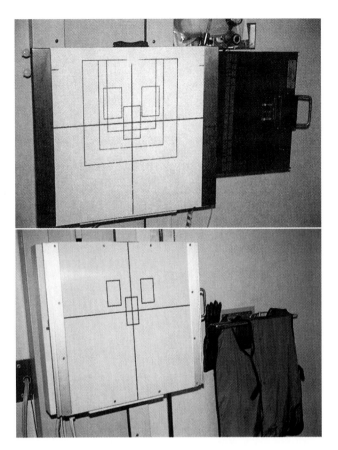

FIGURE 21-19 These vertical chest stands show the position of three independent phototimers. The additional dimensions indicate the standard sizes of the image receptors.

the anatomic part be measured before each examination to determine the appropriate OD selection.

The factors shown in Table 21-10 must be considered when preparing the radiographic exposure chart for an automatic x-ray system. The kVp is selected according to the specific anatomic part being examined. The OD control is positioned according to the part thickness. The specific accessories to be used, such as film, screens, and grids, determine to a great extent the previous selections. It is critical to ensure that collimation confines the x-ray beam to only the anatomic part under investigation or to only the image receptor, whichever is smaller. Excessive scatter radiation affects the response of the automatic-exposure control and reduces image contrast.

Automatic-Exposure Control

Radiation exposure during radiography in most x-ray imagers is determined by **automatic-exposure control (AEC)**. The AEC incorporates a device to sense the amount of radiation falling on the image receptor. Through an electronic feedback circuit the radiation exposure is terminated when a sufficient number of x-rays have reached the image receptor to produce a preset OD.

To image with the use of an AEC, the radiologic technologist selects the appropriate kVp, and the AEC does the rest. Exposure is terminated when the image receptor has received the appropriate radiation exposure to correspond with the preset OD.

AEC devices usually have two or three exposure sensors available for control (Figure 21-19). For instance, three radiation-sensing cells may be available, and the technologist is responsible for selecting which to use for the examination. During a chest examination, if the mediastinum is the region of interest, only the central sensing cell is employed. If the lung fields are of principal importance, the two lateral cells are activated.

Most AECs have a 2-s safety override. If the AEC fails to terminate the exposure, the secondary safety circuit terminates it at 2 s.

In addition to the selection of the exposure cells, the radiologic technologist usually has a three- to seven-position dial labeled *OD* with numerical steps. Each step on the dial is calibrated to increase or decrease the preset average OD of the image receptor by 0.1. This control can be used to accommodate any unusual patient characteristics or to overcome the slowly changing calibration or sensitivity of the AEC.

Programmed Exposure

Microprocessors are being incorporated ever more frequently into operating consoles. A microprocessor allows the operator to digitally select any kVp or mAs, which causes the microprocessor to automatically activate the appropriate mA station and exposure time.

With falling-load generators, the microprocessor begins the exposure at a maximum value and then causes the tube current to be reduced during exposure. The overall objective is to minimize exposure time to reduce motion blur.

Anatomically Programmed Radiography

The ultimate in patient exposure control is termed **anatomically programmed radiography (APR)**. APR also

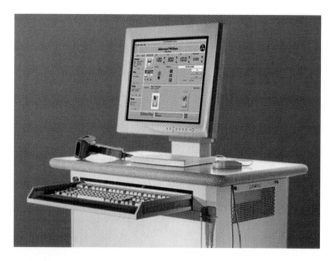

FIGURE 21-20 Anatomically programmed operating console for digital radiography. *(Courtesy Fischer Imaging.)*

uses microprocessor technology. Rather than have the radiologic technologist select a desired kVp and mAs, graphics on the console or on a video touch screen guide the technologist (Figure 21-20).

To produce an image, the radiologic technologist simply touches a picture or a written description of the anatomic part to be imaged and the body habitus. The microprocessor automatically selects the appropriate kVp and mAs. The whole process uses AECs, resulting in near-flawless radiographs. Thus fewer retakes are necessary. However, precise patient positioning relative to the phototiming sensor is still critical in producing quality radiographs.

The principle of APR is similar to that of AEC, with the radiographic-technique chart stored in the microprocessor of the control unit. The service engineer loads the controlling programs during installation and calibrates the exposure-control circuit for the general conditions of the facility. The radiologic technologist need only select the part and its relative size before each exposure. The programmed instructions, however, must be continuously adjusted by the radiologic technologist until the entire panel of examinations is optimized for best image quality.

SUMMARY

Radiographic technique is the combination of factors used to expose an anatomic part to produce a quality radiograph. Radiographic technique is characterized by patient factors, image quality factors, and exposure technique factors.

Patient factors are anatomic thickness, body composition, and any pathology that is present. Body thickness is measured by calipers. Radiographers recognize body habitus of sthenic, asthenic, hyposthenic, and hypers-

thenic as a way to determine body composition and thus proper radiographic technique. Pathologic conditions may be either radiolucent, which requires a reduction in technique, or radiopaque, which requires an increase.

Image quality factors define the quality of the image and are OD, contrast, image detail, and distortion. OD is the blackening of the radiograph and is defined as the log of the incident light divided by the transmitted light. Contrast is the difference in OD between adjacent anatomic structures. A high kVp produces low-contrast images, whereas a low kVp produces high-contrast images. Image detail is the sharpness of the image on the radiograph; to produce the sharpest image detail, use the smallest focal spot, the longest SID, and the least OID. *Distortion* refers to the misrepresentation of object size on the radiograph.

The principal radiographic-technique factors are kVp, mAs, and SID. The two most common technique charts for use by radiographers to produce consistently high-quality radiographs are the fixed-kVp chart and the high-kVp chart. The high-kVp chart is used for barium studies and chest radiographs with kVp from 120 to 135. The fixed-kVp chart uses approximately 60 kVp for extremity radiography and approximately 80 kVp for examinations of the trunk.

Even with AECs, radiographic exposure charts are required. APR uses microprocessor technology to program the technique chart into the control unit. The radiographer selects an anatomic display of the part under examination, and the microprocessor selects the appropriate kVp and mAs automatically.

CHALLENGE QUESTIONS

1. Define or otherwise identify:
   a. Fifteen-percent rule
   b. Body habitus
   c. Radiographic technique
   d. Gray scale of contrast
   e. Radiographic-technique chart
   f. Radiolucency/radiopacity
   g. Five-percent rule
   h. Anatomically programmed radiography
   i. Visibility of image detail
   j. The four principal radiographic image quality factors

2. List and discuss the exposure-technique factors. How does each affect OD?

3. Explain how kVp influences the scale of contrast?

4. A radiographic technique calls for 82 kVp at 400 mA, 200 ms, and an SID of 90 cm. What is the mAs?

5. A radiographic technique of 150 mA and 200 ms is used, but there is motion blur. If the exposure time is reduced to 25 ms, what should be the mA?

6. An acceptable chest radiograph was taken at 180-cm SID with 10 mAs. If the 400-mA station is used, what will be the new exposure time at 90-cm SID?

7. Identify the range of ODs that are too light, too dark, and just right.

8. When a change in OD is required, what exposure-technique factor should be changed and why?

9. When a change in radiographic contrast is required, what exposure-technique factor should be changed and why?

10. List and discuss the nature of the four types of radiographic exposure charts.

11. What are the three groups of variables or factors that determine the quality of the finished radiograph?

12. How does body habitus affect the selection of technical factors?

13. Describe the two classifications of pathology and ways that technical factors may be affected by each classification.

14. Name the tool used to measure the thickness of an anatomic part when a radiographer is determining technical factor selection.

15. How does the radiographer determine the type of pathologic condition a patient may have before a radiographic examination?

16. Write the formula for OD.

17. Identify the numerical equivalent range of ODs from black to clear.

18. What is the relationship between OD and mAs?

19. Define *contrast*. Give an example of tissues with high contrast and an examples of tissues with low contrast.

20. List the three ways to produce the sharpest image detail.

PART IV

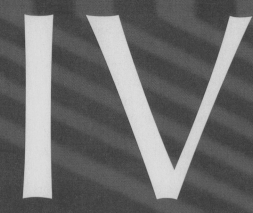

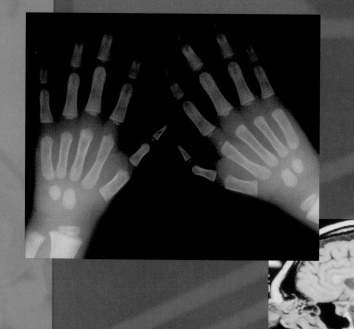

SPECIAL X-RAY IMAGING

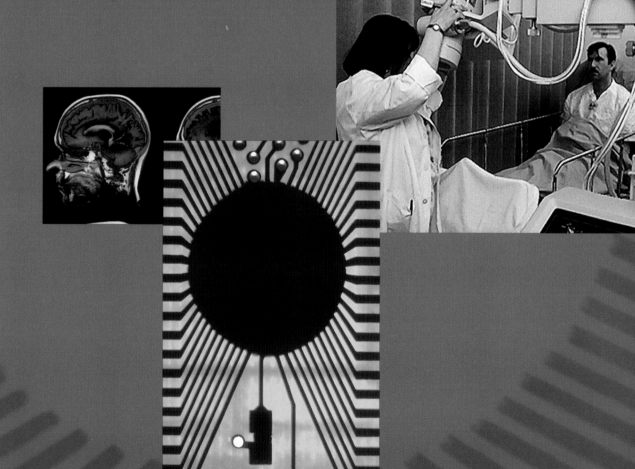

Special Radiographic Procedures

OBJECTIVES

At the completion of this chapter, the student should be able to:

1. List the directional movements of a conventional tomographic imaging system
2. Explain the theory for tomographic motion blur
3. Discuss the relationship between tomographic angle and section thickness
4. Describe magnification radiography and its use

OUTLINE

Many areas of x-ray diagnosis require special equipment and specialized techniques to obtain the required information. Such procedures are designed to visualize more clearly a given anatomic structure, usually at the expense of nonvisualization of other structures. The equipment and procedures discussed in this chapter include tomography, stereoradiography, and magnification radiography. These x-ray examinations are not routine and therefore require the radiologic technologist to be specially trained.

TOMOGRAPHY

A conventional radiograph of the chest or abdomen images all structures contained in these parts of the body with approximately equal fidelity. The structures, however, are superimposed on one another, and often this superimposition results in a masking of the structure of interest. When this occurs, a procedure called **tomography** may be necessary.

The tomographic examination is designed to bring into focus only that anatomic structure lying in a plane of interest while blurring structures on either side of that plane. Actually, the object is not focused in the normal sense, but rather its radiographic contrast is enhanced by the blurring of the anatomic structures above and below.

A tomographic x-ray imager appears similar to a conventional radiographic imager in most features (Figure 22-1). Note the vertical rod that fixes the x-ray tube above the table; that is the feature unique to tomography. The rod links the tube to the radiographic image receptor to enable both to move at the same time.

 The principal advantage of tomography is improved contrast resolution.

Since the introduction of computed tomography (CT) and magnetic resonance imaging (MRI) with their excellent contrast resolution, tomography is used with less frequency. Tomography is now applied principally to high-contrast procedures, such as imaging calcified kidney stones. Table 22-1 lists the more common tomographic examinations and their representative techniques.

During the tomographic examination, the radiographic tube moves in a precise fashion while the image receptor moves synchronously. There are five types of tomographic movement: linear, circular, elliptical, hypocycloidal, and trispiral. Only the linear motion is now used with any regularity because of the dedicated equipment requirements of the others and the common availability of CT and MRI.

Linear Tomography

The simplest tomographic examination is linear tomography. During **linear tomography** (Figure 22-2), the x-ray tube is mechanically attached to the image receptor and moves in one direction while the image receptor moves in the opposite direction.

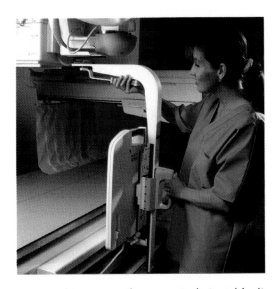

FIGURE 22-1 This tomography system is designed for linear movement with a general-purpose R&F imaging system. *(Courtesy General Electric Medical Systems.)*

TABLE 22-1	Representative Linear Tomographic Techniques			
Examination	**Projection**	**kVp**	**mAs***	**Section Thickness**
Cervical spine	Anterior-posterior	75	60	3-5 mm
	Lateral	77	60	2 mm
Thoracic spine	Anterior-posterior	77	80	5 mm
Lumbar spine	Anterior-posterior	77	140	5 mm
Chest	Anterior-posterior	96	80	2-5 cm
Intravenous pyelogram	Anterior-posterior	70	140	1 cm
Wrist	Anterior-posterior	48	20	2 mm
*Usually automatic-exposure control.				

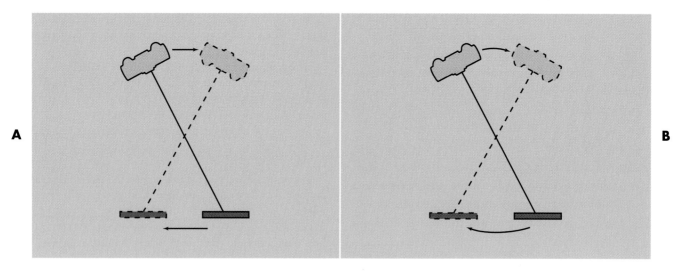

FIGURE 22-2 **A,** Cassette tray and tube head of a general-purpose x-ray table altered for tomography to move in a plane. **B,** Those of a table designed specifically for tomography to move in an arc.

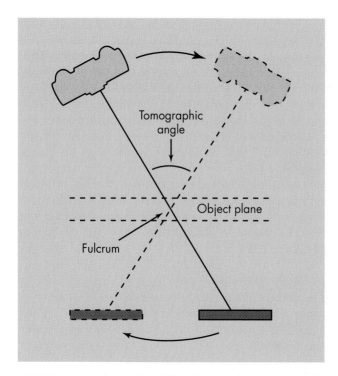

FIGURE 22-3 Relationship of the fulcrum, object plane, and tomographic angle.

The ability to perform tomography can be obtained inexpensively by altering a conventional radiographic imaging system to accommodate x-ray tube and image receptor motion. With this type of linear tomography, the x-ray tube and the image receptor remain in the same plane during motion (Figure 22-2, *A*). Some equipment specially designed for linear tomography is constructed so that the x-ray tube and the image receptor move in simi-

lar arcs during the examination (Figure 22-2, *B*). This method of linear tomography results in higher-quality tomographs, but it is more expensive and has limited use.

Other aspects of the linear tomographic examination are shown in Figure 22-3. The **fulcrum** is the imaginary pivot point about which the x-ray tube and the image receptor move. The fulcrum lies in the **object plane,** and only the anatomic structures in this plane are clearly imaged. The plane of the section is determined by adjusting the height of the x-ray tube from the table or by repositioning the table height between exposures.

The angle of movement is known as the **tomographic angle.** The tomographic angle determines the **section thickness,** or the thickness of tissue that will not be blurred. The determination of the section thickness is made by selecting the proper tomographic angle.

Figure 22-4 illustrates how anatomic structures in the object plane are imaged but structures above and below this plane are not. The examination begins with the x-ray tube and the image receptor positioned on opposite sides of the fulcrum. The exposure begins as the x-ray tube and image receptor move simultaneously in opposite directions. The image of an anatomic structure lying in the object plane, such as the arrow, will have a fixed position on the radiograph throughout the tube travel.

On the other hand, the images of structures lying above or below the object plane, such as the ball and box, will have varying positions on the image receptor during the tomographic movement (Figure 22-4). Consequently the ball and box will be blurred. The larger the tomographic angle, the more blurred the images of structures above and below the object plane appear. The farther from the object plane an anatomic structure, the more blurred its image.

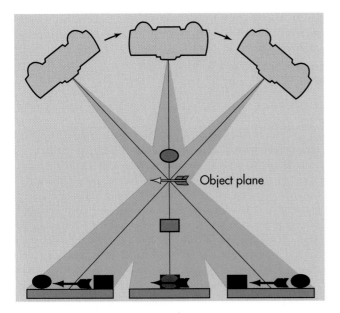

FIGURE 22-4 Only objects lying in the object plane are properly imaged. Objects on either side of this plane are blurred because they are imaged across the film.

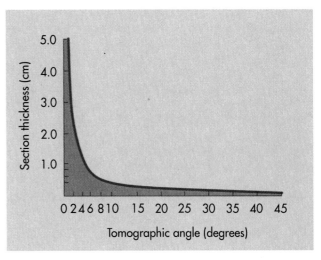

FIGURE 22-6 Section thickness becomes thinner as the tomographic angle is increased.

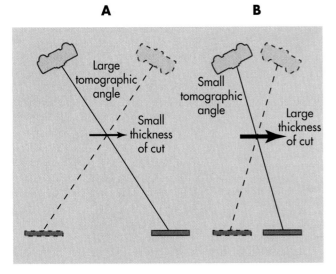

FIGURE 22-5 Section thickness is determined by the tomographic angle. **A,** A large tomographic angle results in a small section thickness. **B,** A small tomographic angle results in a large section thickness.

TABLE 22-2	Section Thickness During Linear Tomography as a Function of Tomographic Angle	
Tomographic Angle (Degrees)		Section Thickness* (mm)
Zero		Infinity
2		31
4		16
6		11
10		6
20		3
35		2
*Approximate values.		

> The larger the tomographic angle, the thinner the section.

The blurring of anatomic structures lying outside the object plane is simply an example of motion blur caused by the moving x-ray source. In theory, only objects lying precisely in the object plane, which is the plane of the fulcrum, are properly imaged. Objects lying outside this plane exhibit increasing motion blur with increasing distance from the object plane. Objects within a section of tissue between two parallel planes are in focus. This thickness of tissue imaged is called the **tomographic layer,** and its width is described numerically by the section thickness (Figure 22-5).

The section thickness is controlled by the tomographic angle. Table 22-2 shows the approximate relationship between tomographic angle and section thickness. This relationship is shown graphically in Figure 22-6. When the tomographic angle is very small (for example, zero degrees), the section thickness is the entire anatomic structure, resulting in a conventional radiograph. When the tomographic angle is 10 degrees, the section thickness is approximately 6 mm; structures lying farther than approximately 3 mm from the object plane appear blurred.

A linear anatomic structure can be imaged with less blur if the length of the structure is positioned parallel to the x-ray tube motion. The tomographic phantom in Figure 22-7 illustrates this point. Conversely, Figure 22-8 shows how linear structures that lie perpendicular to the x-ray tube motion are more easily blurred. These foot tomographs were taken parallel to the long axis of the patient (Figure 22-8, *A*) and perpendicular to the long axis of the patient (Figure 22-8, *B*).

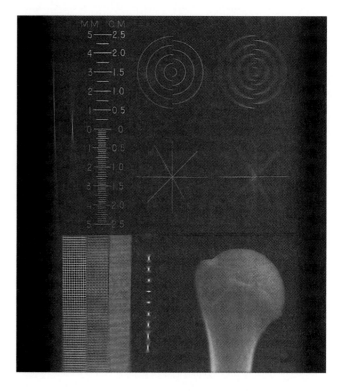

FIGURE 22-7 This phantom image shows properly calibrated elevation and increased blur of objects perpendicular to the motion of the x-ray tube. *(Courtesy Sharon Glaze.)*

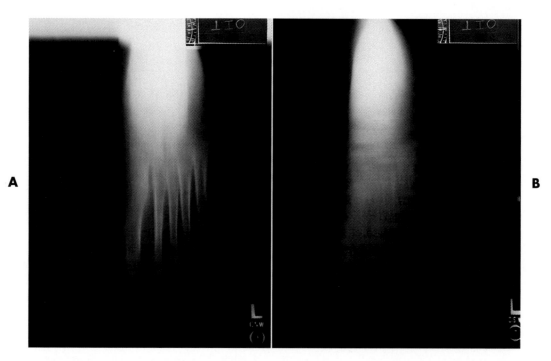

FIGURE 22-8 Foot tomographs obtained with the x-ray tube motion. **A,** Parallel with the body axis. **B,** Perpendicular to the body axis. *(Courtesy Rees Stuteville.)*

Zonography

If the tomographic angle is less than about 10 degrees, the section thickness will be quite large (Table 22-2). This type of tomography is called **zonography** because a relatively large zone of tissue is imaged. Zonography is used when the subject contrast is so low that thin-section tomography would result in a poor image. Zonography is applied most often in chest and renal examination in which tomographic angles of 1 to 5 degrees are usually used.

Panoramic Tomography

Panoramic tomography was first developed for a fast dental survey but is increasingly used to image the curved bony structures of the head, such as the mandible. For this procedure the x-ray tube and image receptor move around the head as shown in Figure 22-9. The x-ray beam is collimated to a slit as shown. The image receptor is likewise slit collimated. During the examination, the image receptor translates behind the slit collimator so that it is exposed for several seconds along its length. Figure 22-10 shows a clinical example of panoramic tomography.

Practical Considerations

The principal advantage of tomography is improved radiographic contrast. By blurring overlying and underlying tissues, the subject contrast of the tissues of the tomographic layer is enhanced. The more irregular the movement of the x-ray tube and image receptor, the

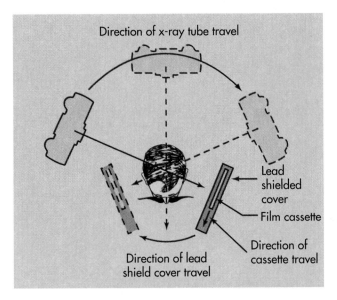

FIGURE 22-9   X-ray source image receptor motion for panoramic tomography.

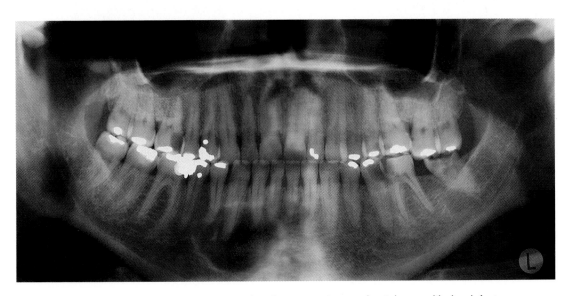

FIGURE 22-10   Panoramic tomogram showing restorations and a right mandibular defect. *(Courtesy Kenneth Abramovitch.)*

greater the contrast enhancement. Multidirectional movement of the x-ray tube and image receptor does not affect the section thickness of the tomographic layer. Only the tomographic angle does.

The principal disadvantage of tomography is increased patient dose. The x-ray tube is on during the entire period of tube travel, which can be several seconds.

A single tomographic exposure of the kidneys, for example, can result in a patient dose of 1000 mrad (10 mGy_t). Furthermore, most tomographic examinations require several exposures to make certain that the section plane of interest is imaged. A 16-film tomographic examination can result in a patient dose of several rad (Gy_t).

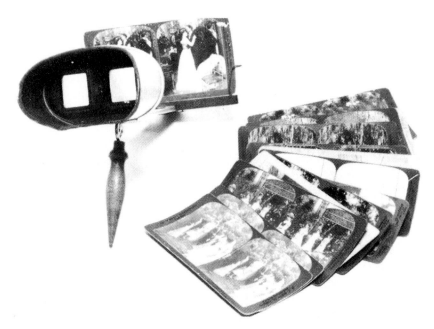

FIGURE 22-11 Early twentieth-century stereoscope. *(Courtesy Sharon Glaze.)*

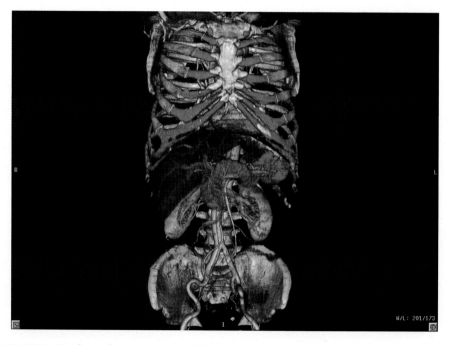

FIGURE 22-12 Three-dimensional spiral CT images such as this one have rendered stereoradiography obsolete. *(Courtesy Vital Images, Inc.)*

During tomography, linear grids must be used, and the grid lines must be oriented in the same direction as the x-ray tube movement.

Grids are used during a tomographic examination for the same reason that they are used during radiography. For linear tomography, this usually means that the grid is positioned with its grid lines parallel with the length of the table.

STEREORADIOGRAPHY

Stereoradiography is the practice of making two radiographs of the same object and viewing them through a device called a *stereoscope,* which allows each eye to view a different radiograph (Figure 22-11). The effect of viewing these radiographs stereoscopically is that they appear as a three-dimensional image. At one time, stereoradiography was prominent, but the ability now to reconstruct three-dimensional CT and MR images with special computer-assisted techniques (Figure 22-12) has made stereoradiography obsolete. On the other hand,

x-ray holography and CT and MR stereograms may become routine for future three-dimensional imaging. The first stereogram was created in 1979 by Christopher Taylor, and they are now a common sight in novelty shops (Figure 22-13). To see this three-dimensional image, hold up your book, cross your eyes and focus on an object across the room. While so focused, slowly bring your eyes down to this image. A ram should appear! Approximately 2% of the population—including this author—is stereoblind and never see the ram.

MAGNIFICATION RADIOGRAPHY

Because magnification radiography enhances the visualization of small vessels, it is used principally by vascular radiologists and neuroradiologists. Conventional radiography strives to minimize the object-to-image receptor distance (OID), but magnification radiography deliberately increases it.

Magnification radiography uses the principles of magnification from Chapter 20. Obtaining a magnified radiograph requires that the OID be increased while the source-to-image receptor distance (SID) is held constant

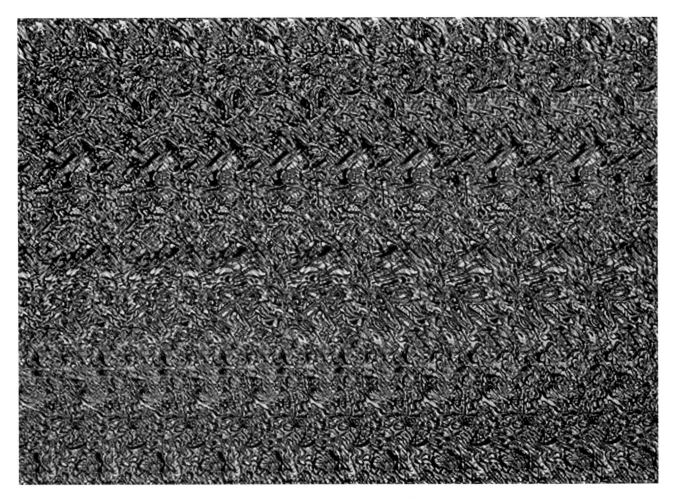

FIGURE 22-13 See text for directions on how to see the ram in this stereogram.

Mammography

OBJECTIVES

At the completion of this chapter, the student should be able to:

1. Discuss the differences between soft tissue radiography and conventional radiography
2. Describe the anatomy of the breast
3. Identify the recommended intervals for self-examination, physical examination, x-ray examination of the breast
4. Describe the unique features of a mammographic imaging system
5. Discuss the requirement for compression in mammography
6. Describe the image receptors used in mammography and the spatial resolution obtained
7. Describe the differences between diagnostic and screening mammography

OUTLINE

Breast cancer is the second leading cause of death from cancer in women. Each year about 175,000 new cases are reported in the United States, with one quarter of these cases resulting in death. These statistics indicate that one of every eight women will develop breast cancer during her life. It is widely believed that early detection of breast cancer can lead to more effective treatment and fewer deaths. X-ray mammography has proved to be an accurate and simple method for breast cancer detection but is not simple to perform. It requires of the radiographer and support staff exceptional knowledge, skill, and caring. The federal government has mandated regulations in the Mammography Quality Standards Act (MQSA), which set standards for image quality, radiation dose, personnel, and examination procedures.

This chapter discusses the imaging technique, equipment, and procedures used in mammography.

MAMMOGRAPHY
Soft Tissue Radiography

Radiographic examination of soft tissues, called **soft tissue radiography,** requires selected techniques that differ from conventional radiography. This is due to the substantial differences in the anatomy being imaged. In conventional radiography, the subject contrast is great because of the large differences in mass density and atomic number among bone, muscle, fat, and lung tissue. In soft tissue radiography, only muscle and fat structures are imaged, and these tissues have similar effective atomic numbers and similar mass densities (see Tables 13-1 and 13-2). Consequently, in soft tissue radiography, the techniques used are designed to enhance differential absorption in these very similar tissues.

History and Development of Mammography

A prime example of soft tissue radiography is **mammography:** radiographic examination of the breast. As a distinct type of radiographic examination, mammography was first attempted in the 1920s. The lack of adequate equipment, however, prevented its development at that time. In the late 1950s, Robert Egan renewed interest in mammography with his demonstration of a successful technique using low kVp, high mAs, and direct film exposure.

In the 1960s, Wolf and Ruzicka showed that xeromammography was superior to direct film exposure because it produced better diagnostic quality images using lower patient dose. Detail and contrast were much improved because of the spatial characteristic **edge en-**

hancement, the accentuation of the interface between different tissues. This characteristic is frequently enhanced in the postprocessing of digital images. Xeromammography was replaced by 1990 with screen-film mammography, which provided even better images using an even lower patient dose.

Mammography has undergone many changes. It now enjoys widespread application, first through the efforts of the American College of Radiology (ACR) volunteer accreditation program and then through the federally mandated the MQSA enacted in 1991.

Breast Cancer

The principal motivation for continuing the development and improvement of mammography is the high incidence of breast cancer. Breast cancer is the leading cancer in women. Each year approximately 175,000 new cases are reported in the United States, and this number is growing. One quarter of these new cases results in death. Several factors, including age, family history, and genetics, have been identified as increasing a woman's risk of developing breast cancer (Box 23-1).

 One of every eight women will develop breast cancer during her life.

Fortunately, early detection and treatment have increased the survival rate of those with breast cancer. In 1995, the National Cancer Institute reported the first reduction in the mortality rate for breast cancer in 50 years, and this trend continues. With early mammographic diagnosis, more than 90% of patients are cured.

The risk of radiation-induced breast cancer resulting from x-ray mammography has been given a lot of attention. Mammography is considered very safe and effective. Benefit (lives saved) to risk (deaths caused) ratios of 700:1 to 1000:1 have been estimated. There is considerable evidence that the mature breast in the age group screened has very low sensitivity to radiation-induced breast cancer. The dose necessary to produce breast cancer is unknown; however, the dose used in mammography is well known and is covered in Chapter 40. Radiation carcinogenesis (the induction of cancer) is discussed in Chapter 37.

BOX 23-1   Risk Factors for Breast Cancer

Age (The older you are, the higher the risk)
Family history: mother or sister with breast cancer
Genetics: presence of *BRCA1* or *BRCA2* genes
Menstruation onset before age 12
Menopause onset after age 55
Prolonged use of estrogen
Late age at birth of first child or not having children
Education (risk increases with higher education)
Socioeconomics (risk increases with higher status)

TABLE 23-2	Features of a Dedicated Mammography System for Use with Screen-Film
High-voltage generator	High frequency, 5 to 10 kHz
Target/filter	Tungsten/60 μm molybdenum
	Molybdenum/30 μm molybdenum
	Molybdenum/50 μm rhodium
	Rhodium/50 μm rhodium
kVp	20 to 35 kVp in 1-kVp increments
Compression	Low anatomic number, autoadjust and release
Grids	Ratio of 3:1 to 5:1, 30 lines/cm
Exposure control	Automatic to account for tissue thickness, composition, and reciprocity law failure
Focal spot: large/small	0.3 mm/0.1 mm
Magnification	Up to 2 times
Source-to-image receptor distance	50 to 80 cm

changes the power to high frequency, typically 5 to 10 kHz, that is then capacitive smoothed. The resulting voltage ripple seen by the x-ray tube is approximately 1%, essentially constant potential. Compared with earlier single- and three-phase mammography generators, high-frequency generators are smaller and less expensive to manufacture. They provide exceptional exposure reproducibility, which contributes to improved image quality.

Target Composition

Mammographic x-ray tubes are manufactured with a tungsten (W), a molybdenum (Mo), or a rhodium (Rh) target. Figure 23-4 shows the x-ray emission spectrum from a tungsten-target tube filtered with 0.5 mm of Al operating at 30 kVp. Note that the bremsstrahlung spectrum predominates and that only the 12-keV characteristic x-rays from L-shell transitions are present. These x-rays are all absorbed and contribute only to patient dose, not to the image. Tungsten L-shell x-rays are of no value in mammography because their 12-keV energy is too low to penetrate the breast. The x-rays most useful for enhancing differential absorption in breast tissue and for maximizing radiographic contrast are those in the 17- to 24-keV range. The tungsten target supplies sufficient x-rays in this energy range but also an abundance of x-rays above and below this range.

Figure 23-5 shows the emission spectrum from a molybdenum-target tube filtered with 30 μm of molybdenum with its near absence of bremsstrahlung x-rays. The most prominent x-rays are characteristic, having en-

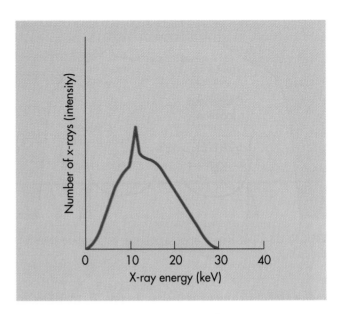

FIGURE 23-4 X-ray emission spectrum for a tungsten-target x-ray tube with 0.5 mm Al filter operated at 30 kVp.

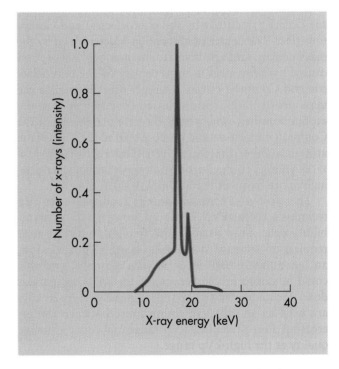

FIGURE 23-5 X-ray emission spectrum for a molybdenum-target x-ray tube with a 30-μm Mo filter operated at 26 kVp.

ergy of approximately 19 keV from K-shell interactions. Molybdenum has an atomic number of 42, compared with 74 for tungsten, and this difference is responsible for the differences in emission spectra.

The x-ray emission spectrum from a rhodium target filtered with rhodium appears similar to that from a molybdenum target (Figure 23-6). However, rhodium

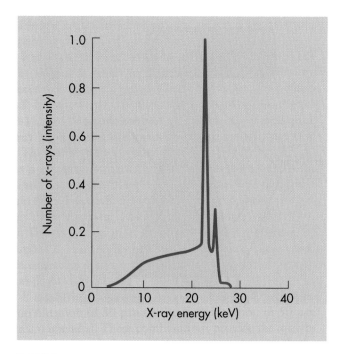

FIGURE 23-6 X-ray emission spectrum for a rhodium-target x-ray tube with a 50-μm Rh filter operated at 28 kVp.

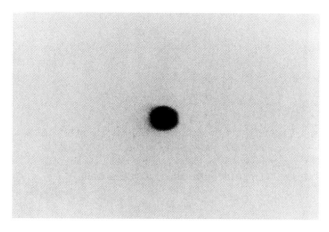

FIGURE 23-7 Pinhole camera images of a circular focal spot. *(Courtesy Donald Jacobson.)*

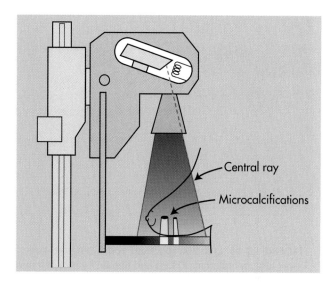

FIGURE 23-8 When the x-ray tube is tilted in its housing, the effective focal spot is small, the x-ray intensity is more uniform, and tissue against the chest wall is imaged.

has a slightly higher atomic number (Z = 45) and therefore a slightly higher K-edge (23 keV) and more bremsstrahlung x-rays. Bremsstrahlung x-rays are produced more easily in target atoms with high atomic number than with low anatomic number. Molybdenum and rhodium K-characteristic x-rays have energy corresponding to their respective K-shell electron binding energy. This is within the range of energies that are most effective for mammographic imaging. All currently manufactured mammography imagers have target/filter combinations of molybdenum/molybdenum. Many are also equipped with molybdenum/rhodium and rhodium/rhodium combinations.

Focal Spot

Focal-spot size is an important characteristic of mammographic x-ray tubes because of the higher demands for spatial resolution. The imaging of microcalcifications requires small focal spots. Mammographic x-ray tubes usually have stated focal-spot sizes: large/small of 0.3/0.1 mm.

In general, the smaller the focal spot, the better; however, the shape of the focal spot is also important (Figure 23-7). A circular focal spot is preferred, but rectangular shapes are common. Manufacturers shape the focal spot through clever cathode design and focusing-cup voltage bias. A considerable variance is allowed for the stated nominal focal-spot size, and therefore medical physics acceptance testing of focal-spot size is essential.

To obtain such small focal-spot size and adequate

x-ray intensity over the entire breast, manufacturers take advantage of the line focus principle, heel effect, and the x-ray tube (Figure 23-8). The effective focal spots, 0.3/0.1 mm, are obtained with an anode angle of approximately 23-degree and a tube tilt of 6-degree. Normally, the cathode is positioned to the chest wall. This allows for easier patient positioning as well as smaller effective focal spots. Tilting the x-ray tube to achieve smaller effective focal spots also ensures that tissue next to the chest wall is imaged. When the tube is tilted, the central ray parallels the chest wall, and no tissue is missed. A relatively long SID can also reduce focal-spot blur (Figure 23-9).

Filtration

At the low kVp used for mammography, it is important that the x-ray tube window not attenuate the x-ray beam relatively long source-to-image receptor distance (SID), 60 to 80 cm, with the cathode to the chest wall and the x-ray tube tilted. This is considered the best arrangement because the focal spot is made effectively smaller and tissue at the chest wall is imaged.

One consequence of the heel effect is the variation in focal-spot size over the image receptor. However, the use of a long SID and vigorous compression makes this change in effective focal-spot size clinically insignificant.

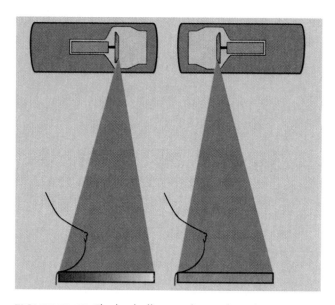

FIGURE 23-12 The heel effect can be used to advantage in mammography by positioning the cathode toward the chest wall to produce a more uniform optical density.

Compression

Compression, the act of flattening soft tissue to improve optical density (OD), is important in many aspects of conventional radiology but it is of particular importance in mammography. Several advantages result from the use of vigorous compression (Figure 23-13). A compressed breast is of more uniform thickness, and therefore the OD of the image will be more uniform. Tissues near the chest wall are less likely to be underexposed, and tissues near the nipple are less likely to be overexposed.

 Vigorous compression must be used in x-ray mammography.

When vigorous compression is used, all tissue is brought closer to the image receptor, and focal-spot blur is reduced. Absorption blur and scatter radiation are also reduced by compression. All dedicated mammographic x-ray imaging systems have a built-in stiff compression device that is parallel with the surface of the image receptor. Vigorous compression of the breast is necessary for the best image quality (Table 23-3). Compression immobilizes the breast, holds it still, and therefore reduces motion blur. It also spreads out the tissue and thus reduces superimposition of tissue structures. Compression results in thinner tissue and therefore less scatter radiation and improved contrast resolution. The overall result of compression on the image is improved ability to detect small, low-contrast lesions and high-contrast microcalcifications. In addition, vigorous compression results in a lower patient dose.

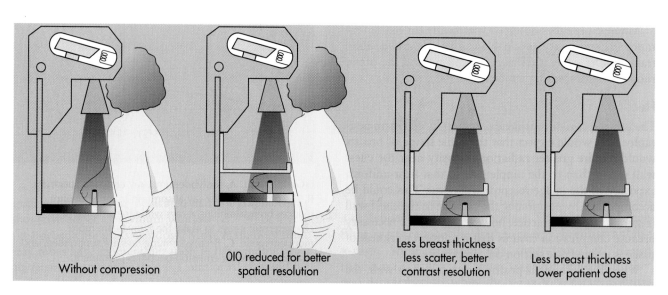

Without compression | OIO reduced for better spatial resolution | Less breast thickness less scatter, better contrast resolution | Less breast thickness lower patient dose

FIGURE 23-13 The use of compression in mammography has three principal advantages: improved spatial resolution, improved contrast resolution, and lower patient dose.

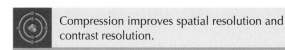

Compression improves spatial resolution and contrast resolution.

Although the optimal degree of compression is unknown, compression of the breast is essential for a quality mammogram. It appears that the more vigorous the compression, the better the image and the lower the patient dose. Unfortunately, vigorous compression does increase patient discomfort. A skillful mammographer compresses the breast until it is taut or just less than painful, whichever occurs first.

Grids

The use of grids during mammography is routine. Although mammographic image contrast is high because of the low kVp used, it is not high enough. Many imaging systems now use moving grids with a ratio of 4:1 to 5:1 focused to the SID to increase image contrast. Grid frequencies of 30 to 50 lines/cm are typical. The use of such grids does not compromise spatial resolution, but it does increase patient dose. The use of a 4:1 ratio grid approximately doubles the patient dose when compared with nongrid contact mammography. However, the dose is acceptably low, and the improvement in contrast is significant.

A unique grid developed specifically for mammography is the high transmission cellular (HTC) grid (Figure 23-14). This grid has the clean-up characteristics of a crossed grid by reducing scatter radiation in two directions, rather than the one direction of a linear or focused grid. The HTC grid has copper as grid strip material and air for the interspace, and its physical dimensions result in a 3.8:1 grid ratio.

Automatic Exposure Control

Phototimers for mammography are designed to measure not only x-ray intensity at the image receptor but also x-ray quality. These phototimers are referred to as *automatic-exposure control (AEC) devices,* and they are positioned after the image receptor to minimize OID

(Figure 23-15). Two types are used: an ionization chamber and a solid-state diode. Each type has at least two detectors or a single detector, which can be positioned from the chest wall, to the nipple. Some AECs incorporate many detectors to cover the entire breast.

The detectors are filtered differently so that the AEC can estimate the beam quality after passing through the breast. This allows an assessment of breast composition

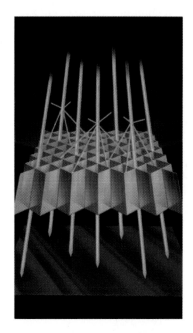

FIGURE 23-14 An HTC grid designed specifically for mammography. *(Courtesy Hologic Imaging.)*

TABLE 23-3	Advantages of Vigorous Compression
Effect	**Result**
Immobilized breast	Reduced motion blur
Uniform thickness	Uniform OD on mammogram
Reduced scatter radiation	Improved contrast resolution
Shorter object-to-image receptor distance	Improved spatial resolution
Thinner tissue	Reduced radiation dose

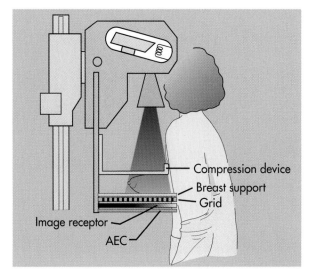

FIGURE 23-15 Relative position of an AEC device.

and selection of the correct target/filter combination. Thick, dense breasts are imaged better with rhodenium/rhodenium, and thin, fatty breasts are imaged better with molybdenum/molybdenum.

Accurate performance of the AEC is necessary to ensure reproducible images at a low radiation dose. The AEC should be able to hold OD within ±0.1 as voltage is varied from 23 to 32 kVp and as breast thickness varies from 2 to 8 cm regardless of breast composition.

Magnification Mammography

Magnification techniques are frequently used in mammography, producing images up to twice normal size. Special equipment, such as microfocus tubes and adequate compression and patient-positioning devices, is required for magnification mammography. Effective focal-spot size should not exceed 0.1 mm.

 Magnification mammography should not be routinely used.

Normal mammograms are adequate for most patients, so magnification mammography is usually unnecessary. The purpose of magnification mammography is to investigate small suspicious lesions or microcalcifications seen on normal mammograms. The breast may not be completely imaged, and patient dose will be approximately doubled.

SCREEN-FILM MAMMOGRAPHY

Four types of image receptors have been used for mammography: direct-exposure film, xeroradiography, screen-film, and digital detectors. Only screen-film and digital detectors are used today. Xeromammography and direct-exposure mammography are no longer used.

Radiographic intensifying screens and films have been especially designed for x-ray mammography. The films are single emulsion and matched with a single back screen. Because of this arrangement, there is no light crossover. The tabular grain emulsion has been replaced by a cubic grain emulsion in many films (Figure 23-16). The result is somewhat higher contrast, especially in the toe region, which is particularly useful in mammography. Regardless of the type of film, it must be matched for the light emission of the associated intensifying screen. Special emulsions coupled with rare earth screen material are available.

The screen-film combination is placed in a specially designed cassette that has a front cover with a low atomic number for low attenuation. The latching/spring mechanism is designed to produce especially good screen-film contact.

The use of the radiographic intensifying intensifying screen significantly increases the speed of the imaging system, resulting in a low patient dose. The use of screens also enhances the radiographic contrast compared with that from direct-exposure examination.

 The emulsion surface of the film must always be next to the screen, and the film must be closer to the x-ray tube than the radiographic intensifying screen.

The position of the radiographic intensifying screen and film in the cassette is important (Figure 23-17). X-rays interact primarily with the entrance surface of the screen. If the screen is between the x-ray tube and the

FIGURE 23-16 The size of cubic grains in mammographic film emulsions ranges from 0.5 to 0.9 μm to produce a higher contrast. *(Courtesy Fujifilm Medical Systems.)*

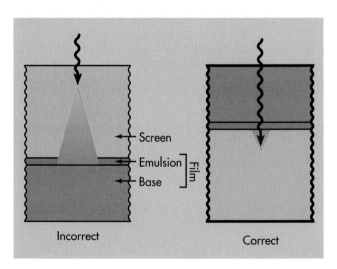

FIGURE 23-17 Correct way to load mammography film and position the cassette. Spatial resolution improves when the x-ray film is placed between the x-ray tube and the radiographic intensifying screen.

film, excess screen blur will result. If, on the other hand, the film is between the x-ray tube and the screen, with the emulsion side to the screen, spatial resolution is better.

Processing and viewing the mammogram are critical stages of mammography. These will be dealt with in Chapter 24, but when properly conducted, image receptor speeds of approximately 200 are obtained. This results in an average glandular dose of approximately 100 mrad (1.0 mGy_t). Image receptor contrast—average gradient—is approximately 3.5.

DIGITAL MAMMOGRAPHY

A recent development that promises improved digital radiographic imaging has special application for digital mammography. The image receptor is a **charged couple device (CCD),** a remarkable solid-state device that charge coupled visible light photons to electrons (Figure 23-18).

 A charged couple device (CCD) converts visible light photons to electrons.

As with screen-film mammography, the remnant x-ray beam interacts with an intensifying screen. However, the similarity ceases there (Figure 23-19). The light from the intensifying screen is captured either by a fiber optic bundle or a lens system and is directed to the CCD. The electron signal is read in pixel fashion to form an image.

Because the CCD is small and has limited coverage, several may be coupled, to image the entire breast. Spatial resolution of 8 to 10 lp/mm is achievable. Although this does not come close to the 20 lp/mm available with screen-film, even 5 lp/mm with digital imaging seems adequate because of the enhanced contrast resolution and postprocessing techniques.

The use of direct or indirect x-ray capture using amorphous selenium or silicon fabricated into thin-film transistors (TFTs) is also available for digital mammography. These devices are discussed more completely in Chapter 28.

Most digital image receptors that are based on phosphor interaction use thallium-activated cesium iodide. This phosphor can be grown as parallel needle–like light pipes for improved spatial resolution. Because these digital detectors are electronic, they have electronic noise. The noise can be reduced by cooling the detector to improve contrast resolution. Digital detectors have image

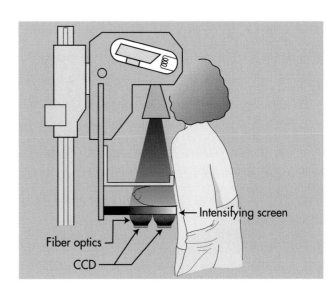

FIGURE 23-19 Multiple CCDs are necessary to image the entire breast.

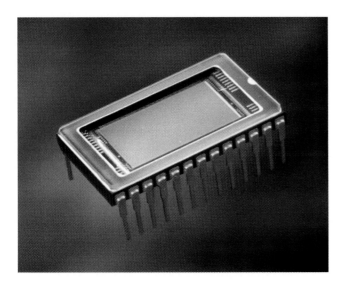

FIGURE 23-18 A CCD. *(Courtesy Swiss Ray.)*

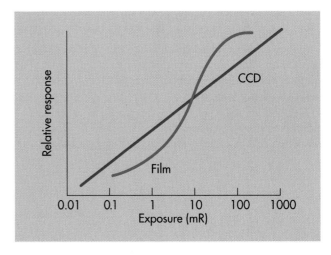

FIGURE 23-20 A CCD has a linear response, not the curvilinear response of screen-film.

characteristics similar to those of screen-film except that the response to x-rays is linear (Figure 23-20). Once the image has been converted into digital, or numerical, data, the computer can enhance contrast resolution. This postprocessing image enhancement is the principal advantage of digital imaging.

The spatial resolution of any of these digital mammography images is limited by the discrete pixel size of the CCD or TFT. Current pixel size ranges from approximately 40 to 100 μm, and this results in limiting spatial frequencies of 12.5 lp/mm and 5 lp/mm, respectively.

SUMMARY

Breast cancer is the leading cause of death in women between 40 and 50 years of age. Because of the rising incidence of breast cancer, improvements in mammography equipment and techniques have developed and the MQSA was instituted.

Anatomically, the breast consists of three different tissues: fibrous, glandular, and adipose. Premenopausal women have breasts composed mainly of fibrous and glandular tissue surrounded by a thin layer of fat. These breasts are dense and difficult to image. In postmenopausal women, the glandular tissue turns to fat. Because of its predominant fatty content, the older breast is easier to image.

It is important for you to know the recommended intervals of BSE, physician examination of the breasts, and mammographic examination for women of various age groups so that you can advise female patients. Diagnostic x-ray mammography is often performed every 6 months on women who have an elevated risk of breast cancer or who have a known lesion.

Compression is an important factor in producing high-quality mammograms.

Radiographic imaging systems are specially designed for mammographic examination. Mammographic x-ray tube targets are tungsten, molybdenum, or rhodium. A low kVp is used to maximize radiographic contrast of soft tissue. The x-ray beam should be filtered with 30 to 60 μ of molybdenum or rhodium to accentuate the characteristic x-ray emission.

Because of the demand for increased spatial resolution when imaging microcalcifications, small focal spots are used. Moving grids and the use of single-emulsion screen-film systems further increase radiographic contrast and image detail. AEC accommodates imaging of various sizes of breast tissue.

CHALLENGE QUESTIONS

1. Define or otherwise identify:
   a. Minimum filtration for mammography
   b. Mammographic grid ratio
   c. Microcalcifications
   d. CCD
   e. Breast cancer incidence
   f. Mammography SID
   g. Edge enhancement
2. Describe the anatomy of the breast, including the types of tissue and structural sizes.
3. Discuss changes in image quality and patient dose in mammography as the kVp is increased. Why is a low-kVp technique necessary?
4. Graphically compare the x-ray emission of a tungsten-target x-ray tube operated at 30 kVp with a molybdenum-target x-ray tube operated at 26 kVp.
5. What is the purpose for tilting the mammographic x-ray tube?
6. Discuss the influence of the heel effect on image quality in mammography.
7. Why should mammography be performed with a molybdenum- or rhodium-target tube?
8. How did Robert Egan help to advance the development of mammographic technique in the 1950s?
9. How is soft tissue radiography different from conventional radiography?
10. To what do the terms *ACR* and *MQSA* refer?
11. What is the difference between diagnostic and screening mammography?
12. List the recommended intervals for high-risk x-ray mammography.
13. List the advantages of mammographic compression.
14. Name the three materials used for mammographic x-ray tube targets.
15. What sizes of focal spots are used for mammography? Why?
16. What is the best target filter combination for imaging dense breast tissue?
17. What grid ratio and grid frequency are used for mammography imaging?
18. What feature of a dedicated mammographic imaging system is important for imaging microcalcifications?

Mammography Quality Control

OBJECTIVES

At the completion of this chapter, the student should be able to:

1. Define *quality control* and discuss its relationship to quality assurance
2. List the members of the quality-control team in radiology
3. Describe role of the radiologist and medical physicist in the quality control
4. Itemize the mammographer's quality-control duties on a weekly, monthly, and annual basis
5. List the processor quality-control steps

OUTLINE

ammography has been a screening and diagnostic tool for breast disease for many years, but there are challenges in producing high-quality mammographic images while keeping patient radiation dose low. A team that includes the radiologist, medical physicist, and mammographer works together using a quality-control program to produce excellence in mammographic imaging. Each member of the team has specific tasks that relate to quality control. This chapter identifies the team responsibilities in maintaining mammographic quality control.

QUALITY-CONTROL TEAM

The American College of Radiology (ACR) and subsequently the Mammography Quality Standards Act (MQSA) have endorsed a quality-control (QC) program of specific duties required of the **radiologist,** a physician specializing in radiology; the **medical physicist,** a physicist who examines and monitors the performance of imaging equipment; and the **mammographer,** a radiologic technologist specializing in breast x-ray imaging (Figure 24-1). A QC program is a program designed to ensure that the radiologist is provided with the best possible image resulting from good equipment performance. Each of these individuals

plays an important role in ensuring that the patient is receiving the best available care with the least radiation exposure. While the responsibilities of each of these three positions are addressed here, the duties of the mammographer are emphasized. The specific evaluation and monitoring tests for any QC program are described in detail in Chapter 31.

Radiologist

The ultimate responsibility for mammographic QC lies with the radiologist. These responsibilities often fall under the more broad area of **quality assurance (QA),** an administrative program designed to fuse the different aspects of QC as well as to ensure that all activities are being carried out at the highest level. It is the responsibility of the radiologist to select qualified medical physicists and mammographers and to oversee the activities of these team members on a regular basis.

 The radiologist's principal responsibility is supervision of the entire QA program.

Another responsibility of the radiologist is the supervision of patient communication and tracking. Quality patient care is the ultimate goal of any mammographic facility, and the final responsibility to see that this goal is met lies with the radiologist. The level of any QA/QC program directly reflects the radiologist's attitude and appreciation for the need of such a program. The MQSA mandates daily "clinical image evaluation" by the radiologist. **Continuous quality improvement (CQI)** is an extension of any QA/QC program, including administrative protocols for the continuous improvement of mammographic quality.

Medical Physicist

The role of the medical physicist as a member of the mammographic QC team is multidimensional. One such aspect is performing QC evaluation of the physical equipment used to produce an image of the breast. This evaluation should be performed annually or whenever a major component has been replaced. The evaluation consists of a number of measurements and tests that are summarized in Box 24-1.

The medical physicist should have an understanding of how the different technical aspects of the imaging chain effect the resulting image and therefore should be able to identify existing or potential problems in image quality. Occasionally, the medical physicist may pass information directly to the service engineer or serve as an intermediary between the facility and the service engineer. The aim of this portion of the QC program is to ensure that equipment functions properly and provides the highest-quality images with the lowest patient dose.

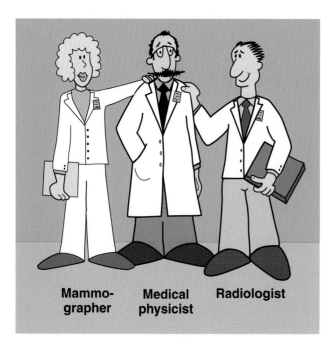

Mammo-grapher   Medical physicist   Radiologist

FIGURE 24-1 The three members of the mammography QC team.

The medical physicist's principal responsibility is an annual performance evaluation of the imaging equipment.

Another role of the medical physicist is serving as an advisor to the mammographer. The medical physicist should understand all of the tests expected of the mammographer well enough to predict likely problems or complications. Thus one responsibility is assisting with the mammographer's portion of the comprehensive QC program. An additional responsibility is evaluating the QC program at least annually. All procedures should be reviewed to ensure that they comply with current recommendations and standards. Charts and records should be thoroughly reviewed to check for compliance as well as to ensure that they are prepared properly and contain all necessary information.

The medical physicist is an integral part of the QC team whose full cooperation and attention should be expected. The very achievable goal of this relationship is a first-class QC program being maintained by a competent mammographer. The mammographer must know to call the medical physicist when a substantial change in images or the imaging system has occurred.

Mammographer

The mammographer plays an extremely important role in a mammographic QC program. The mammographer is the most hands-on member of the QC team, since he or she is responsible for the day-to-day execution of QC and for producing and monitoring all control charts and logs for any trends that might indicate a potential problem. In imaging facilities with several mammographers, one should be assigned the responsibility of **QC mammographer.** The 12 specific tasks required of the QC mammographer may be broken into categories reflecting the frequency with which they should be performed. Table 24-1 outlines these tasks and gives an estimate of the time it takes to perform them.

QC PROGRAM FOR MAMMOGRAPHERS

The 12 tasks required of the mammographer are well defined, and recommended performance standards exist for each. A full understanding of these tasks, as well as the reasons for the recommended performance standards, is absolutely necessary for the mammographer to maintain a thorough and accurate QC program.

Daily Tasks

Darkroom cleanliness. The first task each day is to wipe the darkroom clean. This is done to minimize artifacts on mammograms by maintaining the cleanest possible conditions in the darkroom (Figure 24-2). First, the floor should be mopped with a damp mop. Next, all unnecessary items should be removed from counter tops and work surfaces. A clean, damp towel should be used to wipe off the processor feed tray and all counter tops and work surfaces.

BOX 24-1 Annual QC Evaluation to be Performed by the Medical Physicist

Inspection of the mammographic unit assembly
Collimation assessment
Evaluation of spatial resolution
Accuracy and reproducibility of kVp
Beam quality assessment (half-value layer)
Performance assessment of automatic-exposure control
Reproducibility of automatic-exposure control
Uniformity of screen speed
Breast entrance exposure
Average glandular dose
Image quality evaluation
Artifact evaluation
Radiation output intensity
Measurement of viewing conditions

TABLE 24-1 Elements of a Mammographic QC Program

Task	Minimum Frequency	Approximate Time to Carry Out Procedures (min)
Darkroom cleanliness	Daily	5
Processor QC	Daily	20
Screen cleanliness	Weekly	10
Viewboxes and viewing conditions	Weekly	5
Phantom images	Weekly	30
Visual checklist	Monthly	10
Repeat analysis	Quarterly or 250 pts	60
Analysis of fixer retention in film	Quarterly	5
Conference with radiologist	Quarterly	45
Darkroom fog	Semiannually	10
Screen-film contact	Semiannually	80
Compression	Semiannually	10
TOTAL ANNUAL TIME		160 hrs

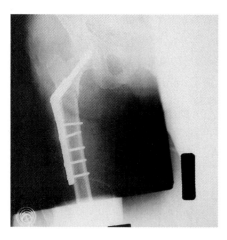

FIGURE 24-2 These white specks were produced by dust trapped between the film and screen. *(Courtesy Linda Shields.)*

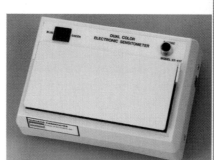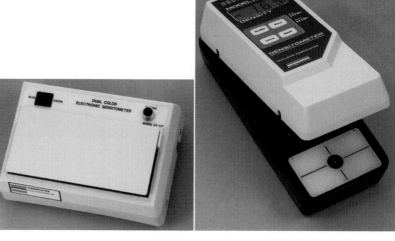

FIGURE 24-3 Sensitometer and densitometer for mammographic QC. *(Courtesy Nuclear Associates.)*

If a passbox is present, it should be cleaned daily as well. Hands should be kept clean to minimize fingerprints and handling artifacts. Overhead air vents and safelights should be wiped or vacuumed weekly before the other cleaning procedures are performed. Even the ceiling tiles should be cleaned to prevent flaking.

 Daily cleaning of the darkroom reduces image artifacts.

Smoking, eating, or drinking in the darkroom is prohibited. Food or drink should not be taken into the darkroom at any time. Nothing should be on the counter top except for items used for loading and unloading cassettes because it would only collect dust. There should be no shelves above the counter tops in the darkroom, since these too serve as a site for dust collection; the dust will eventually fall onto the work surfaces.

Processor QC. Before any films are processed, it should be verified that the processor chemical system is working according to preset specifications. The first step in a processor QC program is establishing operating control levels. First, a new dedicated box of film should be set aside to carry out the future daily processor QC. The processor tanks and racks should be cleaned and the processor supplied with the developer replenisher, fixer, and developer starter fluids specified by the manufacturer. The developer temperature, as well as the developer and fixer replenishment rates, should also be set to the levels specified by the manufacturer. A mercury thermometer should never be used. If the thermometer breaks, mercury contamination could render the processor permanently useless.

Once the processor has been allowed to warm up and the developer is at the correct temperature and stable, testing may continue. In the darkroom, a sheet of control film should be exposed with a sensitometer, such as that shown in Figure 24-3. The semsitometric strip should always be processed in exactly the same manner. The least exposed end is fed into the processor first. The same side of the feed tray is used, and the emulsion side should face down. The time between exposure and processing should be similar each day.

Next a densitometer is used to measure and record the optical densities (ODs) of each step on the sensitometric strip. This process should be repeated each day for 5 consecutive days. The average OD is then determined for each step from the five different strips.

Once the averages have been determined, the step that has an average OD closest to, but not less than, 1.2 should be found and marked as the **mid-density (MD)** step for future comparison. This is sometimes referred to as the **speed index.**

Next, the step with an average OD closest to 2.2 and the step with an average OD closest to, but not less than, 0.5 should be found and marked for future comparison. The difference between these two steps is recorded as the **density difference (DD)**, which is sometimes referred to as the **contrast index.**

Finally, the average OD from an unexposed area of the strips is recorded as the **base plus fog (B+F)**. The three values that have now been determined should be recorded on the center lines of the appropriate control chart. An example of a control chart is shown in Figure 24-4.

Once the control values have been established, the daily processor QC begins. At the beginning of each day,

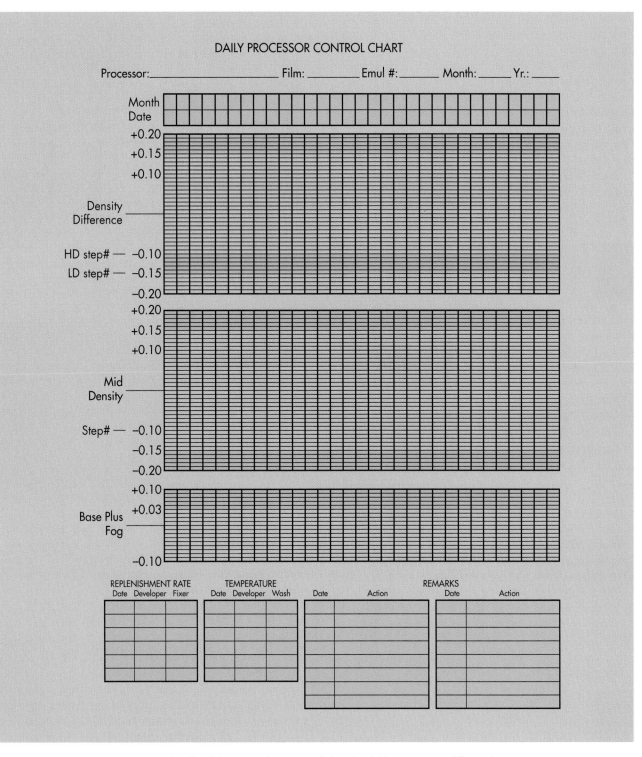

FIGURE 24-4 Example of the type of QC record that should be maintained for each processor.

before any films are processed, a sensitometric strip should be exposed and processed following the guidelines previously discussed. The MD, DD, and B+F are each determined from the appropriate predetermined steps and plotted on the control charts.

The MD is determined to evaluate the constancy of image receptor speed, and the DD is determined to evaluate the constancy of image contrast. These values are allowed to vary within 0.15 of the control values. If either value is out of this control limit, the point should be circled on the graph, the cause of the problem found and corrected, and the test repeated. No clinical images should be processed until the value is brought within 0.15 of the control value.

 If the value of the MD or the DD cannot be brought within the 0.15 variance of control, *no clinical images should be processed.*

If either value falls ±0.1 outside the range of the control value, the test should be repeated. If the value continues to remain outside this range, the processor may be used for clinical processing but should be monitored closely while attempting to identify the problem.

The B+F is determined to evaluate the level of fog present in the processing chain. This value is allowed to vary within +0.03 of control. Anytime the value exceeds this limit, steps should be taken as described for the MD and DD values.

Weekly Tasks

Screen cleanliness. Screens are cleaned to ensure that mammographic cassettes and intensifying screens are free of dust and dirt particles, which can resemble microcalcifications and may result in misdiagnoses. Intensifying screens should be cleaned using the material and methods suggested by the screen manufacturer. If a liquid cleaner is used, screens should be allowed to air-dry while standing vertically, as shown in Figure 24-5, before the cassettes are closed or used. If compressed air is used, the air supply should be checked to ensure that no moisture, oil, or other contaminants are present.

 If dust or dirt artifacts are noticed, the screens should be cleaned immediately.

Each screen cassette combination needs to be clearly labeled. The identification should be on the exterior of the cassette as well as on a lateral border of the screen so that it will be legible on the processed film. This will enable the mammographer to identify specific screens that have been found to contain artifacts.

Viewboxes and viewing conditions. Cleaning ensures that the viewboxes and viewing conditions are main-

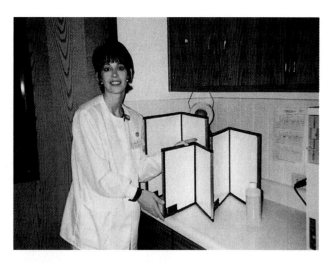

FIGURE 24-5 The proper way to dry screens after cleaning is to position them vertically. *(Courtesy Linda Joppe.)*

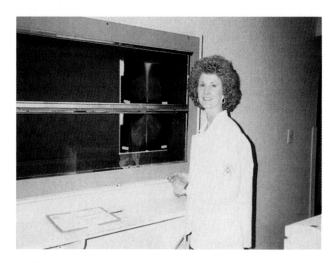

FIGURE 24-6 Mammograms must be masked for proper viewing. *(Courtesy Lois Depouw.)*

tained at an optimal level. Viewbox surfaces should be cleaned with window cleaner and soft paper towels, ensuring that all marks have been removed. The viewboxes should be visually inspected to ensure uniform luminance and to ensure that all masking devices are functioning properly. Room illumination levels should be visually checked as well so that no sources of bright light are present or are being reflected onto the viewbox surface.

Any marks that are not easily removed should be removed with cleaner that will not damage the viewbox. If the viewbox luminance appears to be nonuniform, all of the interior lamps should be replaced. Mammography viewboxes have considerably higher luminance levels than conventional viewboxes. A luminance of at least 3000 nit (candela per square meter) is required.

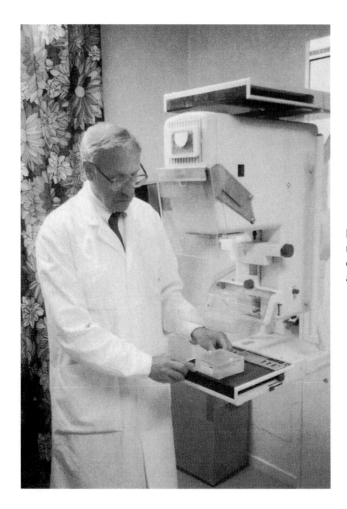

FIGURE 24-7 Analysis of an image of the ACR mammography phantom by a medical physicist scores the detection limits of the system for fibriles, microcalcifications, and nodules. *(Courtesy Art Haus.)*

All mammograms and mammography test images should be completely masked for viewing so that no extraneous light from the viewbox enters the viewer's eyes. **Masking** can be provided simply by cutting black paper to the proper size (Figure 24-6). Commercially adjustable masks are available.

Ambient light in the area of the viewbox should also be diffuse and reduced to approximately that reaching the eye through the mammogram. Sources of glare must be removed and surface reflections eliminated.

Phantom images. Phantom images are taken to ensure that OD, contrast, uniformity, and image quality of the x-ray imaging system and film processor are maintained at optimal levels. Using a standard film and a cassette designated as the control or phantom cassette, an image should be taken of an MQSA accreditation phantom.

The phantom should be placed on the image receptor assembly so that its edge is aligned with the chest wall edge of the receptor as shown in Figure 24-7. The compression device should be brought into contact with the phantom, and the automatic-exposure control sensor should be positioned in a location that will be used for all future phantom images.

The technique selected for imaging the phantom should be the same as that used clinically for a 50% fatty–50% dense, 4.5-cm compressed breast. When the exposure is made, the time or mAs is recorded. The film should then be processed just like a clinical mammogram.

A densitometer is used to determine the OD for the density disk and for the background immediately adjacent to the density disk. The time or mAs recorded earlier, the background OD, and the DD should be plotted on a phantom-image control chart, such as the one in Figure 24-8. The exposure time or mAs should stay within a range of ±15%. The background OD of the film should be approximately 1.4, with an allowed range of ±0.2. A good target value is approximately 1.6. The DD should be approximately 0.4 with an allowed range of ±0.05. However, this is defined for 28 kVp, so slightly different ODs should be expected at other kVps.

The next step is to score the phantom image, which involves determining the number of fibers, speck groups, and masses visible in the phantom image. A radiograph and conceptual drawing of the ACR accreditation phantom are shown in Figure 24-9. These results should also be plotted on the phantom-image control chart.

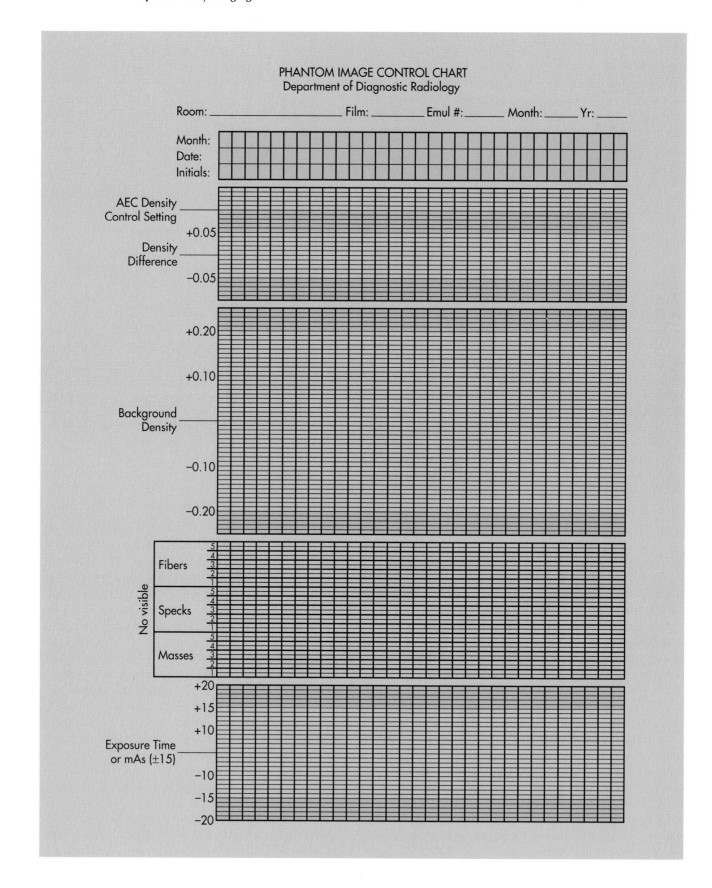

FIGURE 24-8 Phantom image control chart.

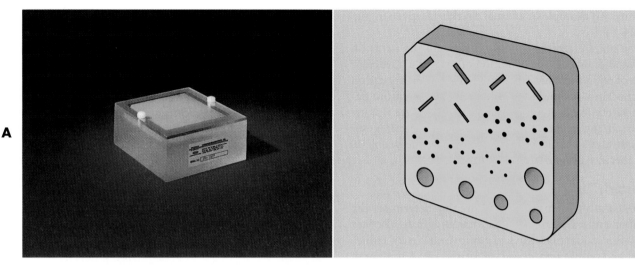

FIGURE 24-9 **A,** ACR accreditation phantom. **B,** Its schematic image. *(Courtesy Gammex RMI.)*

Scoring the objects requires that they always be counted from the largest to the smallest object, with each object group receiving a score of 1.0, 0.5, or zero. A fiber may be counted as 1.0 if its entire length is visible at the correct location and with the correct orientation. A fiber may be given a score of 0.5 if at least half of its length is visible at the correct location and with the correct orientation. The score is zero if less than half of the fiber is visible.

A speck group may be counted as a full point if four or more of the six specks are visible with a magnifying glass. A score of 0.5 may be given to a speck group if at least two of the six specks are visible. If fewer than two specks in group are visible, the score is zero.

A mass may be counted as a full point if a density difference is seen at the correct location with a generally circular border. A score of 0.5 may be given to a mass if a DD is seen at the correct location but the shape is not circular. If there is only a hint of a DD, the score is zero.

Next, the magnifying glass is used to check the image for nonuniform areas or artifacts (Figure 24-10). If any artifacts that resemble the phantom objects are found, they should be subtracted from the score given for that object. Never subtract below the next full integer point. For example, if a score of 3.5 or 4 was given, the score cannot be subtracted below 3.

The score of phantom objects counted on subsequent phantom images for each type of object should not decrease by more than 0.5. The minimum number of objects required to pass ACR accreditation is four fibers, three speck groups, and three masses.

Phantom images should be taken after equipment installation to determine the control values of the phantom objects for future comparison. Phantom images should also be taken after any maintenance is performed on the imaging equipment.

When the phantom image results in any of the factors exceeding control values, the cause should be investi-

FIGURE 24-10 These really gross artifacts are caused by processor rollers that have not been cleaned. *(Courtesy Cristl Thompson.)*

gated and corrected as soon as possible. The phantom images should always be viewed by the same person on the same mammography viewbox under the same viewing conditions, using the same type of magnifier used for mammograms and at the same time of day.

Monthly Tasks

Visual checklist. The monthly visual check ensures that the imaging system lights, displays, and mechanical locks and detents are functioning properly and confirms the optimal level of the equipment's mechanical rigidity and

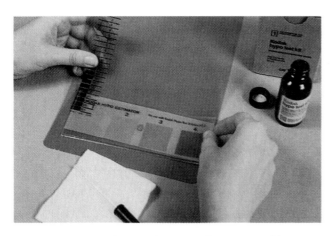

FIGURE 24-13 Analysis to determine the amount of fixer retained on the film. *(Courtesy Eastman Kodak Co.)*

The repeat rate for each category is determined by dividing the number of repeated films in a given category by the total number of repeats. The overall repeat rate should be ≤2%, and the rates for each category should also be ≤2%. If there is a high overall rate or a single category is higher than the others, the problem should be investigated. It is important to note that *all* repeat films should be included in the analysis, not just those rejected by the radiologist.

Question: A mammographic service examined 327 patients during the third calendar quarter of 2000. A total of 719 films were exposed during this period, 8 of which were repeats. What is the repeat rate?

Answer: $\text{repeat rate} = \frac{8}{719} \times 100 = 1.1\%$

Analysis of fixer retention in film. An analysis of fixer retention in film is done to determine the amount of residual fixer in the processed film. The result is used as an indicator of archival quality.

One sheet of unexposed film is processed. Next, one drop of residual hypo test solution should be placed on the emulsion side of the film and allowed to stand for 2 minutes. The excess solution should blotted off and the stain compared with a hypo estimator, which comes with the test solution. A white sheet of paper is used as background. The matching number from the hypo estimator is then recorded. The comparison should be made immediately after blotting, since a prolonged delay allows the spot to darken.

The hypo estimator provides an estimate of the amount of residual hypo in grams per square meter. If the comparison results in an estimate of more than 0.05 gm/m^2, the test must be repeated. If elevated residual hypo is then indicated, the source of the problem should be investigated and corrected. Figure 24-13 shows the result from one such test.

Semiannual Tasks

Darkroom fog. Darkroom fog analysis ensures that darkroom safelights and other sources of light inside and outside of the darkroom do not fog mammographic films. Fog results in a loss of contrast and therefore a loss of diagnostic information. This test should also be performed for a new darkroom and any time that safelight bulbs or filters are changed.

Safelight filters should be checked to ensure that they are those recommended by the film manufacturer and that they are not faded or cracked. The wattage and distance of the bulbs from work surfaces should also be checked against the recommendations of the film manufacturer.

Next, all lights should be turned off for 5 minutes, allowing the eyes to adjust to the darkness. Then, light leaks are sought around the door, passbox, and processor and in the ceiling. Light leaks are often visible from only one perspective, so you may have to move around the darkroom. Any leaks should be corrected before proceeding.

If fluorescent lights are present, they should be turned on for at least 2 minutes and then turned off. A piece of film should then be loaded into the phantom cassette in total darkness, and a phantom image should be taken as previously described. The film should be taken to the darkroom and placed emulsion side up on the counter top, covering one half of the image (left or right) with an opaque object. The safelights should then be turned on for 2 minutes with the half covered film on the countertop.

After 2 minutes, the film should be processed and the OD measured very near both sides of the line separating the covered and uncovered portions of the film. The difference in the two ODs represents the amount of fog created by the safelights or by fluorescent light afterglow. This value should be recorded.

The level of this type of fog should not exceed 0.05 OD. Excessive fog levels should be investigated to find the source so that corrective action can be taken. The background OD (unfogged) of the phantom should be in the range specified previously (1.4 to 1.6).

Screen-film contact. An evaluation of screen-film contrast is done to ensure that close contact is maintained between the screen and the film in each cassette. Poor screen-film contact results in image blur, again causing a loss of diagnostic information in the mammogram.

New cassettes should always be tested before being placed into service. All cassettes and screens should be completely cleaned and allowed to air-dry for at least 30 minutes before being loaded with film for this test. After loading, the cassettes should be allowed to sit upright for 15 minutes to allow any trapped air to escape.

The cassette to be tested should be placed on top of the cassette holder assembly, with the test tool being placed directly on top of the cassette. An appropriate test tool is fabricated of copper wire mesh of at least 40 wires per inch grid density (Figure 24-14). The compression

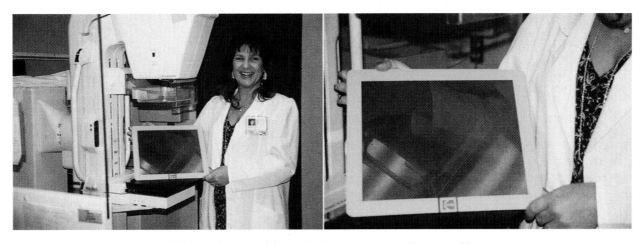

FIGURE 24-14 Wire mesh test tool for evaluating mammographic screen-film contact. *(Courtesy Susan Sprinkle.)*

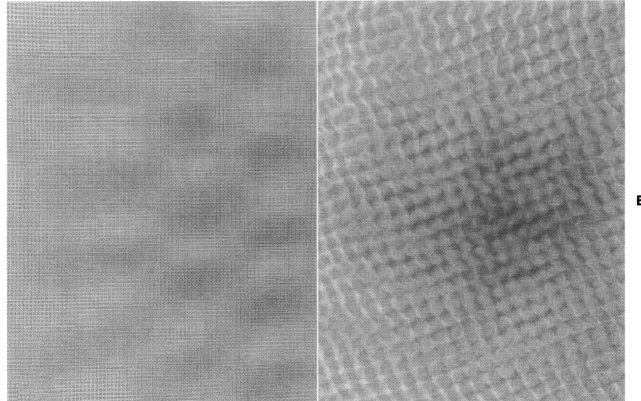

A   B

FIGURE 24-15 Images of a high-frequency wire mesh phantom showing good **(A)** and poor **(B)** screen-film contact. *(Courtesy Sharon Glaze.)*

paddle should be raised as high as possible. A manual technique should be selected between 25 and 28 kVp, which will result in an OD between 0.7 and 0.8 near the chest wall. The exposure time should be at least 500 ms.

A piece of acrylic should be placed between the x-ray tube and cassette if these parameters cannot be met under normal circumstances. If this is done, the acrylic should be placed as close as possible to the x-ray tube to reduce the scatter radiation reaching the cassette.

The film should be processed regularly and viewed from at least 3 feet. Dark areas on the film indicate poor screen-film contact (Figure 24-15). If any cassettes are found to have such poor screen-film contact, they should be cleaned and tested again. If the poor contact persists at the same spot, the problem should be investigated and the cassette removed from service until corrections can be made.

Compression check. A compression check is done to ensure that the mammographic system can provide adequate compression in the manual and power-assisted modes for an adequate amount of time. It must also be shown that the equipment does not allow too much compression to be applied.

To check the compression device, place a towel, tennis balls, or a similar cushioning material on the cassette holder assembly, followed by a flat, bathroom scale centered under the compression device. Another towel should be placed over the scale without covering the readout area (Figure 24-16). The compression device should be engaged automatically until it stops, the degree of compression should be recorded and the device then released.

The procedure should be repeated using the manual drive, again recording the compression. You should

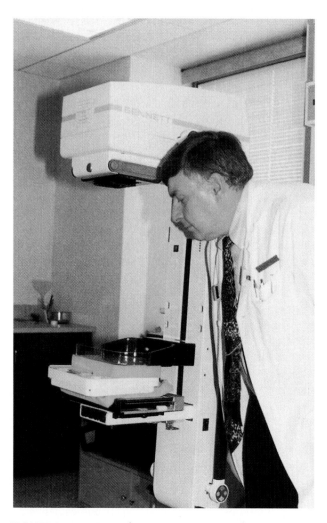

FIGURE 24-16 Testing breast compression with a conventional bathroom scale. *(Courtesy Edward Nickoloff.)*

never exceed 40 lb of compression in the automatic mode. If this is possible, the equipment should be recalibrated so that 40 lb of compression cannot be exceeded. Both modes should be able to compress between 25 and 40 lb and hold this compression for at least 15 s. If either mode fails to reach these levels, the equipment should be properly adjusted.

Firm compression is absolutely necessary for high-quality mammography. Compression reduces the thickness of tissue that the x-rays must penetrate and thus reduces scatter radiation, resulting in increased image contrast at reduced patient dose. Spatial resolution is improved with compression through the reduction of focal-spot blur and patient motion. Finally, compression makes the thickness of the breast more uniform, resulting in a more uniform OD and making the image easier to read.

Nonroutine Tasks

Film crossover check. When a new box of film must be opened and dedicated for processor QC, a crossover must be performed with the old film. This is actually a very difficult and time-consuming activity. More detailed references should be consulted before attempting this exercise.

Five strips from each of the old and new boxes of film should be exposed and processed at the same time. The OD should be read on each film for the three predetermined steps and the B+F. The five values for each of the old and new set of films are then averaged for each of the predetermined steps.

The difference between the old and new values of MD, DD, and B+F should be determined and the values adjusted to the new values on the control chart. If the B+F of the new film exceeds the B+F of the old film by more than 0.02, the cause should be investigated and remedied.

The use of strips exposed with the sensitometer more than an hour or two before processing is unacceptable, since these strips may be less sensitive to changes in the processor. The proper combination of film, processor, chemistry, developer temperature, immersion time, and replenishment rate should be used, as recommended by the film manufacturer. QC should also be performed on the densitometer, sensitometer, and thermometer so that their proper calibrations can be maintained. A log of these evaluations should be kept.

SUMMARY

QC in mammography is part of an overall evaluation analysis and includes performance monitoring, record keeping, and evaluation of results. The three QC team members are the radiologist, who has specific duties of administration and tracking diagnostic results; the medical physicist, who examines and monitors the performance of imaging equipment; and the mammographer, who performs many tests and evaluations involving equipment, processing, and mammographic images.

The many duties and responsibilities of the QC mammographer are listed by time intervals. Daily routines include maintaining darkroom cleanliness and performing processor QC. Processor QC includes sensitometry and densitometry, as well as daily graphing of the results. Weekly routines include cleaning intensifying screens and viewbox illuminators and producing phantom images and performing equipment checks.

Four times a year a repeat analysis is done based on at least 250 mammographic examinations. A repeat rate of less than or equal to 2% is required. Greater repeat rates should be investigated. Also, an archival check of film quality is performed quarterly.

Semiannually, the darkroom fog check is conducted and screen-film contact tests are performed. Finally, the compression test is done using a bathroom scale under the compression paddle. Compression should never exceed 40 lb of pressure. The automatic and manual modes should compress between 25 and 40 lb of compression for 15 s. Annually, the medical physicist evaluates the performance of the mammography imaging system.

CHALLENGE QUESTIONS

1. Define or otherwise identify:
   a. Quality assurance (QA)
   b. CQI
   c. Quality control (QC)
   d. Crossover
   e. MQSA
2. List two aspects of the radiologists' duties involving mammographic QC.
3. What task of the mammographic QC radiographer takes up the greatest amount of time?
4. Which member of the QC team would track patients' positive diagnoses?
5. Which member of the QC would notice a temperature error in the developer solution?
6. What do the fibrils of the ACR accreditation phantom simulate?
7. Describe how to clean radiographic intensifying screens. How often is this task performed?
8. Explain how mammographic viewboxes are different from conventional viewboxes.
9. What is masking?
10. What are the three objects on the mammographic phantom?
11. List the process for scoring the phantom objects.
12. How do you check for light leaks in the darkroom?
13. What is the acceptable fog value for 2 min of safelight exposure of film?
14. Describe the device used to check screen-film contact.
15. What is the maximum pressure allowed for the compression device?
16. How do you ensure darkroom cleanliness?
17. What is the speed index and how is it determined?
18. What is the minimum luminance required of a mammography viewbox?
19. When producing phantom images, what technique should be used?
20. Show how repeat rate is calculated.

CHAPTER

25

Fluoroscopy

OBJECTIVES

At the completion of this chapter, the student should be able to:

1. Discuss the development of fluoroscopy
2. Explain visual physiology and its relationship to fluoroscopy
3. Describe the components of an image intensifier
4. Calculate brightness gain and identify its units
5. List the approximate kilovolt peak levels for common fluoroscopic examinations
6. Discuss the role of the television monitor and television image in forming the fluoroscopic image

OUTLINE

The primary function of the fluoroscope is to provide real-time viewing of anatomic structures. Dynamic studies are examinations that show the motion of circulation or that show the motion of hollow internal structures. During fluoroscopy, the radiologist generally uses contrast media to highlight the anatomic structures and then views a continuous image of the internal structure while the x-ray tube is energized. If the radiologist observes something during the fluoroscopic examination and would like to preserve that image for further study, a radiograph called a *spot film* can be taken with little interruption of the dynamic examination.

The recent introduction of computer technology into fluoroscopy and radiography is placing increasing demands on the training and performance of radiologic technologists. The basic principles of these subjects are presented here. Later chapters more completely explain the emerging role of computer science in radiology.

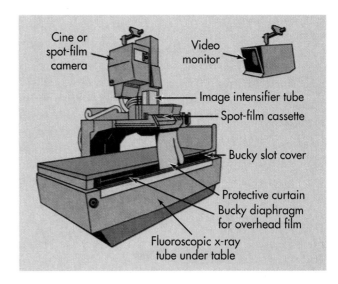

FIGURE 25-1 Fluoroscope and associated parts.

OVERVIEW OF FLUOROSCOPY

Since Thomas A. Edison invented the fluoroscope in 1896, it has been a valuable tool in the practice of radiology. The primary function of the fluoroscope is to perform dynamic studies. During **fluoroscopy**, the radiologist views a continuous image of the motion of internal structures while the x-ray tube is energized.

The fluoroscope is used for the examination of moving internal structures and fluids.

If something is observed that the radiologist would like to preserve for later study, a permanent image can be made with little interruption of the examination. One such commonly used method is known as a **spot film,** a static image in a small-format image receptor. Cineradiography, video imaging, and digital images are other examples.

Fluoroscopy is actually a rather routine type of x-ray examination except for its application in the visualization of vessels, called **angiography.** The two main areas where angiography is performed are neuroradiology and vascular radiology. These areas are now known as *cardiovascular* and *interventional radiology (CVIR).* Spot-film radiographs may also be obtained in these fluoroscopic procedures.

The layout of a fluoroscopic imaging system is shown in Figure 25-1. The x-ray tube is usually located under the patient table. Over the patient table is the image in-

tensifier and other image-detection devices. Some fluoroscopes have the x-ray tube over and the image receptor under the patient table. Some fluoroscopes are operated remotely from outside the x-ray room. There are many different arrangements for fluoroscopy, and the radiologic technologist must become familiar with each.

During image-intensified fluoroscopy, the radiologic image is displayed on a television monitor. The image-intensifier tube and the television chain are described later.

During fluoroscopy, the x-ray tube is operated at less than 5 mA, unlike a radiographic examination, in which the x-ray tube current is measured in hundreds of milliamperes. However, the patient dose during fluoroscopy is considerably higher than that resulting from radiographic examination because the x-ray beam is emitted for considerably longer times.

The kVp of operation depends entirely on the section of the body being examined. Fluoroscopic equipment allows the radiologist to select an image brightness level that is subsequently maintained automatically by varying the kVp, the mA, or sometimes both. Such a feature of the fluoroscope is called **automatic brightness control (ABC),** automatic brightness stabilization (ABS), or automatic gain control (AGC).

SPECIAL DEMANDS OF FLUOROSCOPY

Since fluoroscopy is a dynamic process, the radiologist must adapt to moving images that are sometimes dim. This requires some knowledge of image illumination and the physiology of the human eye.

Illumination

The principal advantage of image-intensified fluoroscopy over earlier fluoroscopy is the increased image brightness. Just as it is much more difficult to read a book in dim than bright illumination, it is much harder to interpret a dim fluoroscopic image than it is to interpret a bright one.

Illumination levels are measured in units of lambert (L) and millilambert (mL) (1 L = 1000 mL). It is not necessary to know the precise definition of a lambert; its importance lies in demonstrating the wide range of illumination levels over which the human eye is sensitive. Figure 25-2 lists some approximate illumination levels for familiar objects. Radiographs are visualized under illumination levels of 10 to 1000 mL; image-intensified fluoroscopy is performed at similar illumination levels.

Human Vision

The structures in the eye responsible for the sensation of vision are called *rods* and *cones*. Figure 25-3 is a cross section of the human eye, identifying its principal parts and its appearance on magnetic resonance imaging. Light incident on the eye must first pass through the cornea, a transparent protective covering, and then through the lens, where the light is focused onto the retina.

Between the cornea and the lens is the iris, which behaves like the diaphragm of a photographic camera to control the amount of light admitted to the eye. In the presence of bright light, the iris contracts and allows only a small amount of light to enter through the pupil. During low-light conditions, such as a darkened movie theater, the iris dilates (that is, opens up) and allows more light to enter. In digital fluoroscopy, there is an iris between the image-intensifier tube and the television-camera tube that functions in a similar fashion.

When light arrives at the retina, it is detected by the rods and the cones. Rods and cones are small structures; there are more than 100,000 of them per square millimeter of retina. The cones are concentrated at the center of the retina in an area called the *fovea centralis*. Rods, on the other hand, are most numerous on the periphery of the retina. There are no rods at the fovea centralis.

The rods are sensitive to low light levels and are stimulated during dim light situations. The threshold for rod vision is approximately 10^{-6} mL. Cones, on the other hand, are less sensitive to light; their threshold is only approximately 10^{-2} mL, but they are capable of responding to intense light levels, whereas rods cannot. Consequently, cones are used primarily for daylight vision called *photopic vision,* and rods are used for night vision called *scotopic vision.* This aspect of visual physiology explains why dim objects are more readily viewed if they are not looked at directly. Astronomers and radiologists are familiar with the fact that a dim object can be seen better if viewed peripherally where rod vision dominates.

The ability of cones to perceive small objects is much better than that of rods. This ability to perceive fine detail is called *visual acuity.* Cones are also much more able

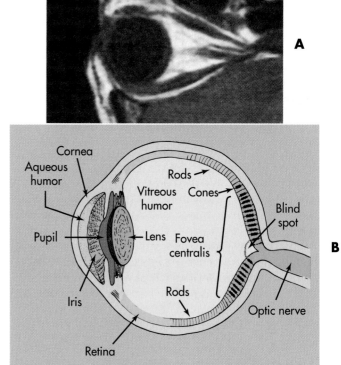

FIGURE 25-3 The human eye's appearance on a magnetic resonance image (**A**) and the parts responsible for vision (**B**). (**A** *courtesy Helen Schumpert.*)

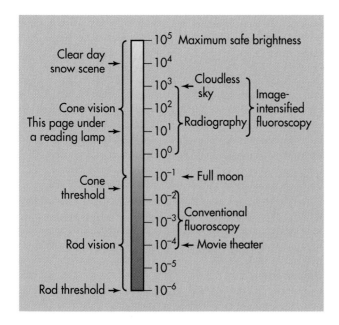

FIGURE 25-2 The range of human vision is wide; it covers 11 orders of magnitude.

to detect differences in brightness levels than rods. This property of vision is termed *contrast perception.* Furthermore, cones are sensitive to a wide range of wavelengths of light. Cones perceive color, but rods are essentially colorblind.

FLUOROSCOPIC TECHNIQUE

During fluoroscopy, maximal image detail is desired, so image brightness must be high. The image intensifier was developed principally to replace the conventional fluorescent screen. The fluorescent screen had to be viewed in a darkened room after 15 minutes of dark adaptation. The image intensifier raises the illumination into the cone vision region, where visual acuity is greatest.

The brightness of the fluoroscopic image depends primarily on the anatomy being examined, the kVp, and the mA. The patient's anatomy cannot be controlled by the radiologic technologist; fluoroscopic kVp and mA can. The influence of kVp and mA on fluoroscopic image quality is similar to their influence on radiographic image quality. Generally, high kVp and low mA are preferred.

The precise fluoroscopic technique is determined by the training and experience of the radiologist and radiologic technologist. Table 25-1 relates representative fluoroscopic kVp for several common examinations. The fluoroscopic mA is not given because it varies according to patient characteristics and the response of the ABS system.

FLUOROSCOPIC IMAGE INTENSIFICATION
Image-Intensifier Tube

The image-intensifier tube is a complex electronic device that receives the image-forming x-ray beam and converts it into a visible light image of high intensity. Figure 25-4 is a rendition of an x-ray image-intensifier tube. The tube components are contained within a glass or metal envelope that provides structural support but more important, maintains a vacuum. When installed, the tube is mounted inside a metal container to protect it from rough handling and breakage.

X-rays that exit the patient and are incident on the image-intensifier tube are transmitted through the glass

envelope and interact with the input phosphor, which is cesium iodide (CsI). When an x-ray interacts with the input phosphor, its energy is converted into visible light similar to the effect of radiographic intensifying screens. The CsI crystals are grown as tiny needles and tightly packed as a 300- to 500-μm layer (Figure 25-5). Each crystal is approximately 5 μm in diameter. This results in microlight pipes with little dispersion and improved spatial resolution.

The next active element of the image-intensifier tube is the photocathode, which is bonded directly to the input phosphor with a thin, transparent adhesive layer. The photocathode is a thin metal layer usually composed of cesium and antimony compounds that respond to the stimulation of input-phosphor light by the emission of electrons. This process is known as **photoemission,** electron emission after light stimulation. The term is similar to thermionic emission, which refers to electron emission after heat stimulation.

The photocathode emits electrons when illuminated by the input phosphor.

It takes a large number of light photons to cause one electron to be emitted. The number of electrons emitted by the photocathode is directly proportional to the intensity of light reaching it. Consequently, the number of electrons emitted is proportional to the intensity of the incident image-forming x-ray beam.

The image-intensifier tube is approximately 50 cm long. A potential difference of about 25,000 V is maintained across the tube between the photocathode and the anode so that the electrons produced by photoemission will be accelerated to the anode.

The anode is a circular plate with a hole in the middle

TABLE 25-1	Representative Fluoroscopic and Spot-Film kVp for Common Examinations	
Examination	**kVp**
Gallbladder study	65-75
Nephrostography	70-80
Myelography	70-80
Barium enema (air contrast) study	80-90
Upper gastrointestinal tract	100-110
Small bowel study	110-120
Barium enema study	110-120

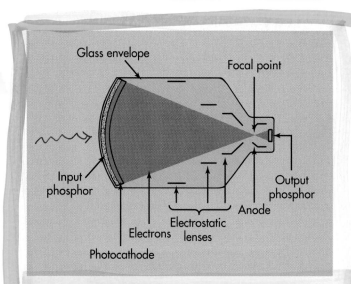

FIGURE 25-4 The image-intensifier tube converts the pattern of the x-ray beam into a bright, visible light image.

to allow the electrons through to the output phosphor, which is just the other side of the anode, and is usually made of zinc cadmium sulfide. The output phosphor is where the electrons interact and produce light.

If there is to be an accurate image pattern, the electron path from photocathode to output phosphor must be precise. The engineering aspects of maintaining proper electron travel are called **electron optics** because the electrons emitted over the face of the image-intensifier tube must be focused just like visible light.

The devices responsible for this control, called *electrostatic focusing lenses,* are located along the length of the image-intensifier tube. The electrons arrive at the output phosphor with high kinetic energy and contain the image of the input phosphor in minified form.

When these high-energy electrons interact with the output phosphor, a considerable amount of light is produced. Each photoelectron that arrives at the output phosphor results in approximately 50 to 75 times as many light photons as were necessary to create it. The entire sequence of events from initial x-ray interaction to output image is summarized in Figure 25-6. This ratio

of the number of light photons at the output phosphor to the number of x-rays at the input phosphor is the **flux gain,** as follows:

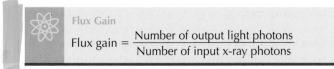

$$Flux\ gain = \frac{Number\ of\ output\ light\ photons}{Number\ of\ input\ x\text{-}ray\ photons}$$

The increased illumination of the image is due to the multiplication of the light photons at the output phosphor compared with the x-rays at the input phosphor and the image minification from input phosphor to output phosphor. The ability of the image intensifier to increase the illumination level of the image is called its **brightness gain.** The brightness gain is simply the product of the minification gain and the flux gain, as follows:

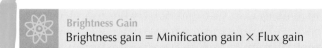

Brightness gain = Minification gain × Flux gain

The **minification gain** is the ratio of the square of the diameter of the input phosphor to the square of the diameter of the output phosphor. Output-phosphor size is fairly standard at 2.5 or 5 cm. Input-phosphor size varies from 10 to 35 cm and is used to identify image-intensifier tubes.

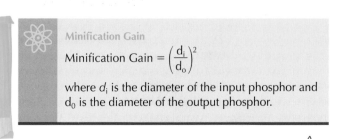

$$Minification\ Gain = \left(\frac{d_i}{d_o}\right)^2$$

where d_i is the diameter of the input phosphor and d_o is the diameter of the output phosphor.

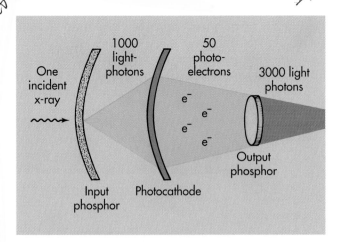

FIGURE 25-6 In an image-intensifier tube, each incident x-ray that interacts with the input phosphor results in a large number of light photons at the output phosphor. The image intensifier shown here has a gain of 3000.

FIGURE 25-5 Celsium iodide crystals for image-intensifier input phosphors are grown as linear filaments and tightly packed as shown in these photomicrographs. **A,** Cross section. **B,** Face. *(Courtesy Philips Medical Systems.)*

Question: What is the brightness gain for a 17-cm image-intensifier tube having a flux gain of 120 and a 2.5-cm output phosphor?

Answer:
$$\text{Brightness gain} = \left(\frac{d_i}{d_o}\right)^2 \times \text{Flux gain}$$
$$= \frac{17^2}{2.5^2} \times 120$$
$$= 46 \times 120$$
$$= 5520$$

The brightness gain of most image intensifiers is 5000 to 30,000, and it decreases with tube age and use. As an image intensifier ages, the patient dose increases to maintain brightness. Ultimately, the image intensifier must be replaced.

When image intensifiers were first introduced, brightness gain was the increased illumination compared to the standard conventional fluorescent screen at that time, a Patterson B-2 screen. Now it is defined as the ratio of the illumination intensity at the output phosphor, measured in candela per meter squared (cd/m^2) to the radiation intensity incident on the input phosphor, measured in milliroentgen per second (mR/s). This quantity is called the **conversion factor** and is approximately 0.01 times the brightness gain. The proper quantity for expressing the intensification is conversion factor, as follows:

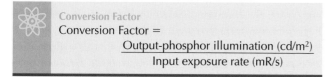

Conversion Factor

$$\text{Conversion Factor} = \frac{\text{Output-phosphor illumination } (cd/m^2)}{\text{Input exposure rate } (mR/s)}$$

Image intensifiers have conversion factors ranging from 50 to 300. This corresponds to brightness gains of 5000 to 30,000.

Figure 25-7 demonstrates some of the modes of operation that can be accommodated with the image-intensifier tube. Fluoroscopic images are viewed on a television monitor. The spot-film camera uses 105-mm film and is becoming increasingly popular. The cineradiography camera is used almost exclusively in cardiac catheterization, but digital images are increasingly being obtained.

Multifield Image Intensification

Most image intensifiers are of the multifield type. These multifield image intensifiers provide for considerably more flexibility for all fluoroscopic examinations and are standard components in digital fluoroscopy. Dual field tubes come in a variety of sizes, but perhaps the most popular is the 25- to 17-cm (25/17) design. Trifield tubes of 25/17/12 or 23/15/10 are also often used. These numeric dimensions refer to the diameter of the input phosphor of the image-intensifier tube. The operation of a typical multifield tube is illustrated by the 25/17 type shown in Figure 25-8. In the 25-cm mode, the photoelectrons from the entire input phosphor are accelerated to the output phosphor. When switched to the 17-cm mode, the voltage on the electrostatic focusing lenses is increased, causing the electron focal point to move farther from the output phosphor. Consequently, only electrons from the center 17-cm diameter of the input phosphor interact with the output phosphor.

The principal result of this change in focal point is to reduce the field of view and thereby magnify the image. Use of the smaller dimension of a multifield image-intensifier tube always results in a magnified im-

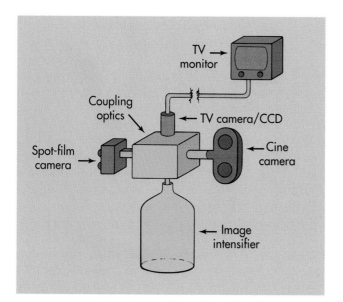

FIGURE 25-7 Some possible modes of operation with an image-intensifier tube. *CCD,* Charge coupled device.

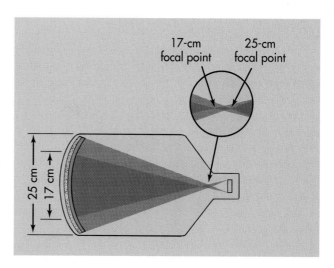

FIGURE 25-8 A 25/17 image-intensifier tube produces a magnified image in the 17-cm mode.

age, with a magnification factor in direct proportion to the ratio of the diameters. A 25/17 tube operated in the 17-cm mode produces an image magnified 1.5 times larger than the image produced in the 25-cm mode.

Question: How magnified is the image of a 25/17/12 image intensifier in the 12-cm mode compared to the 25-cm mode?

Answer: Magnification factor $= \dfrac{25}{12} = 2.1$ magnification

This magnified image comes at a price. In the magnified mode, the minification gain is reduced, and there are fewer photoelectrons incident on the output phosphor. A dimmer image results.

To maintain the same level of brightness, the x-ray tube mA is increased by the ABS, and this increases the patient dose. The increase in dose is equal to the ratio of the area of the input phosphor used, or approximately four times ($25^2 \div 12^2 \simeq 4.34$) the dose obtained in the wide field of view mode.

Question: A 23/15/10 image-intensifier tube is used in the 10-cm mode. How much higher is the patient dose in this mode compared with the 23-cm mode?

Answer: $23^2/10^2 = 5.3$ times as high!

This increase in patient dose results in better image quality. The patient dose is higher because more x-rays per unit area are required to form the image. This results in lower noise and improved contrast resolution.

Magnification mode results in better spatial resolution, better contrast resolution, and higher patient dose.

The portion of any image resulting from the periphery of the input phosphor is inherently unfocused and suffers from **vignetting,** a reduction in brightness at the periphery of the image.

Because only the central region of the input phosphor is used in the magnification mode, spatial resolution is also improved. In the 25-cm mode, a CsI image-intensifier tube can image approximately 0.125-mm objects (4 lp/mm); in the 10-cm mode, the resolution is approximately 0.08 mm (6 lp/mm).

The concept of spatial resolution as measured in line pairs per millimeter was first introduced in Chapter 16 and is discussed more completely in Chapter 29. At this stage, it is sufficient to know that good spatial resolution is associated with more line pairs per millimeter.

FLUOROSCOPIC IMAGE MONITORING
Television Monitoring

When a television-monitoring system is used, the output phosphor of the image-intensifier tube is coupled directly to a television camera tube. The **vidicon** (Figure 25-9) is the television-camera tube most often used in television fluoroscopy. It has a sensitive input surface the same size as the output phosphor of the image-intensifier tube. The television-camera tube converts the light image from the output phosphor of the image intensifier into an electrical signal that is sent to the television monitor, where it is reconstructed as an image on the television screen.

A significant advantage of television monitoring is that brightness level and contrast can be controlled electronically. With television monitoring, several observers can view the fluoroscopic image at the same time. It is even common to place monitors outside the examination room for others to observe.

Television monitoring also allows for storage of the image in its electronic form for later playback and image manipulation. Television monitoring is an essential part of the digital fluoroscopic equipment described in Chapter 28.

Television camera. The television camera consists of a cylindric housing approximately 15 mm in diameter by 25 cm in length, which contains the heart of the camera: the television-camera tube. It also contains electromagnetic coils for properly steering the electron beam inside the tube. A number of such television-camera tubes are available for television fluoroscopy, but the vidicon and its modified version, the Plumbicon, are used most often.

Figure 25-10 shows a typical vidicon. The glass envelope serves the same function that it does for the x-ray

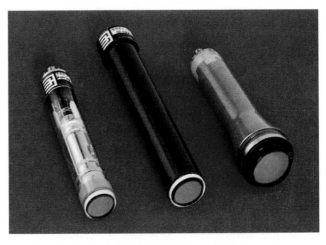

FIGURE 25-9 These three variations of a vidicon television-camera tube have a diameter of approximately 1 inch and a length of 6 inches. The right tube uses electrostatic rather than electromagnetic electron beam deflection. *(Courtesy Marconi Medical Systems.)*

tube: to maintain a vacuum and provide mechanical support for the internal elements. The internal elements are the cathode, its electron gun, assorted electrostatic grids, and a target assembly that serves as an anode.

The electron gun is a heated filament that supplies a constant electron current via thermionic emission. These electrons are formed into an electron beam by the control grid, which also helps accelerate the electrons to the anode. The electron beam is further accelerated and focused by additional electrostatic grids. The size of the electron beam and its position are controlled by external electromagnetic coils known as *deflection coils, focusing coils,* and *alignment coils.*

At the anode end of the tube the electron beam passes through a wire mesh–like structure and interacts with the target assembly. The target assembly consists of three layers sandwiched together. The outside layer is the face

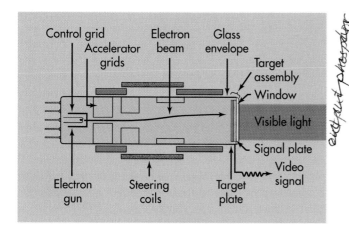

FIGURE 25-10 Vidicon television camera tube and its principal parts.

plate or window, the thin part of the glass envelope. Coated on the inside of the window is a thin layer of metal or graphite, called the *signal plate.* The signal plate is thin enough to transmit light, yet thick enough to be an efficient electrical conductor. Its name derives from the fact that it conducts the video signal out of the tube into the external video circuit.

A photoconductive layer of antimony trisulfide is applied to the inside of the signal plate. This layer is called the *target* or *photoconductive layer,* and the electron beam interacts with this layer. Antimony trisulfide is photoconductive because when illuminated, it conducts electrons; when dark, it behaves as an insulator.

The mechanism of the target assembly is complex but can be described simplistically. When light from the output phosphor of the image-intensifier tube strikes the window, it is transmitted through the signal plate to the target. If the electron beam is incident on the same part of the target at the same time, some of its electrons will be conducted through the target to the signal plate and conducted from there out of the tube as the video signal. If that area of the target is dark, there will be no video signal. The magnitude of the video signal is proportional to the intensity of light (Figure 25-11).

Coupling the Television Camera. Image intensifiers and television-camera tubes are manufactured so that the output phosphor of the image-intensifier tube is the same diameter as the window of the television-camera tube, usually 2.5 or 5 cm. Two methods are commonly used to attach, or couple, the television-camera tube to the image-intensifier tube (Figure 25-12).

The simplest method is to use a bundle of fiber optics. The fiber-optic bundle is only a few millimeters thick and contains thousands of glass fibers per square millimeter of cross section. One advantage of this type of coupling

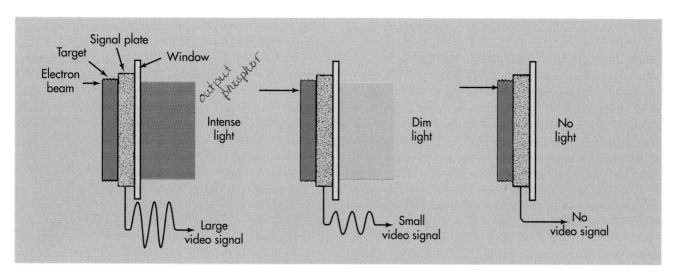

FIGURE 25-11 The target of a television-camera tube conducts electrons, creating a video signal only when illuminated.

A   **B**

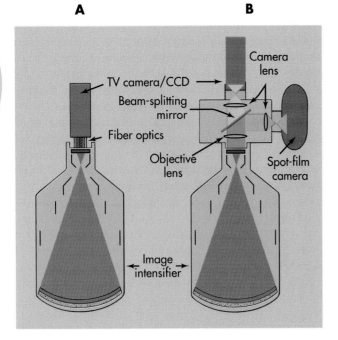

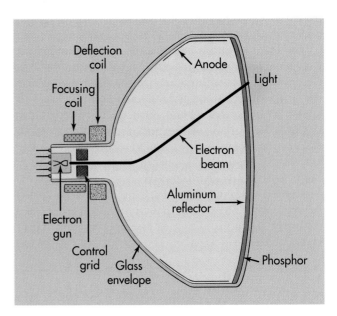

FIGURE 25-12 Television-camera tubes are coupled to an image-intensifier tube in two ways. **A,** Fiber optics. **B,** Lens system. *CCD,* Charge coupled device.

FIGURE 25-13 Television picture tube (CRT) and its principal parts.

is its small, compact assembly, making it easy to move the image-intensifier tower. This coupling is also rugged and can withstand relatively rough handling. The principal disadvantage is that it cannot accommodate auxiliary imaging devices such as cine or photospot cameras. With this type of coupling, cassette-loaded spot films are necessary.

For a cine or photospot camera to be accepted, lens coupling is required. This type of coupling results in a much larger assembly that should be handled with care. It is absolutely essential that the lenses and mirror remain precisely adjusted. Malpositioning results in a blurred image.

The objective lens accepts the light from the output phosphor and converts it into a parallel beam. When an image is being recorded on film, this beam is interrupted by a beam-splitting mirror so that only a portion is transmitted to the television camera, as the remainder is reflected to a film camera. The amount of reflected image is determined by the film and camera system used. Such a system allows the fluoroscopist to view the image while it is being recorded.

Usually, the beam-splitting mirror is retracted from the beam when a film camera is not in use. Both the television camera and the film camera are coupled to lenses that focus the parallel light beam onto the film and target of the respective cameras. These camera lenses are the most critical elements in the optical chain in terms of alignment. Although the lenses are shown as simple convex lenses, it should be understood that each is a compound lens system consisting of several separate lens elements.

Television monitor. The video signal is amplified and transmitted by cable to the television monitor, where it is transformed back into a visible image. The television monitor forms one end of a closed-circuit television system. The other end is the television camera. There are two immediately obvious differences between closed-circuit-television fluoroscopy and a home television set: no audio and no channel selection. There are usually only two controls that the radiologic technologist manipulates: contrast and brightness.

The heart of the television monitor is the television-picture tube, or cathode ray tube (CRT) (Figure 25-13). It has many similarities to the camera tube: a glass envelope, an electron gun, and external coils for focusing and steering the electron beam. It is different from a camera tube in that it is much larger and its anode assembly consists of a fluorescent screen and graphite lining.

The video signal received by the picture tube is modulated. **Modulation** means that the magnitude of the video signal is directly proportional to the light intensity received by the television-camera tube. Unlike the television camera, the electron beam of the television picture tube varies in amplitude in accordance to the modulation of the video signal.

The intensity of the electron beam is modulated by a control grid, which is attached to the electron gun. This electron beam is focused onto the output fluorescent screen by the external coils. There, the electrons interact with an output phosphor and produce a burst of light. The phosphor is composed of linear crystals aligned perpendicularly to the glass envelope to reduce lateral dispersion. It is usually backed by a thin layer of aluminum, which transmits the electron beam but reflects the light.

Television image. The image on the television monitor is formed in a complex way, but it can be described rather simply. It involves transforming the visible light image of the output phosphor of the image-intensifier tube into an electrical video signal that is created by a continuous electron beam in the television-camera tube. The video signal then modulates, or varies, the electron beam of the television-picture tube and transforms that electron beam into a visible image at the fluorescent screen of the picture tube.

Both electron beams, the continuous one of the television-camera tube and the modulated one of the television-picture tube, are finely focused pencil beams that are precisely and synchronously directed by the external electromagnetic coils of each tube. The beams are synchronous because they are always at the same position at the same time and move in precisely the same fashion.

The movement of these electron beams produces a **raster pattern** on the screen of a television picture tube (Figure 25-14). Although the following discussion relates to a picture tube, remember that the same electron beam pattern is occurring in the camera tube.

The electron beam begins in the upper left corner of the screen and moves to the upper right corner, creating a line of varying intensity of light as it moves. This is called an active trace. The electron beam then is blanked, or turned off, and it returns to the left side of the screen as shown. This is the horizontal retrace. There follows a series of active traces followed by horizontal retraces until the electron beam is at the bottom of the screen. This is much like the action of a typist who processes a line of information (the active trace); the cursor returns (the horizontal retrace) and continues this sequence to the bottom of the page. Whereas the typist completes a page, the electron beam completes a television field.

The similarity stops there, however, because the typist would continue word processing. The electron beam is blanked again and undergoes a vertical retrace to the top of the screen. It now transmits a second television field, the same as the first except that each active trace lies between two adjacent active traces of the first field. This movement of the electron beam is termed *interlace,* and two interlaced television fields form one television frame.

In the United States, power is supplied at 60 Hz, therefore there are 60 television fields per second and 30 television frames per second. This is fortunate because the flickering of home movies shown at 16 frames per second or of old time movies—the "flicks"—does

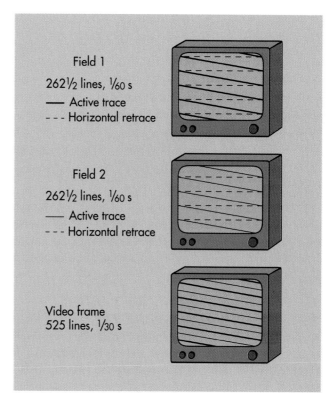

FIGURE 25-14 A video frame is formed from a raster pattern of two interlaced video fields.

not appear on the television image. Flickering is not detectable by the human eye at rates above approximately 20 frames per second. At a frame rate of 30 per second, each frame is 33 ms long.

 Video monitoring uses a rate of 30 frames per second.

In the television-camera tube, as the electron beam reads the optical signal, the signal is erased. In the television-picture tube, as the electron beam creates the television optical signal, it immediately fades: hence the term **fluorescent screen.** Therefore each new television frame represents 33 ms of new information.

Standard broadcast and closed-circuit televisions are called *525-line systems* because they have 525 lines of active trace per frame. Actually, there are only about 480 lines per frame because of the time required for retracing. Other special-purpose systems have 875 or 1024 lines per frame and therefore have better spatial resolution. These high-resolution systems are particularly important for digital fluoroscopy.

The vertical resolution is determined by number of scan lines. The horizontal resolution is determined by a property called bandpass. **Bandpass,** expressed in frequency (Hz), describes the number of times per second that the electron beam can be modulated, or changed.

A 1-MHz bandpass would indicate that the electron beam intensity could be changed a million times each second. The higher the bandpass, the better the horizontal resolution.

The objective of television designers is to create a television frame having equal horizontal and vertical resolution. Commercial television systems have a bandpass of about 3.5 MHz. Those used in fluoroscopy are approximately 4.5 MHz; 1000-line, high-resolution systems have a bandpass of approximately 20 MHz.

The television monitor remains the weakest link in image-intensified fluoroscopy. The spatial resolution of a 525-line system is approximately 2 lp/mm, but the image intensifier is good to about 5 lp/mm. Therefore to take advantage of the superior resolution of the image intensifier the radiographer must record the image on film through an optically coupled photographic camera.

FLUOROSCOPIC IMAGE RECORDING

The conventional **cassette-loaded spot film** is one method used with image-intensified fluoroscopes. The spot film is positioned between the patient and the image intensifier (Figure 25-15). During fluoroscopy the cassette is encased in a lead-lined shroud so that it is not unintentionally exposed. When a cassette spot-film exposure is desired, the radiologist must actuate a control that properly positions the cassette in the x-ray beam and changes the operation of the x-ray tube from low fluoroscopic mA to high radiographic mA. Sometimes a second or two is required for the rotating anode to be energized to a higher speed.

The cassette-loaded spot film is masked by a series of lead diaphragms to allow several image formats. When the entire film is exposed at one time, that is called the

one-on-one mode. When only half of the film is exposed at a time, two images result; that is called the *two-on-one mode.* Four-on-one and six-on-one modes are also available, with the images becoming successively smaller.

Exposures with cassette-loaded spot films require more patient dose, and the delay necessary before exposure can be made is sometimes a nuisance. Cassette-loaded spot films, however, provide a familiar format for the radiologist and have high image quality.

The **photospot camera** is similar to a movie camera except that it exposes only one frame when activated. It receives its image from the output phosphor of the image intensifier tube and therefore requires less patient exposure than the cassette-loaded spot film. It does not require significant interruption of the fluoroscopic examination, nor is there the additional heat load on the x-ray tube associated with cassette-loaded spot films.

The photospot camera uses film sizes of 70 and 105 mm. In general, the larger film format results in better image quality but at increased patient dose. Even with 105-mm spot films, however, the patient dose is only approximately half of that with cassette-loaded spot films.

The trend in spot filming is to use the photospot camera. The photospot camera provides adequate image quality without interruption of the fluoroscopic examination and at a rate of up to 12 images per second. See Table 25-2 for a comparison of the cassette spot vs. the photospot camera.

SUMMARY

The original fluoroscope, invented by Edison, had a zinc–cadmium sulfide screen placed in the x-ray beam directly above the patient. The radiologist stared directly into the screen and viewed a faint yellow-green fluoroscopic image. It was not until the 1950s that the image intensifier was developed.

In the past, fluoroscopy required radiologists to adapt their eyes to the dark before the examination. Under dim viewing conditions, the human eye uses rods, which have low visual acuity, for vision. The image from today's fluoroscope is bright enough to be perceived by cone vision. Cone vision has superior visual acuity and contrast perception. When viewing the fluoroscopic image, the radiologist is able to see fine anatomic detail and differences in brightness levels of anatomic parts.

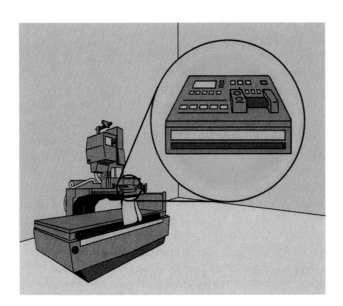

FIGURE 25-15 The cassette-loaded spot film is positioned between the patient and the image intensifier.

TABLE 25-2	Cassette Spot vs. Photospot	
	Cassette Spot	**Photospot**
Spatial resolution	8 lp/mm	5 lp/mm
Frame rate	1/s	12/s
Patient entrance skin exposure	200 mR	100 mR

The image intensifier is a complex device that receives the image-forming x-ray beam, converts it to light, and increases the light intensity for better viewing. The input phosphor converts the x-ray beam into light. When stimulated by light, the photocathode then emits electrons, and the electrons are accelerated to the output phosphor.

The following relationships define several characteristics of image-intensified fluoroscopy:

$$\text{Flux gain} = \frac{\text{Number of output light photons}}{\text{Number of input x-ray photons}}$$

$$\text{Minification gain} = \frac{(\text{Diameter of input phosphor})^2}{(\text{Diameter of output phosphor})^2}$$

$$\text{Brightness gain} = \text{Minification gain} \times \text{Flux gain}$$

Brightness gain or intensification is also expressed as the following conversion factor:

$$\text{Conversion factor} = \frac{\text{Output-phosphor illumination (candela/m}^2)}{\text{Input exposure rate (mR/s)}}$$

The fluoroscopic television camera is attached to the image intensifier with a lens coupling to accommodate a cine or a spot-film camera. When an image is being recorded on film, a beam-splitting mirror separates the beam so that only a portion is transmitted to the television camera and the remainder is reflected to a spot-film camera.

CHALLENGE QUESTIONS

1. Define or otherwise identify:
   a. Fluoroscopy
   b. Automatic brightness control
   c. Flux gain, brightness gain, and minification gain
   d. Angiography
   e. Vidicon
   f. Photoemission
   g. Electron optics
   h. Spot film
   i. Modulation

2. Diagram the relationship among the x-ray tube, the patient table, and the image intensifier.

3. What is the difference between rod and cone vision? When is visual acuity greater?

4. What is the approximate kVp for the following fluoroscopic examinations: barium enema, gallbladder, and upper gastrointestinal tract?

5. Explain the difference between photoemission and thermionic emission.

6. Diagram the image-intensifier tube, label its principle parts, and discuss the function of each.

7. A 23-cm image-intensifier has an output phosphor size of 2.5 cm and flux gain of 75. What is its brightness gain?

8. What is vignetting?

9. Why is the television monitor considered the weakest link in image-intensified fluoroscopy?

10. What is the primary function of the fluoroscope?

11. What determines the image frame rate in video fluoroscopy?

12. What limits the vertical and horizontal resolution of a video monitor?

13. When viewing in the magnification mode compared to normal mode, is there a change in spatial resolution? Explain.

14. What is meant by a *trifield image intensifier*?

15. Draw the approximate raster pattern for a conventional video monitor.

16. When switching the image intensifier from 15- to 25-cm mode, what happens to patient dose and contrast resolution?

17. Trace the path of the information-carrying elements in a fluoroscopic system from incident x-rays to video image.

18. What is the principal difference between a standard video system for fluoroscopy and a high-resolution system?

Cardiovascular and Interventional Radiology

OBJECTIVES

At the completion of this chapter, the student should be able to:

1. Discuss the Seldinger technique for vascular access
2. Describe the most common routes of vascular access
3. Name the five catheters most commonly used in cardiovascular and interventional radiography
4. Discuss the types of contrast media used during cardiovascular and interventional procedures
5. Identify the risks of arteriography
6. Describe the types of equipment in the cardiovascular and interventional suite

OUTLINE

There continues to be rapid development in the area of cardiovascular imaging and therapeutic angiographic intervention. Suites of x-ray rooms contain complex equipment specially designed for cardiovascular and interventional radiology (CVIR). Radiologic technologists trained in these areas can now be certified by the American Registry of Radiologic Technologists as vascular technologists, which is written as RT (CV) (ARRT) after their name. This chapter describes the various CVIR procedures and the special x-ray equipment necessary to perform such procedures.

CARDIOVASCULAR AND INTERVENTIONAL TECHNOLOGIST

As imaging technology has developed so has the way we identify ourselves. First, we were called *x-ray operators,* then *technicians,* and now *radiologic technologists* or more specifically, *radiographers.* A radiologic technologist can be a radiographer, a nuclear medicine technologist, or another type of imaging technologist as shown in Figure 26-1.

In the same way that radiologic technology has become more precisely divided into disciplines, so have our imaging tasks become more specialized. Radiographers used to perform special procedures, such as pneumoencephalography, myelography, and neuroangiography. The rapid development of vascular imaging and aggressive therapeutic intervention through vessels has resulted in rooms and equipment designed especially for cardiovascular and interventional procedures. The radiologic technologists who perform these procedures are cardiovascular and interventional technologists. The radiographer who specializes in angiointerventional radiography is highly skilled. The American Registry of Radiologic Technologists offers an examination in cardiovascular and interventional radiography. Once the examination is passed, the radiographer may add (CV) after the RT (R).

CARDIOVASCULAR AND INTERVENTIONAL PROCEDURES
History

CVIR procedures began in the 1930s with **angiography,** an imaging technique that uses needles and contrast media to enter and highlight an artery. The early 1960s saw the introduction of transbrachial selective coronary angiography—entering select coronary arteries through an artery of the arm—a procedure pioneered by Mason Jones.

Also during the 1960s, transfemoral angiography— entering via an artery in the thigh—of selective visceral, heart, and head arteries was developed. The femoral approach to angiography was introduced by Melvin Judkins for coronary angiography, Charles Dotter for visceral angiography, and Vincent Hinck for neuroangiography.

Angiography refers to the imaging of vessels after the injection of contrast media. Angioplasty, thrombolysis, embolization, vascular stents, and biopsy are interventional therapeutic procedures conducted in and through vessels. Box 26-1 lists the types of imaging and interventional procedures likely to be conducted in a CVIR suite.

Basic Principles

Arterial access. In 1953, Sven-Ivar Seldinger described a method of arterial access that uses a needle and catheter and makes cutdown of the vessel unnecessary. The Seldinger needle is an 18-gauge hollow needle with a stylet. Once the Seldinger needle is inserted into the femoral artery and pulsating, arterial blood returns, and the stylet is removed. A guidewire is then inserted through the needle into the arterial lumen. With the guidewire in

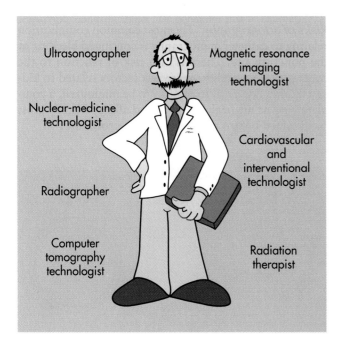

FIGURE 26-1 A radiologic technologist can specialize in many types of imaging.

BOX 26-1	Representative Procedures Conducted in a CVIR Suite
Imaging Procedures	**Interventional Procedures**
Angiography	Stent placement
Aortography	Embolization
Arteriography	Intravascular stent
Cardiac catheterization	Thrombolysis
Myelography	Balloon angioplasty
Venography	Atherectomy

TABLE 26-1	Specifications for a Typical CVIR X-Ray Tube	
Feature	**Size**	**Reason**
Focal spot	1.0 mm/0.3 mm	Is large for heat load and small for magnification
Disc size	15-cm diameter, 5 cm thick	Accommodates heat load
Power rating	80 kW	Is used for rapid sequence, serial radiography
Anode heat capacity	3 MHU	Accommodates head load

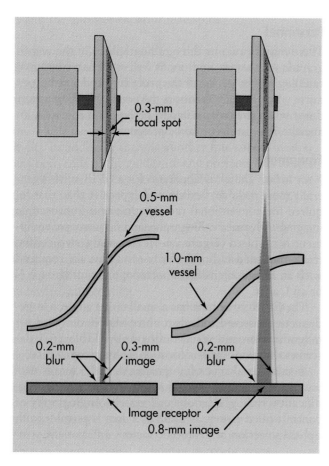

FIGURE 26-5 For a given geometry, such as this resulting in a 0.5-mm focal-spot blur, the vessels must be twice the size of the focal-spot blur.

tioning. With a source-to-image receptor distance (SID) that equals 100 cm and an object-to-image receptor distance (OID) that equals 40 cm, the radiographer can take advantage of the air gap to improve image contrast. Using a 0.3-mm focal spot results in a focal-spot blur of 1.2 mm.

Question: A left cerebral angiogram is performed with a 0.3-mm focal spot at 100-cm SID. The artery to be imaged is 20 cm from the image receptor. What is the magnification factor (MF) and focal-spot blur (FSB)? (*SOD* is the source-to-object distance.)

Answer:
$$MF = \frac{100\text{-cm SID}}{80\text{-cm SOD}} = 1.25$$

$$FSB = 0.3\left(\frac{20\text{-cm OID}}{80\text{-cm SOD}}\right) = 0.075$$

Spatial resolution for this procedure can be approximated by multiplying the focal-spot blur by two. Figure 26-5 shows geometry that results in 0.5-mm focal-spot blur images of a 1.0-mm vessel. A 0.5-mm vessel is too blurred to be seen. Any vessel larger than 1.0 mm will be imaged.

All the other essential characteristics of a CVIR x-ray tube are based on required tube loading. The size and construction of the anode disc determines the anode heat capacity, which in turn influences the power rating. An x-ray tube with a minimum 80-kW rating with 3-MHU heat capacity is required.

High-voltage generator. High-frequency generators are increasingly popular in all x-ray examinations, including CVIR. However, some CVIR procedures require higher power than may be available with high-frequency generators. High-voltage generators with three-phase, 12-pulse power capable of at least 100 kW with low ripple are needed for such high-power requirements.

Patient table. Whereas most general fluoroscopy imagers have a tilt-table, CVIR imagers do not. During general fluoroscopy head-down and head-up tilting of the patient is often necessary for manipulating contrast. Only myelography as a CVIR procedure requires a tilt-table, and therefore that procedure is often done in general fluoroscopy.

Other CVIR procedures do not require a tilt-table. They use a stationary patient table with a floating or moveable tabletop (Figure 26-6). Controls for table positioning are located on the side of the table and duplicated on a floor switch. The floor switch is necessary to accommodate patient positioning while maintaining a sterile field.

The patient table may also have a computer-controlled **stepping** capability. This feature is necessary to allow imaging from the abdomen to the feet after a single injection of contrast medium. An additional requirement of this stepping feature is the ability to preselect the time and position of the patient couch to coincide with the image receptor.

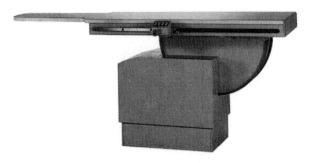

FIGURE 26-6 Typical CVIR patient table with a floating, rotating, and tilting top. *(Courtesy Odelft Corp.)*

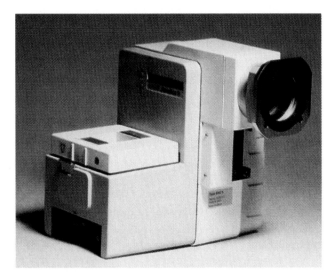

FIGURE 26-7 This 105-mm photofluorographic spot-film camera captures images from the output phosphor of an image intensifier in either single or rapid serial fashion. *(Courtesy Odelft Corp.)*

Image receptor. Three different types of image receptors are used in CVIR. The cinefluorographic camera is used during cardiac catheterization. The serialographic changer has been the principal image receptor for many years, but digital fluoroscopy is rapidly making these devices obsolete (see Chapter 28). Photofluorographic cameras (Figure 26-7) have been described (see Chapter 25).

Cinefluorographic camera (cine). In **cinefluorography** the television-camera tube is replaced with a movie camera that records the image on film for later playback. Cinefluorography is used most often in certain angiographic procedures, especially those associated with cardiac catheterization. The patient dose is much higher than that required for recording images electronically, but the image quality is also better.

Both 16- and 35-mm film movie cameras are used for cinefluorography. The 35-mm film format requires more

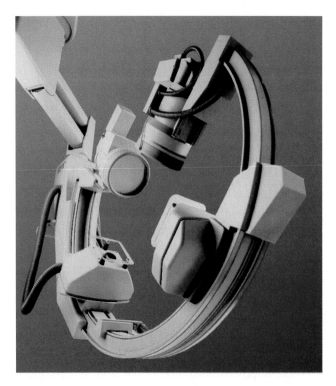

FIGURE 26-8 Ceiling-mounted flexible biplane imaging system. *(Courtesy Fischer Imaging.)*

patient exposure than the 16-mm film format, but the projected image is larger.

Cine cameras are driven by synchronous motors controlled by the line voltage, which is 60 Hz. Therefore they have rates of 7.5, 15, 30, and 60 frames per second. Naturally, the higher the frame rate, the higher the radiation dose. High frame rates are necessary for cardiac studies, but 7.5 frames per second may be adequate for other examinations.

Cinefluorographic systems are synchronized; that is, the x-ray tube is energized only during the time when the cine film is in position for exposure. The x-ray tube is not energized during the time between frames when the film is advancing because this would result in excessive and unnecessary patient exposure.

Serialographic (serial) changer. The serial changer has been the principal unique CVIR image receptor since the 1950s. Production of these devices has dwindled because of the emergence of digital fluoroscopy. Serial changers, referred to as *rapid film changers* or simply *film changers*, are often used in pairs with two orthogonal x-ray sources in a configuration called **biplane imaging** (Figure 26-8). There are two types of serialographic changers: roll film and cut film.

The roll-film changer predates automatic processing and was designed to replace bulky cassette changers. Up to 12 images per second are possible, but processing, viewing, and storage of the roll of images are difficult. Because of this deficiency, this type of film changer was quickly replaced by cut-film changers.

Cut-film changers incorporate a supply magazine of sheets of film, an exposure chamber, and a receiving magazine for exposed film. The supply and receiving magazines are lined with lead to protect the unexposed and unprocessed film from radiation.

The exposure chamber contains two radiographic intensifying screens to accommodate 35 × 35 cm double-emulsion film. Before exposure, the screens are separated while a film from the supply magazine is moved into position. During exposure, the screens are pressed against the film to ensure good screen-film contact. After exposure, the screens separate, and the exposed film is moved to the receiving magazine. Precise mechanical and electrical synchronization with the x-ray generator, exposure timer and x-ray tube are essential.

Normally, up to four images-per second can be made, and an 8:1 or 10:1 carbon-fiber focused grid is used. Alternately, a 10-cm air gap may be used. An 800-speed screen-film combination is also normal. The two standard cut-film changers are identified as AOT or Puck.

The AOT film changer is contained in a large, cumbersome cabinet that is usually positioned on the floor under the patient couch (Figure 26-9). The Puck film changer is much smaller and simpler than the AOT film changer. It is mounted on the image-intensifier tower and rotated into the x-ray beam for serial radiography (Figure 26-10).

Charge coupled device. Charge coupled devices (CCDs) are photosensitive silicon chips that are rapidly replacing the television-camera tube in the fluoroscopic chain (Figure 26-11). CCDs are similar in appearance to a computer chip and can be used anywhere that light will be converted to a digital video image. Mammography and CVIR procedures were the first medical imaging applications of CCDs.

The sensitive component of a CCD is a layer of amorphorous silicon. When the silicon is illuminated, an electrical charge is generated, which is then sampled, pixel by pixel, and used to produce a digital image. The CCD is mounted on the output phosphor of the image-intensifier tube and is coupled by fiber optics or a lens system or is directly coupled (Figure 26-12).

The principal advantages of CCDs in most applications, such as camcorder, are its small size and its ruggedness. The principal advantages for medical imaging are listed in Box 26-2.

The spatial resolution of a CCD is determined by its physical size and pixel count. Systems incorporating a 1024 matrix can produce an image with a spatial resolu-

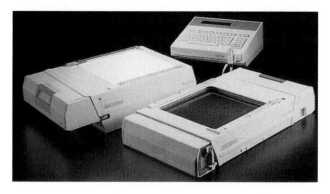

FIGURE 26-10 The Puck film changer can be mounted on the image intensifier and rotated into the x-ray beam or positioned on an independent stand during use. *(Courtesy Elena-Schonander.)*

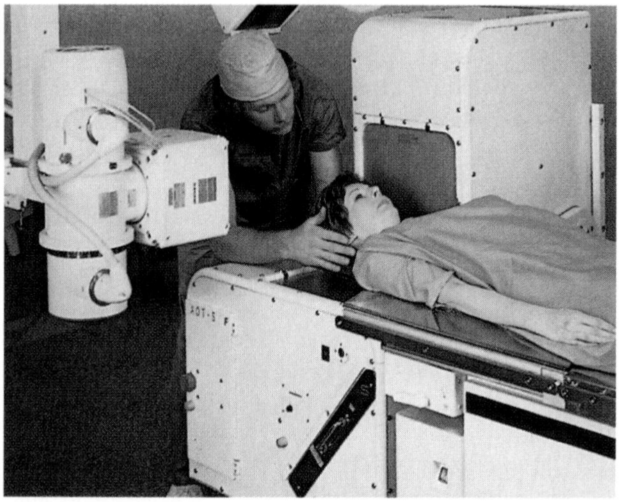

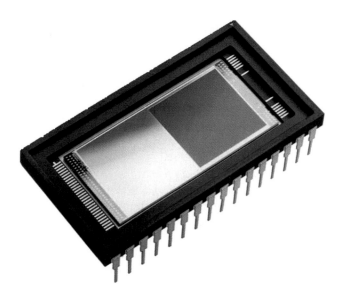

FIGURE 26-11 This CCD can be used in many imaging devices, including x-ray fluoroscopy. *(Courtesy EEV.)*

FIGURE 26-9 The AOT film changer may be positioned with difficulty for vertical or horizontal imaging. *(Courtesy Elema Schonander.)*

tion of 10 lp/mm, which exceeds that of the video chain. Mammographic applications are reaching 15 lp/mm, which is superior to film. Television-camera tubes can show spatial distortion in what is described as *pincushion* or *barrel artifact*. There is no such distortion with a CCD.

The CCD has a higher sensitivity to light (detective quantum efficiency) and lower electron noise than a television camera. The result is a higher signal-to-noise ratio and better contrast resolution. These characteristics also result in substantially lower patient dose.

The response of the CCD to light is very stable. Warmup of the CCD is not required. Neither image lag nor blooming occurs. The CCD has an essentially unlimited life expectancy and requires no maintenance.

Perhaps the single most important feature of CCD imaging is its linear response (see Figure 23-20). Other image receptors have a sigmoid-shaped response, which makes it difficult to image either very dim or very bright objects. Information in the toe and shoulder region of

such a response is lost. This feature is particularly helpful for subtraction imaging. The result is improved dynamic range and better contrast resolution.

The next improvement in this type of imaging will probably be flat-panel imagers composed of silicon pixel detectors (SPD). Such direct x-ray detectors exist in laboratories at this time. Perhaps about the time all television camera tubes are replaced by CCDs, CCDs will begin to be replaced by SPDs.

Filming. After catheter placement during the CVIR procedure, a test injection is done under fluoroscopy before filming to check that the catheter tip is not wedged and is in the correct vessel. Injection rates of the automatic power injector are gauged by the test flow speed. A scout film is obtained by the radiologic technologist to check positioning and exposure factors.

SUMMARY

Angiography refers to the many methods of imaging contrast-filled vessels. Sven-Ivan Seldinger described a method of arterial access that uses an 18-gauge hollow needle with a stylet. Using a guidewire and catheter, radiologists have access to the vascular network without surgery. The common femoral artery is most often used for arterial access in angiography.

There are many catheter-tip designs, and each is used to access specific arteries. The contrast media used are generally nonionic, which reduces the incidence of physiologic problems and adverse reactions in patients undergoing angiographic procedures. During the procedure, the patient's vital signs must be carefully monitored. The most common risk is continued bleeding at the puncture site.

The typical CVIR x-ray tube is designed for magnification, high resolution, and massive heat loads. The patient table is a floating tabletop with a stepping capability to automatically allow imaging from the abdomen to the feet after a single injection of contrast medium.

Cine cameras with 16- or 35-mm frames are used in cardiovascular imaging procedures. Serial changers or digital imaging is generally used for CVIR procedures. With both serial changers and digital imaging, power injection of contrast media and imaging are synchronized to obtain optimal visualization of the vessel of interest.

BOX 26-2   Advantages of CCDs for CVIR

High spatial resolution
High signal-to-noise ratio
High detective quantum efficiency (DQE)
Lack of warm up requirements
Lack of lag or blooming
Lack of spatial distortion
Lack of maintenance requirements
Unlimited life expectancy
Freedom from influence of magnetic fields
Linear response
Lower dose

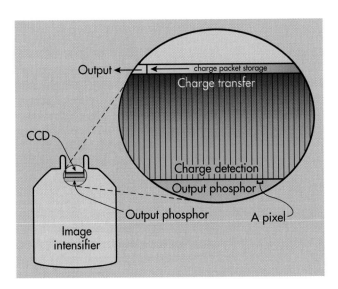

FIGURE 26-12 The CCD is much smaller than a television camera tube and can be coupled directly to the output phosphor of the image-intensifier tube in several ways.

CHALLENGE QUESTIONS

1. Define or otherwise identify:
   a. Contrast media
   b. Angiography
   c. Guidewire
   d. Cinefluorography
   e. Biplane imaging
   f. Stepping

2. Describe cardiac catheterization.

3. What is the Seldinger method for arterial access?

4. Which artery is most commonly used for arterial access in angiography?

5. Why is a guidewire used for arterial access of catheters?

6. List four types of catheters and the vessels for which they are designed.

7. Name two reasons why the radiologist visits the patient before a CVIR procedure.

8. What is the most common problem patients encounter after the CVIR procedure?

9. What are thrombolysis and embolization?

10. What is the required heating capacity of the CVIR x-ray tube?

11. List the focal-spot requirements for the CVIR x-ray tube. For what procedure is the small focal spot used?

12. Name the frame rates for a cine camera.

13. What are the frame rates for the cut-film serial changer?

14. Discuss how subtraction films are obtained during filming of a CVIR procedure.

15. Why are some catheters fenestrated?

16. How does osmolity affect the action of a contrast agent?

17. What initials may an ARRT with a specialty in CVIR place as a title postscript?

CHAPTER

27

Introduction to Computer Science

OBJECTIVES

At the completion of this chapter, the student should be able to:

1. Discuss the history of computers and the role of the transistor
2. Explain the differences among a microcomputer, a minicomputer, and a mainframe computer
3. List and define the components of computer hardware
4. Define *bit*, *byte*, and *word* as used in computer terminology
5. Contrast the two classifications of computer programs: systems software and applications programs
6. List and explain various computer languages
7. Discuss four computer-processing methods

OUTLINE

It is hard to imagine life without computers, or personal computers, to be more exact. From ATMs to supermarket checkouts to automobile ignition systems, computers are integrated into our daily lives.

Computer applications in radiology also continue to grow. The first large-scale radiology application was computed tomography (CT). Computers are used in magnetic resonance imaging (MRI) and diagnostic ultrasound in the same way they are used in CT. Computers control x-ray generators and radiographic control panels, making digital fluoroscopy and radiography routine. Telecommunication systems have provided for the development of teleradiology: the transfer of images and patient data to remote locations for interpretation and filing. Teleradiology has also changed the way that human resources are allocated for these tasks.

HISTORY OF COMPUTERS

The earliest calculating tool, the abacus (Figure 27-1), was invented thousands of years ago in China and is still used in some parts of Asia. In the seventeenth century, two mathematicians, Blaise Pascal and Gottfried Leibniz, built mechanical calculators using pegged wheels that could perform the four basic arithmetic functions of addition, subtraction, multiplication, and division. In 1842, Charles Babbage designed an analytical engine that performed general calculations automatically. Herman Hollerith designed a tabulating machine to record census data in 1890. The tabulating machines stored information as holes on cards that were interpreted by machines with electrical sensors. Hollerith's company later grew to become IBM.

In 1939, John Atanasoff and Clifford Berry designed and built the first electronic digital computer. The first general-purpose modern computer was developed in 1944 at Harvard University. Originally called the *Automatic Sequence Controlled Calculator (ASCC)*, it is now known simply as the *Mark I*. It was an electromechanical device and was exceedingly slow and prone to malfunction.

The first general-purpose electronic computer was developed in 1946 at the University of Pennsylvania by J. Presper Eckert and John Mauchly at a cost of $500,000. This computer called *ENIAC (Electronic Numerical Integrator And Calculator)* contained over 18,000 vacuum tubes that failed at an average of one every 7 minutes. Neither the Mark I nor the ENIAC had its instructions stored in a memory device.

In 1948, scientists led by William Shockley at the Bell Telephone Laboratories developed the transistor. A transistor is an electronic switch that alternately allows or does not allow electronic signals to pass. It also made possible the development of the "stored-program" computer and thus the continuing explosion in computer science.

The transistor allowed Eckert and Mauchly, of the Sperry-Rand Corporation, to develop the UNIVAC (UNIVersal Automatic Computer). It appeared in 1951 as the first commercially successful general-purpose, stored-program electronic digital computer.

Computers have undergone four generations of development distinguished by the technology of their electronic devices. First-generation computers were vacuum-tube machines (1939 to 1958). Second-generation computers, which became generally available in about 1958, were based on individually packaged transistors. Third-generation computers used integrated circuits. Integrated circuits consist of many transistors and other electronic elements fused onto a **chip,** a tiny piece of semiconductor material, usually silicon. They were introduced in 1964. The microprocessor, which used chips, was developed in 1971 by Ted Hoff of Intel Corporation.

The fourth generation of computers, which first appeared in 1975, was an extension of the third generation and incorporated large-scale integration (LSI), now replaced by very-large-scale integration (VLSI), which places hundreds of thousands of circuit elements on a chip less than 1 cm in size (Figure 27-2).

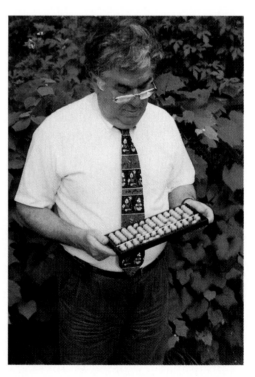

FIGURE 27-1 The abacus is the earliest calculating tool. *(Courtesy Robert J. Wilson.)*

MODERN COMPUTERS

Computer refers to any general-purpose, stored-program electronic digital computer; however, today the word *computer* identifies the personal computer (PC) to most of us. This device is made of both electronic and electromechanical components. *General-purpose* identifies a computer as able to solve any solvable problem. This is unlike *special-purpose* computers, which are designed for a particular singular task, such as control of an assembly-line robot or an automobile ignition switch.

All modern computers are stored program because they have their instructions (programs) and data stored in their memory. These stored-program computers are laid out so that the sequence of steps to be followed during any calculation is already established. *Electronic* implies that the computer is powered by electrical and electronic devices, rather than by a mechanical device.

Today, digital computers have replaced analog computers and the word *digital* is almost synonymous with computer. A timeline showing the evolution of computers shows how rapidly this technology is advancing (Figure 27-3).

 Analog refers to a continuously varying quantity; *digital* quantities vary discretely.

The difference between analog and digital is illustrated in Figure 27-4, which shows two kinds of watches. An analog watch is mechanical and has hands that move continuously around a dial face. A digital watch contains a computer chip and indicates time with numbers. Analog and digital meters are used in many commercial and scientific applications. Digital meters are easier to read and can be more precise.

Computers are distinguished from calculators by their functionality. Calculators can handle only arithmetic functions, whereas computers can handle arithmetic and logic functions: "do," "if," "then," and "else." **Logic functions** evaluate an intermediate result and perform

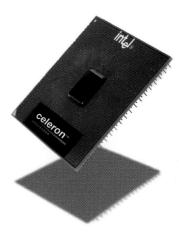

FIGURE 27-2 This Celeron microprocessor incorporates over 1 million transistors on a chip of silicon less than 1 cm on a side. (*Courtesy Intel.*)

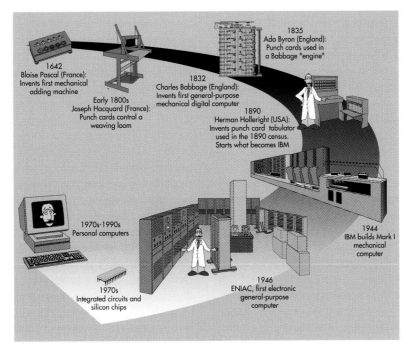

FIGURE 27-3 Timeline of the evolution of the computer.

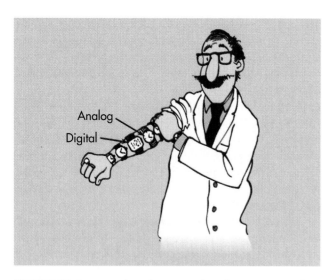

FIGURE 27-4 Two styles of wristwatches demonstrate analog vs. digital.

subsequent computations depending on that result. However, new technology has brought advanced calculators with graphing and limited programming abilities. Now, calculators can execute logic functions, solve equations, draw lines, and transmit data to other calculators via cords or infrared beams.

Computers are also often classified according to size, processing speed, and storage capacity. Distinguishing these types has become more difficult as technology improves, but they are defined as the following categories: supercomputers, mainframe computers, workstations, microcomputers, and microcontrollers.

Supercomputers are the fastest and highest-capacity computers, containing hundreds to thousands of microprocessors. They are often used for research in fields, such as weather forecasting, oil exploration, and mathematics. **Mainframe computers** are fast, medium-sized to large, large-capacity systems that also have multiple microprocessors. They can support a few hundred to thousands of users and are found in airlines, banks, universities, and government. **Workstations** were introduced in the early 1980s and are powerful desktop systems, often used by scientists and engineers. They are often connected to larger computer systems so that users can transfer and share data and information. **Microcomputers**, best known as PCs, also describe electronic organizers and personal data assistants (PDAs), such as palmtop and hand-held systems. **Microcontrollers** are tiny computers installed in calculators and "smart" appliances such as microwave ovens.

A radiographic operating console is controlled by a microcomputer that can consider and control many characteristics of an examination. For example, when body part, size of patient, and image receptor is selected, the microcomputer logically selects the proper radiographic technique.

ANATOMY OF A COMPUTER

There are two principal parts to a computer—hardware and software—each of which have several components. The **hardware** is everything about the computer that is visible: the nuts, bolts, and chips of the system that form the **central processing unit** (CPU) and the various input and output devices. Hardware is usually categorized according to which operation it performs. These operations are input processing, memory, storage, output, and communications. The software is invisible. It consists of the computer programs that tell the hardware what to do and how to store data. Software is discussed later in this chapter.

Hardware

Input. The process of transferring information into primary memory is known as **input.** Input hardware includes keyboards, pointing devices, and source–data entry devices. A keyboard includes the standard typewriter keys that are used to enter words and numbers and specialized keys or functions keys that enter specific commands. Digital fluoroscopy (see Chapter 28) uses function keys for masking, reregistration and time-interval-difference imaging.

 Input hardware converts data into a form that the computer can use.

A mouse is a pointing device that the user rolls on a desktop or mouse pad to direct a pointer on the computer's display screen. The pointer is a symbol, often an arrow, that selects items from lists and menus or positions the cursor on the screen. The cursor indicates the insertion point on the screen where data may be entered next. A trackball is a variant of a mouse, usually found in portable computers. A joystick is a pointing device used primarily in video games and computer-aided design systems. Special joysticks are also available for people with certain disabilities.

Touchpads are small, rectangular devices that allow you to control the cursor with your finger. A light pen connects by a wire to a computer display and when pressed to the screen, identifies that screen position to the computer. Pen-based systems use a penlike instrument to input handwriting and marks into a computer. Pen-based systems are being used in hospitals to enter comments into patient records.

Source–data entry devices include scanners, fax machines, imaging systems, audio and video devices, electronic cameras, voice-recognition systems, sensors, and biologic input devices. Scanners translate images of text, drawings, or photographs into a digital format recognizable by the computer. Bar-code readers, which translate the vertical, black-and-white striped codes on retail products into digital form, are a type of scanner.

An audio input device translates analog sound into digital format. Similarly, video images, such as those from a VCR or camcorder, are digitized by a special video card that can be installed in a computer. The newest cameras and video recorders capture images in digital format that can easily be transferred to computer for immediate access.

Voice-recognition systems add a microphone and audio sound card to a computer and can convert speech into digital format. Radiologists are beginning to use these systems to rapidly produce diagnostic reports and send findings to remote locations via teleradiology.

Sensors collect data directly from the environment and transmit it to a computer. Sensors are used to detect things such as wind speed or temperature.

Human-biology input devices detect specific movements and characteristics of the human body. Security systems that identity a person through a fingerprint or retinal print are examples of these devices.

Processing. The electronic circuitry that does the actual computations and the memory that supports this are called the processing hardware, or **processor.** In large computers, such as mainframes, the processing hardware is the **central processing unit** or **(CPU).** In microcomputers, it is often referred to as the *microprocessor.* Figure 27-5 is a photomicrograph of the Pentium microprocessor manufactured by the Intel Corporation. The Pentium processor is designed for large, high-performance, multiuser and/or multitasking systems.

A computer's processor consists of a control unit and an arithmetic/logic unit (ALU). These two components are connected by an electrical conductor called a *bus* (Figure 27-6). The control unit tells the computer how to perform software instructions, which direct the hardware to perform a task. The control unit directs data to the ALU or to the memory. It also controls data transfer between the main memory and the input and output hardware (Figure 27-7).

The speed of these tasks are determined by an internal system clock. The faster the clock, the faster the processing. Microcomputer processing speeds are usually defined in megahertz (MHz), where 1 MHz equals 1 million cycles per second. Today's microcomputers commonly run at up to 1 gigahertz (GHz), where 1 GHz equals 1000 MHz.

Workstations, microcomputers, and mainframes measure processing speeds as MIPS (millions of instructions per second). Speeds can range from 100 MIPS in a workstation to 1200 MIPS (1.2 BIPS [billions of instructions per second]) in a mainframe. Supercomputer processing is measured in flops (floating-point operations per second) and is represented as megaflops (mflops), gigaflops, and teraflops, which correspond to millions, billions, and trillions of flops.

The ALU performs arithmetic or logic calculations, temporarily holds the results until they can be transferred to memory, and controls the speed of these oper-

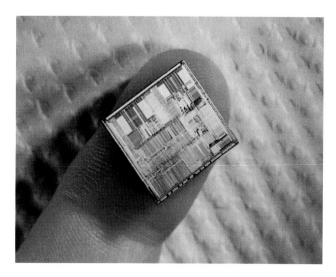

FIGURE 27-5 The width of the conductive lines and spacing in this microprocessor chip is 1.5 μm. *(Courtesy Intel.)*

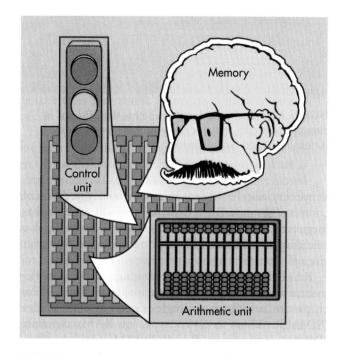

FIGURE 27-6 The CPU contains a control unit, an arithmetic/logic unit, and sometimes memory.

ations. The speed of the ALU is also controlled by the system clock.

Memory. The CPU contains two types of memory: **storage memory,** otherwise known as *main memory,* in which the program and data files are stored, and **active memory.** Active memory is also referred to as **random access memory (RAM),** which means that data can be stored or accessed at random from anywhere in main memory in approximately equal amounts of time, regardless of where the data is located. RAM contents are

process of designing a macro is called recording. The programmer turns the macro recorder on, carries out the steps he wants the macro to carry out and stops the recorder. The macro now knows exactly what the programmer wants implemented and can run the same series of steps over and over.

Other program languages have been developed for other purposes. LOGO is a language designed for children. ADA is the official language approved by the U.S. Department of Defense for software development. It is used principally for military applications and artificial intelligence.

PROCESSING METHODS

Regardless of the operating software or the application programs in use, the essential modes of computer processing are batch, on-line, time-sharing, and real-time systems. The modes often operate together as interactive systems when a short response time between issuing a command and receiving a response is of major importance. Such processing methods are different from batch processing, which offers a relatively long turnaround time but aims at lowering computing costs.

Batch Processing

When a computer is performing operations on defined data without human input or intervention, the computer is said to be *batch processing* data. Depending on the amount of data involved and the operation, the computer could run by itself for weeks.

A batch operating system is the most widely used mode of processing with mainframe computers. The users submit the complete job, which includes the program, the data, and the control statements. After a relatively long time, minutes to hours, the results are available. Normally, the jobs in a batch are processed in sequence, one after the other. This method does not require the user to attend to the system once the batch has started. Batch processing can be handled by a remote job-entry (RJE) system in which users submit their batch jobs to a remote terminal connected to the computer by a cable or modem.

On-Line Systems

In an on-line system, certain transactions are processed immediately. In such a system, the users have multiple access terminals from which they may introduce one or a few of the transactions exclusively. The response comes within seconds. Examples of on-line systems include airline reservation systems, automatic bank tellers, and supermarket checkout systems.

Time-Sharing Systems

The goal of time-sharing systems is to provide the illusion of having the computer dedicated exclusively to each user. Several hundred users, the maximum number depending on the system, may simultaneously interact with the computer.

The time between the user's sign-on and sign-off is called a session. During a typical session, the user does the following:

1. Signs onto the system by presenting a password
2. Enters a program under the control of a text editor
3. Usually saves this program under an assigned name
4. Has the program compiled
5. Runs the program

While the program is being run, the user may interact with it. For example, the user may request the result of a partial execution of a program, or the computer may make a request of the user and then proceed based on the result. This type of system is in use in most large research and development institutions, where multiple user groups must be accommodated.

Real-Time Systems

Real-time systems are most often designed as special-purpose operating systems to provide for fast management of the system hardware. This is the case in most radiologic imaging departments. The processing of the incoming data (for example, from the detectors of a CT imager) is completed in a matter of seconds.

Real-time systems often use special-purpose, high-speed hardware to perform computationally intensive tasks such as image reconstruction and filtering. Pipeline processors work like an assembly line. Different parts of the data are processed by different parts of the processor at the same time. The data move through the processor ("down the pipe") and are fully processed by the time they reach the output device. Array processors perform the same computations in parallel on many items of data at once.

SUMMARY

The word *computer* is used as an abbreviation for any general-purpose, stored-program electronic digital device. *General purpose* means the computer can solve problems. *Stored-program* means the computer has instructions and data stored in its memory. *Electronic* means the computer is powered by electrical and electronic devices. *Digital* means that the display is in discrete values.

There are two principal parts of a computer: the hardware and the software. The hardware is the computer's nuts and bolts. The software is the computer's programs, which tell the hardware what to do.

There are several types of hardware: CPU, control unit, arithmetic logic unit (ALU), memory unit, input and output devices, VDTs, secondary memory devices, printers, and modems.

The basic parts of the software are the bits, bytes, and words. In computer language, a single binary digit, either 0 or 1, is called a *bit*. Bits grouped in bunches of eight are called *bytes*. A word is two bytes. Computer capacity is expressed in bytes or megabytes.

Computers have a specific language for communicating within the software systems and programs. Computers operate on the simplest number system of all: the binary system. There are only two digits: 0 and 1. The computer performs all operations by converting alphabetic characters, decimal values, and logic functions into binary values. Other computer languages allow the programmer to write instructions in a form approaching that of human language.

CHALLENGE QUESTIONS

1. Define or otherwise identify:
   a. Logic function
   b. Modem
   c. Pixel
   d. Teleradiology
   e. Operating system
   f. Input, output
   g. Binary number system

2. Name three computerized operations in diagnostic imaging departments.

3. What is the difference between a calculator and a computer?

4. Explain the differences among the microcomputer, the workstation, and the mainframe computer.

5. What are the two principal parts of a computer and the distinguishing features of each?

6. List and define the several parts of computer hardware.

7. Define *bit, byte,* and *word* as used in computer terminology.

8. Distinguish systems software from applications programs.

9. List several types of computer languages.

10. What is the difference between a CD and a DVD?

11. A memory chip is said to have 256 Mbytes of capacity. If each byte is 8 bits, what is the total bit capacity?

12. What is a high-level computer language?

13. What computer language was the first modern programmers' language?

14. List and define the four computer-processing methods.

15. Describe a CPU. Include its three principal parts and their functions.

16. What input and output devices are commonly used in radiology?

17. Convert the decimal number 147 into binary form.

18. Convert the binary number 110001 into decimal form.

CHAPTER

28

Digital X-Ray Imaging

OBJECTIVES

At the completion of this chapter, the student should be able to:

1. Discuss the use of digital modalities in today's imaging department
2. Relate the research and development of digital imaging
3. Explain the characteristics of digital images, specifically image matrix and dynamic range
4. Discuss the components and use of a digital radiographic system
5. Describe the parts of a digital fluoroscopic system and their functions
6. Explain the picture-archiving and teleradiology systems used in diagnostic imaging departments

OUTLINE

Conventional radiographic and fluoroscopic imaging systems have provided increasingly better diagnostic images for many years, but both systems have limitations. Static radiographic images require processing time that can delay the completion of the examination. Once an image is obtained, there is very little that can enhance the information content. When the examination is complete, the images are in the form of hardcopy film that must be cataloged and stored for future review.

Another and perhaps more severe limitation is the noise inherent in these images. Radiography and fluoroscopy both use area beams (that is, large rectangular beams of x-rays). The Compton-scattered portion of the remnant x-ray beam increases with increasing field size, which increases the noise of the image and severely degrades contrast resolution.

These limitations can be overcome somewhat by incorporating computer technology into diagnostic x-ray imaging. Computer technology is based on transforming the conventional analog images into digital form, processing the digital data, and displaying the images so that they look like conventional images. Such data conversion and manipulation would be impossible if it were not for advanced computer technology.

This chapter introduces the current technology of digital radiography and digital fluoroscopy.

DIGITAL IMAGING

Medical imaging is undergoing a revolutionary change. Since Roentgen's discovery of x-rays, anatomic images have been obtained in basically the same fashion. Now, this is changing very rapidly.

A conventional static radiographic image is made like a shadowgraph: using an x-ray beam that forms an image pattern after transmission through the patient. The image receptor, a screen-film combination, is a device that records this transmitted image directly. Figure 28-1 diagrams the imaging chain for conventional radiography.

Likewise, conventional fluoroscopy produces a shadowgraph-type image on a receptor that directly produces an image from the transmitted x-ray beam. Until the 1960s, a fluoroscopic screen was the image receptor used for this type of dynamic examination. Currently, image-intensifier tubes serve as the image receptor. These tubes are usually electronically coupled to a television monitor for remote viewing, as described in Chapter 25. Figure 28-2 diagrams the components used in conventional fluoroscopy.

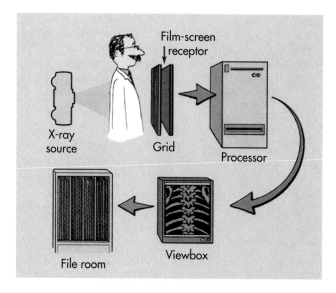

FIGURE 28-1 Imaging chain in conventional radiography.

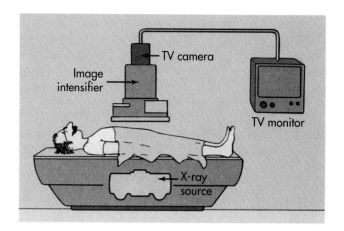

FIGURE 28-2 Imaging chain in conventional fluoroscopy.

 Radiography and fluoroscopy both use large area beams of x-rays.

These conventional radiographic and fluoroscopic systems have served us well for many years, providing increasingly better diagnostic images. However, they both have several limitations. Static radiographic images require processing time that can delay the completion of the examination. This can be particularly bothersome during cardiovascular and interventional procedures and when image-subtraction techniques are required. Once these images are obtained, very little can be done to enhance their information content. When the examination is complete, the images are in the form of hardcopy film that must be cataloged and stored for future review.

Another and perhaps more severe limitation is the noise inherent in these images. The Compton-scattered portion of the remnant x-ray beam increases with increasing field size. This increases the noise of the image and severely degrades low-contrast resolution. The use of grids is only marginally helpful in improving this situation.

These limitations can be overcome somewhat by the incorporation of computer technology into diagnostic x-ray imaging. This approach to imaging is based on transforming the conventional analog images into digital form, processing the digital data in useful ways while displaying it in a manner that makes it appear very much like a conventional image. Such data conversion and manipulation would be impossible if it were not for advanced computer technology.

Digital imaging techniques are applied to computed tomography (CT), diagnostic ultrasound, radioisotope studies, magnetic resonance imaging (MRI), digital radiography, and digital fluoroscopy. Digital radiography and digital fluoroscopy are under continuing development and increasing clinical application. As computer technology advances, so will digital x-ray imaging. Many predict that digital x-ray imaging will replace conventional x-ray imaging in the near future.

Standard nomenclature for identifying the methods of obtaining digital images has not yet been uniformly adopted. Terms such as *digital vascular imaging, digital subtraction angiography, computed radiography, computed fluoroscopy, digital videoangiography, scan beam digital radiography,* and others appear frequently.

Digital fluoroscopy and *digital radiography* are terms that include many different types of image receptors. In the following discussions ***digital fluoroscopy (DF)*** identifies a digital x-ray imaging system that produces a series of dynamic images obtained with an area x-ray beam and an image intensifier. ***Digital radiography (DR)*** refers to the static images produced with either a fan x-ray beam intercepted by a linear array of radiation detectors or an area x-ray beam intercepted by a photostimulable phosphor plate or a direct-capture solid-state device.

Development of Digital Imaging

The development of digital imaging equipment was limited until sufficient computer technology became available to process the large quantities of data generated. The microprocessor and semiconductor memory made this development possible. Digital imaging, first investigated in the early 1970s, developed along two independent lines and became a clinical reality by 1980.

The medical physics groups at the University of Wisconsin and the University of Arizona independently initiated studies of DF in the early 1970s. These studies were continued through the decade by the research and development groups of most manufacturers of x-ray equipment. They used fluoroscopic equipment and placed a computer between the television camera and the television monitor. The video signal from the television camera was routed through the computer, manipulated

in various ways, and transmitted to the television monitor in a form ready for viewing. The initial investigators of DF demonstrated that nearly instantaneous, high-contrast subtraction images could be obtained after intravenous injection of contrast media. Although the intravenous route is still widely used, intraarterial injections are also used with DF. ***The two distinct advantages of DF over conventional fluoroscopy are the speed of image acquisition and the postprocessing that can enhance image contrast.***

DR has enjoyed a similar path of development by a number of different investigators. One approach, developed in the late 1970s to complement CT, uses a narrow fan beam of x-rays that intercepts a linear array of radiation detectors and is called **scanned projection radiography (SPR)**. The signal from each detector is computer manipulated to reconstruct an image. A second approach to DR was developed by Fuji, also in the late 1970s, and has been advanced and marketed by a number of x-ray companies. Referred to as **computed radiography (CR)**, it uses a photostimulable phosphor as the image receptor and an area beam. (Both SPR and CR are discussed later in this chapter.) Currently, much research is devoted to the development of direct-capture solid-state devices such as selenium, silicon, and thin-film transistors (TFTs), which eliminate screen-film but not grids.

Although the image in digital x-ray techniques may appear as a conventional video or radiographic image, it is not. It is formed of individual image elements.

Image Characteristics

The image obtained in digital x-ray procedures is unlike that obtained in conventional fluoroscopy or radiography, in which x-rays form an image directly on the image receptor. With digital techniques, x-rays form an electronic latent image on a radiation detector array. The latent image is then manipulated by a computer, temporarily stored in memory, and displayed as a matrix of intensities, each having a dynamic range of values. Dynamic range is the range of values over which a system can respond (also known as *gray-scale range*).

Image matrix. The term **image matrix** refers to a layout of cells in rows and columns. Each cell corresponds to a specific location in the image. The number in the cell represents the brightness or intensity at that location. Figure 28-3 shows a 10×10 matrix of cells, a 5×5 matrix of cells, and a 5×5 matrix of numbers in imaginary cells, and Figure 28-4 shows the associated image. Each digital image consists of a matrix of cells having various brightness levels on the video monitor. The brightness of a cell is determined by the computer-generated number stored in that cell.

Each cell of the image matrix is called a **pixel** (*picture element*). In digital x-ray imaging, the value of the pixel

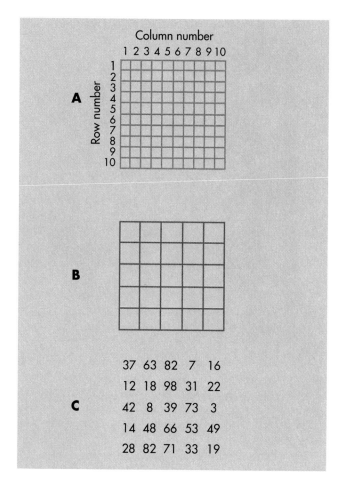

FIGURE 28-3 *Matrix* refers to an arrangement of columns and rows. Three matrices are shown. **A,** 10 × 10 matrix of cells. **B,** 5 × 5 matrix of cells. **C,** 5 × 5 matrix of numbers in imaginary cells.

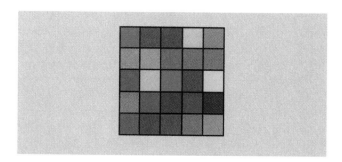

FIGURE 28-4 Associated image of the matrix in Figure 28-3, **C.**

determines pixel brightness. The value is relative and is used to provide subtraction images and define the image contrast. In CT imaging, the numerical value of each pixel is a CT number, or **Hounsfield unit (HU)**. The value of the HU can be manipulated to judge the composition of the tissue represented. In MRI, diagnostic ultrasound, and nuclear medicine the numeric value of the

TABLE 28-1	Pixel Value as a Function of Tissue Characteristics
Image Modality	**Tissue Characteristic**
Radiography and fluoroscopy	Atomic number, mass density
CT	Atomic number, mass density
Nuclear medicine	Radionuclide uptake
Diagnostic ultrasound	Interface reflectivity
MRI	Spin density, spin relaxation

pixel also has a relationship to the composition of the tissue imaged (Table 28-1).

The size of the image matrix is determined by characteristics of the imaging equipment and by the capacity of the computer. Matrix size can usually be selected by the operator. Most digital x-ray imaging systems provide image matrix sizes, or **fields of view (FOV)** of 512 × 512 and 1024 × 1024. For the same FOV, spatial resolution is better with a larger image matrix.

Question: How many pixels are contained in an image matrix described as 256 × 256?

Answer: 256 × 256 = 65,536 pixels

A 1024 × 1024 image matrix is sometimes described as a 1000-line system. In DF the spatial resolution is determined both by the image matrix and by the size of the image intensifier. A rough estimate of the theoretic limits of spatial resolution can be obtained by dividing the size of the input phosphor of the image intensifier tube by the matrix size, as follows:

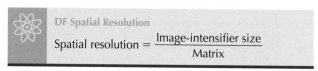

DF Spatial Resolution
$$\text{Spatial resolution} = \frac{\text{Image-intensifier size}}{\text{Matrix}}$$

Question: What is the pixel size of a 1000-line DF system operating in the 5-in mode?

Answer: A total of 5 in equals 127 mm (5 × 25.4 mm/in). Therefore the size of each pixel is as follows:
$$\frac{127 \text{ mm}}{1024} = 0.124 \text{ mm}$$

Figure 28-5 illustrates the influence of matrix size on image quality. A 32 × 32 image matrix appears definitely "boxy," whereas a 512 × 512 image is a good representation of the original analog image.

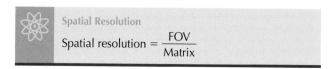

Spatial Resolution
$$\text{Spatial resolution} = \frac{\text{FOV}}{\text{Matrix}}$$

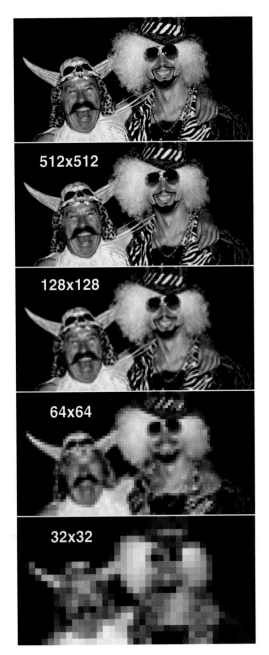

FIGURE 28-5 This Zulu king and his Mardi Gras consort (actually Louisiana RTs) posed to illustrate the improvement in spatial resolution with larger matrix size. *(Courtesy Reanette Lejeune.)*

The size of the image matrix and FOV determines the spatial resolution for direct digital images, such as CT, MRI, and digital ultrasound. **Spatial resolution in digital imaging can be no better than the size of a pixel.**

The future of total digital imaging is dictated by the requirements of chest imaging. There has been much effort to define these requirements. With a 14 × 14 in chest image as the standard, the accepted minimal spatial resolution requires an image matrix size of 2048

× 2048. If there is less than that, spatial resolution may be unacceptable.

Question: What is the pixel size for a 14 × 14 in digital image reconstructed on a 2048 × 2048 matrix?

Answer: 14 in × 25.4 mm/in = 355.6 mm

$$\frac{355.6 \text{ mm}}{2048 \text{ pixels}} = 0.17 \text{ mm/pixel}$$

Dynamic range. An imaging system that could display only black or white would have a dynamic range of 2^1, or 2. Such an image would be very high contrast but would display very little information. Although the actual value of each pixel is important, the range of values is extremely important in determining the final image.

> The range of values over which a system can respond is called its *gray-scale range* or *dynamic range.*

Dynamic range in a digital system corresponds to the numerical range of each pixel. Visually, *dynamic range* refers to the number of shades of gray that can be represented.

The dynamic range of the human eye is approximately 2^5, or 32, shades of gray stretching from white to black. The dynamic range of the x-ray beam as it exits the patient is in excess of 2^{10}. Although humans cannot visualize such a dynamic range, a computer with sufficient capacity can.

The larger the dynamic range, the more gradual the gray scale representing the range from maximal to minimal x-ray intensity. The greater the dynamic range therefore the better the contrast resolution. This is particularly true of images from **subtraction techniques,** the process of removing stationary tissue from an image and leaving only constant-enhanced anatomy.

Digital x-ray imaging systems are characterized by their dynamic range, which is determined by the capacity of the computer and the software. Most use an 8-, 10-, or 12-bit dynamic range, meaning a 2^8, 2^{10}, or 2^{12} dynamic range. The signal that characterizes the x-ray intensity of the image is converted into digital form. The digital form is displayed as an image matrix, where each pixel is capable of a range of 2^8 (0 to 256), 2^{10} (0 to 1024), or 2^{12} (0 to 4096).

> For acceptable contrast resolution on radiographic, CT, and MR images, a 12-bit dynamic range is usually required.

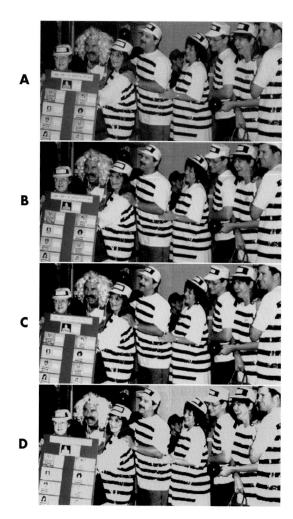

FIGURE 28-6 Image of Texas jailbirds illustrates the concept of dynamic range. **A,** Original image. **B,** 12-bit dynamic range. **C,** 10-bit dynamic range. **D,** 8-bit dynamic range.

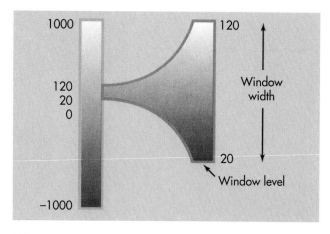

FIGURE 28-7 Windowing a digital image controls the image contrast and OD.

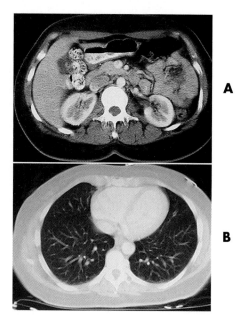

FIGURE 28-8 The selection of window level depends on the anatomy imaged. **A,** The soft tissues of the abdomen require a low window level (level, 50; width, 400). **B,** The lung fields require a very negative window level (level, 500; width, 1500). *(Courtesy Nancy Adams.)*

Figure 28-6 illustrates the effect of dynamic range on the image. Clearly a system with low dynamic range is high contrast but only over a limited portion of the image. A high dynamic range allows for a wide image latitude. The contrast of a region of interest (ROI) of the image can be enhanced if the computer system has sufficient dynamic range. When a subtraction examination is undertaken, the information contained in the final image is far greater for a system with high dynamic range.

Because some radiologists are reluctant to diagnose from a console with a cathode ray tube (CRT), the radiologic technologist is responsible for producing film images from the CRT of proper optical density and contrast. This is done by using a postprocessing computer, which allows one to see only a "window" of the entire dynamic range. This technique is called **windowing.**

The two characteristics of the window are window level and window width (Figure 28-7). **Window level** identifies the type of tissue to be imaged. For instance, a CT window level of approximately 50 best images abdominal tissue, whereas a window level of approximately −500 best images lung tissue (Figure 28-8). **Window width** determines the gray-scale rendition of that tissue and therefore image contrast. The wider the window width, the longer the gray scale. Narrow window widths produce high contrast (Figure 28-9).

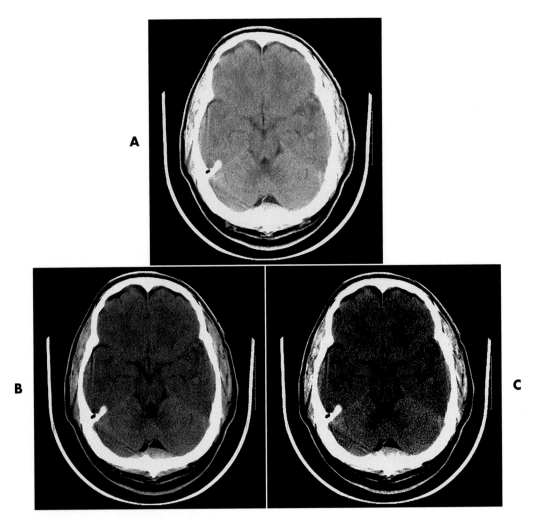

FIGURE 28-9 These brain scans show the loss of contrast with increasing window width. **A,** Level, 40; width 44. **B,** Level, 40; width, 80. **C,** Level, 40; width, 168. *(Courtesy Mike Enrique.)*

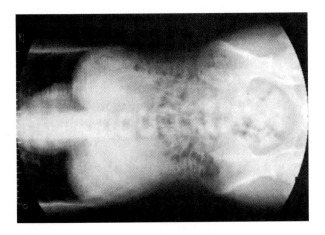

FIGURE 28-10 This CR is typical of SPRs obtained with CT scanners. *(Courtesy Larry Rothenberg.)*

DIGITAL RADIOGRAPHY

DR is developing along several paths. It differs from conventional radiography because film is not the image receptor. It uses radiation detectors whose electrical output is proportional to the radiation intensity. Initially, this output signal is in analog form, but it is converted to digital form. The image is displayed on a video monitor after computer processing.

Scanned Projection Radiography

Perhaps the first clinically useful application of DR was a complement to CT developed by General Electric Medical Systems. This has come to be known as *scanned projection radiography (SPR)*. Basically, SPR involves the use of the existing CT gantry and computer to generate an image that looks surprisingly like a conventional radiograph (Figure 28-10).

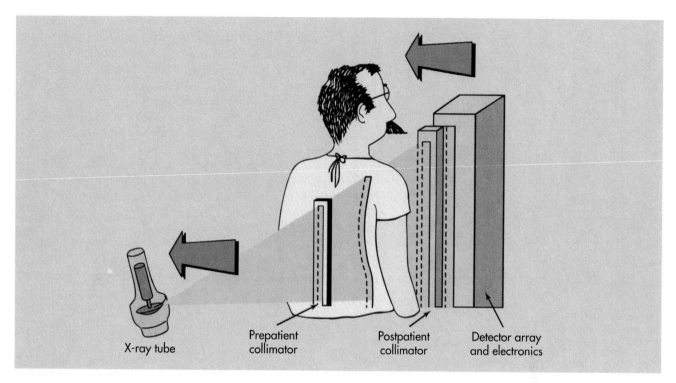

FIGURE 28-11 Components of an SPR system. *(Courtesy Gary Barnes.)*

This image is similar to a conventional radiographic image because there is superposition of tissues through the body. It differs from a conventional image in that it is virtually free of scatter radiation and is digital in form. This reduced scatter radiation results from the fan beam collimation and produces enhanced radiographic contrast. The digital form of the image permits subtraction techniques as described for DF and provides for other types of image manipulation.

The basic component of an SPR system is an x-ray beam shaped into a fan by collimators that confine the beam to a 2- to 10-mm thickness through an arc of 30 to 45 degrees (Figure 28-11). There are two collimators. The prepatient collimators shape the beam, reduce scatter radiation, and control patient dose. The postpatient collimators further reduce scatter radiation.

On passing through the patient and postpatient collimators, the image-forming x-rays are intercepted by a detector array. Each detector responds with a signal that is related to the body part through which the x-ray beam passed. The response of the total detector array thus represents an attenuation profile of that body section.

Another way to view the production of the high-contrast image in DR is to consider that the reduction in scattered x-rays decreases the noise in the image. Remember that Compton-scattered x-rays carry no useful information but simply contribute to the background noise of an image. Consequently, in DR the radiographic contrast is high, and the detection of low-contrast objects is improved.

 In any imaging system, noise is the principal limitation to imaging low-contrast objects.

The principal disadvantage with DR is its poor spatial resolution. Whereas a conventional screen-film system can image 100-μm objects, SPR cannot image objects smaller than approximately 500 μm. However, this degree of resolution is adequate for most examinations. In DR, resolution is controlled principally by the design of the detector array and the speed with which the patient or x-ray beam is translated, or moved.

 The more detectors there are per degree of fan x-ray beam, the better the spatial resolution.

As the speed of translation, or sweeping movement, is increased, fewer x-rays are detected because the translation of the patient through the x-ray beam or the translation of the beam across the patient decreases the resulting image quality by reducing high- and low-contrast resolution.

Obtaining enough profiles for a complete image requires that the source-detector assembly remain stationary and the patient be translated through the x-ray beam. Alternatively, the patient may remain stationary while the source-detector assembly translates. During translation, either the x-ray beam is pulsed, or each detector is sampled intermittently. The sequential profiles

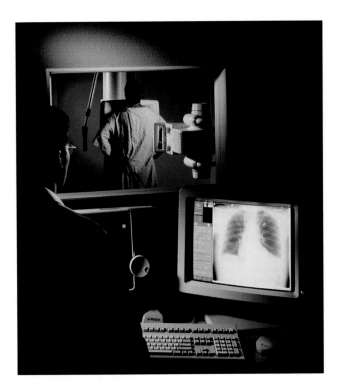

FIGURE 28-12 Dedicated DR chest unit. *(Courtesy GE Medical Systems.)*

obtained during translation are computer-processed to form an image resembling a radiograph.

SPR designs with patient translation are incorporated into most CT scanners. After proper positioning of the x-ray tube detector array, anterior-posterior, posterior-anterior, lateral, and oblique views can be obtained.

X-Ray Tube and Detector Assembly

An x-ray tube used for DR must have a high heat capacity. A heat capacity in excess of 1 MHU is usually required. The requirement for high heat capacity occurs because of two characteristics of the system: imaging time and detector efficiency. Usually 20 to 50 cm of the patient is imaged at a translation speed of 1 to 2 cm/s. The detectors may not be intrinsically as efficient as a screen-film receptor, and because of the precise beam collimation, few scattered x-rays reach the detectors. Consequently, techniques of 500 to 2000 mAs are required.

Two basic designs are used in the detector array: a gas-filled detector assembly and scintillation detectors coupled to solid-state photodiodes. Similar designs are described in relation to CT (see also Chapter 29).

The gas-filled detector array usually contains xenon under high pressure in many small chambers. Xenon is used because of its high atomic number, 53, which results in high photoelectric absorption. The individual detector chamber can be made as small as 0.5 mm with an even smaller interspace.

The solid-state scintillation detector array incorporates individual crystal-photodiode assemblies. Such an array usually presents an active area to the x-ray beam of 5 × 20 mm with an interspace between detectors of 1 mm. This results in a limit to the number of detectors that can be incorporated.

The scintillation crystal used is cadmium tungstate ($CdWO_4$), although bismuth germinate (BGO), cesium iodide (CsI), and sodium iodide (NaI) have also been used. The photodiode is a semiconductor material, usually silicon or germanium, whose output signal is proportional to the intensity of light striking it.

Area Beam and Fan Beam

A principal limitation of the SPR mode of DR is the time required to obtain an image. In conventional radiography a latent image is produced in a matter of milliseconds. When a fan beam, an x-ray beam pattern projected as a slit, is used in DR, an exposure of several seconds may be required, and thus image blur may be increased because of patient motion.

The image-acquisition time in DR can be reduced by decreasing the translation time in SPR or by using an area beam (an x-ray beam pattern projected as a square or rectangle) with an image receptor, as in conventional radiography. There is nothing special in providing an area beam. It is difficult, however, to fabricate an area image receptor that will retain the rapid response time required.

Three approaches are available for the use of an area beam for DR. An assembly of solid-state detectors formed in matrix fashion can be used. The electronics associated with the enormous number of detectors required is quite sophisticated, and therefore the expense can be excessive. The use of charge coupled device (CCD) is described in Chapter 26, and it can be used for DR. The use of a photostimulable phosphor as a replacement for screen-film was the first application of an area beam for DR. A dedicated DR imager is shown in Figure 28-12.

Computed Radiography

Directly acquired DR images with a photostimulable phosphor as a solid-state image receptor in plate form can also be used as a detector. This process is called *computed radiography (CR)* and is shown schematically in Figure 28-13. The image receptor resembles a conventional radiographic intensifying screen and is exposed in a cassette with conventional x-ray equipment. It is composed of europium-activated barium fluorohalide compounds, which are energized when exposed to x-rays. The sensitivity is approximately equal to that of a 200-speed screen-film combination and can be much greater when contrast resolution is sacrificed. The latent image consists of valence electrons stored in high-energy traps.

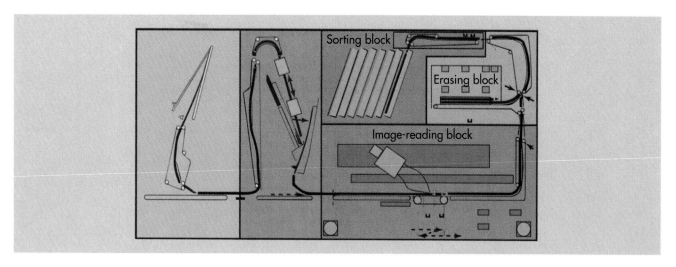

FIGURE 28-13 Process of CR using photostimulable phosphors. *(Courtesy Fuji Photo Company.)*

The latent image is made manifest by exposure to a very narrow beam from a high-intensity laser. The laser beam causes the trapped electrons to return to the valence band with the emission of blue light. This is called *optically stimulated luminescence* and is described in Chapters 16 and 40.

The blue emission is viewed by an ultrasensitive photomultiplier tube. The electronic signal, which is the output of the photomultiplier tube, is digitized and stored for subsequent display on a console with a CRT or a hardcopy from a laser printer.

The spatial resolution of CR is not quite as good as that of conventional radiography, but the contrast resolution is better because of image postprocessing modes. The latitude of the system is exceptional, and for many examinations, patient dose is considerably less.

Direct-Capture Radiography

CR has been in use in clinics for nearly 20 years. In the late 1990s, two totally new approaches to direct-capture DR appeared. It is too early to tell which will prevail or whether the two approaches will complement each other.

Both direct-capture systems are based on TFTs fashioned as an active matrix array (AMA). The result is a flat-panel image receptor the size of conventional screen-film receptors. Direct-capture technology can perform fluoroscopically as well as radiographically.

The first approach of direct-capture radiography uses a CsI scintillation phosphor coated over an AMA of amorphous silicon (a-Si) photo diodes (Figure 28-14). The term *amorphous* describes a noncrystalline state of an otherwise crystalline material. In the amorphous state, the silicon is easily coated on the AMA at controlled thickness. Image-forming x-rays interact with the CsI, producing light, which in turn interacts with the a-Si to produce a signal (Figure 28-15). The TFT stores the signal until readout, one pixel at a time.

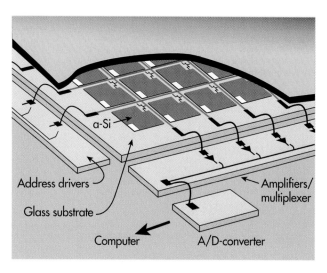

FIGURE 28-14 Direct-capture DR images can be formed from the CsI phosphor light detected by silicon photodiodes.

The second approach does not use a phosphor coating. Image-forming x-rays interact directly with a thin layer of amorphous selenium (a-Se), creating electron-hole pairs (Figure 28-16). The electron-hole pair is the signal that charges the AMA of TFTs. The advantage of the a-Se approach is that there is no spreading of light in the phosphor and therefore there is improved spatial resolution (Figure 28-17). On the other hand, the CsI phosphor has a high detective quantum efficiency, and therefore it results in lower dose.

With both systems, the latent image is electronic and is stored in the TFT array. This array is read sequentially from one TFT to another through precise electronic control (Figure 28-18). The array of TFTs is such that each TFT and its x-ray detector represents a pixel. Consequently, spatial resolution is limited by the pixel size. Available pixel size is limited to approximately 100

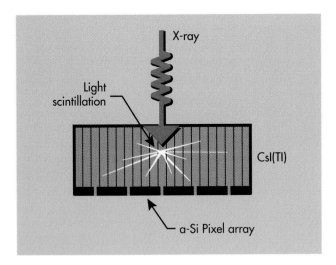

FIGURE 28-15 The CsI phosphor in DR image receptors is in the form of crystalline channels to better confine light dispersion.

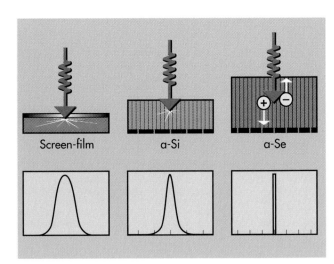

FIGURE 28-17 CsI phosphor detection has better dose efficiency, whereas a-Se can provide better spatial resolution.

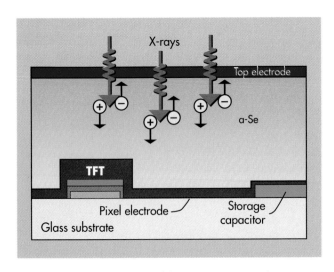

FIGURE 28-16 In this type of direct-capture DR, electron-hole pairs are generated and detected by the active matrix array of thin-film transistors.

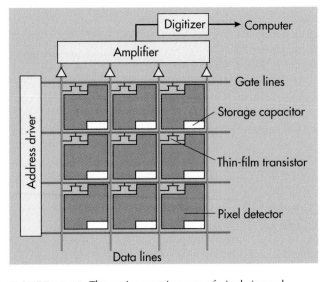

FIGURE 28-18 The active matrix array of pixels is read sequentially one pixel at a time.

μm, which is equivalent to a spatial resolution of 5 lp/mm (Figure 28-19). Much smaller pixels are being developed.

Although the detective quantum efficiency, and therefore patient dose, is determined principally by atomic number of the detector, $Z_{CsI} = 55/53$, $Z_{Se} = 34$, the geometry of each pixel is also very important (Figure 28-20). A portion of the pixel face is occupied by electronic conductors and the TFT. The "filling factor" is the percentage of the pixel face that contains the x-ray detector. The filling factor is approximately 80%.

Direct-capture radiography has all of the advantages of other digital imaging techniques: postprocessing, a

picture archiving and communications system, and teleradiology. The future is very bright for this modality.

DIGITAL FLUOROSCOPY

A DF examination is conducted in much the same manner as a conventional study. To the casual observer the equipment used is the same, but this is not the case (Figure 28-21). DF requires a computer, two video monitors, and a more complex operating console.

Figure 28-22 shows a representative digital fluoroscopic operating console, which controls examination technique and displays the results of image manipulation. The operating console contains alphanumeric

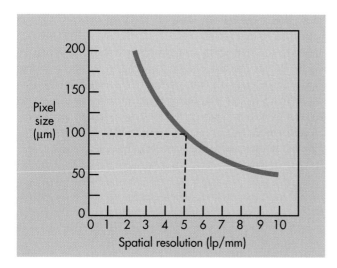

FIGURE 28-19 The pixel size is approximately 100 μm square, which results in limiting spatial resolution of 5 lp/mm.

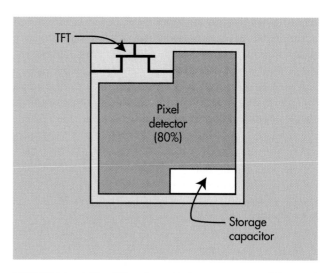

FIGURE 28-20 The filling factor is the percentage of the pixel element occupied by the sensitive image receptor.

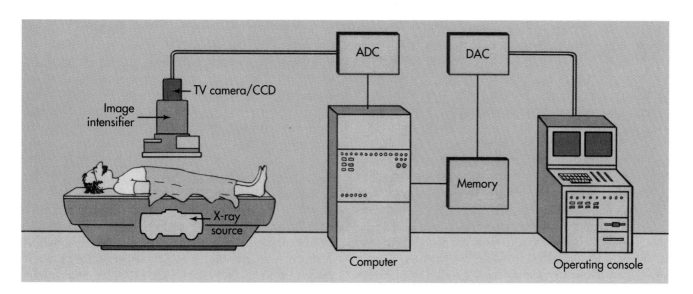

FIGURE 28-21 Components of a DF system.

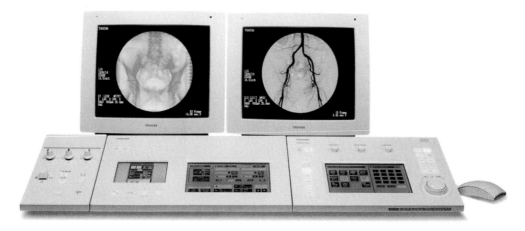

FIGURE 28-22 Operating console for a DF system. *(Courtesy Toshiba.)*

and special function keys for entering patient data and communicating with the computer. The console also contains additional special function keys for data acquisition, image display, and image postprocessing.

Two video screens are needed; one screen is used to edit patient and examination data and to annotate final images, and the other displays subtracted images.

High-Voltage Generator

During DF, the undertable x-ray tube actually operates in the radiographic mode. The tube current is measured in hundreds of milliamperes instead of less than 5 mA, as in image-intensifying fluoroscopy. This is not a problem, however, because the tube is not energized continuously. (If the tube were energized continuously, it would fail because of thermal overloading, and the patient dose would be exceedingly high.) Images from DF are obtained by pulsing the x-ray beam in much the same fashion that rapid film changer images are obtained in cardiovascular and interventional radiology (see Chapter 26).

 During DF, the x-ray tube operates in the radiographic mode.

Image acquisition rates of 1 to 10 per second are common in many examinations. Since it requires 33 ms to produce one video frame, x-ray exposures longer than that can result in unnecessary patient dose. That is a theoretic limit, however, and longer exposures may be necessary to ensure low noise and good image quality. Consequently, the x-ray generator must be capable of switching on and off very rapidly. The time required for the x-ray tube to be switched on and reach the selected level of kVp and mA is called the **interrogation time.** The time required for the x-ray tube to be switched off is the **extinction time.** It is necessary that DF systems incorporate three-phase or high-frequency generators with interrogation and extinction times of less than 1 ms.

Video System

The video system used in conventional fluoroscopy is usually a 525-line system. Such a system is adequate for DF, although higher spatial resolution can be obtained with 1000-line systems. Conventional video, however, has two limitations that restrict its application in digital techniques. First, the interlaced mode of reading the target of the television camera can significantly degrade a digital image. Second, conventional television-camera tubes are relatively noisy. They have a signal-to-noise (SNR) ratio of about 200:1, whereas an SNR ratio of 1000:1 is necessary for DF.

Interlace vs. progressive mode. In Chapter 25, the method by which a conventional television-camera tube reads its target assembly is described. That method is called an *interlace mode,* in which two fields of 262½

lines each were read in $\frac{1}{60}$ s (17 ms) to form a 525-line video frame in $\frac{1}{30}$ s (33 ms).

In DF the television-camera tube reads in progressive mode. When the video signal is read in the progressive mode, the electron beam of the television-camera tube sweeps the target assembly continuously from top to bottom in 33 ms (Figure 28-23). The video image is similarly formed on the television monitor. There is no interlace of one field with another, which results in a sharper image with less flicker.

Signal-to-noise ratio. All electronic devices are inherently noisy. Because of heated filaments and voltage differences, there is always a very small electric current flowing in any circuit. This is called *background electronic noise.* It is similar to the noise (fog) on a radiograph in that it conveys no information and serves only to obscure the electronic signal.

Since conventional television-camera tubes have an SNR of about 200:1, the maximum output signal will be 200 times greater than the background electronic noise. This is not sufficient for DF because the video signal is rarely at maximum and lower signals become even more lost in the noise, especially when subtraction techniques are used. Image contrast resolution is severely degraded by a system with a low SNR.

Figure 28-24 illustrates the difference between the output of a 200:1 and a 1000:1 television-camera tube. At 200:1, the dynamic range is less than 2^8, and at 1000:1, it is about 2^{10}. The tube with a 1000:1 SNR contains five times the useful information and is more compatible with computer-assisted image enhancement.

Computer

Minicomputers are widely used by DF systems. The capacity of the computer is an important factor in determining image quality, the manner and speed of image acquisition, and image processing and manipulation. Important characteristics of a DF system that are computer controlled are the image matrix size, the system dynamic range, and the image acquisition rate.

The output signal from the television-camera tube is transmitted by cable to an analog-to-digital converter

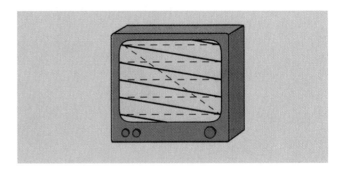

FIGURE 28-23 Progressive mode of reading a video signal.

(ADC). The ADC accepts the continuously varying analog signal of the television camera and converts it to digital numbers.

To be compatible with the computer, the ADC must have the same dynamic range as the computer. An 8-bit ADC would convert the analog signal into values of 0 to 255. A 10-bit ADC would be more precise, with an analog-to-digital conversion range of 0 to 2^{10}, or 0 to 1023.

The output of the ADC is then transferred to the main memory and manipulated so that a digital image in matrix form is stored. The dynamic range of each pixel, the number of pixels, and the method of storage determine the speed at which the image can be acquired, processed, and transferred to an output device.

If image storage is in primary memory, which is usually the case, then data acquisition and transfer occur as rapidly as 30 images per second. In general, if the image matrix is doubled (for example, from 512 × 512 to 1024 × 1024), the image acquisition rate will be reduced by a factor of four. A representative system might be capable of acquiring 30 images per second in the 512 × 512 mode. However, if a higher spatial resolution image is required and the 1024 × 1024 mode is requested, then only 8 images per second can be acquired. This limitation on data transfer is imposed because of the time required to conduct the enormous quantities of data from one segment of memory to another.

Image Formation

The principal advantages of DF examinations are the image-subtraction techniques that are possible and the ability to visualize vasculature with a venous injection of contrast material. Unfortunately, an area beam must be used, which reduces image contrast because of the associated scatter radiation. Image contrast, however, can be enhanced electronically. Image contrast is improved by subtraction techniques that provide instantaneous viewing of the subtracted image during the passage of a bolus of contrast medium.

 DF provides better contrast resolution via postprocessing image subtraction.

Two methods, temporal subtraction and energy subtraction, can be used to enhance image contrast in DF. Each has distinct advantages and disadvantages (Table 28-2.) Temporal subtraction techniques are most frequently used because of the limitations of the high-voltage generator in the energy-subtraction mode. When the two techniques are combined, the process is called *hybrid subtraction*. Image contrast is enhanced still further by hybrid subtraction because of reduced patient motion between subtracted images.

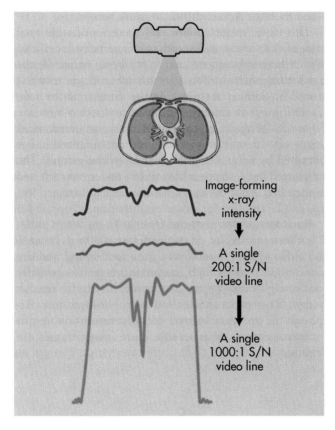

FIGURE 28-24 The information content of a video system with a high SNR is greatly enhanced. Shown here are a single video line through an object and the resulting signal at 200:1 and 1000:1 SNRs.

TABLE 28-2	Comparison of Temporal and Energy Subtraction
Temporal Subtraction	**Energy Subtraction**
A single kVp is used.	Rapid kVp switching is required.
Normal x-ray beam filtration is adequate.	X-ray beam filter switching is preferred.
A contrast resolution of 1 mm at 1% is achieved.	Higher x-ray intensity is required for comparable contrast resolution.
Simple arithmetic image subtraction is necessary.	Complex image subtraction is necessary.
Motion artifacts are a problem.	Motion artifacts are greatly reduced.
Total subtraction of common structures is achieved.	Some residual bone may survive subtraction.
Subtraction possibilities are limited by the number of images.	Many more types of subtraction images are possible.

Reregistration can be a tedious process. Often, when one area of an image is reregistered, another area becomes misregistered. This can be controlled on some systems by ROI reregistration. Most systems can reregister not only in increments of pixel widths but also down to one tenth of a pixel width.

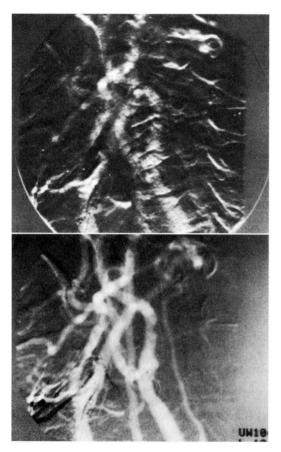

FIGURE 28-29 Misregistration artifacts. *(Courtesy Ben Arnold.)*

FIGURE 28-30 Photoelectric absorption in iodine, bone, and muscle.

Energy subtraction. Temporal-subtraction techniques take advantage of changing contrast media during the time of the examination and require no special demands on the high-voltage generator. **Energy subtraction** uses two x-ray beams alternately to provide a subtraction image resulting from differences in photoelectric interaction. The basis for this technique is similar to that described in Chapter 16 for rare earth screens. It is based on the abrupt change in photoelectric absorption at the K edge of the contrast media compared with that for soft tissue and bone.

Figure 28-30 shows the probability of x-ray interaction with iodine, bone, and muscle as a function of x-ray energy. The probability of photoelectric absorption in all three decreases with increasing x-ray energy. At an energy of 33 keV, there is an abrupt increase in the absorption in iodine and a modest decrease in soft tissue and bone.

This energy corresponds to the binding energy of the two K-shell electrons of iodine. When the incident x-ray energy is sufficient to overcome the K-shell electron binding energy of iodine, there is an abrupt and large increase in absorption. Graphically, this increase is known as the *K absorption edge.*

If monoenergetic x-ray beams of 32 and 34 keV (E_1 and E_2, respectively, in Figure 28-30) could be used alternately, the difference in absorption in iodine would be enormous, and the resulting subtraction images would have very high contrast. Such is not the case, however, since every x-ray beam contains a wide spectrum of energies.

Energy subtraction has the decided disadvantage of requiring some method of providing an alternating x-ray beam of two different emission spectra. Two methods have been devised: (1) alternately pulsing the x-ray beam at 70 kVp and then 90 kVp and (2) introducing dissimilar metal filters into the x-ray beam alternately on a fly wheel.

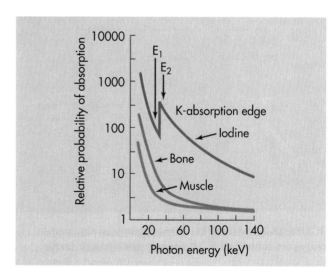

Hybrid subtraction. Some DF systems are capable of combining temporal- and energy-subtraction techniques into what is called **hybrid subtraction** (Figure 28-31). Image acquisition follows the mask-mode procedure as previously described. In hybrid subtraction, however, the mask and each subsequent image are formed by an energy-subtraction technique. If patient motion can be controlled, hybrid imaging can theoretically produce the highest-quality DF images.

Patient Dose

One potential advantage of DF is reduced patient dose. DF images appear to be continuous, but in fact they are discrete. Most DF x-ray beams are pulsed to fill one or more 33-ms video frames; therefore the fluoroscopic dose rate is lower than that for continuous analog fluoroscopy even though the mA may be higher.

Static images with DF are also made with a lower dose per frame than with a 105-mm spot-film camera. Both the television-camera tube and a CCD have higher sensitivity than the spot film. Table 28-3 compares a representative fluoroscopic study performed conventionally vs. digitally.

Digital spot images are so easy to acquire that it is possible to make more exposures than is necessary. If the fluoroscopist gets carried away, any patient dose savings will disappear.

PICTURE ARCHIVING AND COMMUNICATION SYSTEM

Radiology is adopting digital imaging at the expense of analog images on film. Estimates of the present level of digitally acquired images range up to 70%. These images come from nuclear medicine, digital ultrasound, DR, DF, CT, and MRI. Analog images, such as conventional radiographs, also can be digitized (Figure 28-32). Film digitizers are based on laser beam technology.

A picture archiving and communication system (PACS), when fully implemented, allows not only the acquisition but also the interpretation and storage of each medical image in digital form without resorting to film. The projected savings in time and money are enormous. The three principal components of a PACS are the display system, the network, and the storage system.

Display System

The heart of a PACS display system is the CRT monitor of a video workstation (Figure 28-33). To truly replace film viewing, the CRT monitors must be high resolution, at least 2048 × 2048. Present image matrices used with most digitally acquired images range from 256 × 256 to 1024 × 1024, which is considerably less than that required to equal the spatial resolution of film; however, PACS are equipped with a keyboard control for the various image-processing modes.

TABLE 28-3	Approximate Patient Dose in a Representative Fluoroscopic Examination	
	PATIENT DOSE	
Imaging Mode	**Conventional**	**Digital**
5-minute fluoroscopy	20 rad	10 rad
3 spot films: normal mode	0.6 rad	0.15 rad
3 spot films: magnified mode	1.0 rad	0.3 rad
TOTAL DOSE	21.6 rad	10.45 rad

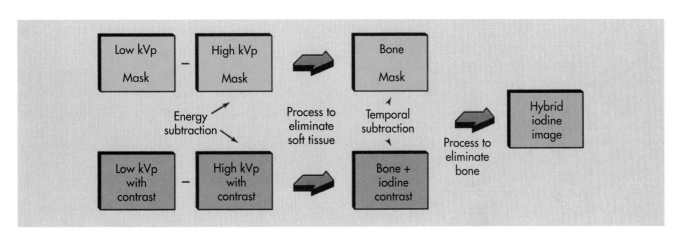

FIGURE 28-31 Hybrid subtraction involves both the temporal- and the energy-subtraction techniques.

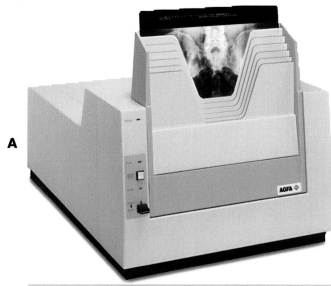

A

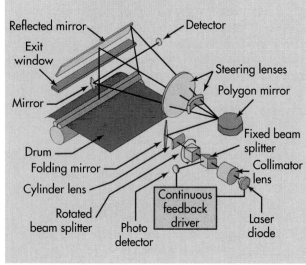

B

FIGURE 28-32 **A,** This film digitizer uses a laser beam to convert an analog radiograph into a digital image. **B,** Schematic of a digitizer. (***A*** *courtesy Agfa.* ***B*** *courtesy B, Courtesy Imation.*)

Some relaxation of the spatial resolution requirements of the workstation is allowed because of the following electronic image processing modes: (1) subtraction of one image from another, which emphasizes vascular structures; (2) edge enhancement, which is effective for fractures and small, high-contrast objects; (3) windowing, which is useful for amplifying soft tissue differences; (4) highlighting, which can be effective in identifying diffuse nonfocal disease; and (5) pan, scroll, and zoom, which allow for careful visualization of precise regions of an image. To be truly effective, each of these image-processing modes must be quick and easy to use. This requires that every workstation be microprocessor controlled and that it interact with each imaging device and the central computer. To provide for such interaction, a network is required.

Network

Computer scientists use the term *network* to describe the manner in which many computers can be connected to interact with one another. In a business office, for instance, each clerical worker might have a microprocessor-based workstation, which is interfaced with a central office computer so that information can be transferred from one workstation to another or to and from the main computer memory.

In radiology, in addition to clerical workstations, the network may consist of various types of images, PACS workstations, remote PACS workstations, a departmental mainframe, and a hospital mainframe (Figure 28-34). Each of these devices is called a *node* of the network. Nodes are interconnected, usually by cable within a building, by telephone or cable-television lines among buildings, and by microwave or satellite transmission to remote facilities.

The name *teleradiology* has been given to the process of remote transmission and viewing of images. To facilitate this transfer of data, The American College of Radiology (ACR), in cooperation with the National Elec-

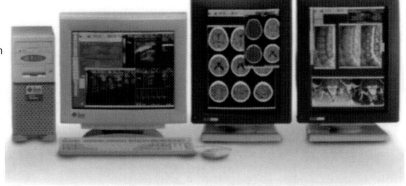

FIGURE 28-33 The PC-based PACS workstation supports filmless (soft copy) digital image interpretation, transfer, and storage. (*Courtesy Canon Medical Systems.*)

trical Manufacturers Association (NEMA), has produced a standard imaging and interface format.

The network begins operation at the imager, where data are acquired in digital form. The images reconstructed from the data are processed at the console of the imager or transmitted to a PACS workstation for processing. At any time, such images can be transferred to other nodes inside or outside the hospital. Instead of running films up to surgery for viewing on a viewbox, you simply transfer the image electronically to the PACS workstation in surgery.

When a radiologist is not immediately available for image interpretation, the image can be transferred to a PACS workstation in the radiologist's home. Essentially everywhere that film is required now, electronic images can be substituted. Time is essential when considering image manipulation, and therefore very large, fast computers are required for this task.

Time requirements are relaxed for the information-management and database portion of PACS. Such lower-priority functions include message and mail utilities, calendar reporting, text data, and financial accounting and planning.

From the PACS workstation, any number of coded diagnostic reports can be initiated and transferred to a clerical workstation for report generation. The clerical workstation in turn can communicate with the main hospital computer for patient identification, billing, and accounting and for interaction with other departments.

Similarly, a clerical workstation at the departmental reception desk can interact with a departmental computer for scheduling of patients, technologists, and radiologists and for analysis of departmental statistics. Finally, at the completion of an examination, PACS allows for more efficient image archiving.

Storage System

One justification for PACS is archiving. How often are films checked out from the file room and never returned? How many films disappear from jackets? How many jackets disappear? How often are films for clinicians copied? Just the cost of the hospital space to accommodate a film file may be sufficient to justify PACS.

With PACS, a film file room is replaced by a magnetic or optical memory device. The future of PACS, however, depends on the continuing development of the optical disc. Optical discs can accommodate tens of gigabytes of data and images and when positioned in a jukebox, will accommodate terabytes. An entire hospital file room can be accommodated by a storage device the size of a desk (Figure 28-35). Electronically, images can be recalled from this archival system to any workstation in seconds.

Question: How much computer capacity is required to store a single chest image having a 4096 × 4096 matrix size and a 12-bit dynamic range (considered by many as minimally acceptable)?

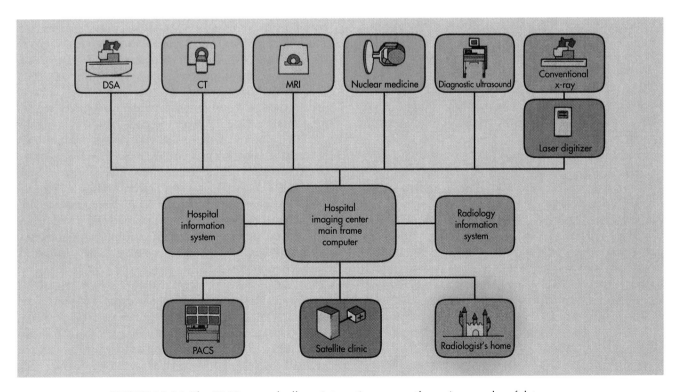

FIGURE 28-34 The PACS network allows interaction among the various modes of data acquisition, image processing, and image archiving.

Answer: This is a 4096 × 4096 matrix with 1024 shades of gray.

Size of matrix	Shades of gray
4096 × 4096	12 bit
16,777,216	1.5 byte
= 25,165,824 bytes or approximately 25 Mbytes	

Question: How much computer capacity is required to store an MRI examination consisting of 120 images, each with an image matrix size of 256 × 256 and 256 shades of gray?

Answer:

Size of matrix		Shades of gray
256 × 256	×	256
256 × 256	×	8 bit
65,536	×	1 byte
= 65,536 bytes		
120 × 65,536 = 7,864,320 bytes or approximately 7.9 MB		

The acceptance of PACS in diagnostic imaging departments is growing. Although image quality is equal to that of film in most instances, the cost is still high, and the acceptance by radiologists and clinicians is slow. Even though diagnosis in many instances is presently made from a CRT, a radiologist still feels more secure with a hard copy. Undoubtedly, that will change with time.

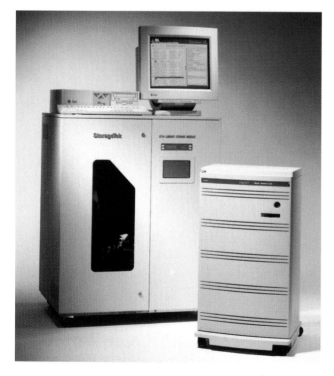

FIGURE 28-35 Image archiving System. *(Courtesy Sun.)*

SUMMARY

Conventional radiography has several limitations. First, images require processing time that can delay completion of an examination. Second, once images are obtained, little can be done to enhance their information content. Most important, however, is that noise is inherent in conventional radiography and fluoroscopy because of Compton-scattered radiation from the large rectangular x-ray beam.

The development of digital imaging equipment stalled in the 1970s. In the 1980s the microprocessor and semiconductor memory systems were developed; they were designed to process large amount of data. Digital images are displayed as a matrix of pixels of various gray-scale values. Postprocessing allows the radiologic technologist to optimize the digital image for optical density and contrast.

One type of DR results in a fan-shaped beam to reduce scatter and enhance radiographic contrast. The primary disadvantage of DR is poor spatial resolution compared with screen-film radiography. The fan-shaped image-forming x-ray beam is intercepted by a detector array, which is either a gas-filled detector or a solid-state scintillation detector. These devices are expensive. Another image receptor now in use is a solid-state plate. The barium-fluorohalide compounds are energized when exposed to x-rays. The spatial resolution of the digitized image is not as good as that of screen-film images, but it does allow postprocessing modes.

DF has added a computer, two monitors, and a complex operating console to the conventional equipment. The minicomputers in DF control the image matrix size, the system dynamic range, and the image acquisition rate. From 8 to 30 images per second can be acquired with DF depending on the image matrix mode.

Subtraction is a process of removing, or masking, all unnecessary anatomy from an image and enhancing only the anatomy of interest. With DF, subtraction is a process accomplished via either temporal or energy subtraction.

Digital processing can be used in diagnostic imaging departments for PACS. The file room can be replaced by a magnetic or optical memory device about the size of a desk. Teleradiology is the remote transmission of digital images to workstations in other areas of the hospital or offsite.

CHALLENGE QUESTIONS

1. Define or otherwise identify:
   a. Scanned projection radiography
   b. Window level, window width
   c. Mask mode
   d. Time-interval-difference mode

e. Dynamic range

f. Interrogation time

g. Temporal subtraction, energy subtraction, hybrid subtraction

2. Define *image matrix*.

3. What are the principal advantages of DF over conventional fluoroscopy?

4. How many pixels are contained in an image whose matrix size is 256×256?

5. Define *windowing*.

6. A digital image with a 10-bit dynamic range contains how many gray-scale values?

7. Describe the sequence of image acquisition in mask-mode fluoroscopy.

8. Describe the differences between a video system operating in the interlace mode and one operating in the progressive mode.

9. Why are all electronic devices inherently noisy?

10. Briefly describe the processes of temporal and energy subtraction.

11. Describe the process of recording an image with CR.

12. List the postprocessing image enhancements that can take place at the CRT monitor of the video workstation.

13. List three uses of digital imaging at your clinical site.

14. Explain what the dynamic range of values for digital imaging means.

15. What are the principal advantages of DR over conventional radiography?

16. A DF system is operated in a 512×512 image mode with a 23-cm image intensifier. What is the size of each pixel?

17. The dynamic range of certain DF systems is described as being 12 bits deep. What does this mean?

18. What are the components of an SPR system and how is the image produced?

19. How does spatial resolution change with image matrix size and image-intensifier size?

20. What principally determines spatial resolution in digital imaging?

Computed Tomography

OBJECTIVES

At the completion of this chapter, the student should be able to:

1. Discuss the concepts of transverse tomography, translation, and reconstruction of images
2. List and describe the various generations of computed tomographic scanners
3. Relate the system components of a computed tomographic scanner and their functions
4. Describe the image characteristics of image matrix and Hounsfield unit
5. Review image reconstruction
6. Discuss image quality as it relates to spatial resolution, contrast resolution, noise, linearity, and uniformity

OUTLINE

The computed tomographic (CT) scanner is revolutionary. It does not use an ordinary image receptor, such as film or an image-intensifier tube. Instead a well-collimated x-ray beam is directed on the patient, and the attenuated image-forming radiation is measured by a detector whose response is transmitted to a computer. After analyzing the signal from the detector, the computer reconstructs the image and displays it on a monitor. The image can then be photographed for evaluation and filing. The computer reconstruction of the cross-sectional anatomic structures is accomplished with mathematic equations (algorithms) adapted for computer processing.

To perform CT scanning effectively, the radiologic technologist must know something of the development of CT, the system components, and characteristics of the CT image. These topics, as well as a discussion of CT quality control, are presented in this chapter.

HISTORY AND DESCRIPTION OF COMPUTED TOMOGRAPHY

The components to construct a CT scanner were available to medical physicists 20 years before Godfrey Hounsfield, a physicist/engineer with EMI, Ltd., first demonstrated the technique in 1970. In 1982, Hounsfield shared the Nobel Prize in physics with Alan Cormack, a Tufts University medical physicist. Cormack had earlier developed the mathematics used to reconstruct CT images.

The CT scanner is an invaluable radiologic diagnostic tool. Its development and introduction into radiologic practice has assumed importance as significant as the Snook interrupterless transformer, the Coolidge hot-cathode x-ray tube, the Potter-Bucky diaphragm, and the image-intensifier tube. No other development in x-ray apparatus in the past 40 years is as significant. One could argue that magnetic resonance imaging (MRI) or diagnostic ultrasound is equally as significant; however, neither is an x-ray procedure.

The CT scanner is revolutionary in that it does not record an image in the conventional way. There is no ordinary image receptor, such as film or an image-intensifier tube, in a CT scanner. A collimated x-ray beam is directed on the patient, and the attenuated image-forming, radiation is measured by a detector whose response is transmitted to a computer. The computer analyzes the signal from the detector, reconstructs an image, and displays the image on a television monitor. The image can then be photographed for later evaluation and filing. The computer reconstruction of the cross-sectional anatomy is

accomplished with mathematical equations adapted for computer processing called *algorithms*.

The difference in operating characteristics and image quality is far greater over the range of the CT scanners than for a comparable top-to-bottom range of conventional radiographic equipment. It is particularly important to perform a careful evaluation before purchasing a CT scanner because of the many features now available. Scheduled preventive maintenance is a must.

PRINCIPLES OF OPERATION

When the abdomen is imaged with conventional radiographic techniques, the image is created directly on the film image receptor and is relatively low in contrast (Figure 29-1). The image is not as clear as might be expected because of superposition of all the anatomic structures within the abdomen. Scatter radiation further degrades the visibility of image detail.

For better visualization of an abdominal structure such as the kidneys, conventional tomography can be used (Figure 29-1). In nephrotomography, the renal outline is distinct because the overlying and underlying tissues are blurred. In addition, the contrast of the in-focus

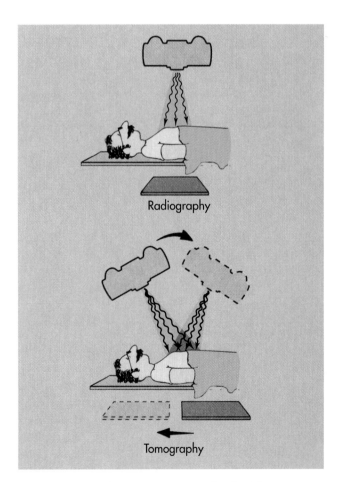

FIGURE 29-1 Equipment arrangement for obtaining a radiograph and a conventional tomograph.

structures has been enhanced. Yet, the image is still rather dull and blurred.

Conventional tomography is **axial tomography,** since the plane of the image is parallel with the long axis of the body and results in sagittal and coronal images. A CT scan is a transaxial or **transverse image.** The image is perpendicular to the long axis of the body (Figure 29-2).

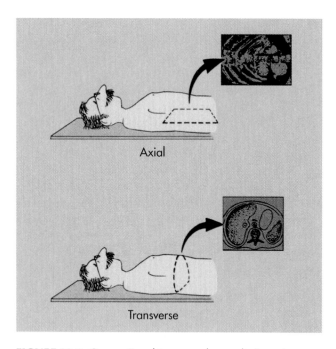

FIGURE 29-2 Conventional tomography results in an image that is parallel to the long axis of the body. CT produces a transverse image.

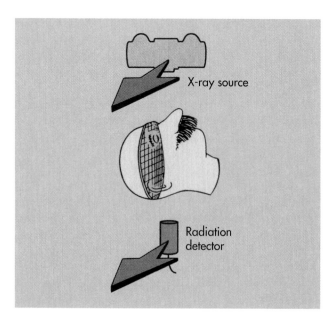

FIGURE 29-3 In its simplest form, a CT scanner consists of a finely collimated x-ray beam and a single detector, both moving synchronously in a translate-rotate mode.

The precise methodology by which a CT scanner produces a cross-sectional image is extremely complicated and requires knowledge of physics, engineering, and computer science. The basic principles, however, can be demonstrated if you consider the simplest of CT systems, consisting of a finely collimated x-ray beam and a single detector (Figure 29-3). The x-ray source and detector are connected so that they move synchronously. When the source-detector assembly makes one sweep, or translation, across the patient, the internal structures of the body attenuate the x-ray beam according to their mass density and effective atomic number as discussed in Chapter 13. The intensity of radiation detected varies according to this attenuation pattern and forms an **intensity profile,** or projection (Figure 29-4).

At the end of this translation, the source-detector assembly returns to its starting position, and the entire assembly rotates and begins a second translation. During the second translation, the detector signal is again proportional to the x-ray beam attenuation of anatomic structures, and a second projection is formed.

If this process is repeated many times, a large number of projections will be generated. These projections are not displayed visually but are stored in digital form in the computer. The computer processing of these projections involves the effective superimposition of each projection to reconstruct an image of the anatomic structures in that slice. The superimposition of the projections does not occur as might be imagined. The detector signal during each translation is registered in increments with values as high as 1000. The value for each increment is related to the x-ray attenuation coefficient of the total path through the tissue. Through the use of simultaneous equations, a matrix of values is obtained that represents a cross section of anatomy.

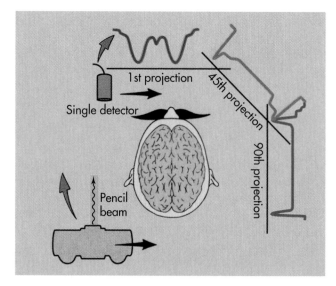

FIGURE 29-4 Each sweep of the source-detector assembly results in a projection that represents the attenuation pattern of the patient profile.

OPERATIONAL MODES
First-Generation Scanners

The previous description of a finely collimated x-ray beam and a single detector assembly translating across the patient and rotating between successive translations is characteristics of **first-generation CT scanners.** The original EMI system required 180 translations, each separated by a 1-degree rotation (Figure 29-5). It incorporated two detectors and split the finely collimated x-ray beam so that two contiguous slices could be imaged during each scan. The principal drawback of these units was that nearly 5 minutes was required to complete one scan.

First-Generation Scanner
Translate-rotate configuration
Pencil-shaped beam
Single detector
5-min scan time

Second-Generation Scanners

First-generation CT scanners can be considered a demonstration project. They demonstrated the feasibility of the functional marriage of the source-detector assembly, the mechanical gantry motion, and the computer to produce an image. **Second-generation scanners** were also of the translate-rotate type. These units incorporated the natural extension of the single detector to a multiple detector assembly intercepting a fan-shaped rather than a pencil x-ray beam (Figure 29-6). One disadvantage of the fan beam was the increased scatter radiation. This affected the final image in much the same way as in conventional radiography. Another disadvantage was the in-

creased intensity toward the edges of the beam because of body shape. A "bow-tie" filter was used to compensate for this problem. The characteristic features of a second-generation CT scanner are shown in Figure 29-7.

The principal advantage of the second-generation CT scanner was speed. These scanners had 5 to 30 detectors in the detector assembly, and therefore shorter scan times were possible. Because of the multiple detector array, a single translation resulted in the same number of data points as several translations with a first-generation CT scanner. Consequently, each translation was separated by rotation increments of 5 degrees or more. With a rotation increment of 10 degrees, only 18 trans-

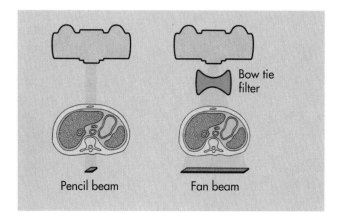

FIGURE 29-6 Profiles of two x-ray beams used in CT scanning. With the fan-shaped beam, a bow-tie filter was sometimes used to equalize the radiation intensity reaching the detector array.

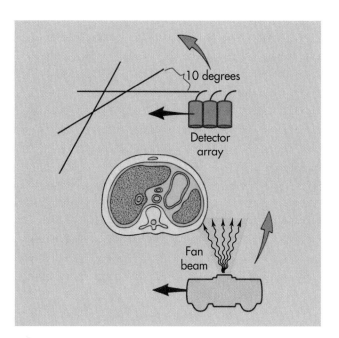

FIGURE 29-7 Second-generation CT scanners operated in the translate-rotate mode with a multiple detector array intercepting a fan-shaped x-ray beam.

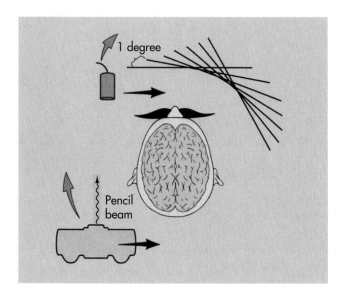

FIGURE 29-5 First-generation CT scanners used a pencil-shaped x-ray beam and a single detector moving in the translate-rotate mode.

lations would have been required for a 180-degree image scan.

Third-Generation Scanners

The principal limitation of second-generation CT scanners was the lengthy examination time. Because of the complex mechanical motion of translate-rotate and the enormous mass involved in the gantry, most units were designed for scan times of 20 s or more. This limitation was overcome by the evolution of the **third-generation scanners.** In these scanners the x-ray tube and detector array are rotated concentrically about the patient (Figure 29-8). As rotate-only units, third-generation scanners can produce an image in 1 s.

The third-generation CT scanner uses a curvilinear array containing many detectors and a fan beam. The number of detectors and the width of the fan beam, between 30 and 60 degrees, are both substantially larger than for second-generation scanners. In third-generation CT scanners, the fan beam and detector array view the entire patient at all times.

The curvilinear detector array results in a constant source-to-detector path length, which was an advantage for good image reconstruction. This feature also allows for better x-ray beam collimation to reduce the effect of scatter radiation. Figure 29-9 compares the detector assembly functions for second- and third-generation CT scanners.

One of the principal disadvantages of third-generation CT scanners is the occasional appearance of ring artifacts. These occur for several reasons. Each detector views a separate ring of an anatomy. If any single detector or a bank of detectors malfunctions, the acquired signal will result in a ring on the reconstructed image (Figure 29-10). Software-corrected image reconstruction algorithms minimize such artifacts.

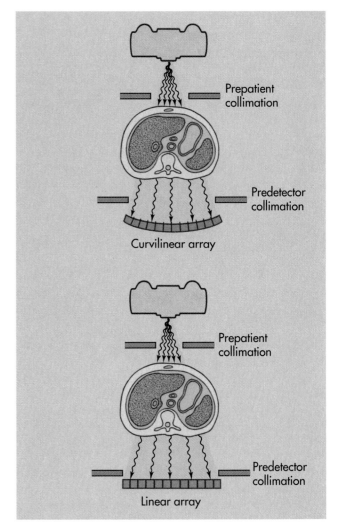

FIGURE 29-9 The linear detector array is characteristic of first- and second-generation CT scanners; the curvilinear array is used in third- and fourth-generation scanners. The collimation is positioned on either side of the section scanned.

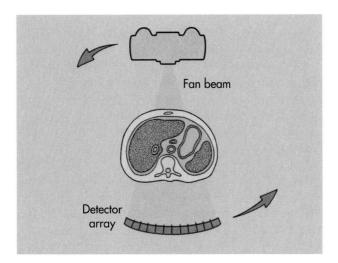

FIGURE 29-8 Third-generation CT scanners operate in the rotate-only mode with a fan x-ray beam and a multiple detector array revolving concentrically around the patient.

Fourth-Generation Scanners

The **fourth-generation design** for CT scanners have a rotate-stationary configuration. The x-ray source rotates, but the detector assembly does not. Radiation detection is accomplished through a fixed circular array (Figure 29-11), which contains as many as 8000 individual elements. The x-ray beam is fan shaped, with characteristics

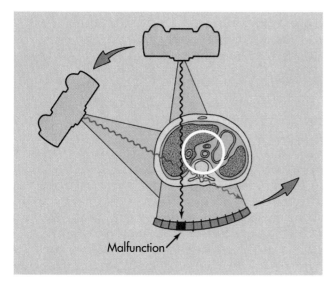

FIGURE 29-10 Ring artifacts occur in third-generation scanners because each detector views an anulus (ring) of anatomy during the examination.

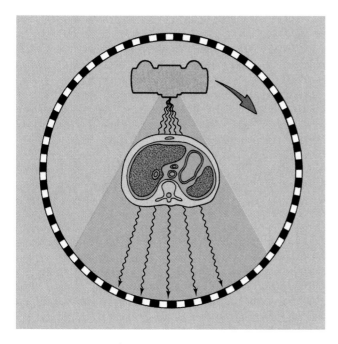

FIGURE 29-11 Fourth-generation CT scanners operate with a rotating x-ray source and stationary detectors.

similar to those of third-generation fan beams. These units are capable of 1-s imaging times, can accommodate variable slice thickness through automatic prepatient collimation, and can provide the image-manipulation capabilities of earlier scanners.

The fixed detector array of fourth-generation CT scanners does not result in a constant beam path from the source to all detectors, but it does allow each detector to be calibrated and its signal normalized during a scan, as was possible with second-generation scanners. Fourth-generation scanners are generally free of ring artifacts.

The principal disadvantage of fourth-generation CT scanners is patient dose, which is somewhat higher than that with other types of scanners. The cost of these units may also be somewhat higher because of the large number of detectors and their associated electronics.

Although many comparisons of image quality have been attempted, no generalizations are possible, and a clear decision regarding the best image is not likely. Much of the final image quality depends on the mathematics of image reconstruction, and these techniques are continually being refined.

Fourth-Generation Scanners
Rotate-stationary configuration
Fan-shaped beam
Detector array
1-s scan time

Fifth-Generation Scanners

Continuing developments in CT scanner design promise still further improvements in image quality at less patient dose. Some incorporate novel motions of either the x-ray tube, the detector array, or both. Some involve patient motion.

Faster imagers have been developed, making cine CT possible. There is continuing development of reconstruction algorithms so that the operator can select one of several for a particular examination. Slip-ring technology is incorporated into spiral CT scanners (see Chapter 30). This allows continuous rotation of the x-ray tube and detectors.

Rotate-nutate scanners. Toshiba has produced a novel extension of fourth-generation scanners. To maintain the x-ray source at the same distance from the patient as the detectors, the detector array nutates, or wobbles, as the x-ray source rotated (Figure 29-12).

Electron-beam CT. Electron-beam CT (EBCT), a fundamentally different way to produce CT images, was pioneered by Imatron for cardiac imaging. The term *Heartscan* is used by many to describe this technique. Currently, EBCT is used to scan all tissues but especially when ultrafast imaging is helpful.

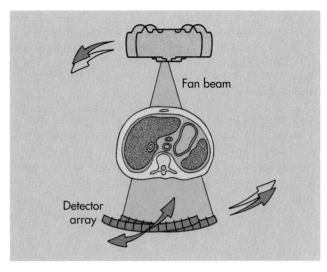

FIGURE 29-12 In this design, the x-ray source rotates while the stationary detector array nutates.

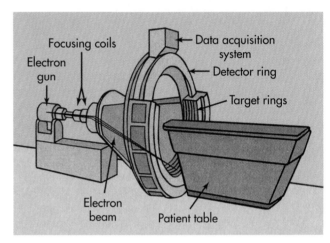

FIGURE 29-13 EBCT has no moving parts in the gantry.

With EBCT, a waveguide accelerates a focused electron beam onto a semicircular tungsten target through a bending magnet (Figure 29-13). Actually, there are four tungsten targets, so four tissue slices are scanned at the same time. Nothing in the EBCT gantry moves except the electron beam. The tungsten target is fixed and so is the detector array. EBCT images are produced in as little as 50 ms.

SYSTEM COMPONENTS

Just as it was convenient to classify the components of a conventional x-ray imaging system according to three major systems—the x-ray tube, the generator, and the operating console—it is also convenient to identify the three major components of a CT scanner: the gantry, the computer, and the operating console (Figure 29-14). Each component has several subsystems.

Gantry

The gantry includes the x-ray tube, the detector array, the high-voltage generator, the patient-support couch, and the mechanical support for each. These subsystems receive electronic commands from the operating console

and transmit data to the computer for image production and analysis.

X-ray tube. The x-ray tubes used in CT scanning have special requirements. Although some operate at a relatively low tube current, for many, the instantaneous power capacity must be high. The anode heating capacity must be at least several million heat units (MHU), and some tubes designed specifically for CT have 8-MHU capacity.

High-speed rotors are used in most tubes for the best heat dissipation. Experience to date has shown that x-ray tube failure is a principal cause of CT scanner malfunction and the principal limitation on sequential scanning frequency.

Focal-spot size is also important in most designs, even though the CT scan is not based on principles of direct geometric imaging. CT scanners designed for imaging using high spatial resolution incorporate x-ray tubes with a small focal spot.

X-ray tubes are energized differently, depending on the design of the CT scanner. Third-generation CT scanners operate with either a continuous or a pulsed x-ray

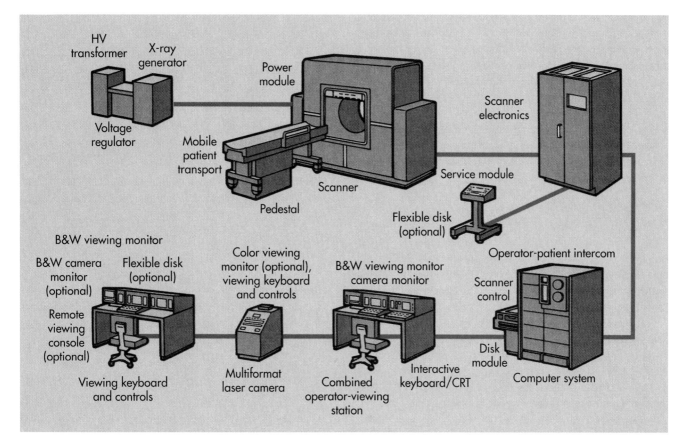

FIGURE 29-14 Components of a complete CT scanning system. *(Courtesy Marconi Medical Systems.)*

beam. Continuous x-ray beams at tube currents up to 400 mA are produced during the entire rotation. Pulsed units produce x-ray beams at tube currents approaching 1000 mA, with pulse widths from 1 to 5 ms at pulse repetition rates of 60 Hz. Fourth- and fifth-generation CT scanners use a continuous x-ray beam.

Detector assembly. Early CT scanners had one detector. Modern CT scanners have multiple detectors in an array numbering up to 8000 in two general classifications: scintillation detectors and gas-filled detectors.

Scintillation detectors. Early scintillation detector arrays contained scintillation crystal–photomultiplier tube assemblies. These detectors could not be packed very tightly together, and they required a power supply for each photomultiplier tube. Consequently, they have been replaced with scintillation crystal–photodiode assemblies. Photodiodes convert light into electronic signal, are smaller and cheaper, do not require a power supply, and are equally efficient as other CT radiation detectors.

Sodium iodide (NaI) was the crystal used in the earliest scanners. It was quickly replaced by bismuth germanate (BGO) and cesium iodide (CsI). Cadmium tungstate ($CdWO_4$) and special ceramics are the current crystals of choice.

The spacing of these detectors varies from one design to another, but generally one to eight detectors per centimeter or one to five detectors per degree are available. The concentration of scintillation detectors is an important characteristic of a CT scanner that affects the spatial resolution of the system.

Scintillation detectors are highly efficient at detecting x-rays. Approximately 90% of the x-rays incident on the detector are absorbed and contribute to the output signal. Unfortunately, it is not possible to pack the detectors so that the space between them is small. The detector interspace may occupy 50% of the total area intercepting the x-ray beam. Consequently, the overall detection efficiency may be only 50%. Approximately 50% of the remnant x-rays exiting the patient contribute to patient dose without contributing to the image.

GAS-FILLED DETECTORS. Gas-filled detectors are also used in CT scanners (Figure 29-15). They are constructed of a large metallic chamber with baffles spaced at approximately 1-mm intervals. The baffles are like grid strips and divide the large chamber into many small chambers. Each small chamber functions as a separate radiation detector. The entire detector array is hermetically sealed and filled under pressure with an inert gas with a high atomic number, such as xenon or a xenon-

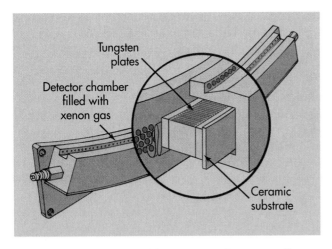

FIGURE 29-15 A gas-filled detector array features small detectors in high concentration with little interdetector dead space. *(Courtesy General Electric Medical Systems.)*

krypton mixture. Ionization of the gas in each chamber is proportional to the radiation incident on the chamber and is detected in much the same way as the ideal gas–filled detector described in Chapter 39.

The intrinsic detection efficiency of a gas-filled detector is only about 45%; however, the detector interspace can be reduced so that very little of the face area of the detector assembly is not used. The geometric efficiency is diagrammed in Figure 29-16, which shows a comparison between the scintillation detector array and the gas-filled detector array. Consequently, the overall total detection efficiency for a gas-filled detector array is approximately 45%, similar to that for the scintillation detector array. Patient dose is about the same for both gas-filled and scintillation detector arrays.

Collimators. Collimation is required during CT scanning for precisely the same reasons it is required in conventional radiography. Proper collimation reduces patient dose by restricting the volume of tissue irradiated. More important, it enhances image contrast by limiting scatter radiation.

In conventional radiography, there is only one collimator: the one mounted on the x-ray tube housing. In CT scanning, there are usually two collimators (Figure 29-17). The first, the **prepatient collimator,** mounted on the x-ray tube housing or adjacent to it, limits the area of the patient that intercepts the useful beam and thereby determines the slice thickness, also called **sensitivity profile,** and patient dose. This collimator usually consists of several sections so that a nearly parallel x-ray beam results. Improper adjustment of prepatient collimators results in most of the unnecessary patient radiation dose during a CT scan.

The **predetector collimator** restricts the x-ray beam viewed by the detector array. This collimator reduces the scatter radiation incident on the detector array and when

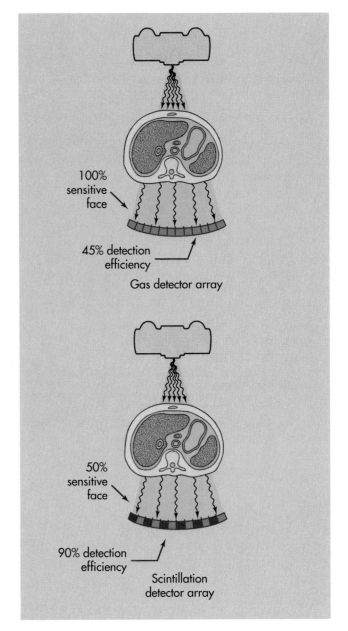

FIGURE 29-16 Overall detection efficiency of a gas-filled detector array is approximately equal to that of the scintillation detector array.

properly coupled with the prepatient collimator, defines the slice thickness. The predetector collimator reduces scatter radiation to the detector array and therefore improves image contrast. The predetector collimator does not affect patient dose.

High-voltage generator. All CT scanners operate on three-phase or high-frequency power. This accommodates the higher rotor speeds of the x-ray tube and the instantaneous power surges characteristic of pulsed systems. Most manufacturers conserve space by building the high-voltage generator into the gantry or even by

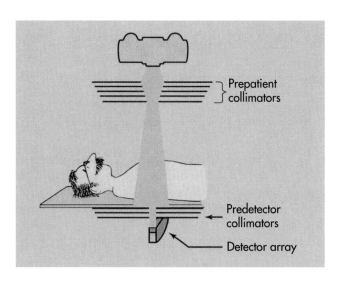

FIGURE 29-17 CT scanners incorporate both a prepatient collimator and a predetector collimator.

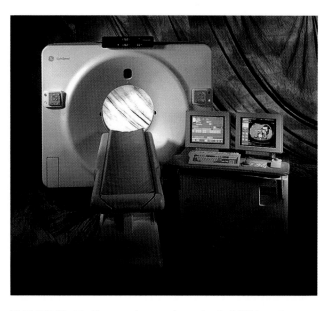

FIGURE 29-18 Operator's console and spiral CT imaging system. *(Courtesy General Electric Medical Systems.)*

mounting it on the rotating wheel of the gantry so that winding and unwinding a power cable is unnecessary.

Patient positioning and support couch. In addition to supporting the patient comfortably, the patient couch must be constructed of a material with a low atomic number, such as carbon fiber, so that it does not interfere with x-ray beam transmission and patient imaging. It should be smoothly and accurately motor driven to allow precise patient positioning. This is particularly important during spiral CT.

When patient couch positioning is not exact, the same tissue can be scanned twice, doubling the dose, or it can be missed altogether. The patient couch should be capable of automatic indexing so that the operator does not have to enter the examination room between each scan. Such a feature reduces the examination time required for each patient.

Computer

The computer is a unique subsystem of the CT scanner. If it were not for the ultra-high-speed digital computer, CT scanning would be impossible. Depending on the image format, as many as 250,000 equations must be solved simultaneously, thus a large-capacity computer is required. Computer costs can easily run to one third the cost of the entire CT scanner, although such costs continue to fall.

At the heart of the computer used in CT are the microprocessor and primary memory. These determine the time between the end of scanning and the appearance of an image: the **reconstruction time**. Subsecond reconstruction times are now common. The efficiency of an

examination is greatly influenced by reconstruction time, especially when a large number of slices are involved.

 Reconstruction time is the time from end of scanning to image appearance.

Many CT scanners use an **array processor** instead of a microprocessor for image reconstruction. The array processor does many calculations simultaneously. It is significantly faster than the microprocessor, and an image can be reconstructed in less than 1 s.

Operating Console

Many CT scanners are equipped with two or three consoles: one for the CT radiologic technologist to operate the scanner, one for another technologist to postprocess images for filming, and one for the physician to view the image and manipulate its contrast, size, and general visual appearance. The operating console contains meters and controls for selecting technique factors for proper imaging, for proper mechanical movement of the gantry and patient couch, and for computer commands that allow image reconstruction and transfer. The physician's viewing console accepts the reconstructed image from the operating console and displays it for viewing and diagnosis.

A typical operating console contains controls and monitors for the various technique factors (Figure 29-18). Operation is generally in excess of 120 kVp. The usual x-ray tube current is 100 mA if the x-ray beam is continuous and several hundred mA if it is a pulsed beam. The length of time required per scan is often selectable and varies from 1 to 5 s. Subsecond CT scanners are available.

The thickness of the tissue slice to be scanned can also be adjusted. Nominal thicknesses are 1 to 10 mm, but some units provide slice thicknesses as thin as 0.5 mm for high-resolution scanning. Slice thickness is selected from the console via automatic collimator adjustment. Controls are also provided for automatic movement and indexing of the patient support couch. This allows the operator to program for contiguous slices, for intermittent slices, or for spiral imaging.

The operating console usually has two television monitors. One is provided so that patient data (for example, hospital identification, name, patient number, age, gender) can be indicated on the scan and identification for each scan (for example, number, technique, couch position) is provided. The second monitor is provided so that the operator can view the resulting scan before transferring it to either hardcopy or the physician's viewing console.

Physician's viewing console. Smaller, less expensive CT scanners may not have a physician's viewing console. If the workload is high and the system fully utilized, however, such a console is essential so that patient scans can be reviewed and reported without interfering with scanner operations. For maximal effectiveness, the physician's viewing console is supported by an independent computer. In scanners without a separate computer for the physician's viewing console, the main computer's priority is image acquisition. Image viewing and postprocessing must be delayed in favor of imaging, considerably slowing the time of examinations.

This console allows the physician to call up any previous image and manipulate it to optimize diagnostic information. The manipulative controls provide for contrast and brightness adjustments, magnification techniques, region of interest (ROI) viewing, and use of on-line computer software packages. This software may include programs to generate CT number histograms along any preselected axis, compute the mean and standard deviations of CT values within an ROI, use subtraction techniques, and perform planar and volumetric quantitative analysis. Reconstruction of images along coronal, sagittal, and oblique planes is also possible.

Image storage. There are a number of useful image storage formats. Current CT scanners store images on either magnetic tapes or discs. If the disc format is used, data from a single patient are transferred to a single disc that can be stored in a jacket with other patient reports and films. If magnetic tape storage is used, data from many patients can be transferred to a single tape. Each tape generally accommodates 150 scans, which is equivalent to 5 to 10 patients. Removable hard discs are also used.

For later viewing and filing, CT scans are usually recorded on film in a laser camera. Typical cameras use 14 × 17 inch films and can provide one, two, four, six, or twelve images to a film. Naturally, the more images per film, the smaller the image.

IMAGE CHARACTERISTICS

The image obtained in CT is unlike that obtained in conventional radiography. In radiography, x-rays form an image directly on the image receptor: the film. With CT scanners, the x-rays form a stored electronic image that is displayed as a matrix of intensities.

Image Matrix

The CT scan format consists of many cells, each assigned a number and displayed as an optical density or brightness level on the video monitor. The original EMI format consisted of an 80 × 80 matrix for a total of 6400 individual cells of information. Current imagers provide matrices of 512 × 512, resulting in 262,144 cells of information.

Each cell of information is a **pixel** (*pi*cture *el*ement) and the numerical information contained in each pixel is a CT number, or **Hounsfield unit (HU)**. The pixel is a two-dimensional representation of a corresponding tissue volume (Figure 29-19).

The diameter of image reconstruction is called the **field of view (FOV)**. When the FOV is increased for a fixed matrix size (for example, from 12 to 20 cm), the size of each pixel is increased proportionately. When the matrix size is increased for a fixed FOV (for example, 512 × 512 to 1024 × 1024), the pixel size grows smaller.

> **Pixel Size**
>
> $$\text{Pixel size} = \frac{\text{FOV}}{\text{Matrix size}}$$

Question: Compute the pixel size for the following characteristics of a CT scanner:
  a. 20-cm FOV, 120 × 120 matrix
  b. 20-cm FOV, 512 × 512 matrix
  c. 36-cm FOV, 512 × 512 matrix

Answer: a. $\dfrac{200 \text{ mm}}{120 \text{ pixels}} = 1.7$ mm/pixel

  b. $\dfrac{200 \text{ mm}}{512 \text{ pixels}} = 0.4$ mm/pixel

  c. $\dfrac{360 \text{ mm}}{512 \text{ pixels}} = 0.7$ mm/pixel

The tissue volume is known as a **voxel** (*vo*lume *el*ement), and the voxel is determined by multiplying the square of the pixel size by the thickness of the CT image slice.

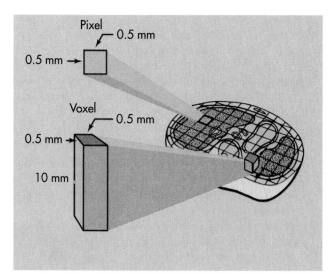

FIGURE 29-19 Each cell in a CT scan matrix is a two-dimensional representation (pixel) of a volume of tissue (voxel).

TABLE 29-1	CT Number for Various Tissues and X-Ray Linear Attenuation Coefficients at Three Operating kVp			
		LINEAR ATTENUATION COEFFICIENT (CM^{-1})		
Tissue	Approximate CT Number	100 kVp	125 kVp	150 kVp
Dense bone	1000	0.528	0.460	0.410
Muscle	50	0.237	0.208	0.184
White matter	45	0.213	0.187	0.166
Gray matter	40	0.212	0.184	0.163
Blood	20	0.208	0.182	0.163
Cerebrospinal fluid	15	0.207	0.181	0.160
Water	0	0.206	0.180	0.160
Fat	−100	0.185	0.162	0.144
Lungs	−200	0.093	0.081	0.072
Air	−1000	0.0004	0.0003	0.0002

Voxel Size
Voxel size = Pixel size × Slice thickness

Question: If each of the three brain scans in the previous question was conducted at a 5-mm slice thickness, what would be the respective voxel sizes?

Answer:
a. $(1.7 \text{ mm})^2 \times 5 \text{ mm} = 14.5 \text{ mm}^3$
b. $(0.4 \text{ mm})^2 \times 5 \text{ mm} = 0.8 \text{ mm}^3$
c. $(0.7 \text{ mm})^2 \times 5 \text{ mm} = 2.5 \text{ mm}^3$

CT Numbers

Each pixel is displayed on the video monitor as a level of brightness and on the photographic image as a level of optical density. These levels correspond to a range of CT numbers from −1000 to +1000 for each pixel. A CT number of −1000 corresponds to air, a CT number of +1000 corresponds to dense bone, and a CT number of 0 indicates water. Table 29-1 shows the CT values for

various tissues along with respective x-ray linear attenuation coefficients.

The precise CT number of any given pixel is related to the x-ray attenuation coefficient of the tissue contained in the voxel. As discussed in Chapter 13, the degree of x-ray attenuation is determined by the average energy of the x-ray beam and the effective atomic number of the absorber and is expressed by the attenuation coefficient. The value of a CT number is given by the following:

CT Number
$$\text{CT number} = k \left(\frac{\mu_t - \mu_w}{\mu_w} \right)$$
where:
μ_t = Attenuation coefficient of the tissue in the pixel under analysis
μ_w = X-ray attenuation coefficient of water
k = Constant that determines the scale factor for the range of CT numbers

This equation shows that the CT number for water is always zero because for water $\mu_t = \mu_w$, so $\mu_t - \mu_w = 0$. For the CT imaging system to operate with precision, detector response must continuously be calibrated so that water is always represented by zero. When k is 1000, the CT numbers are Hounsfield units.

Obviously, an enormous amount of information is wasted when the actual dynamic range of the image is 2000, but the image is displayed on a video screen or film at no more than 32 shades of gray.

IMAGE RECONSTRUCTION

The projections acquired by each detector during CT are stored in the computer's memory. The image is reconstructed from these projections by a process called **filtered back projection**. Here, the term *filter* refers to a mathematical function rather than an aluminum or other metal filter. This process is much too complicated to be discussed here, but a simple example helps explain how it works.

Imagine a box divided into four sections labeled *a*, *b*, *c*, and *d*, with two holes cut in each side for each section (Figure 29-20). There is a Texas-sized cockroach in section *c*. If we now cover the box and look through the four sets of holes, we can devise a way of determining precisely in which section the cockroach resides.

Let *1* represent the presence of the cockroach for each viewing. If you can see through a hole, two empty sections, and the opposite hole, then obviously the cockroach is not there. We indicate the absence of the cockroach with *0*. The path being viewed in Figure 29-20 can be represented symbolically as $c + d = 1$. Examining all possible paths show the following:

$$a + b = 0$$
$$c + d = 1$$
$$a + c = 1$$
$$b + d = 0$$

Thus the simultaneous solution of these four equations is $c = 1$ and *a*, *b*, and $d = 0$. The roach is in section C.

In CT, we would have not four sections (pixels), but rather over 250,000. Consequently, CT image reconstruction requires the solution of over 250,000 simultaneous equations.

IMAGE QUALITY

The image quality of conventional radiographs is expressed in terms of spatial resolution, contrast resolution, and noise. These characteristics are relatively easy to describe but somewhat difficult to measure and express quantitatively.

Since CT images are composed of discrete pixel values that are then converted to film format, image quality is somewhat easier to characterize and quantitate. A number of methods are available for measuring CT image quality, and there are five principal characteristics that are numerically assigned: spatial resolution, contrast resolution, noise, linearity, and uniformity.

Spatial Resolution

If you scan a regular geometric structure that has a sharp interface, the image at the interface will be somewhat blurred (Figure 29-21). The degree of blurring is a measure of the spatial resolution of the system and is controlled by a number of factors. Since the image of the interface is a visual rendition of pixel values, you could analyze these values across the interface to arrive at a measure of spatial resolution.

Suppose the organ in Figure 29-21 were composed of material of a relatively high CT value (for example, 100) and was immersed in water, which has a CT number of 0. This would be a relatively high-contrast interface. The

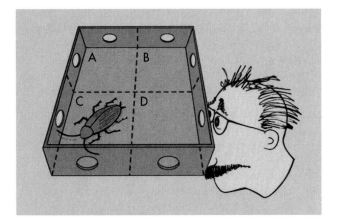

FIGURE 29-20 This four-pixel matrix demonstrates the method for reconstructing a CT scan by back projection.

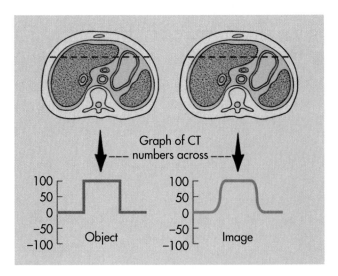

FIGURE 29-21 A CT examination of an object with distinct borders, such as the spine, results in an image with somewhat blurred borders. The actual CT number profile of the object is abrupt, whereas that of the image is smoothed.

CT numbers across the interface might have actual values, such as those shown in the object graph in Figure 29-21.

Since, however, the image is somewhat blurred because of limitations of the CT scanner, the expected sharp edge of CT values is replaced with a smoothed range of CT values across the interface. This smoothing results in reduced spatial resolution because of several features of the CT scanner. The larger the pixel size and the lower the subject contrast, the poorer the spatial resolution. The detector size and design of the prepatient and postpatient collimation affect the level of scatter radiation and influence spatial resolution by affecting the contrast of the system. Even the x-ray tube's focal-spot size influences spatial resolution in CT.

The ability of the CT scanner to reproduce a high-contrast edge with accuracy is expressed mathematically as the **edge-response function (ERF)**. The measured ERF can be transformed into another mathematical expression called the **modulation transfer function (MTF)**. The MTF and its graphic representation are most often cited to express the spatial resolution of a CT scanner.

Although the MTF is a rather complicated mathematical formulation, its meaning is not too difficult to represent. Consider, for instance, a series of bar patterns that are imaged by CT (Figure 29-22). One bar and its equal width interspace are called a **line pair (lp)**. The number of line pairs per unit length is called the **spatial frequency,** and for CT scanners it is expressed in line pairs per centimeter (lp/cm). A low spatial frequency represents large objects, and a high spatial frequency represents small objects.

The image obtained from the low-frequency bar pattern appears more like the object than the image from the high-frequency bar pattern. The loss in faithful reproduction with increasing spatial frequency occurs because of a number of limitations of the imaging system. Characteristics of the CT scanner that contribute to such image degradation are collimation, detector size and concentration, mechanical-electrical gantry control, and the reconstruction algorithm.

In simplistic terms, the MTF is the ratio of the image to the object. If the image faithfully represents the object, the MTF of the CT scanner would have a value of 1. If the image were simply blank and contained no information whatsoever about the object, the MTF would be equal to zero. Intermediate levels of fidelity result in intermediate MTF values.

In Figure 29-22, image fidelity is measured by the optical density along the axis of the image. At a spatial frequency of 1 lp/cm, for instance, the variation in the optical density of the image is 0.88 times that of the object. At 4 lp/cm, it is only 0.1, or 10%, that of the object. A graph of this ratio of image contrast to object contrast at each spatial frequency results in an MTF curve (Figure 29-23).

Figure 29-24 shows the MTF for two different CT scanners and illustrates how such curves should be interpreted. An MTF curve that extends farther to the right indicates a higher spatial resolution, which means that the imaging system is better able to reproduce very small objects. An MTF curve that is higher at low spatial frequencies indicates better contrast resolution (Figure 29-25).

Obviously, MTF is a complex relationship, since it relates the imaging capacity of the system for various-sized objects. Most CT scanners are judged by the spatial frequency at an MTF equal to 0.1, sometimes called the **limiting resolution.** As shown in Figure 29-24, scanner

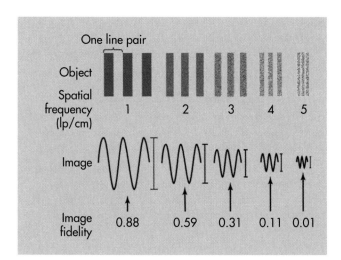

FIGURE 29-22 As you image a bar pattern of increasing spatial frequency, the fidelity of the image decreases. The tracing of optical density across the image reveals the loss of contrast.

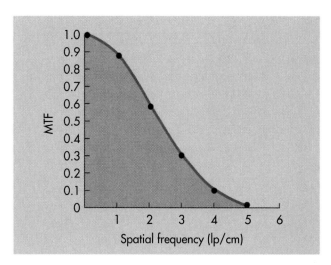

FIGURE 29-23 MTF is a plot of the image fidelity vs. spatial frequency. The six data points plotted here are from the analysis of Figure 29-22.

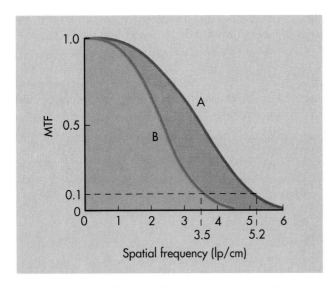

FIGURE 29-24 MTF curves for two representative CT scanners. Scanner *A* has higher spatial resolution than scanner *B*.

A has an MTF of 0.1 at 5.2 lp/cm, whereas scanner *B* can only manage 3.5 lp/cm. Therefore scanner *A* has better spatial resolution than scanner *B*.

Although CT resolution is often expressed by the spatial frequency of the limiting resolution, it is easier to think in terms of the object size that can be reproduced. Figure 29-26 shows the relationship between spatial frequency and object size. The absolute object size that can be resolved by a CT scanner is equal to half the reciprocal of the spatial frequency at the limiting resolution.

> **Spatial Resolution (SR)**
>
> $$SR \ (cm) = \frac{1}{2} \left(\frac{1}{SR \ (1p/cm)} \right)$$
>
> $$SR \ (lp/cm) = \frac{1}{2} \left(\frac{1}{SR \ (cm)} \right)$$

Question: A CT scanner is said to be capable of 5 lp/cm resolution. What size object does this represent?

Answer: The reciprocal of 5 lp/cm = $(5 \ lp/cm)^{-1}$

$$= \frac{1}{5 \ lp/cm}$$

$$= \frac{1 \ cm}{5 \ lp}$$

$$= \frac{10 \ mm}{5 \ lp}$$

$$= \frac{2 \ mm}{lp}$$

Since a line pair consists of a bar and an interspace of equal width, 2 mm/lp represents a 1-mm object separated by a 1-mm interspace. The system resolution is therefore 1 mm.

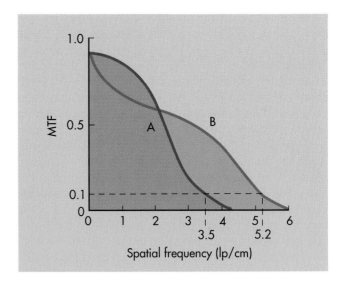

FIGURE 29-25 Scanner *A* has better contrast resolution. Scanner *B* has better spatial resolution.

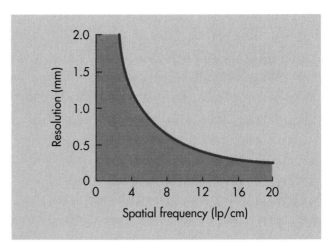

FIGURE 29-26 Increasing spatial frequency means smaller objects and better spatial resolution.

Question: Currently, the best CT scanners have a limiting resolution of approximately 20 lp/cm. What object size does this represent?

Answer: The reciprocal of 20 lp/cm = $\dfrac{1}{20 \ lp/cm}$

$$= \frac{1 \ cm}{20 \ lp}$$

$$= \frac{10 \ mm}{20 \ lp}$$

$$= 0.5 \ mm/lp$$

Therefore the CT resolution is 0.25 mm.

Question: A CT scanner can resolve a 0.65-mm high-contrast object. What spatial frequency does this represent?

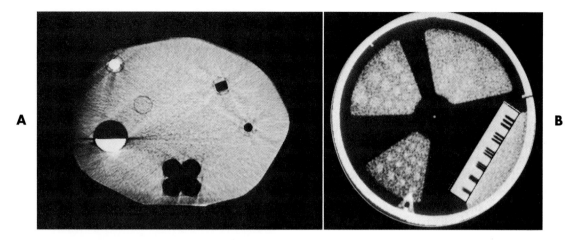

A, B

FIGURE 29-27 **A,** This anthropomorphic phantom for evaluating CT scan quality contains objects simulating a barium-filled stomach, intestinal folds, a rib, and airways. **B,** This phantom is designed to measure both spatial resolution and contrast resolution. *(Courtesy Edwin C. McCullough.)*

Answer: 0.65-mm object +

$$0.65\text{-mm interspace} = 1.3 \text{ mm/lp}$$

$$\frac{1}{1.3 \text{ mm/lp}} = 0.77 \text{ lp/mm}$$

$$= 7.7 \text{ lp/cm}$$

Specially designed phantoms are necessary for evaluating CT scanner performance. Such phantoms are usually fabricated from plastics of different densities in various shapes and configurations. The important measures of scanner performance that can be evaluated with phantoms are artifact generation contrast resolution, and spatial resolution. Figure 29-27, *A,* shows an anthropomorphic phantom designed to test the body mode of a CT scan for generation of artifacts. Figure 29-27, *B,* shows a specially designed phantom containing an array of low-contrast holes and high-contrast bars to test both low and high contrast resolution with a single scan.

 The best possible spatial resolution for a CT scan is the pixel size.

Although MTF and spatial frequency are used to describe CT spatial resolution, no scanner can do better than the size of a pixel. In terms of line pairs, one line and its interspace require at least two pixels.

Contrast Resolution

The ability to distinguish one soft tissue from another without regard for size or shape is called *contrast resolution*. This is an area in which CT excels. The absorption of x-rays in tissue is characterized by the x-ray linear attenuation coefficient. This coefficient, as already seen, is a function of x-ray energy and the atomic number of the tissue. In CT, the amount of radiation penetrating the patient is determined also by the mass density of the body part.

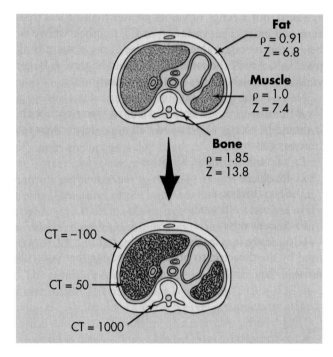

FIGURE 29-28 There are not many differences in mass density and effective atomic number among tissues, but the differences are greatly amplified by CT.

Consider the situation outlined in Figure 29-28, a fat-muscle-bone structure. Not only are the atomic numbers somewhat different (6.8, 7.4, and 13.8, respectively) but the mass densities also are different ($\rho = 0.91$, 1.0, and 1.85, respectively). Although these differences are measurable, they are not imaged well in conventional radiography. The CT scanner can amplify these differences in subject contrast so that the image contrast is high. On computer reconstruction, the range of CT numbers for these tissues is approximately −100, 50, and 1000, re-

In 1989, spiral computed tomography (CT) was introduced with great promise. In some imaging departments, CT use had declined in favor of magnetic resonance imaging (MRI), which has better contrast resolution. However, the future of medicine changes fast. Cost containment and limited reimbursement for high-tech studies such as CT and MRI made it difficult for CT to grow. For CT to grow or at least survive, it had to provide more information than other imaging modalities in a cost-effective, time-efficient manner.

As a result spiral CT has emerged as a new and improved diagnostic tool. Spiral CT improves the imaging of anatomy that would otherwise be compromised by voluntary and involuntary patient motion. In addition, spiral CT can perform conventional transverse imaging for regions of the body where motion is not a problem, such as the head, spine, and extremities. Spiral CT can also image more tissue in a single examination. The early 1990s saw the invention of multislice spiral CT. This chapter discusses the technology, the advantages, and the disadvantages of multislice spiral imaging.

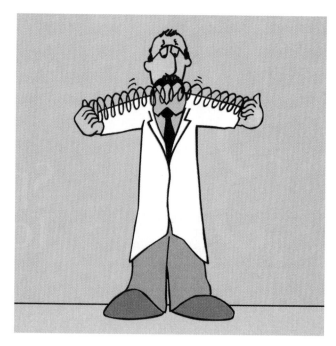

FIGURE 30-1 A Slinky toy is a common example of a spiral.

IMAGING PRINCIPLES

In 1989, spiral CT was introduced with great promise for advanced patient examinations. The term **spiral**—some call it **helical**—was coined because it is the apparent motion of the x-ray tube during the scan. The Slinky toy is an example of a spiral (Figure 30-1); so is the structure of the molecule, DNA (see Chapter 33).

Figure 30-2 shows the difference between the spiral of a Slinky toy and the apparent spiral motion of the x-ray tube during a spiral CT examination. When the examination begins, the x-ray tube rotates continuously without reversing. While the x-ray tube is rotating, the couch moves the patient through the plane of the rotating x-ray beam. The x-ray tube is energized continuously, and data are continuously collected. This data can be reconstructed at any desired z-axis position along the patient (Figure 30-3).

Interpolation Algorithms

The ability to reconstruct an image at any z-axis position is due to **interpolation,** the estimation of a value between two known values. Figure 30-4 presents a graphic representation of interpolation and **extrapolation,** the estimation of a value beyond the range of known values.

During spiral CT, image data are continuously received as shown by the data points of Figure 30-5, *A.*

When an image is reconstructed as in Figure 30-5, *B*, the plane of the image does not contain enough data for reconstruction. Data in that plane must be estimated by interpolation.

Data interpolation is performed by a special computer program called an *interpolation algorithm.* The first interpolation algorithms used 360-degree linear interpolation (Figure 30-6). The plane of the reconstructed image was interpolated from data acquired one revolution apart. The interpolation algorithm is called *linear* because it assumed a straight-line relationship between the two known data points. The result is a transverse image nearly identical with that of conventional CT.

When these images are formatted into sagittal and coronal views, prominent blurring can occur when compared with conventional CT reformatted views. One solution to this problem is interpolation of values separated by 180 degrees, half a revolution of the x-ray tube. This results in improved z-axis resolution and greatly improved reformatted sagittal and coronal views. Different types of interpolation algorithms have been developed: simple linear interpolation and higher-order interpolation. The disadvantage of the 180-degree interpolation algorithms is increased image noise compared with 360-degree interpolation algorithms and conventional CT imaging.

This noise is not bothersome, but the use of some higher-order interpolation algorithms can produce what is called a *breakup artifact* at high-contrast interfaces, such as that of bone and soft tissue. The breakup artifact has a stair-step appearance.

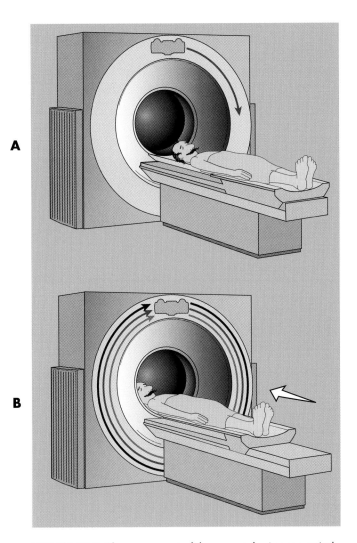

A

B

FIGURE 30-2 The movement of the x-ray tube is not a spiral **(A).** It just appears that way because the patient moves through the plane of rotation during the image **(B).**

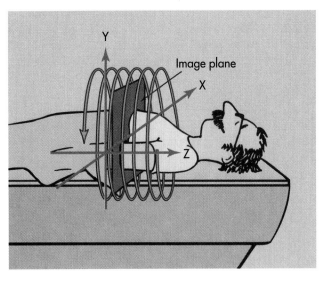

FIGURE 30-3 Transverse images can be reconstructed at any plane along the z-axis.

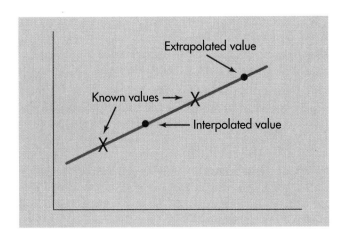

FIGURE 30-4 Interpolation estimates a value between two known values. Extrapolation estimates a value beyond known values.

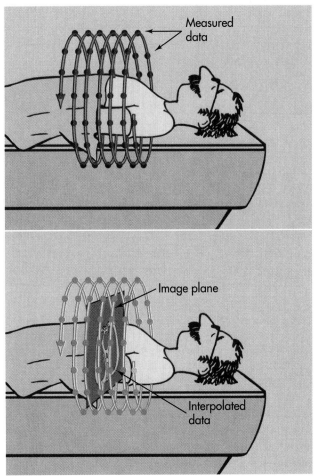

A

B

FIGURE 30-5 **A,** During spiral CT, image data are continuously sampled. **B,** Interpolation of data is performed to reconstruct the image in any transverse plane.

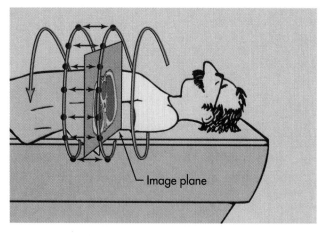

FIGURE 30-6 Interpolation between data points 360 degrees apart was the earliest spiral CT reconstruction algorithm.

 Linear interpolation at 180 degrees provides improvement in z-axis resolution.

Pitch

Spiral pitch ratio, simply referred to as **pitch,** is the relationship between the patient couch movement and x-ray beam collimation. In addition to improved sagittal and coronal reformatted views, 180-degree interpolation algorithms allow imaging at a pitch greater than 1, as follows:

 Spiral Pitch Ratio

$$\text{Pitch} = \frac{\text{Couch movement every 360 degrees (mm)}}{\text{Slice thickness (mm)}}$$

Pitch is expressed as a ratio (for example, 0.5:1, 1.0:1, 1.5:1, 2:1). A pitch of 0.5:1 results in overlapping images and higher patient dose. A pitch of 2:1 results in extended imaging and reduced patient dose.

Question: During a 360-degree x-ray tube rotation, the patient couch moves 8 mm. The section collimation is 5 mm. What is the pitch?

Answer: $\dfrac{8 \text{ mm}}{5 \text{ mm}} = 1.6:1$

Increasing pitch above 1:1 increases the volume of tissue that can be imaged in a given time. This is the principle advantage of spiral CT: the ability to image a larger volume of tissue in a single breathhold. This is particularly helpful in CT angiography, treatment planning for radiation therapy, and imaging of uncooperative patients.

The relationship between the volume of tissue imaged and pitch is given as follows:

Volume Imaging

Tissue imaged = Collimation × Pitch × Imaging time

TABLE 30-1	Tissue Imaged with Changing Pitch			
Section thickness (mm)	10	10	10	10
Imaging time (s)	30	30	30	30
Pitch	1.0:1	1.3:1	1.6:1	2.0:1
Tissue imaged (cm)	30	39	48	60

TABLE 30-2	Tissue Imaged with Changing Pitch and a Gantry Rotation Time of 0.5 s		
Section thickness (mm)	10	10	10
Scan time (s)	30	30	30
Gantry rotation time (s)	0.5	0.5	0.5
Pitch	1.0:1	1.5:1	2.0:1
Tissue imaged (cm)	60	90	120

Table 30-1 shows this relationship for a fixed imaging time and fixed section thickness.

Question: How much tissue will be imaged if collimation is set to 8 mm, imaging time is 25 s, and the pitch is 1.5:1?

Answer: Tissue imaged = 8 mm × 25 s × 1.5
= 300 mm
= 30 cm

If the gantry rotation time is not 360 degrees in 1 s, the volume of tissue imaged is as follows:

Volume Imaging

Tissue imaged =

$$\frac{\text{Collimation} \times \text{Pitch} \times \text{Image time}}{\text{Gantry rotation time}}$$

If the gantry rotation time is reduced to 0.5 s, the information in Table 30-1 is changed to that in Table 30-2. Because of such fast spiral CT, whole-body imaging is now possible within a single breathhold.

Question: How much tissue will be imaged with 5-mm collimation, a pitch of 1.6:1, and a 20-s image time at a gantry rotation time of 2 s?

Answer: Tissue imaged = $\dfrac{5 \text{ mm} \times 1.6 \times 20 \text{ s}}{2 \text{ s}}$
= 80 mm
= 8 cm

Question: You wish to image 40 cm of tissue in 25 s with a slice thickness of 8 mm. If the gantry rotation time is 1.5 s, what should be the pitch?

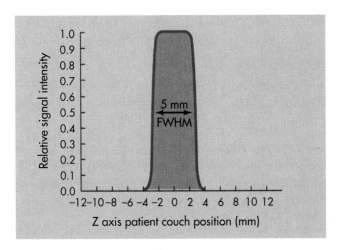

FIGURE 30-7 The SSP for a CT scanner is nearly square and is described by the FWHM.

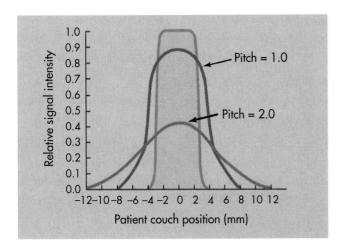

FIGURE 30-8 The SSP for spiral CT widens as pitch increases.

Answer: $\text{Pitch} = \dfrac{\text{Tissue image} \times \text{Gantry rotation time}}{\text{Collimation} \times \text{Image time}}$

$= \dfrac{400 \text{ mm} \times 1.5 \text{ s}}{8 \text{ mm} \times 25 \text{ s}}$

$= \dfrac{600}{200}$

$= 3.0{:}1$

Unfortunately, when the pitch exceeds approximately 2.0:1, the z-axis resolution is very poor because of a wide section sensitivity profile.

Sensitivity Profile

Consider the section sensitivity profile (SSP) (slice thickness) of a 5-mm section obtained with a conventional CT scanner (Figure 30-7). If properly collimated, it will have a **full width at half maximum (FWHM)** of 5 mm. The FWHM, the width of the profile at half of its maximum value, is diagrammed in Figure 30-7. Some report SSP as full width at tenth maximum (FWTM). At a pitch of 1:1, the SSP is only approximately 10% wider than

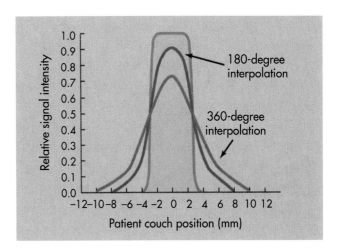

FIGURE 30-9 The SSP is wider for 360-degree interpolation than for 180-degree interpolation.

that of conventional CT (Figure 30-8). However, at a pitch of 2:1, the SSP is approximately 40% wider, and at a pitch of 3:1, it soars.

Pitch influences SSP in the same way that the interpolation algorithm does. The z-axis resolution is worse for a 360-degree compared with a 180-degree interpolation algorithm because the SSP is wider (Figure 30-9).

SCANNER DESIGN

Spiral CT is made possible by slip-ring technology. Continuing development of advanced imaging protocols is also due to improvements in the x-ray tube, the high-voltage generator, and the detector array.

Slip-Ring Technology

Slip rings are electromechanical devices that conduct electricity and electric signals through rings and brushes from a rotating surface onto a fixed surface. One surface is a smooth ring, and the other a ring with brushes that sweep the smooth ring (Figure 30-10). Spiral CT is made possible by the use of **slip-ring technology,** which allows the gantry to rotate continuously without interruption. Conventional CT scanning is performed with a pause between each gantry rotation. During the pause, the patient couch is moved, and the gantry must be rewound to a starting position. In a slip-ring gantry system, power and electric signals are transmitted through stationary rings within the gantry, eliminating the need for the electrical cables that make continuous rotation impossible.

 Slip rings make spiral CT possible.

There are two slip-ring designs in spiral CT scanners: the disc and the cylinder. The disc design incorporates concentric conductive rings in the plane of rotation. In the cylindric design, the conductive rings lie parallel to the axis of rotation, forming a cylinder. The brushes that transmit power to the gantry components glide in con-

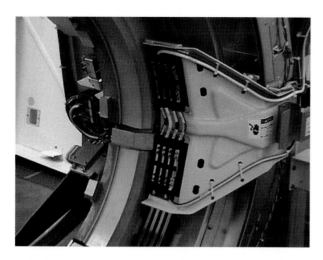

FIGURE 30-10 Slip rings and brushes electrically connect the components on the rotating gantry with the rest of the CT scanner. *(Courtesy Toshiba American Medical Systems.)*

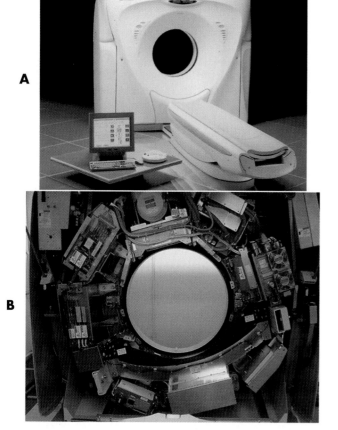

FIGURE 30-11 A, Spiral CT scanner. **B,** Exposed gantry. (**A** Courtesy Marconi Medical Systems; **B** courtesy Toshiba *American Medical Systems.)*

tact grooves on the stationary slip ring. Composite brushes made of conductive material (for example, silver graphite alloy) are used as a sliding contact. The rings should last the life of the scanner. The brushes have to be replaced every year or so during preventive maintenance.

There are usually three slip rings on a gantry. One provides high-voltage power to the x-ray tube or low-voltage power to the gantry-mounted, high-voltage generator. A second provides low-voltage power to control systems on the rotating gantry. The third transfers digital data from the rotating detector array in a third-generation scanner. Some designs now use radiofrequency (RF) for data transfer.

The design of the high-voltage slip ring differs among manufacturers. One approach generates the high voltage off the gantry. In this design, the slip ring must be sealed to insulate the transfer of up to 150 kVp. Another approach transfers a low voltage onto the rotating gantry, where it is increased to the desired kVp. This requires the design of inverters and transformers to produce that high voltage; yet it must be compact enough to fit on the rotating gantry. Intermediate between those two approaches are hybrid designs. Figure 30-11 shows how compact a rotating gantry must be.

X-Ray Tube

In conventional CT, the x-ray tube is energized for one rotation, usually 1 s, every 6 to 10 s. This allows the tube to cool between scans. Spiral CT places a considerable thermal demand on the x-ray tube. The x-ray tube is energized up to 60 s continuously.

Because of the continuous rotation and energization of the x-ray tube for longer exposure times, higher power levels must be sustained. Most systems use an x-ray tube with two focal spots. The small focal spot is used for high-resolution examination, and the large spot is used for high-technique studies of large patients. A high heat capacity and high cooling rates are trademarks of x-ray tubes designed for spiral CT.

Spiral CT x-ray tubes are very large. They have an anode heat capacity of approximately 8 MHU (8 MJ). They have anode-cooling rates of approximately 1 MHU per minute because the anode disc has a larger diameter, and it is thicker, resulting in much greater mass.

The limiting characteristics of spiral CT scanners are focal-spot design and heat dissipation. The small focal spot must be especially robust in design. Manufacturers design focal-spot cooling algorithms to predict the focal-spot thermal state and adjust the mA accordingly. The x-ray tube in Figure 30-12 is designed especially for spiral CT. This x-ray tube is expected to last for at least 50,000 exposures, the approximate x-ray tube life for conventional CT.

X-Ray Detectors

The efficiency of the x-ray detector array reduces patient dose, allows faster scanning time, and improves

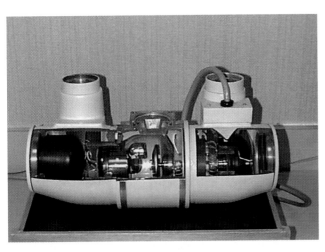

FIGURE 30-12 Cutaway of an x-ray tube with an anode heat capacity of 6.5 MHU designed especially for spiral CT. (*Courtesy Marconi Medical Systems.*)

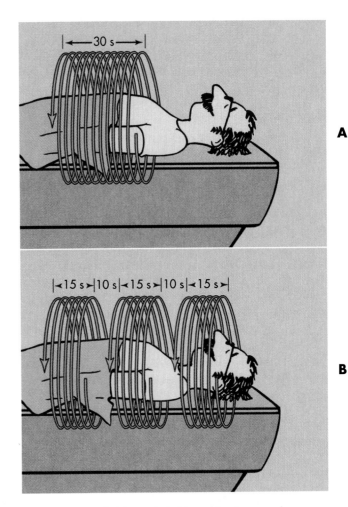

FIGURE 30-13 **A,** Most spiral CT examinations can be completed in a single breathhold. **B,** When patient breathing is limited, a skip-scan technique must be selected.

image quality by increasing the signal-to-noise ratio. Detector array design is especially critical for spiral CT. The total efficiency for solid-state arrays is approximately 80%, whereas that for gas-filled detectors is somewhat less.

High-Voltage Generator

The design constraints placed on the high-voltage generator are the same as those for the x-ray tube. In a properly designed spiral CT scanner, these two pieces of equipment should be matched to maximum capacity. Approximately 50 kW of power is necessary.

Designing such a high-voltage generator to fit onto the rotating gantry is indeed a challenge. Designing the insulated high-voltage slip rings is an equal challenge. Both design requirements have been adequately met.

TECHNIQUE SELECTION

The radiologist and radiologic technologist have more decisions to make and more work to do for spiral CT. The principal advantage of spiral CT is the ability to image a large volume of anatomy in one breathhold. However, the patient's ability at breathholding determines the imaging parameters selected.

The volume of tissue imaged is determined by the examination time, couch travel, pitch, and collimation. In addition, rotation time, reconstruction algorithm, reconstruction index, and skip-scan delay must be selected.

Examination Time

Most spiral CT scanners can perform up to 60 s continuously. Most patients can hold their breath for 40 s. Therefore if 45 s of imaging time is required, as shown in Figure 30-13, *A*, it may be necessary to skip-scan as in Figure 30-13, *B*, with a 10-s interscan delay to allow the patient to breathe.

Z-Axis Resolution

Depending on the spatial resolution requirements of the examination, the **z-axis resolution** must be specified by technique selection. Longitudinal (z-axis) resolution is determined by several technique factors that must be preselected. Transverse resolution is determined by the reconstruction matrix and field of view.

When high z-axis resolution is required, thin-section collimation is selected. A high z-axis resolution also requires the selection of a low pitch, slow couch motion, and 180-degree interpolation reconstruction. Z-axis resolution is determined by section collimation, interpolation algorithm, and pitch.

Examinations requiring high z-axis resolution are those attempting to scan small structures, such as lung calcifications and contrast-filled arteries. Normal resolution would be required for organ imaging, such as that of the liver, spleen, and kidneys. Table 30-3 provides representative technique factors for high-resolution and normal-resolution spiral CT examinations.

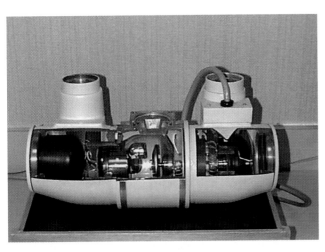

TABLE 30-3	Representative Technique Factors for Scanning Lung Nodules and Renal Parenchyma	
	Lung Nodules	Renal Parenchyma
Slice thickness (mm)	2	10
Pitch	1.0:1	2.0:1
Couch movement (mm)	2	5
Gantry rotation (s)	1.0	1.5

Image Reconstruction

For high-resolution imaging, 180-degree interpolation is required. Transverse, longitudinally reformatted, or both kinds of scans may be needed. If a longitudinally reformatted scan is required, a decision among volume-rendered CT, surface-rendered CT, or CT angiography will be required.

IMAGE CHARACTERISTICS

Image quality in spiral CT, as measured by spatial resolution and contrast resolution, is comparable to that of conventional CT. Since the number of detectors, the detector spacing, and the number of projections in the image plane are generally the same as that in conventional CT, in-plane resolution is the same.

However, although the SSP is worse in spiral CT, there can be notable improvement in the z-axis spatial resolution because there are no gaps in the data and image reconstruction can be made at any position along the z-axis. Reconstructed images can even overlap.

 With spiral CT, image reconstruction can be made at any position along the z-axis.

Overlapping Images

Consider the calcified lung nodule in Figure 30-14. With conventional CT, the nodule may be missed as a result of partial volume averaging if it lies at a section interface. When the transverse image reconstruction is overlapped, the nodule can be brought into the midsection with accompanying improvement in contrast resolution.

In addition to overlapping transverse images for improved contrast resolution, spiral CT excels in three-dimensional **multiplanar reformation (MPR),** in which transverse images are stacked to form a three-dimensional data set that can be rendered as an image in several ways. Three-dimensional MPR algorithms are most frequently used: maximum-intensity projection, shaded surface display, and shaded volume display.

Maximum-Intensity Projection

Maximum-intensity projection (MIP) reconstructs an image by selecting the pixels with the highest value along

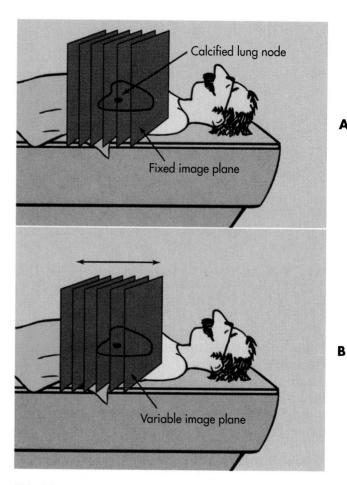

FIGURE 30-14 A very small structure, such as this lung nodule **(A),** will be poorly imaged by conventional CT if the nodule is at the section interface. With spiral CT **(B),** a 50% overlap can be performed in reconstruction to improve the contrast resolution.

any arbitrary line through the data set and exhibiting only those pixels (Figure 30-15). MIP images are widely used in CT angiography because they can be reconstructed very fast.

Only approximately 10% of the three-dimensional data points are used. The result can be a very-high-contrast three-dimensional image of contrast-filled vessels (Figure 30-16). On most computer workstations the image can be rotated to show striking three-dimensional features.

MIP is the simplest form of three-dimensional imaging. It provides excellent differentiation of vasculature from surrounding tissue but lacks vessel depth because superimposed vessels are not displayed. This is accommodated somewhat by image rotation. Small vessels that pass obliquely through a voxel may not be imaged because of partial volume averaging.

Shaded Surface Display

Shaded surface display (SSD) is a computer-aided technique borrowed from computer-aided design and manu-

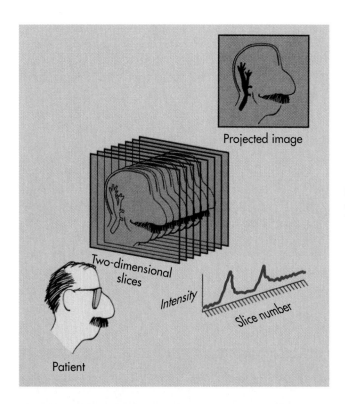

Projected image

Two-dimensional slices

Intensity

Slice number

Patient

FIGURE 30-15 An MIP reconstruction creates a three-dimensional image from multislice two-dimensional data sets. The result is a CT angiogram.

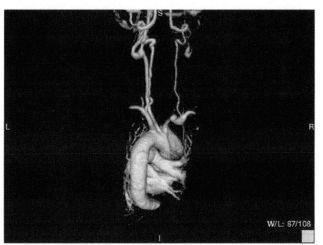

FIGURE 30-16 This cartoid MR angiogram was reconstructed from a volume-acquired MR data set. *(Courtesy Vital Images, Inc., and New York University.)*

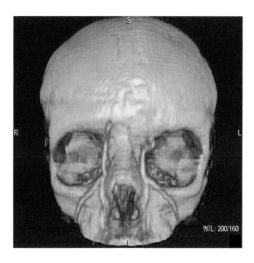

FIGURE 30-17 Volume-rendered image of a head that could be reconstructed to face and rotated. *(Courtesy Vital Images, Inc., and St. Paul Radiology.)*

facturing applications. It was initially applied to bone imaging (Figure 30-17). Shaded surface display identifies a narrow range of values as belonging to the object to be imaged and displays that range. The range displayed will appear as an organ surface that is determined by operator selected values.

The computer capacity required for SSD is comparatively modest. Surface boundaries can be made very distinctive; the image appears very three-dimensional (Figure 30-18).

SSD appears a bit shallow in depth because structures inside or behind the surface are not shown. Volume ren-

dering is another postprocessing technique that provides depth in an image (Figure 30-18). SSD and volume rendering are sensitive to the operator-selected pixel range, which can make imaging of anatomic structures difficult.

MULTISLICE CT

In the early 1990s, the Israeli company El Scint, introduced the use of two detector arrays to produce two spiral slices in the time previously required for one slice (Figure 30-19). This new technology was called **multislice computed tomography.** The advantages were obvious: Scanning the same anatomy in half the time or scan-

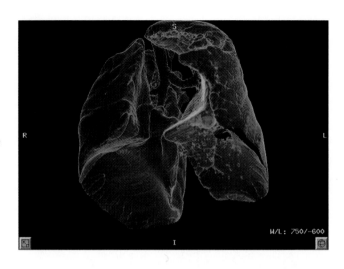

FIGURE 30-18 Volume rendering processing provides additional depth to the spiral CT image, as shown in this view of the lung. *(Courtesy Vital Images, Inc., and Toshiba America Medical Systems.)*

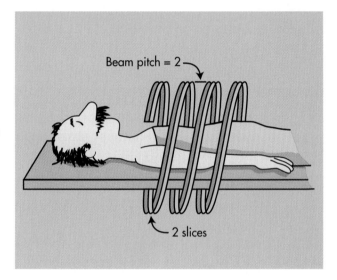

FIGURE 30-19 Dual detector arrays allows twice as much tissue volume to be imaged with no loss of image quality.

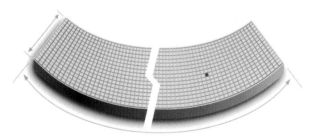

FIGURE 30-20 The multidetector array contains 16 rows of 912 individual detectors, each 1.25 mm wide (14,592 detectors). The side strips are data detectors. *(Courtesy General Electric Medical Systems.)*

ning twice the anatomy in the same time. The latter proved to be more important.

By the end of the millennium, every CT vendor had developed and marketed multislice CT systems. There are two distinguishing features of these scanners. First, instead of a detector array, multislice CT requires several parallel detector arrays containing thousands of individual detectors (Figure 30-20). Second, energizing such a large detector array for quickly scanning large volumes requires an x-ray tube with a very large capacity.

Multislice Detector Array

After the initial demonstration of dual-slice scanning, detector arrays up to 16 rows were developed. The simplest approach to multislice scanning uses four detector arrays, each of equal width. This design is shown in Fig-

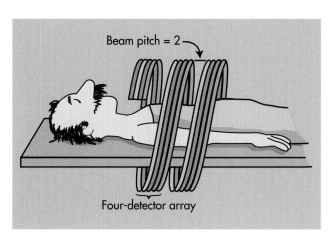

FIGURE 30-21 A four-detector array with a beam pitch of 2.0 covers eight times the tissue volume of single-slice spiral CT.

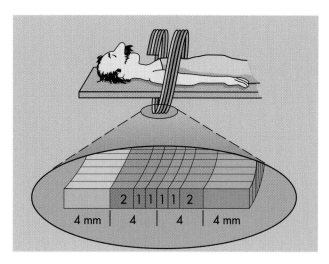

FIGURE 30-23 Asymmetric eight-detector array.

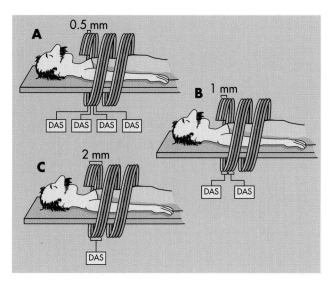

FIGURE 30-22 Four-detector array system. **A,** Four single slices of 0.5 mm each. **B,** Combine two single slices to make 1 mm each. **C,** Combine four single slices to make one slice 2 mm thick.

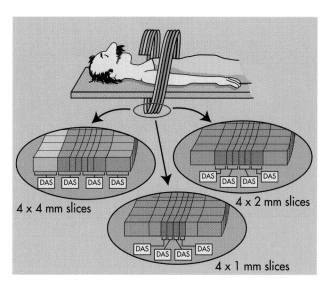

FIGURE 30-24 The asymmetric eight-detector array provides a choice of slice thickness by switching the DAS.

ure 30-21 with a beam pitch of two—the x-ray beam width is half the patient couch movement. The width of each detector array is usually 0.5 mm, resulting in four slices of 0.5-mm width.

The design of such a CT scanner usually allows detected signals from adjacent arrays to be combined to produce two 1-mm slices or one 2-mm slice (Figure 30-22). Wider slice scanning results in better contrast resolution at the same mA because the detected signal is larger. This improvement in contrast resolution is accompanied by a slight reduction in spatial resolution because of increased voxel size. Alternately, a larger tissue volume can be scanned with original contrast resolution at a reduced mA.

 Wider multislices allow more tissue volume to be imaged.

An alternate approach to four-slice scanning is shown in Figure 30-23. This design uses eight detector arrays of different widths. When adjacent arrays are combined, four 0.5-mm slices, four 1-mm slices, four 2-mm slices, or four 4-mm slices can be obtained (Figure 30-24).

 Smaller detector size results in better spatial resolution.

Another design uses 32 detector arrays, each 0.5 mm wide, resulting in a total width of 16 mm. This design produces four contiguous slices ranging from 0.5 mm each to 4 mm each (Figure 30-25). This design allows even better z-axis resolution.

The principle disadvantage of the larger detector size is reduced spatial resolution. With a larger detector size, some of the lost spatial resolution can be regained by the use of an additional predetector collimator (Figure 30-26). However, the detector geometric efficiency is reduced, resulting in wasted x-rays. The patient dose is increased because this mode of imaging requires a higher mA to produce the same signal intensity.

 Higher-resolution multislice spiral CT results in a high patient radiation dose.

Data-Acquisition System

The signal from each radiation detector of a multislice spiral CT scanner is connected to a computer-controlled electronic amplifier and switching device called a **data-acquisition system (DAS)**. It is the DAS that selects the detector combinations for signal summation (Figure 30-27).

Multislice Pitch

As discussed earlier, spiral CT pitch is designed to convey information on image characteristics and pa-

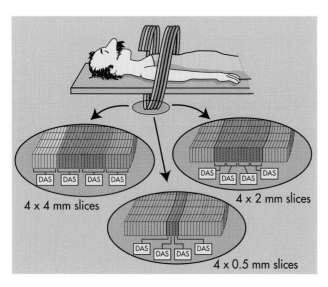

FIGURE 30-25 With 32 detector arrays and a four-channel DAS, z-axis resolution or patient volume can be emphasized.

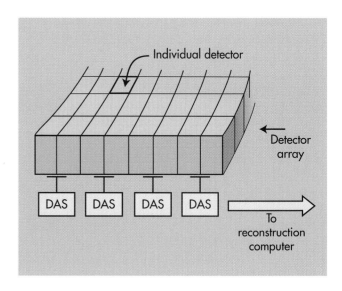

FIGURE 30-27 The DAS selects combinations of detector arrays for various slice thicknesses.

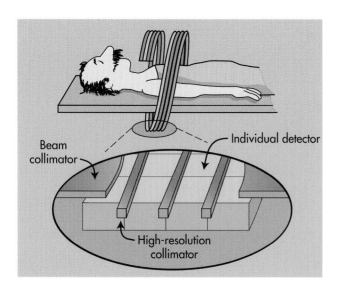

FIGURE 30-26 Additional predetector collimation is used to produce higher spatial resolution.

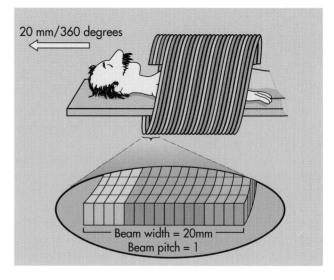

FIGURE 30-28 A 16-detector array collimated to a 20-mm beam width resulting in a beam pitch of 1.0.

tient dose. These relationships are reviewed in Table 30-4.

Pitch in multislice spiral CT must be stated differently, since the entire width of the multidetector array, or at least those rows of detectors used for a particular scanning task, intercepts the collimated x-ray fan beam (Figure 30-28). In fact, there are two designations for pitch in multislice spiral CT.

Beam pitch relates patient translation per 360-degree revolution to the width of the x-ray beam. For example, if you use all of the detectors of a 16-detector array, each of which is 1.25 mm in width, when the patient couch translates 20 mm, the beam pitch will be 1.0 because the beam width is also 20 mm (Figure 30-29). If only the central rows of detectors are used, the beam width will be collimated to 10 mm. Now, if the patient couch translates 20 mm, an extended spiral with a beam pitch of 2.0 will be observed. When the beam is collimated to 5 mm, the beam pitch is 4.0.

Question: The beam width during a multislice spiral CT examination is 16 mm. If the patient couch moves 8 mm per revolution, what is the beam pitch?

Answer: Beam pitch = $\dfrac{\text{Patient movement per 360 degrees}}{\text{Beam width}}$

= 16 mm/8 mm

= 2.0, an extended spiral

Slice pitch has the same form as beam pitch except the denominator is the slice thickness rather than the beam width. For example, if the central four detectors of a 16-detector array, each of which is 1.25 mm wide, are selected and the patient couch translates 20 mm, the slice pitch would be 16.0 and the beam pitch, 4.0. If the patient couch translates only 10 mm, the slice pitch would be 8.0 (Figure 30-30) and the beam pitch 2.0.

Question: The slice width of a multislice spiral CT examination is 0.5 mm. If the patient couch moves 8 mm per revolution, what is the slice pitch?

Answer: Slice pitch = $\dfrac{\text{Patient movement per 360 degrees}}{\text{Slice width}}$

= 8 mm/0.5 mm

= 16.0, a *very* extended spiral

TABLE 30-4	Comparison of Image Characteristics and Patient Dose in Conventional and Spiral CT			
	Conventional Single-Slice CT	Spiral CT Pitch		
		0.5	1.0	2.0
Relative z-axis resolution* (mm)	10	9	10	12
Relative image noise	1.0	0.8	1.0	1.3
Relative patient dose	1.0	2.0	1.0	0.5

*For a 10-mm slice.

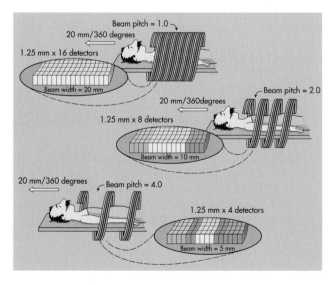

FIGURE 30-29 Beam pitch is the patient couch movement divided by x-ray beam width.

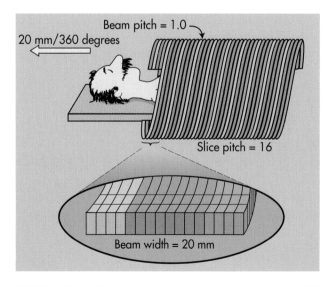

FIGURE 30-30 Slice pitch is not as important in multislice CT as beam pitch.

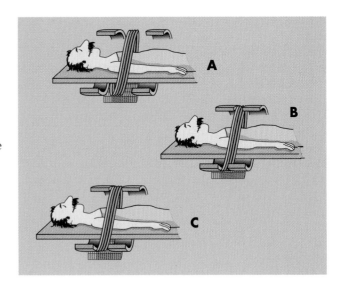

FIGURE 30-31 Improper collimation in multislice spiral CT can result in excessive patient dose. **A,** Wide collimation, high dose. **B,** Narrow collimation, inadequate image. **C,** Proper collimation, normal dose and quality image.

Slice pitch does not have much application in multislice spiral CT because all except the outermost rows of detectors are within the beam width. The outermost detector rows are also within the beam width unless the predetector collimators are not properly adjusted (Figure 30-31).

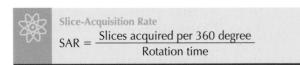

Spiral CT Pitch

Single-slice slice pitch =
$$\frac{\text{Patient movement per 360 degrees}}{\text{Slice width}}$$

Multislice beam pitch =
$$\frac{\text{Patient movement per 360 degrees}}{\text{Beam width}}$$

Multislice slice pitch =
$$\frac{\text{Patient movement per 360 degrees}}{\text{Slice width}}$$

In practice, the beam pitch for multislice spiral CT is 1.0. Since multiple slices are obtained and z-axis location and reconstruction width can be selected after imaging, overlapping images are unnecessary. Because of the multislice capability, more slices are acquired per unit time. This results in a much larger volume of tissue imaged, and therefore extended spirals (beam pitch >1.0) are rarely necessary.

Slice-Acquisition Rate

Multislice spiral CT results in 4, 8, or 16 slices being acquired in the same time previously required for a single slice. The **slice-acquisition rate (SAR)** is one measure of the efficiency of the multislice spiral CT scanner.

Slice-Acquisition Rate

$$\text{SAR} = \frac{\text{Slices acquired per 360 degree}}{\text{Rotation time}}$$

Question: An eight-element multidetector array is used for 0.5-s multislice imaging. What is the SAR?

Answer:
$$\text{SAR} = \frac{\text{Slices acquired per 360 degree}}{\text{Rotation time}}$$
$$= 8/0.5 = 16 \text{ slices/s}$$

Tissue Volume Covered

The principal advantage of multislice spiral CT is the extended volume of tissue that can be covered. It is now possible to scan the entire body—from head to toe—in a single breathhold. Although it is a volume of tissue that is being scanned, this volume is represented by the z-axis coverage, as follows:

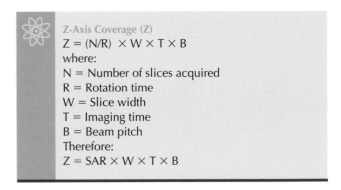

Z-Axis Coverage (Z)

$Z = (N/R) \times W \times T \times B$
where:
N = Number of slices acquired
R = Rotation time
W = Slice width
T = Imaging time
B = Beam pitch
Therefore:
$Z = \text{SAR} \times W \times T \times B$

Question: An eight-slice multislice examination is obtained with a 12-mm x-ray beam and a 20-s examination at 0.5 s per revolution. What z-axis coverage is obtained? The patient couch translates 6 mm each revolution.

Answer:
$Z = (N/R) \times W \times T \times B$
$= (8/0.5) \times (12 \div 8) \times 20 \times (6 \div 12)$
$= (16) \times 1.5 \times 20 \times 0.5$
$= 24 \text{ cm}$

TABLE 30-5	Features of Spiral CT
Feature	**Comment**
Advantages	
Lack of motion artifacts	Spiral CT removes respiratory misregistration.
Improved lesion detection	Spiral CT allows reconstruction at arbitrary intervals.
Reduced partial volume	Spiral CT allows reconstruction at overlapping intervals
	Spiral CT allows reconstructions at a smaller-than-image interval.
Optimized intravenous contrast	Data are obtained during the peak of enhancement.
	There is a reduced volume of contrast agent.
Multiplanar imaging	A higher-quality reconstruction occurs.
Improved patient throughput	Scanning time is reduced.
Limitations	
Increased image noise	Scanner needs higher-HU x-ray tubes.
Reduced z-axis resolution	Resolution increases with pitch.
Increased processing time	More data and more images are obtained.

ADVANTAGES AND LIMITATIONS OF SPIRAL CT

The advantages and limitations of spiral CT are summarized in Table 30-5.

SUMMARY

Spiral CT has the following advantages over conventional CT: (1) motion blur is reduced, and there are fewer motion artifacts, (2) imaging time is reduced, and (3) there is reduced partial volume artifact. These improvements allow CT to compete with the contrast resolution and three-dimensional versatility of MRI.

When the examination begins, the x-ray tube rotates continuously, and the patient couch moves through the plane of the rotating beam. The data collected are reconstructed at any desired z-axis position by interpolation.

The spiral scan pitch ratio is the relationship between the patient couch movement and the x-ray beam collimation. Increasing the pitch above 1:1 increases the volume of tissue that can be imaged at a reduced patient dose.

Spiral CT is made possible by slip-ring technology. Slip rings are electromechanical devices that conduct electric power and signals through brushes across a rotating surface onto a fixed surface. This technology allows the gantry to rotate continuously. Because of the continuous rotation and the need for the x-ray tube to be energized for longer periods, high power levels are required in the spiral CT x-ray tube. Solid-state detector arrays having an overall detection efficiency of 80% are preferred.

The volume of tissue imaged is determined by examination time, couch travel, pitch, and collimation. In addition, rotation time, reconstruction algorithm, reconstruction interval, and skip-scan delay must be selected.

There is improvement in the z-axis spatial resolution with spiral CT because there are no gaps in data and reconstructed images can even overlap. In addition, spiral CT excels in three-dimensional multiplanar reformation.

CHALLENGE QUESTIONS

1. Define or otherwise identify:
   a. Data acquisition system
   b. Z-axis resolution
   c. Spiral pitch ratio
   d. Slice-acquisition rate
   e. Full width at half maximum
   f. Slip-ring technology

2. Discuss the special computer program called the *interpolation algorithm.*

3. Explain the term *linear interpolation at 180 degrees.*

4. Write the formula for the beam pitch ratio.

5. What is the volume of tissue imaged with a section thickness of 10 mm, a scan time of 30 s, and a pitch of 1.6:1?

6. What is the formula for tissue imaged as a function of scan time and gantry rotation time.

7. When 40 cm of tissue is imaged in 25 s with a slice thickness of 8 mm, what would be the pitch if the gantry rotation time is 1.5 s?

8. Explain how slip-ring technology contributed to the development of spiral CT.

9. What special characteristics are required of the x-ray tube for spiral CT?

10. Why is the solid-state detector array preferred over the gas-filled detector array?

11. The volume of tissue imaged in spiral CT is determined by which technique selection?

12. Which examinations require a high z-axis resolution?

13. Define *multiplanar reformation (MPR)*.

14. List the limitations of spiral CT imaging.

15. What is the principal advantage of spiral CT over MRI?

16. What type of high-voltage generator is used for spiral CT?

17. A 10-s spiral CT examination is conducted with a 1.5:1 pitch and 5-mm collimation. How much tissue is imaged?

18. Why is a spiral CT pitch greater than 2:1 rarely used?

19. What happens to the section sensitivity profile of a multislice spiral CT as the pitch is increased?

20. What is the principle advantage of multislice spiral CT?

Quality Control

OBJECTIVES

At the completion of this chapter, the student should be able to:

1. Define *quality assurance* and *quality control*
2. Describe the 10-step quality assurance model recommended for hospitals
3. Name the three steps of quality control
4. List the quality control tests and describe the schedule for quality control programs for radiographic systems
5. List the quality control tests and describe the schedule for the fluoroscopic quality control process
6. Explain the quality control process for conventional and computed tomography
7. Discuss processor quality control

OUTLINE

Every field of medicine and every hospital department is required to develop and conduct programs that ensure the quality of patient care and management.

There are two areas of activity designed to make certain that the patient receives the benefit of the best possible diagnosis at an acceptable level of radiation dose and with minimum cost. These areas of quality management are quality assurance and quality control. This chapter discusses the properties of quality assurance and quality control with special emphasis in radiographic and fluoroscopic imaging systems. Processor quality control is reviewed. (See Chapter 24 for a thorough discussion.)

---

uses a 10-step process to resolve it. To make sure that a health care organization is committed to providing high-quality services and care to patients, accreditation agencies encourage the adoption of a QA model, such as the one developed by the JCAHO.

QUALITY ASSURANCE
Definition

Quality assurance concerns patient care and image interpretation.

A quality assurance (QA) program involves monitoring numerous aspects of radiology. Two important areas are the patient and the interpretation of the image. Patient concerns include areas such as scheduling, reception, and preparation (for example, whether the correct examination has been scheduled or whether the patient had proper instruction before the procedure). Concerns about patient care and management include consideration of whether the patient's belongings have been safely stored and whether the examination results have been properly reported.

QA also involves image interpretation: whether the patient's disease or condition matches the radiologist's diagnosis. Determining this agreement is called **outcome analysis.** Proper record keeping is another important part of QA: whether the report of the diagnosis was promptly prepared, distributed, and filed for subsequent evaluation and whether the clinician or patient was informed in a timely fashion. Although all of these QA activities are principally the responsibility of the radiologist, they require attention from the entire imaging team.

Model

Health care organizations often adopt a formal model of QA. The Joint Commission on Accreditation of Healthcare Organizations (JCAHO) promotes a 10-step monitoring and evaluation process (Box 31-1). This QA model identifies a patient care problem and

QUALITY CONTROL
Definition

Quality control concerns imaging instrumentation and equipment.

Quality control (QC) is more tangible and obvious than QA. A program of QC is designed to ensure that the radiologist is provided with an optimal image resulting from good equipment performance.

QC begins with the x-ray equipment used to produce the image and continues with the routine evaluation of the image-processing facilities. QC concludes with a dedicated analysis of each image to identify deficiencies and artifacts and their cause and to minimize reexamination.

In addition to patient care, there are other reasons for conducting a QC program in radiology. Our litigious society demands QC records. Some insurance carriers pay for services only from facilities with approved QC programs. The JCAHO will not place its seal of approval on facilities that do not have an ongoing QC program. Most states, through their Department of Health and with guidance from the Council of Radiation Control Program Directors (CRCPD), require QC by regulation.

Three Steps of Quality Control

Three steps are necessary for an acceptable QC program: (1) acceptance testing, (2) routine performance monitoring, and (3) maintenance. Each new piece of radiologic equipment, whether it be x-ray producing or image processing, should be acceptance tested before clinical application. The acceptance test must be performed by someone other than the manufacturer's representative

TABLE 31-1	Characteristics of Various Diagnostic Imaging Systems				
	Spatial Resolution	Contrast Resolution	Temporal Resolution	Signal-to-Noise Ratio	Artifacts
Radiography	E	F	E	E	F
Mammography	E	G	G	E	F
Fluoroscopy	G	F	E	G	F
Digital radiography & fluoroscopy	G	E	G	G	G
Computed tomography	F	E	G	F	G
Magnetic resonance imaging	F	E	F	F	F
Ultrasound	F	G	G	G	F
Nuclear medicine	F	G	F	F	F

E, Excellent; F, fair; G, good.

TABLE 31-2	Elements of a QC Program for Radiographic Systems	
Measurement	Frequency*	Tolerance
Filtration	Annually	>2.5 mm Al
Collimation	Semiannually	±2% SID
Focal-spot size	Annually	±50%
Calibration of peak kilovoltage	Annually	±10%
Exposure timer accuracy	Annually	±5% > 10 ms / ±20% ≤ 10 ms
Exposure linearity	Annually	±10%
Exposure reproducibility	Annually	±5%
Radiographic intensifying screens	Semiannually	Zero defects/blur
Protective apparel	Annually	Zero defects/cracks
Film illuminators	Annually	≥1500 cd/m^2 ±10%

SID, Source-to-image receptor distance.
Evaluation should follow any major equipment modification.

because it is designed to show that the equipment is performing within the manufacturer's specifications.

With use, the performance characteristics of all such equipment change and may deteriorate. Consequently, periodic monitoring of equipment performance is required. On most systems, annual monitoring is satisfactory unless there has been a replacement of a major component, such as an x-ray tube.

When periodic monitoring shows that equipment is not performing as it was intended, maintenance or repair is necessary. Preventive maintenance usually makes repair unnecessary.

An acceptable QC program includes three steps:
1. Acceptance testing
2. Routine performance monitoring
3. Maintenance

As with QA, QC is also a team effort, but it is principally the responsibility of the medical physicist. In private offices, clinics, and hospitals the medical physicist, as a consultant, establishes the QC program and oversees its implementation at a frequency determined by the activity of the institution.

In a large medical center where the medical physicist is a member of the professional staff, he or she performs many of the routine activities and supervises other activities. With the help of the QC technologist and the radiologic engineers, the medical physicist sees that all necessary monitoring measurements and observations are performed.

The nature of a QC program is determined somewhat by the characteristics of the image produced. Table 31-1 summarizes the characteristic features of most imaging systems. Usually, the QC program focuses on the strengths of the image to ensure that those strengths are maintained.

RADIOGRAPHIC QUALITY CONTROL

Organizations such as the American College of Medical Physics (ACMP) and the American Association of Physicists in Medicine (AAPM) have developed guidelines for QC programs in radiography and other imaging modalities. Table 31-2 presents the essentials of such a program, the recommended frequency of evaluation, and the tolerance limit for each assessment. Figure 31-1 shows a medical physicist preparing dosimetry equipment for QC measurements.

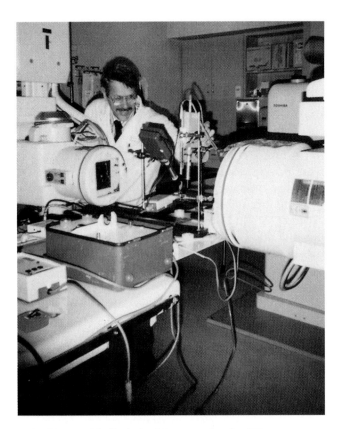

FIGURE 31-1 Medical physicist preparing for QC measurements. *(Courtesy Louis Wagner.)*

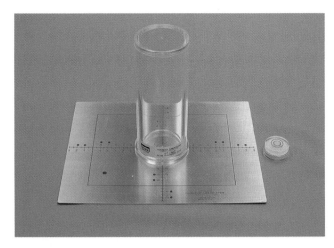

FIGURE 31-2 Test tool for monitoring x-ray beam, light-field coincidence. *(Courtesy Nuclear Associates.)*

TABLE 31-3	Minimum HVL Required to Ensure Adequate X-Ray Beam Filtration				
Minimum	OPERATING PEAK KILOVOLTAGE				
HVL (mm Al)	30	50	70	90	120
Single phase	0.3	1.2	1.6	2.6	3.6
Three phase/high frequency	0.4	1.5	2.0	3.1	4.2

Filtration

Perhaps the most important patient-protection characteristic of a radiographic unit is x-ray beam filtration. State statutes require that general-purpose radiographic units have a minimum total filtration of 2.5 mm Al. It is normally not possible to measure filtration directly, so a measurement of the half-value layer (HVL) of the x-ray beam is used as described in Chapter 12. The measured HVL must meet or exceed the value shown in Table 31-3 for the total filtration to be considered adequate. This determination of filtration should be made annually or after a change in the x-ray tube or tube housing.

Collimation

It is essential that the x-ray field coincide with the light field of the variable-aperture light-localizing collimator.

If these fields are misaligned, the intended anatomy will be missed and unintended anatomy irradiated. Determination of adequate collimation can be performed with any of a number of test tools designed for that purpose (Figure 31-2).

 Misalignment must not exceed ±2% of the source-to-image receptor distance (SID).

Most systems today are equipped with **positive-beam-limiting collimators (PBLs).** These devices are automatic collimators that sense the size of the image receptor and adjust the collimating shutters to that size. Since different sizes of image receptors must be accommodated, the PBL function must be evaluated for all possible receptor sizes. With a PBL collimator, the x-ray beam must be no larger than the image receptor except in the override mode.

Distance and centering indicators must be accurate to within 2% and 1% of the SID, respectively. The distance indicator can be checked simply with a tape measure. The location of the focal spot is marked on the x-ray tube housing. Centering is checked visually for the light field and with markers for the exposure field.

Question: The distance from the Bucky tray to the dot on the x-ray tube housing indicating focal-spot position is measured at 98.4 cm. The automatic distance indications show an SID of 100 cm. Is this acceptable?

Answer: $\dfrac{100 - 98.4}{100} = \dfrac{1.6}{100} = 1.6\%$, yes

Focal-Spot Size

The spatial resolution of a radiographic imaging system is determined principally by the focal-spot size of the x-ray tube. When new equipment or a replacement x-

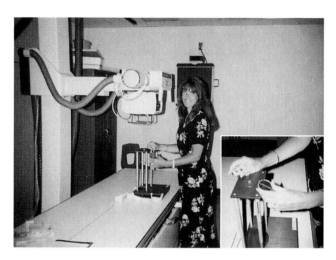

FIGURE 31-3 The pinhole camera, star pattern, and slit camera may be used to measure focal-spot size. *(Courtesy Teresa Rice.)*

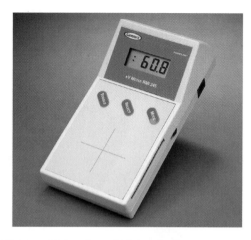

FIGURE 31-4 High voltage (kVp) and other generator functions can be evaluated with compact test devices. *(Courtesy Gammex RMI.)*

ray tube is installed, the focal-spot size must be measured (Figure 31-3). Thereafter, it should be evaluated annually.

 Three tools are used for measuring focal-spot size: the pinhole camera, the star pattern, and the slit camera.

The pinhole camera is difficult to use and requires excessive exposure time. The star pattern is easy to use but has significant limitations for focal-spot sizes smaller than 0.3 mm. The standard for measuring effective focal-spot size is the slit camera.

The fabrication of an x-ray tube is an exceptionally complex process. Specification of focal-spot size depends not only on the geometry of the tube but also on the focusing of the electron beam. Consequently, vendors are permitted a substantial variance from their advertised focal-spot sizes (see Table 10-2).

Kilovolt Peak Calibration

Kilovolt peak (kVp) is selected for every examination by the radiologic technologist. The radiologic technologist goes to exceptional lengths to determine the appropriate kVp; therefore the x-ray generator should be properly calibrated.

A number of methods are available for evaluating the accuracy of kVp. Today, most medical physicists use one of a number of devices based on filtered ion chambers or filtered photodiodes (Figure 31-4). Other methods using voltage diodes and oscilloscopes are more accurate but require an exceptional amount of time.

The kVp calibration should be evaluated annually or at any time there has been a significant change in the components of the high-voltage generator. In the diagnostic range, any change in kVp affects patient

dose. A variation of approximately 3% in kVp is necessary to effect image optical density and radiographic contrast.

 The measured kVp should be within ±10% of the indicated kVp.

Exposure Timer Accuracy

Exposure time is operator selectable on most radiographic consoles. Although many radiographic systems are phototimed or mAs controlled, exposure time is still the responsibility of the radiologic technologist. This parameter is particularly responsible for patient dose and image optical density.

There are a number of ways to assess exposure time accuracy. The spinning top is sufficiently effective with single-phase radiographic equipment, and the synchronous spinning top may be used with three-phase and high-frequency equipment. Most medical physicists, however, use one of several commercially available products that measure exposure time based on the irradiation time of an ion chamber or photodiode assembly (Figure 31-5).

 Exposure timer accuracy should be within ±5% of the indicated time for exposure times greater than 10 ms.

The accuracy of the exposure timer should be assessed annually or more frequently if there has been a major change or repair to a component of the operating console or the high-voltage generator. An accuracy

TABLE 31-5	ESE with Cassette-Loaded Spot Film*
kVp	ESE (mR)
60	450
70	270
80	170
90	150
100	130

*These values were obtained with a 10:1 grid using a 400-speed image receptor; nongrid exposures are approximately half these values.

TABLE 31-6	ESE with Photofluorospot Imaging Systems	
	ESE (mR)	
kVp	15-cm II	25-cm II
60	90	50
70	65	35
80	50	30
90	40	25
100	30	20

*II, Image intensifier.

of the image intensifier, particularly the diameter of the input phosphor. Table 31-6 shows a representative ESE for two input-phosphor sizes and no grid. They are substantially lower than those with cassette spot films.

As the active area of the input phosphor of the image-intensifier tube is increased, patient dose is reduced in approximate proportion to the change in the diameter of the input phosphor. The use of a grid during photofluorospot imaging approximately doubles the ESE.

 Fluoroscopic ABS should be evaluated annually.

Question: A photofluorospot image is made at 80 kVp in the 15-cm mode without a grid, as seen in Table 31-6. The measured ESE is 50 mR. What would be the expected ESE if the 25-cm mode was used?

Answer:
$$\frac{x}{50} = \frac{15}{25}$$
$$x = 50\left(\frac{15}{25}\right)$$
$$= 30 \text{ mR}$$

Automatic Exposure Systems

All fluoroscopes are equipped with some sort of automatic brightness stabilization (ABS), automatic brightness control, or automatic exposure control. Each system functions like the AEC of a radiographic imager, producing constant image brightness on the video monitor regardless of the thickness or composition of the

TABLE 31-7	Exposure Technique and ESE During Conventional Tomography	
Examination	Technique (kVp/mAs)	ESE (mR)
Temporomandibular joint study	90/300	2300
Cervical spine study	76/200	1300
Thoracic and lumbar spine study	78/250	1700
Chest study	110/8	75
Intravenous pyelogram	70/300	1800
Nephrotomogram	74/350	2200

anatomy. These systems are prone to deteriorate or fail with use.

 An ESE of approximately 100 mR may be assumed for a photofluorospot imaging system.

Performance monitoring of an ABS is conducted by determining that the radiation exposure to the input phosphor of the image-intensifier tube is constant regardless of the thickness of anatomy. When a test object is in place, the image brightness on the video monitor should not change perceptibly as various thicknesses of patient-simulating material are inserted in the beam. A measurement of the input exposure rate to the image-intensifier tube is made and should be in the range of 10 to 40 μR/s (0.1 to 0.4 μGy$_a$/s).

TOMOGRAPHIC QUALITY CONTROL

In addition to the evaluations performed in the course of QC of a radiographic system, several other measurements are required for systems that can also perform conventional tomography. Precise performance standards do not exist for conventional tomography. QC measurements are designed to ensure that the characteristics evaluated remain constant.

Patient exposure should be measured for the most frequent type of tomographic examinations. Table 31-7 is a sample of the results from a three-phase system and six representative tomographic examinations.

The geometric characteristics of a tomogram can be evaluated with any number of phantoms designed for this use. Agreement between the indicated section level and the measured level should be within ±5 mm. When incrementing from one tomographic section to the next, the section level should be accurate to within ±2 mm. A constancy of ±1 mm from one QC evaluation to the next should be achieved.

Section uniformity is evaluated by imaging a hole in a lead sheet. The optical density of the image tracing of the hole should be uniform with no perceptible variations, no gaps, and no overlaps (Figure 31-7).

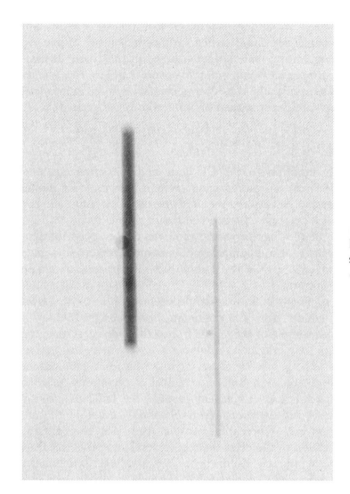

FIGURE 31-7 Images of a pinhole in a lead attenuator during linear tomography. The larger pinhole image shows modest staggering motion resulting in a variation in optical density. *(Courtesy Sharon Glaze.)*

TABLE 31-8	Elements of a QC Program for CT	
Measurement	**Frequency***	**Tolerance**
Noise	Weekly	±10 HU
Uniformity	Weekly	±10 HU
Linearity	Semiannually	≥0.96%, or ±2 standard deviations
Spatial resolution	Semiannually	Within vendor specifications
Contrast resolution	Semiannually	5 mm at 0.5%
Slice thickness	Semiannually	≥5 mm for 1-mm slice; <5 mm for 0.5-mm slice
Couch incrementation	Semiannually	±2 mm
Laser localizer	Semiannually	±1 mm
Patient dose	Annually	†
Dose profile	Annually	±10%

*Evaluation should follow any major equipment modification.
†Within manufacturer's specifications.

COMPUTED TOMOGRAPHIC QUALITY CONTROL

CT imagers are subject to all the misalignment, miscalibration, and malfunction difficulties of conventional x-ray imaging systems. They have the additional complexities of the multimotional gantry, the interactive console, and the associated computer. Each of these subsystems increases the risk of drift and instability that could result in degradation of image quality. Consequently, a dedicated QC program is essential for each CT imager. Such a program includes daily, weekly, monthly, and annual monitoring, in addition to an ongoing preventive maintenance program.

Table 31-8 identifies the measurements and their required frequencies for an adequate CT imager QC program. Figure 31-8 shows a popular phantom for CT measurements. The measurements specified for an annual performance should also be conducted on all new

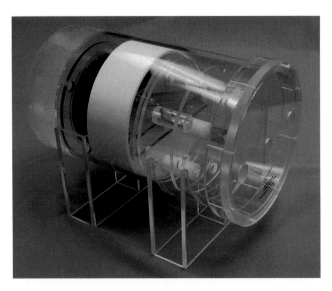

FIGURE 31-8 This CT test object is used to evaluate noise, spatial resolution, contrast resolution, slice thickness, linearity, and uniformity. *(Courtesy Nuclear Associates.)*

equipment and on all existing equipment after the replacement or repair of a major component.

Noise and Uniformity

A 20-cm water bath should be imaged weekly, and the average value for water should be within ±10 HU of zero. Furthermore, the uniformity across the image should not vary by more than ±10 HU from center to periphery.

Nearly all CT imagers easily meet these performance specifications. If, however, a system is used for quantitative CT, tighter specifications may be appropriate. When this assessment is performed, one or more of the following should be changed: CT scan parameters, slice thickness, reconstruction diameter, and reconstruction algorithm.

Linearity

Linearity is assessed with an image of the AAPM five-pin insert. Analysis of the values of the five pins should show a linear relationship between Hounsfield unit and electron density. The coefficient of correlation for this linear relationship should equal or exceed 0.96%, or two standard deviations.

This feature of the QC program should be conducted semiannually. It is particularly important for systems used for quantitative CT in which the precise value of tissue in Hounsfield units is determined.

Spatial Resolution

Monitoring spatial resolution is the most important component of the QC program. Constant spatial resolution ensures that not only the detector array and reconstruction electronics but also the mechanical components are performing properly.

Spatial resolution is assessed by imaging a wire or an edge to get the point-spread function or edge-response function, respectively. These functions are then mathematically transformed to obtain the modulation transfer function. This process, however, requires considerable time and attention. Most medical physicists find it acceptable to image a bar pattern or hole pattern. Spatial resolution should be assessed on a semiannual basis and should be within the manufacturer's specifications.

Contrast Resolution

CT excels as an imaging modality because of its superior contrast resolution. The performance specifications of the various CT imagers differ from one manufacturer to another and form one model to another, depending on the design of the imager. All imagers should be capable of resolving 5-mm objects at 0.5% contrast.

Contrast resolution should be assessed semiannually. It is performed with any one of a number of low-contrast phantoms with the built-in analytical schemes available on all CT imagers (Figure 31-9).

Slice Thickness

Slice thickness (sensitivity profile) is measured with a specially designed test object that incorporates a ramp, a spiral, or a step wedge. This assessment should be performed semiannually; the slice thickness should be within 1 mm of the intended slice thickness for a thickness of 5 mm or greater. For intended slice thickness of less than a 5 mm, the acceptable tolerance is 0.5 mm.

Couch Incrementation

With the automatic maneuvering of the patient through the CT gantry, it is essential that the patient couch position be precise. This easy evaluation should be performed monthly. During a clinical examination with a patient-loaded couch, the position of the couch is noted at the beginning and at the end of the examination, using tape measure and a straight edge on the couch rails. These values are compared with the intended couch movement. The difference should be within ±2 mm.

Laser Localizer

On most CT imagers, internal and external laser localizing lights are available for patient positioning. The accuracy of these lasers can be determined with any number of specially designed test objects. Their accuracy should be assessed at least semiannually, and this is usually done at the same time as the evaluation of couch incrementation.

Patient Dose

No recommended limits are specified for patient dose during CT examination. Furthermore, the dose varies considerably according to the scan parameters. High-resolution imaging requires more dose. Multislice CT imagers can result in even higher dose.

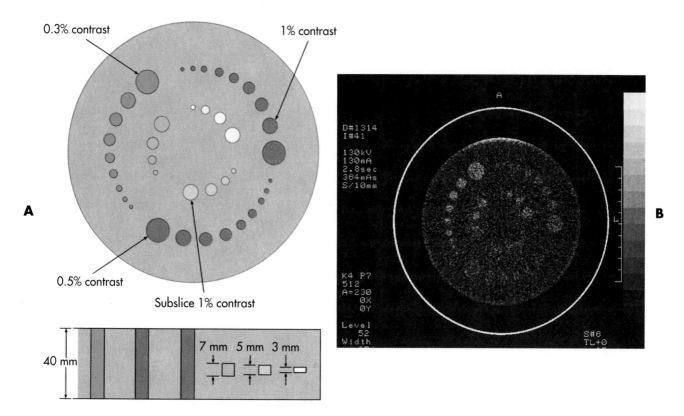

FIGURE 31-9 Schematic drawing **(A)** of a low-contrast object and its image **(B)**. This test object is designed especially for spiral CT. *(Courtesy The Phantom Laboratory.)*

When a fixed technique is used, patient dose should not vary by more than ±10% from one assessment to the next. Such assessment should be made on a semiannual basis or after replacement of the x-ray tube.

Patient dose, specified as the computed tomography dose index (CTDI), can be monitored with specially designed pencil ionization chambers or thermoluminescent dosimeters. Not only is it necessary to measure patient dose but also dose profile for the most common slice thicknesses. Figure 31-10 illustrates these measurements in progress.

PROCESSOR QUALITY CONTROL

QC in any activity involves routine and special procedures developed to ensure that the final product is of consistently high quality. QC in diagnostic radiology requires a planned, continuous program of evaluation and surveillance or radiologic equipment and procedures. When applied to automatic processing, such a program involves periodic cleaning, system maintenance, and daily monitoring. Table 31-9 lists an approximate processor QC program.

Processor Cleaning

The first automatic processor had a dry-to-drop time of 7 min. Soon, this was shortened to 3 min because of double-capacity processors. A further reduction in pro-

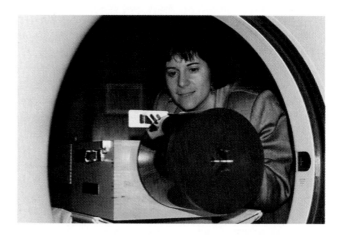

FIGURE 31-10 Medical physics evaluation of CT performance requires a number of measurements using specifically designed test objects. *(Courtesy Cynthia McCollough.)*

cessing time was made with the fast-access system, which is today's popular 90-s processor.

Such a processor can handle up to 500 films per hour but requires a high concentration of processing chemistry, a high development temperature (95° F [35° C], and a developer immersion time of 22 s. The wash water temperature should be 87° F (31° C). Earlier automatic processors were supplied with hot and cold water, so the primary control of wash temperature was through a

TABLE 31-9	QC Program for the Radiographic Processor	
Activity	**Procedure or Item**	**Schedule**
Processor cleaning	Cleaning of crossover racks	Daily
	Cleaning of entire rack assembly and processing ranks	Weekly
Scheduled maintenance	Observation and adjustment of belts, pulleys, and gears	Weekly
	Lubrication	Weekly or monthly
Processor monitoring	Planned replacement of parts	Regularly
	Check of developer temperature	Daily
	Check of wash water temperature	Daily
	Check of replenishment tanks	Daily
	Sensitometry and densitometry	Daily

mixing valve. Current processors are supplied with only cold water. Temperature control is maintained with a thermostatically controlled heater.

This rapid activity performed at high temperature with concentrated chemistry tends to wear and corrode the mechanism of the transport system and contaminate the chemistry with processing sludge. A deposit of sludge and debris on the rollers may result. This can severely affect film quality and cause artifacts if the processor is not properly cleaned at appropriate intervals.

In most hospitals, weekly cleaning is the appropriate frequency and records of such cleaning should be maintained. The cleaning procedure is rather simple. The transport and crossover racks are removed and cleaned in the processing tanks. This takes no more than a few minutes, reduces processor wear, and ensures consistent production of high-quality radiographs that are artifact free. When the racks are reassembled, sensitometric levels must be reestablished.

Processor Maintenance

As with any electromechanical device, maintenance is essential. If equipment is not properly maintained, then when least expected or when the workload is the heaviest, the processor may fail. There are three types of maintenance programs that should be a part of the QC program for an automatic processor.

Scheduled maintenance refers to procedures performed on a routine basis, usually weekly or monthly. Such maintenance includes observation of all moving parts for wear; adjustment of all belts, pulleys, and gears; and application of proper lubrication to minimize wear. When a processor is lubricated, it is especially important to keep the lubricant off of the hands, thereby keeping it away from film and rollers and of course out of processor chemistry.

Preventive maintenance is a planned program of parts replacement at regular intervals. Preventive maintenance requires that a part be replaced before its failure. With such a program, unexpected downtime should not occur.

Nonscheduled maintenance involves a nonscheduled failure in the system that necessitates processor repair. A proper program of scheduled maintenance and preventive maintenance ensures that nonscheduled maintenance is kept to a minimum.

Processor Monitoring

At least once a day, the operation of the processor should be observed and certain measurements recorded. The temperature of the developer and wash water should be noted. The developer and fixer replenishment rates should be observed and recorded. The replenishment tanks should be checked to determine whether the floating lids are properly positioned and whether fresh chemistry is needed. It is often appropriate to check the pH and specific gravity of the developer and fixer solutions. Residual hypo should be determined.

A sensitometric strip should be passed through the processor, and appropriate measurements of fog, speed, and contrast are determined and recorded. Most film suppliers provide forms and assistance in establishing and conducting a program of processor monitoring. The written record of the results of such a program is important.

The processor monitoring described in Chapter 24 for the dedicated mammographic processor can be applied to all other processors in the health care facility.

SUMMARY

In diagnostic imaging, QA involves the assessment and evaluation of patient care. QC is the measurement and performance evaluation of imaging equipment. Both processes ensure that the radiologist is provided with an optimal image for proper diagnosis. The QA/QC team includes radiologic technologists, management and secretarial personnel, the equipment manufacturer's representative, the medical physicist, radiologic engineers, and radiologists. The JCAHO does not accredit health care facilities unless proper QA and QC programs are evident.

The three steps of QC are (1) acceptance testing, (2) routine performance monitoring, and (3) maintenance. Radiographic QC evaluates filtration, collimation, focal-spot size, kVp, timers, linearity, and reproducibility.

Intensifying screens are evaluated regularly for cleanliness and screen-film contact. All protective apparel is checked for cracks, tears, and holes. Finally, viewboxes or film illuminators are examined for intensity and cleanliness.

Because fluoroscopy has the highest patient dose of all x-ray procedures, fluoroscopic equipment is evaluated regularly for exposure rate. Under federal law, the ESE must not exceed 10 R/min. Section sensitivity in conventional tomography is also evaluated regularly, with each of the subsystems of CT checked for misalignment and miscalibration.

Radiographic processor QC is essential for optimal image quality. Sensitometry and densitometry are important daily functions of the QC radiographer as discussed in Chapter 24 on mammographic QA.

CHALLENGE QUESTIONS

1. Define or otherwise identify:
   a. Quality assurance
   b. Quality control
   c. CT linearity
   d. Outcome analysis
   e. Minimum half-value layer
   f. CRCPD
   g. CT section sensitivity
   h. Exposure linearity

2. Describe the QA model recommended by the JCAHO and explain its effectiveness.

3. Discuss the three steps of QC for radiographic equipment.

4. Identify the members of the diagnostic imaging QC team.

5. How is filtration measured in radiographic imaging equipment?

6. Why is it important to have proper x-ray beam alignment and collimation?

7. What are the radiographic x-ray beam misalignment limitations?

8. What are three QC tools used to measure focal-spot size?

9. What is the permitted variation of radiographic x-ray beam reproducibility?

10. What test is performed on intensifying screens and cassettes to check for proper screen-film contact?

11. What products are used to clean radiographic intensifying screens?

12. How often should protective apparel be checked for integrity?

13. What is the average ESE during a fluoroscopic examination?

14. Describe the process of monitoring the spatial resolution in a CT imaging system.

15. List and briefly describe the eight parts of CT QC.

16. What is the importance of preventive maintenance for a radiographic processor?

17. A high-frequency radiographic generator requires how much x-ray beam filtration?

18. What is the allowed radiographic collimator misalignment?

19. When should defective protective apparel be discarded?

20. Which procedure results in a lower patient radiation dose: cassette-loaded spot films or 105-mm photofluorospot images?

Image Artifacts

OBJECTIVES

At the completion of this chapter, the student should be able to:

1. Visually identify the radiographic artifacts shown in this chapter
2. List and discuss the three categories of artifacts
3. Explain the causes of exposure artifacts
4. Describe the types of artifacts caused during film processing
5. Discuss how improper handling and storage of film can cause artifacts

OUTLINE

One of the most interesting areas of study for student radiographers is the identification of image artifacts. Most schools or clinical sites have an extensive file of film artifacts, and it is fun to assess such a film to determine the cause of the artifact. However, preventing artifacts is a critical responsibility of the practicing radiographer. Artifacts can compromise the radiologist's ability to make a diagnosis from a radiographic image, thereby necessitating a repeat examination and increased patient dose.

It is important for every radiographer to be alert to artifacts and their origin so that quality control personnel and managers can be informed. The cause of an artifact must be identified and eliminated to prevent the same problem from occurring in subsequent radiographs. Records of artifacts must be kept to indicate trends. For example, if sludge artifacts occur more than once before a scheduled processor cleaning, the processor may need to be cleaned more frequently.

DEFINITION OF IMAGE ARTIFACTS

An artifact is any undesirable optical density on an image that does not properly show the anatomy being examined. More simply put, artifacts are undesirable optical densities (ODs) or blemishes on a radiograph. Artifacts can interfere with visualization of the anatomic structure being imaged and can lead to misdiagnosis. Fortunately, artifacts can be controlled when their cause is properly identified. The cause can be narrowed down to when an artifact was created: (1) when the film is being exposed, (2) when the film is being processed, and (3) when the film is being handled and stored, either before or after

processing. Figure 32-1 provides a classification of the artifacts likely to be seen.

 An artifact is unwanted optical density on an image that can obscure anatomy.

EXPOSURE ARTIFACTS

Exposure artifacts are usually easy to detect and correct. They are generally associated with the manner in which the radiographer conducts the examination. Incorrect screen-film match, poor screen-film contact, warped cassettes, and improper positioning of the grid can all lead to artifacts. Improper patient position, patient motion, double exposure, and incorrect radiographic technique can result in poor images that may be considered to have artifacts. Such poor technique results in the largest number of repeat examinations.

Improper preparation of the patient immediately before exposure can lead to disturbing artifacts such as the jewelry, eyeglasses, and other items in Figure 32-2. These artifacts could easily have been prevented. Double exposures are also avoidable. They occur when radiographers mix up cassettes and a film that has already been exposed is exposed again.

A radiograph with motion appears blurred. The patient may have moved or may not have breathed according to the radiographer's instructions. It is important to communicate clear instructions to the patient to encourage understanding and cooperation.

Positioning errors can also cause artifacts. If the patient is placed under the x-ray tube when the tube is not centered to the table or Bucky tray, grid cutoff artifacts may occur.

Artifacts can occur if the wrong film is loaded into a cassette. If high contrast, single-emulsion mammographic film is loaded into a radiographic cassette, the resulting image will be underexposed. Cassettes that

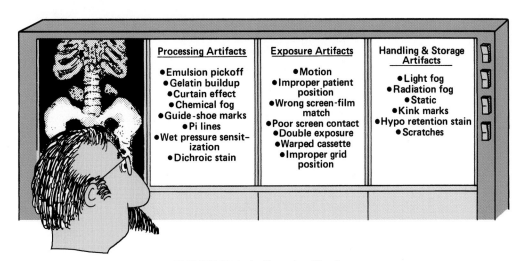

Processing Artifacts	Exposure Artifacts	Handling & Storage Artifacts
• Emulsion pickoff	• Motion	• Light fog
• Gelatin buildup	• Improper patient position	• Radiation fog
• Curtain effect	• Wrong screen-film match	• Static
• Chemical fog	• Poor screen contact	• Kink marks
• Guide-shoe marks	• Double exposure	• Hypo retention stain
• Pi lines	• Warped cassette	• Scratches
• Wet pressure sensitization	• Improper grid position	
• Dichroic stain		

FIGURE 32-1 Artifact classification.

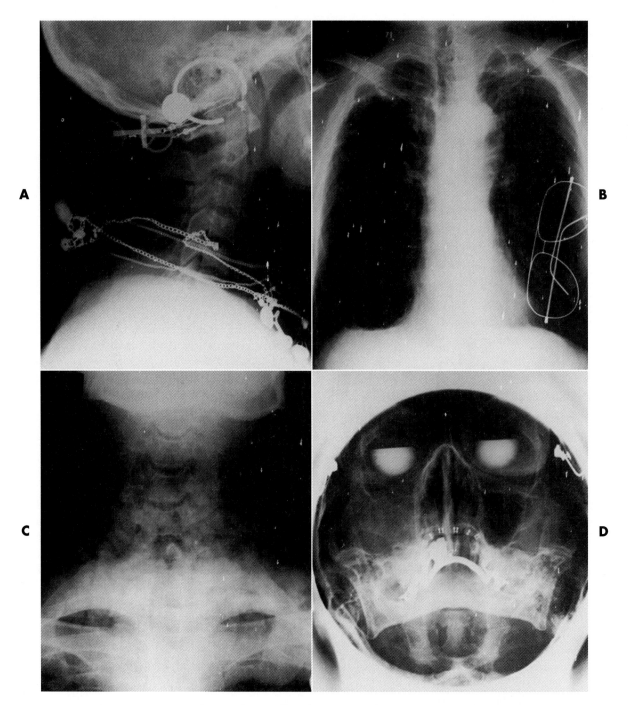

FIGURE 32-2 A, Lateral cervical spine film of a patient with a "Mr. T starter set." **B,** The patient's glasses were not removed from the shirt pocket. **C,** The ice bag under the neck was not removed during this anterior-posterior cervical spine study. **D,** This Waters' view was properly coned, but the bifocals, earrings, and dental apparatus should have been removed. *(Courtesy Paul Laudicina.)*

TABLE 32-1	Common Exposure Artifacts
Appearance on Radiographic Film	**Cause**
Unexpected foreign objects such as jewelry	Improper patient preparation
Double exposure	Reuse of cassettes already exposed
Blur	Improper patient movement, including breathing
Grid cutoff artifacts	Improper patient positioning
Obscured detail	Poor screen-film contact

TABLE 32-2	Common Processing Artifacts
Appearance on Radiographic Film	**Cause**
Guide-shoe marks	Improper position or springing of guide shoes in turn-around assembly
Pi lines	Dirt or chemical stains on rollers
Sharp increase or decrease in OD	Dirty or warped rollers, which can leave sludge deposits on film
Uniform dull, gray fog	Improper or inadequate processing chemistry
Dichroic stain or "curtain effect"	Improper squeezing of processing chemicals from film
Small, circular patterns of increased OD	Pressure caused by irregular or dirty rollers
Yellow-brown drops on film	Oxidized developer
Milky appearance	Unreplenished fixer
Greasy appearance	Inadequate washing
Brittle appearance	Improper dryer temperature or hardener in the fixer

have not been checked for proper screen-film contact cause a smoothness in the area of poor contact, which obscures detail and is an artifact.

An artifact is not produced by a swallowed object when the purpose of the examination is to locate that object. On the other hand, if such an object appears on an image unexpectedly, it is an artifact because it is not the object that was intended to be imaged. Table 32-1 summarizes the exposure artifacts discussed here.

PROCESSING ARTIFACTS

During processing, any number of artifacts can be produced. Most are pressure-type artifacts caused by the transport system of the processor. Pressure-type artifacts usually sensitize the emulsion and appear as a higher OD. Those that scrape or remove emulsion appear as a lower OD. Table 32-2 summarizes the processing artifacts discussed here and includes some others that commonly occur.

Roller Marks

Guide-shoe marks occur when the guide shoes in the turn-around assembly of the processor are sprung or improperly positioned (Figure 32-3, *A*). If the guide shoe is before the developer, the ridges in the guide shoes press against the film, sensitize it, and leave a characteristic mark. Guide-shoe marks can be found on the leading edge or the trailing edge of the film parallel to the direction of film travel through the processor.

Pi lines occur at 3.1416 inch (π) intervals because of dirt or a chemical stain on a roller, which sensitizes the emulsion (Figure 32-3, *B*). Since the rollers are 1 inch in diameter, 3.1416 inches represent one revolution of a roller, and the artifact appears perpendicular to the way that film travels through the processor.

Dirty Rollers

Dirty or warped rollers can cause emulsion pick-off and gelatin buildup, which result in **sludge** deposits on the film. These artifacts usually appear as sharp areas of ei-

ther increased or reduced OD. Occasionally, particles of sludge are transported through the processor and are actually dried on the film in the dryer.

Chemical Fog

Chemical fog looks like light or radiation fog and is usually a uniform, dull gray. Improper or inadequate processing chemistry can result in a special type of chemical fog called a **dichroic stain**. The dichroic stain appears as a curtain effect on the radiograph (Figure 32-4). *Dichroic stain* is a term generally applied to all chemical stains. *Dichroic* means "two colors."

The chemical stains seen on a radiograph can appear yellow, green, blue, or purple. In slow processors, the chemistry may not be properly squeezed from the film, and it either runs down the leading edge of the film or runs up the trailing edge. Both are called a *curtain effect*.

Wet-Pressure Sensitization

Wet-pressure sensitization is a common artifact produced in the developer tank. Irregular or dirty rollers cause pressure during development and produce small, circular patterns of increased OD.

HANDLING AND STORAGE ARTIFACTS

A number of artifacts are caused by improper film storage. *Image fog can result if the temperature or the humidity is too high or if the film bin does not have adequate radiation shielding.* Pressure marks can occur if film is stacked too high. Table 32-3 summarizes the storage artifacts discussed here.

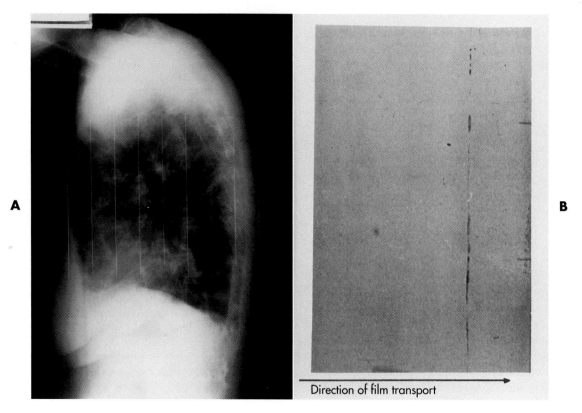

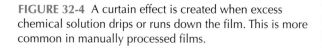
Direction of film transport

FIGURE 32-3 **A,** Guide-shoe marks. **B,** Pi lines.

FIGURE 32-4 A curtain effect is created when excess chemical solution drips or runs down the film. This is more common in manually processed films.

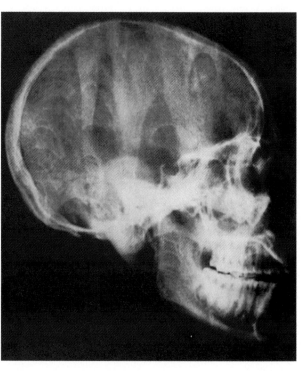

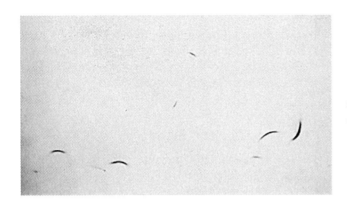

FIGURE 32-5 Preprocessing pressure artifacts can appear as scratches caused by heavy finger pressure on the feed tray and as "fingernail" marks caused by kinking of the film.

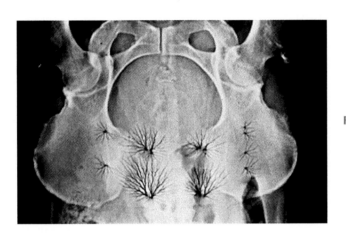

FIGURE 32-6 Tree static.

TABLE 32-3	Common Handling and Storage Artifacts
Appearance on Radiographic Film	**Cause**
Fog	The temperature or humidity is too high.
	The film bin is inadequately shielded from radiation.
	The safelight is too bright, is too close to the processing tray, or has an improper filter.
	The film has been left in the x-ray room during other exposures.
Pressure or kink marks	The film is improperly or roughly handled.
	The film is stacked too high in storage. (The weight causes marks.)
Streaks of increased OD	There are white-light leaks in the darkroom or cassette.
Crown, tree, and smudge static	The temperature or humidity is too low.
Yellow-brown stains	Thiosulfate is left on the film because of inadequate washing.

Safelight or Radiation Fog

White-light leaks in the darkroom or within the cassette cause streaklike artifacts of increased OD. If the safelight has an improper filter, if the safelight is too bright, or if the safelight is too close to the film-processing tray, fog will be evident on the image. Films left in the x-ray room during other exposures can become fogged by radiation. Radiation fog and safelight fog look alike.

Kink Marks

Characteristic artifacts can be caused by improper handling or storage, either before or after processing. Rough handling before processing can cause scratches and kink marks, such as those shown in Figure 32-5. Although the kink mark may appear as a fingernail mark, it is not. It is caused by the kinking or abrupt bending of film. Both usually appear as increased OD.

Static

Static is probably the most obvious artifact. It is caused by the buildup of electrons in the emulsion and is most noticeable during the winter or during periods of extremely low humidity. The following are three kinds of distinct patterns of static: crown, tree, and smudge. Tree static is illustrated in Figure 32-6.

Hypo Retention

The yellow-brown stain slowly appearing on a radiograph after long storage indicates a problem with hypo retention from the fixer. Not all of the residual thiosulfate from fixing was removed during washing, and silver sulfide slowly built up, appearing yellow in the stored radiograph.

SUMMARY

An artifact is an undesirable OD that appears on the radiograph. Artifacts occur (1) when the film is being exposed, (2) when the film is being processed, (3) when the film is being handled and stored either before or after processing. Causes include patient motion, positioning errors, wrong screen-film combinations, double expo-

sures, and improper grid positioning. Processing artifacts are mostly pressure marks on the film emulsion caused by the roller-transport system in the processor. They include sludge from dirty rollers, chemical fog, roller marks, and wet-pressure sensitization.

CHALLENGE QUESTIONS

1. Define or otherwise identify:
   a. Exposure artifact
   b. Guide-shoe marks
   c. Pick-off
   d. Pressure mark
   e. Kink mark
   f. Hypo retention
   g. Safelight

h. Curtain effect

i. Pi line

j. Processing artifact

2. Why must records be kept when artifacts are seen by the quality-control technologist?

3. List the three times when artifacts tend to occur.

4. Name three examples of exposure artifacts.

5. How would a radiographer correct a radiograph blurred by patient motion?

6. Why does double exposure occur?

7. Name three types of processing artifacts?

8. What is dichroic stain?

9. How do guide-shoe marks occur?

10. Explain what 3.1416 inches has to do with pi lines.

11. Describe the cause of wet-pressure sensitization marks.

12. Explain three ways that fog can occur on a radiograph.

13. What is the cause of a static artifact on the processed radiograph?

14. List the three kinds of static artifact patterns.

15. Why is it important for radiographers to be alert to film artifacts?

16. How can processor artifacts be avoided?

17. What causes grid cutoff artifacts?

18. How do pressure-type artifacts appear?

19. What type of artifact does hypo retention cause?

PART

V

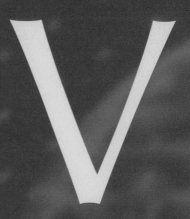

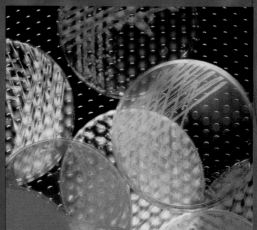

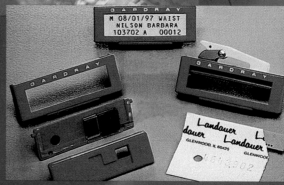

RADIATION
PROTECTION

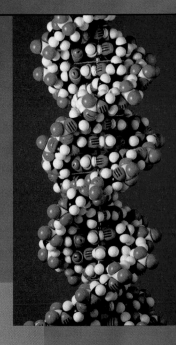

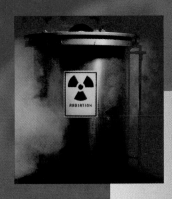

PREGNANT?

or you think you might be...

tell your doctor before getting an x-ray or prescription

Distributed by the Food and Drug Administration and the American College of Obstetricians and Gynecologists
DEPARTMENT OF HEALTH, EDUCATION, AND WELFARE • PUBLIC HEALTH SERVICE SERVICE
FOOD AND DRUG ADMINISTRATION, ROCKVILLE, MD 20857
HEW PUBLICATIONS NO. (FDA) 78-1045

CHAPTER

33

Human Biology

OBJECTIVES

At the completion of this chapter, the student should be able to:

1. Discuss the cell theory of human biology
2. List and describe the molecular composition of the human body
3. Explain the parts and function of the human cell
4. Describe the processes of mitosis and meiosis
5. Evaluate the radiosensitivity of tissues and organs

OUTLINE

W hen sufficiently intense, x-radiation has harmful effects such as skin burns, cancer, and leukemia. What is not known for certain is what degree of harmful effect, if any, follows diagnostic levels of x-radiation. There is no dispute, however, that the benefits derived from the diagnostic application of x-rays in medicine are enormous. It is therefore the job of the radiologic technologist, working with the radiologist and medical physicist, to produce high-quality x-ray images with a minimum of radiation exposure. This approach works to gain the highest diagnostic benefit with the lowest risk to patients and radiation workers. This chapters examines the basics of human biology and establishes a basis for understanding how x-radiation affects biologic tissue.

HUMAN RESPONSE TO IONIZING RADIATION

The effect of x-rays on humans is the result of interactions at atomic levels (see Chapter 13). These atomic interactions take the form of ionization, or excitation of orbital electrons, and result in the deposition of energy in tissue. The deposited energy can result in a molecular change, the consequences of which can be measurable if a critical molecule is involved.

When an atom is ionized, its chemical binding properties change. If the atom is a constituent of a large molecule, the ionization may result in breakage of the molecule or relocation of the atom within the molecule. The abnormal molecule may in time function improperly or cease to function, which can result in serious impairment or death of the cell. This process is reversible: ionized atoms can become neutral again by attracting a free electron. Molecules can be mended by repair-enzymes. Cell and tissues can regenerate and recover from the radiation injury. If the radiation response occurs within minutes or days after the radiation exposure, it is classified as an immediate or **early effect of radiation.** On the other hand, if the human injury is not observed for six months or more, it is termed a delayed or **late effect of radiation.**

Box 33-1 summarizes a general classification scheme of the possible early and late human responses to radiation. In addition, many other radiation responses have been observed in animals during experiments. Most of the human responses have been observed after rather large radiation doses. However, radiographers must be cautious and assume that even small doses are harmful. Table 33-1 lists some of the human population groups in which many of these radiation responses have been observed.

BOX 33-1 Human Responses to Ionizing Radiation

Early effects of radiation on humans

Acute radiation syndrome
  Hematologic syndrome
  Gastrointestinal syndrome
  Central nervous system syndrome
Local tissue damage
  Skin
  Gonads
  Extremities
Hematologic depression
Cytogenetic damage

Late effects of radiation on humans

Leukemia
Other malignant disease
  Bone cancer
  Lung cancer
  Thyroid cancer
  Breast cancer
Local tissue damage
  Skin
  Gonads
  Eyes
Shortening of lifespan
Genetic damage
  Cytogenetic damage
  Doubling dose
  Genetically significant dose

Effects of fetal irradiation

Prenatal death
Neonatal death
Congenital malformation
Childhood malignancy
Diminished growth and development

 Radiobiology is the study of the effects of ionizing radiation on biologic tissue.

The ultimate goal of radiobiologic research is the accurate description of the effects of radiation on humans so that radiation can be used more safely in diagnosis and more effectively in therapy. Most radiobiologic research is designed to develop dose-response relationships so that the effect of planned doses can be predicted and the response to accidental exposure better managed. Figure 33-1 illustrates the sequence of events in human tissue after radiation exposure.

COMPOSITION OF THE BODY

The composition of the human body has its basis in atoms, and it is at the atomic level that radiation interacts. The atomic composition of the body determines the character and degree of the radiation interaction, and the molecular and tissue composition defines the nature of

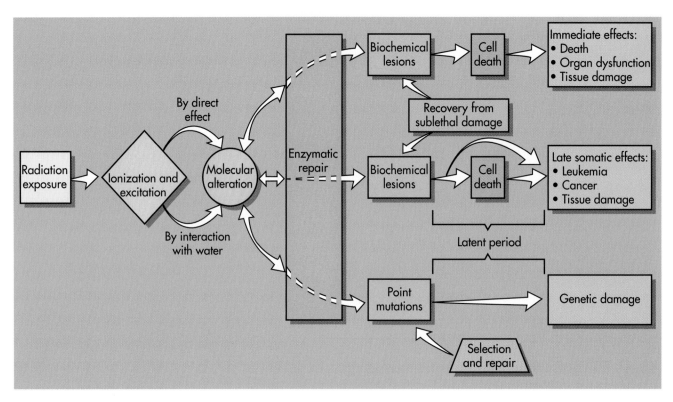

FIGURE 33-1 The sequence of events after radiation exposure of humans can lead to several radiation responses. At nearly every step, mechanisms for recovery and repair are available.

TABLE 33-1	Human Populations in Which Radiation Effects Have Been Observed
Population	**Effect Observed**
American radiologists	Leukemia, shortened life-span
Atomic bomb survivors	Malignant disease
Radiation accident victims	Acute death
Marshall Islanders	Thyroid cancer
Uranium miners	Lung cancer
Radium watch-dial painters	Bone cancer
Patients treated with ^{131}I	Thyroid cancer
Children treated for enlarged thymus	Thyroid cancer
Patients with ankylosing spondylitis	Leukemia
Patients treated with thorotrast	Liver cancer
Patients who had irradiation in utero	Childhood malignancy
Volunteer convicts	Fertility impairment
Cyclotron workers	Cataracts

BOX 33-2 Atomic Composition of the Body
60.0% hydrogen
25.7% oxygen
10.7% carbon
2.4% nitrogen
0.2% calcium
0.1% phosphorus
0.1% sulfur
0.8% trace elements

the radiation response. Box 33-2 summarizes the atomic composition of the body and shows that over 85% of the body is hydrogen and oxygen.

Cell Theory

Radiation interaction at the atomic level results in molecular change, and this in turn can produce a cell deficient in its normal growth and metabolism. Robert Hooke, an English schoolmaster, determined in 1665 that the **cell** is the biologic building block. Shortly thereafter, in 1673, Anton van Leeuwenhoek accurately described a living cell based on his microscopic observations. It was more than 100 years later, however, in 1838, that Matthias Schleiden and Theodor Schwann conclusively showed that all plants and animals contain

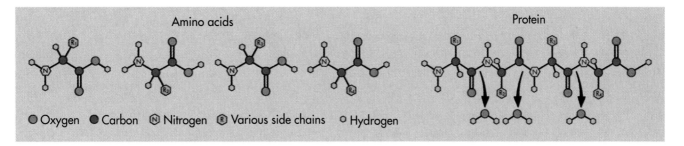

Amino acids   Protein

● Oxygen ● Carbon Ⓝ Nitrogen Ⓡ Various side chains ○ Hydrogen

FIGURE 33-2 Proteins consist of amino acids linked by peptide bonds. The creation of the peptide bond requires that a molecule of water be removed.

BOX 33-3   Molecular Composition of the Body
80% water
15% protein
2% lipids
1% carbohydrates
1% nucleic acid
1% other

cells as their basic functional units. This was the beginning of the **cell theory.**

The most significant milestone in recent studies of the living cell was the Watson and Crick description in 1953 of the molecular structure of deoxyribonucleic acid, the genetic substance of the cell.

Molecular Composition

There are five principal types of molecules in the body (Box 33-3). Four—proteins, lipids (fats), carbohydrates (sugars and starches), and nucleic acids—are macromolecules. Proteins, lipids, and carbohydrates are the principal classes of **organic molecules.** An **organic molecule** is life supporting and contains carbon. One of the rarest molecules, a nucleic acid concentrated in the nucleus of a cell, is DNA.

 Macromolecules are very large molecules, sometimes consisting of hundreds of thousands of atoms.

Water is the most abundant molecule in the body and also the simplest. Water, however, plays a particularly important role in delivering energy to the target molecule, thereby contributing to radiation effects. In addition to water and the macromolecules, there are some trace elements and inorganic salts that are essential to proper metabolism.

Water. The most abundant molecular constituent of the body is water. It consists of two atoms of hydrogen

and one atom of oxygen (H_2O) and constitutes approximately 80% of human substance. Humans are basically made of structured water. The water molecules exist both in the free state and in the bound state (that is, bound, or attached, to other molecules). They provide some form and shape for the cell, assist in maintaining body temperature, and enter into some biochemical reactions.

During vigorous exercise, water is lost through perspiration to stabilize the body's temperature and respiration. The water lost must be replaced to maintain **homeostasis,** which is the concept of the relative constancy of the internal environment of the human body. Water and carbon dioxide are end products in the **catabolism** (breaking down into smaller units) of macromolecules. **Anabolism,** the production of large molecules from small, and catabolism are collectively termed **metabolism.** Anabolic steroids are used by some athletes to build muscle mass, but harmful side effects may occur.

Proteins. Approximately 15% of the molecular composition of the body is protein. Proteins are long-chain macromolecules that consist of a linear sequence of amino acids connected by peptide bonds. There are 22 amino acids used in **protein synthesis,** the metabolic production of proteins. The linear sequence, or arrangement, of these amino acids determines the precise function of the protein molecule.

 Protein = AA — AA — AA — AA . . . where AA is amino acid and — is the peptide bond.

Figure 33-2 shows the general chemical form of a protein molecule. The generalized formula for a protein is $C_nH_nO_nN_nT_n$, where the subscript *n* refers to the number of atoms of each element in the molecule and T represents trace elements. In general, 50% of the mass of a protein molecule is carbon (C), 20% is oxygen (O), 17% is nitrogen (N), 7% is hydrogen (H), and 6% is other (trace) elements.

Proteins have a variety of uses in the body. They provide structure and support. Muscles are very high in protein content. Proteins also function as enzymes, hormones, and antibodies. **Enzymes** are molecules that are necessary in small quantities to allow a biochemical reaction to continue, even though they do not directly enter into the reaction. They function much like the catalyst in a chemical interaction. **Hormones** are molecules that exercise regulatory control over some body functions, such as growth and development or metabolic rate. Hormones are produced and secreted by the endocrine glands: the pituitary, adrenal, thyroid, parathyroid, pancreas, and gonads. **Antibodies** constitute a primary defense mechanism of the body against infection and disease. The molecular configuration of an antibody may be precise for attacking a particular type of invasive or infectious agent, called an **antigen.**

Lipids. **Lipids** are organic macromolecules composed solely of carbon, hydrogen, and oxygen. They have the general formula $C_nH_nO_n$. Structurally, lipids have the form shown in Figure 33-3, and it is this structure that distinguishes them from carbohydrates like the one shown in Figure 33-4. In general, lipids are composed of two kinds of smaller molecules: glycerol and fatty acids.

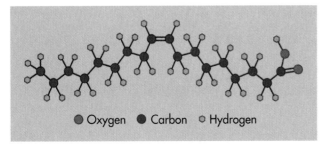

● Oxygen ● Carbon ○ Hydrogen

FIGURE 33-3 Structural configuration of a lipid is represented by a molecule of oleic acid: $CH_2(CH_2)_7CH = CH(CH_2)_7COOH$.

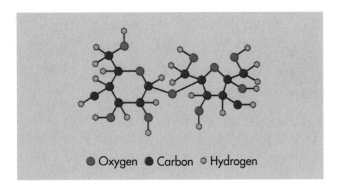

● Oxygen ● Carbon ○ Hydrogen

FIGURE 33-4 Carbohydrates are structurally different from lipids, even though their composition is similar. This is a molecular of sucrose, or ordinary table sugar: $C_{12}H_{22}O_{11}$.

Each lipid molecule is composed of one molecule of glycerol and three molecules of fatty acid.

Lipids are present in all tissues of the body and are the structural components of cell membranes. Lipids often are concentrated just under the skin and serve as a thermal insulator from the environment. Polar bears, for instance, have a particularly thick layer of subcutaneous fat (blubber) to protect them from the cold. Lipids also serve as fuel for the body by providing energy stores. It is more difficult, however, to extract energy from lipids than from the other major fuel source, carbohydrates; this relationship, of course, is associated with one of the major dilemmas in modern nutrition: obesity.

Carbohydrates. Carbohydrates, like lipids, are composed solely of carbon, hydrogen, and oxygen, but their structure is different (Figure 33-4). This structural difference determines the contribution of the carbohydrate molecule to body biochemistry. The ratio of the number of hydrogen atoms to oxygen atoms in a carbohydrate molecule is 2:1, like in water, and a large fraction of this molecule consists of water. Consequently, carbohydrates were once considered to be watered, or hydrated, carbons: hence their name.

Carbohydrates are also called **saccharides. Monosaccharides** and **disaccharides** are sugars. The chemical formula for glucose, a simple sugar, is $C_6H_{12}O_6$. These molecules are relatively small. **Polysaccharides** are large and include plant **starches** and animal **glycogen.** The chemical formula for a polysaccharide is $(C_6H_{10}O_5)_n$, where n is the number of simple sugar molecules in the macromolecule.

 The chief function of carbohydrates in the body is to provide fuel for cell metabolism.

Some carbohydrates are incorporated into the structure of cells and tissues to provide shape and stability for them. The human polysaccharide, glycogen, is stored in the tissues of the body and is used as fuel only when the simple sugar, glucose, is not present in adequate quantities.

Glucose is the ultimate molecule that fuels the body. Lipids can be catabolized into glucose for energy but only with great difficulty. Polysaccharides are much more readily transformed into glucose. This explains why a chocolate bar, which is high in glucose, can provide a quick burst of energy for an athlete.

Nucleic acids. There are two principal nucleic acids of importance to human metabolism: **deoxyribonucleic acid (DNA)** and **ribonucleic acid (RNA).** Located principally in the nucleus of the cell, DNA serves as the command or control molecule for cell function. It contains all the hereditary information representing a cell and, of course, if the cell is a **germ cell** (sperm or egg), all the hereditary information of the whole individual.

Located principally in the cytoplasm, RNA is also

found in the nucleus. There are two types: messenger RNA (mRNA) and transfer RNA (tRNA). They are distinguished according to their biochemical functions. These molecules are involved in the growth and development of the cell through a number of biochemical pathways, notably protein synthesis.

The nucleic acids are very large and extremely complex macromolecules. Figure 33-5 shows the structural composition of DNA and the manner in which the component molecules are joined. DNA consists of a backbone composed of alternating segments of deoxyribose (a sugar) and phosphate. For each deoxyribose-phosphate conjugate formed, a molecule of water is removed.

 DNA is the principal radiation-sensitive molecule.

Attached to each deoxyribose molecule is one of four different nitrogen-containing or nitrogenous, organic bases: adenine, guanine, thymine, or cytosine. Adenine and guanine are classified as purines; thymine and cytosine are classified as pyrimidines.

The base-sugar-phosphate combination is called a **nucleotide,** and the nucleotides are strung together in one long-chain macromolecule. Human DNA exists as two of these long chains attached together in ladder fashion (Figure 33-6). The side rails of the ladder are the alternating sugar-phosphate molecules, and the rungs of the ladder consist of bases joined by hydrogen bonds.

To complete the picture, the ladder is twisted about an imaginary axis like a spring. This produces a molecule having the **double-helix** configuration (Figure 33-7). The sequence of base bonding is limited to adenines bonded to thymines and cytosines bonded to guanines. No other base-bonding combinations are possible.

RNA resembles DNA structurally. The sugar component is ribose rather than deoxyribose, and uracil replaces thymines as a base component. In contrast, RNA forms a single spiral, not a double helix.

The Human Cell

The principal molecular components of the human body are made of intricate cellular structures. The structures are distributed throughout the cell in assembled fashion much like the parts of an automobile. This assembly ensures proper growth, development, and function of the

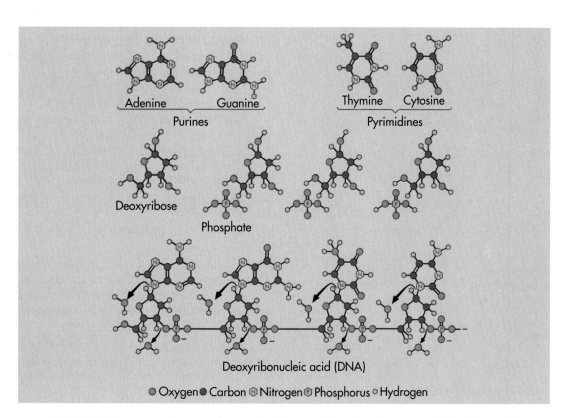

Adenine   Guanine   Thymine   Cytosine
    Purines   Pyrimidines

Deoxyribose

Phosphate

Deoxyribonucleic acid (DNA)

○ Oxygen ● Carbon ⊛ Nitrogen ⊚ Phosphorus ○ Hydrogen

FIGURE 33-5 DNA is the control center for life. A single molecule consists of a backbone of alternating sugar (deoxyribose) and phosphate molecules. Each sugar molecule has one of the four organic bases attached to it.

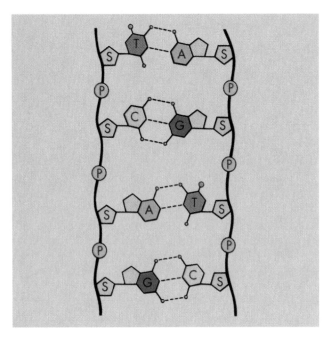

FIGURE 33-6 DNA consists of two long chains of alternating sugar and phosphate molecules fashioned like the side rails of a ladder with pairs of bases as rungs.

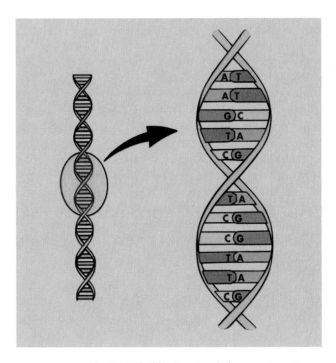

FIGURE 33-7 The DNA ladder is twisted about an imaginary axis to form a double helix.

cell. Figure 33-8 is a cutaway view of a human cell with its principal structures labeled.

The two major structures of the cell are the nucleus and the cytoplasm. The principal molecular component of the **nucleus** is DNA, the genetic material of the cell.

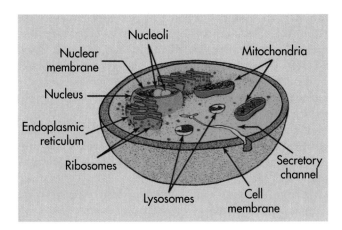

FIGURE 33-8 Schematic view of a human cell showing the principal structural components.

The nucleus also contains some RNA, protein, and water. Most of the RNA is contained in a rounded structure within the nucleus: the **nucleolus.** The nucleolus is often attached to the nuclear membrane, a double-walled structure that at some locations is connected to the endoplasmic reticulum. The nature of this connection controls the passage of molecules, particularly RNA, from nucleus to cytoplasm.

The **cytoplasm** makes up the bulk of the cell and contains all the molecular components in great quantity, except DNA. Found in the cytoplasm are a number of intracellular structures. The **endoplasmic reticulum** is a channel or series of channels that allows the nucleus to communicate with the cytoplasm.

The large bean-shaped structures are **mitochondria.** Macromolecules are digested in the mitochondria to produce energy for the cell. The mitochondria are therefore called the *engine of the cell.*

The small dotlike structures are ribosomes. **Ribosomes** are the site of protein synthesis and therefore are essential to normal cellular function. Ribosomes are found scattered in the cytoplasm or on the endoplasmic reticulum.

The small pealike sacs are lysosomes. The **lysosomes** contain enzymes capable of digesting cellular fragments and in some situations the cell itself. Lysosomes are helpful in the control of intracellular contaminants.

All these structures, including the cell itself, are surrounded by membranes. These membranes consist principally of lipid-protein complexes that selectively allow small molecules and water to diffuse from one side to the other. Of course, these cellular membranes also provide structure and form for the cell and its components.

When the critical macromolecular cellular components by themselves are irradiated, a dose of approximately 1 Mrad (10 kGy$_t$) is required to produce a measurable change in any physical characteristic of the molecule. When such a molecule is incorporated into the apparatus of a living cell, only a few rad are necessary to produce a measurable biologic response. The dose necessary to produce lethality in some single-cell organisms, such as bacteria, is measured in kilorads, whereas human cells can be killed with a dose of less than 100 rad (1 Gy_t).

A number of experiments have been conducted to show that the nucleus is much more sensitive to the effects of radiation than the cytoplasm. Such experiments are conducted by focusing and directing precise microbeams of electrons to a particular cell part or by incorporating the radioactive isotopes ^{3}H and ^{14}C into cellular molecules that localize exclusively either in the cytoplasm or in the nucleus.

Cell function. Every human cell has a specific function in supporting the total body. Some differences are obvious, as with nerve cells, blood cells, and muscle cells. The similarities are also somewhat obvious.

In addition to its specialized function, each cell to some extent performs the function of absorbing all molecular nutrients through the cell membrane and using these nutrients in the production of energy and in molecular synthesis. If the synthesis of molecules is damaged by radiation exposure, the cell may malfunction and die.

Protein synthesis is a good example of a cellular function necessary for survival (Figure 33-9). Located in the nucleus of a cell, DNA contains a molecular code that identifies what proteins that cell will make. This code is determined by the sequence of the base pairs, adenine-thymine and cytosine-guanine. A series of three base pairs, called a **codon**, identifies one of the 22 human amino acids available for protein synthesis. This genetic message is transferred in the nucleus to a molecule of mRNA. The mRNA leaves the nucleus by way of the endoplasmic reticulum and makes its way to a ribosome, where the genetic message is transferred to tRNA. The tRNA searches the cytoplasm for the amino acids for which it is coded. It attaches to the amino acid and carries it to the ribosome, where it is joined with other amino acids by peptide bonds to form the required protein molecule.

Interference with any phase of this procedure for protein synthesis could result in damage to the cell. Radiation interaction with the molecule having primary control over protein synthesis, DNA, is more effective in producing a response than radiation interaction with the other molecules involved in protein synthesis.

Cell proliferation. Although many thousands of rad *in vitro* are necessary to produce physically measurable disruption of macromolecules, single ionizing events at a particularly sensitive site of a critical target molecule are thought to be capable of disrupting cell proliferation.

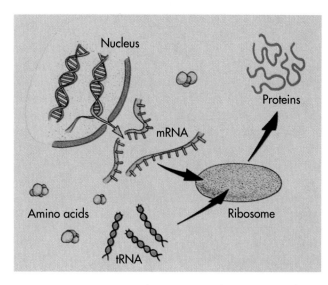

FIGURE 33-9 Protein synthesis is a complex process and involves many different molecules and cellular structures.

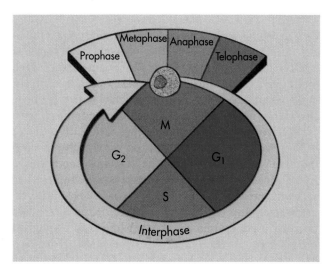

FIGURE 33-10 As the cell progresses through one growth cycle, several phases are observed. The cell biologist and the geneticist identify each phase differently.

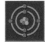 Cell proliferation is the act of a single cell or group of cells reproducing and multiplying in number.

Two general types of cells exist in the human body: **genetic cells** and **somatic cells**. The **genetic cells** are the oogonium of the female and the spermatogonium of the male. All other cells of the body are **somatic cells**. When somatic cells undergo proliferation, or cell division, they undergo **mitosis**. Genetic cells undergo **meiosis**.

Mitosis. The cell cycle is visualized differently by the cell biologist than by the geneticist (Figure 33-10). Each cycle includes the various states of cell growth, develop-

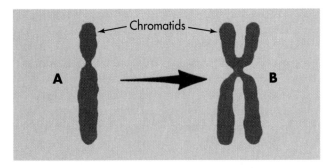

FIGURE 33-11 During the synthesis portion of interphase, the chromosomes replicate from a two-chromatid structure (A) to a four-chromatid structure (B).

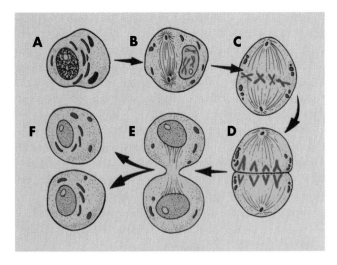

FIGURE 33-12 Mitosis is the phase of the cell cycle during which the chromosomes become visible, divide, and migrate to daughter cells. **A,** Interphase. **B,** Prophase. **C,** Metaphase. **D,** Anaphase. **E,** Telophase. **F,** Interphase.

ment, and division. The geneticist considers only two phases of the cell cycle—**mitosis** and **interphase.**

Mitosis, the division phase, is characterized by four subphases: prophase, metaphase, anaphase, and telophase. The portion of the cell cycle between mitotic events is termed **interphase.** Interphase is the period of growth of the cell between divisions.

The cell biologist usually identifies four phases of the cell cycle: M (mitosis), G_1 (first growth), S (synthesis), and G_2 (second growth). These phases are characterized by the structure of the chromosomes, which contain the genetic material DNA. The gap in cell growth between M and S is G_1, which is the pre–DNA synthesis phase.

The DNA synthesis phase is S. During this period, each DNA molecule is replicated into two identical daughter DNA molecules. The chromosome is transformed from a structure with two chromatids attached to a centromere to a structure with four chromatids attached to a centromere (Figure 33-11). The result is two pairs of homologous chromatids (that is, chromatids having precisely the same DNA content and structure). The G_2 phase is the post–DNA synthesis gap of cell growth.

During interphase, the chromosomes are not visible; however, during mitosis, the DNA slowly takes the form of the chromosomes as seen microscopically. Figure 33-12 shows the process of mitosis schematically. During **prophase,** the nucleus swells, and the DNA becomes more prominent and begins to take structural form. At **metaphase,** the chromosomes appear and are lined up along the equator of the nucleus. It is during metaphase that mitosis can be stopped and chromosomes studied carefully under the microscope.

 Radiation-induced chromosome damage is analyzed during metaphase.

During **anaphase,** each chromosome splits at the centromere so that a centromere and two chromatids are connected by a fiber to the poles of the nucleus. These poles are called **spindles,** and the fibers are called **spindle**

fibers. The number of chromatids per centromere has been reduced by half, and these newly formed chromosomes migrate slowly toward the spindle.

The final segment of mitosis, **telophase,** is characterized by the disappearance of the structural chromosomes into a mass of DNA and the closing off of the nuclear membrane like a dumbbell into two nuclei. At the same time the cytoplasm is divided into two equal parts, each accompanying one of the new nuclei.

Cell division is now complete. The two daughter cells look precisely like the parent and contain exactly the same genetic material.

Meiosis. Changes in genetic material can occur during the division process of genetic cells, which is called **meiosis.** The genetic cells begin with the same number of chromosomes as somatic cells: 23 pairs (46 chromosomes). However, for a genetic cell to be capable of "marriage" with another genetic cell, its complement of chromosomes must be reduced by half to 23 so that after conception and the union of two genetic cells, the daughter cells will contain 46 chromosomes (Figure 33-13).

 The process of reduction and division in genetic cells is meiosis.

The genetic cell begins meiosis with 46 chromosomes, appearing as a somatic cell having completed the G_2 phase. It then progresses through the phases of mitosis into two daughter cells, each containing 46 chromosomes of two chromatids each. The names of the subphases of meiosis and mitosis are the same.

Each daughter cell of this first division now progresses through a second division in which all the cellular mate-

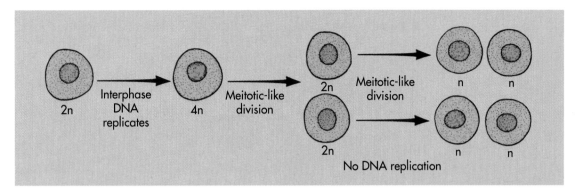

FIGURE 33-13 Meiosis is the process of reduction and division, and it occurs only in germ cells. *n,* Number of similar chromosomes.

rial is divided, including the chromosomes. However, the second division is not accompanied by an S phase, and therefore there is no replication of DNA and consequently no duplication of the chromosomes. The resulting granddaughter cells contain only 23 chromosomes each.

Each parent has undergone two division processes, resulting in four daughter cells. During the second division, there is some exchange of chromosomal material among chromatids by a process called **crossing over.** Crossing over results in changes in genetic constitution and changes in inheritable traits.

Tissues and Organs

During the development and maturation of a human from the two united genetic cells, a number of cell types evolve. Collections of cells of similar structure and function form **tissues.** Box 33-4 is a breakdown of the composition of the body according to its tissue constituents.

These tissues are in turn bound together in precise fashion to form **organs.** The tissues and the organs of the body serve as discrete units with specific functional responsibilities. Some tissues and organs combine into an overall integrated organization known as an **organ system.**

The principal organ systems of the body are the nervous, digestive, endocrine, respiratory, and reproductive systems. The effects of radiation that appear at the whole-body level result from damage to organ systems, which in turn is a result of radiation injury to the cells of that system.

The cells of a tissue system are identified by their rate of proliferation and their stage of development. Immature cells are called **undifferentiated cells, precursor cells,** or **stem cells.** As a cell matures through growth and proliferation, it can pass through various stages of differentiation into a fully functional and mature cell.

 Stem cells are more sensitive to radiation than mature cells.

BOX 33-4	Tissue Composition of the Body

43% muscle
14% fat
12% organs
10% skeleton
8% blood
6% subcutaneous tissue
4% bone marrow
3% skin

TABLE 33-2	Response to Radiation is Related to Cell Type

Radiosensitivity	Cell Type
High	Lymphocytes
	Spermatogonia
	Erythroblasts
	Intestinal crypt cells
Intermediate	Endothelial cells
	Osteoblasts
	Spermatids
	Fibroblasts
Low	Muscle cells
	Nerve cells

The sensitivity of the cell to radiation is determined to some degree by its state of maturity and its functional role. Table 33-2 is a list of a number of different types of cells in the body according to their degree of radiosensitivity.

The tissues and organs of the body consist of both stem cells and mature cells. There are several types of tissue, and they can be classified according to structural or functional features. These features influence the degree of radiosensitivity of the tissue.

The **epithelium** is the covering tissue, and it lines all exposed surfaces of the body, both exterior and interior. Epithelium covers the skin, blood vessels, abdominal and chest cavities, and gastrointestinal tract.

TABLE 33-3	Relative Radiosensitivity of Tissues and Organs	
Level of Radiosensitivity*	**Tissue or Organ**	**Effect**
High: 200 to 1000 rad	Lymphoid tissue	Atrophy
	Bone marrow	Hypoplasia
	Gonads	Atrophy
Intermediate: 1000 to 1500 rad	Skin	Erythema
	Gastrointestinal tract	Ulcer
	Cornea	Cataract
	Growing bone	Growth arrest
	Kidney	Nephrosclerosis
	Liver	Ascites
	Thyroid	Atrophy
Low: >5000 rad	Muscle	Fibrosis
	Brain	Necrosis
	Spinal	Transection

*The minimum dose delivered at the rate of approximately 200 rad/day that will produce a response.

Connective and **supporting tissues** are high in protein and are composed principally of fibers that usually have a high degree of elasticity. **Connective tissue** binds tissues and organs together. Bone ligaments and cartilage are examples of connective tissue.

Muscle is a special type of tissue that is capable of contracting. It is found throughout the body and also is high in protein content.

Nervous tissue consists of specialized cells called **neurons** that have long, thin extensions from the cell to distant parts of the body. **Nervous tissue** is the avenue through which electrical impulses are transmitted throughout the body for control and response.

When these various types of tissue are combined to form an organ, they are identified according to two parts of the organ. The **parencyhmal** part contains tissues that are representative of that particular organ, whereas the **stromal** part is composed of connective tissue and vasculature, which provide structure to the organ. When the early effects of high doses of radiation are considered, it is organ damage that ultimately results in observable effects. The various organs of the body exhibit a wide range of sensitivity to radiation. This radiosensitivity is determined by the function of the organ in the body, the rate at which cells mature in the organ, and the inherent radiosensitivty of the cell type. A precise knowledge of these various organ radiosensitivities is unnecessary; however, knowledge of the general levels of radiosensitivity is helpful in understanding the effects of whole-body radiation exposure and, in particular, the acute radiation syndrome (Table 33-3).

SUMMARY

After radiation exposure, the human body responds in predictable ways. Radiobiology is the study of the effects of ionizing radiation on biologic tissue to refine knowledge of the expected response. If a response occurs within minutes or days of exposure, it is called an *early effect of radiation*. If the injury is not observable within 6 months, it is termed a *late effect of radiation exposure.*

The cell theory describes the cell as the basic functional unit of all plants and animals. Radiobiology studies radiation's effects at the cellular and molecular levels. At the molecular level, the human body is composed of mostly water, protein, lipid, carbohydrates, and nucleic acid. The two important nucleic acids in human metabolism are DNA and RNA. DNA contains all the hereditary information in the cell. If the cell is a genetic cell, the DNA contains the hereditary information of the whole individual. DNA is a macromolecule made up of two long chains of base-sugar-phosphate combinations twisted in a double-helix configuration.

Major cellular function consists of protein synthesis and cell division. Mitosis is the growth, development, and division of cells. *Meiosis* is the term for the division of genetic cells.

Cells of similar structure bind together to form tissue, and tissue binds together to form organs. An integrated organization of tissue and organs is called an *organ system*. The principal systems of the body are the nervous, digestive, endocrine, respiratory, and reproductive systems. The radiosensitivity of various tissue and organ systems varies widely. Reproductive cells are highly radiosensitive, whereas nerve cells are less radiosensitive.

CHALLENGE QUESTIONS

1. Define or otherwise identify:
   a. Cell theory
   b. Anabolism
   c. Carbohydrate
   d. M, G_1, S, and G_2
   e. Epithelium

   f. Cytoplasm
   g. Enzyme
   h. Homeostasis
   i. Late effect of radiation

2. At what structural level do x-rays interact to produce a radiation response in humans?

3. How does ionizing radiation affect an atom within a large molecule?

4. Describe the radiation effects observed in five different human populations.

5. Who first named the cell the building block of biologic tissue?

6. Who won a Nobel Prize for describing the molecular structure of DNA?

7. Why are humans basically a structured aqueous suspension?

8. How do proteins function in the human body?

9. What do carbohydrates do for humans?

10. DNA is the abbreviation for what molecule?

11. Which molecule is considered the genetic material of the cell?

12. What is the function of the endoplasmic reticulum?

13. Approximately what dose of radiation is required to produce a measurable physical change in a macromolecule?

14. List the stages of cell division in a somatic cell.

15. List the stages of cell reduction division in a genetic cell.

16. Which type of cell is more radiosensitive: stem cells or mature cells?

17. What type of tissue has the lowest sensitivity to radiation?

Fundamental Principles of Radiobiology

OBJECTIVES

At the completion of this chapter, the student should be able to:

1. State the law of Bergonie and Tribondeau
2. Describe the physical factors affecting radiation response
3. Describe the biologic factors affecting radiation response
4. Explain dose-response relationships
5. List and describe the types of dose-response relationships

OUTLINE

Some types of tissue respond more quickly and to lower doses of radiation than others. Such tissues are said to be more sensitive to radiation exposure. For example, reproductive tissue is more sensitive than nervous tissue. Radiation sensitivity is one radiobiologic concept that was detailed in 1906 by the two French scientists, Jean Bergonie and Louis Tribondeau. Both physical and biologic factors affect radiosensitivity in biologic tissue. Although most of these discoveries come from the field of radiation oncology, it is important for radiologic technologists to understand the effects of low-dose radiation exposure. The study of radiobiology is directed principally to the establishment of radiation dose-response relationships. A dose-response relationship is a mathematic function expressed as a graph that relates radiation dose to observed response.

LAW OF BERGONIE AND TRIBONDEAU

In 1906, two French scientists, Bergonie and Tribondeau, theorized and observed that radiosensitivity was a function of the metabolic state of the tissue being irradiated. This has come to be known as the *law of Bergonie and Tribondeau* and has been verified many times. Basically, the law states that the radiosensitivity of living tissue varies with maturation and metabolism, as follows:

1. Stem cells are radiosensitive. The more mature a cell, the more resistant to radiation it is.
2. The younger the tissue and organs, the more radiosensitive they are.
3. When the level of metabolic activity is high, radiosensitivity is also high.
4. As the proliferation rate for cells and the growth rate for tissues increase, the radiosensitivity also increases.

Box 34-1 summarizes the law of Bergonie and Tribondeau.

This law is of interest principally as a historical note in the development of radiobiology. It has found some application in radiotherapy. In diagnostic imaging, it reminds us that the fetus is considerably more sensitive to radiation exposure than the child or the adult.

PHYSICAL FACTORS AFFECTING RADIOSENSITIVITY

When tissue is irradiated, the response of that tissue is determined principally by the amount of energy deposited per unit mass: the dose in rads (Gy_1). Even under controlled experimental conditions, however, when equal doses are delivered to equal specimens, the response may not be the same because of other modifying

> **BOX 34-1 Law of Bergonie and Tribondeau**
> Stem cells are radiosensitive; mature cells are radioresistant.
> Younger tissues and organs are radiosensitive.
> Tissues with high metabolic activity are radiosensitive
> A high proliferation rate for cells and a high growth rate for tissues result in increased radiosensitivity.

factors. A number of physical factors, including linear energy transfer, relative biologic effectiveness, and fractionation and protraction, affect the degree of radiation response.

Linear Energy Transfer

Linear energy transfer (LET) is a measure of the rate at which energy is transferred from ionizing radiation to soft tissue. It is another method of expressing radiation quality and determining the value of the tissue weighting factor (W_T) used in radiation protection. The tissue weighting factor accounts for the relative radiosensitivity of various tissues and organs (see Chapter 38). LET is expressed in units of kiloelectron volts of energy transferred per micrometer of track length in soft tissue (keV/μm).

The ability of ionizing radiation to produce a biologic response increases as the LET of the radiation increases. When the LET is high, ionizations occur frequently, so the probability of interaction with the target molecule is higher.

 The LET of diagnostic x-rays is approximately 3 keV/μm.

Relative Biologic Effectiveness

As the LET of radiation increases, the ability to produce biologic damage also increases. This is quantitatively described as the **relative biologic effectiveness (RBE)**:

$$RBE = \frac{\text{Dose of standard radiation necessary to produce a given effect}}{\text{Dose of test radiation necessary to produce the same effect}}$$

The standard radiation, by convention, is orthovoltage x-radiation in the 200- to 250-kVp range. This type of x-ray beam was used for many years in radiation oncology and in essentially all early radiobiology research. Diagnostic x-rays have an RBE of 1. Radiation with a lower LET than that of diagnostic x-rays has an RBE less than 1, whereas radiation with a higher LET has a higher RBE.

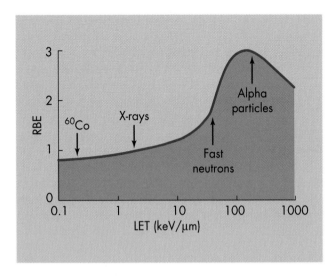

FIGURE 34-1 As the LET increases, the RBE increases also, but a maximum value is reached beyond which the RBE can increase no further.

TABLE 34-1	LET and RBE of Various Types of Radiation	
Type of Radiation	LET (keV/μm)	RBE
25-MV x-rays	0.2	0.8
^{60}Co rays	0.3	0.9
1-MeV electrons	0.3	0.9
Diagnostic x-rays	3.0	1.0
10-MeV protons	4.0	5.0
Fast neutrons	50.0	10
5-MeV alpha particles	100.0	20
Heavy nuclei	1000.0	30

RBE, Relative biologic effectiveness.

Figure 34-1 shows the relationship between RBE and LET and identifies some of the more common types of radiation. The maximum value of the RBE is approximately 3. Table 34-1 lists the approximate LET and RBE of various types of ionizing radiation.

 The RBE of diagnostic x-rays is 1.

Question: When mice are irradiated with 250-kVp x-rays, 650 rad (6.5 Gy$_t$) is necessary to produce death. If similar mice are irradiated with fast neutrons, only 210 rad (2.1 Gy$_t$) is needed. What is the RBE for the fast neutrons?

Answer:
$$RBE = \frac{650 \text{ rad}}{210 \text{ rad}}$$
$$= 3.1$$

Fractionation and Protraction

If a dose of radiation is delivered over a long time rather than quickly, the effect of that dose will be less. Stated differently, if the time of irradiation is lengthened, a higher dose will be required to produce the same effect. This lengthening of time can be accomplished in two ways.

If the dose is delivered continuously but at a lower dose rate, it is said to be **protracted.** A total of 600 rad (6 Gy$_t$) delivered in 3 minutes (200 rad/min [2 Gy$_t$/min]) is lethal for a mouse. However, when 600 rad is delivered at the rate of 1 rad/hr (10 mGy$_t$/hr) for a total of 600 hours, the mouse survives. Dose protraction causes less effect because of the lower dose rate, which allows time for intracellular repair and tissue recovery.

If the 600-rad dose is delivered at the same dose rate, 200 rad/min, but in 12 equal fractions of 50 rad (500

mGy$_t$), each separated by 24 hours, the mouse will survive. In this situation the dose is said to be **fractionated.** Dose fractionation causes less effect because intracellular repair and recovery occur between doses. Dose fractionation is used routinely in radiation oncology.

BIOLOGIC FACTORS AFFECTING RADIOSENSITIVITY

In addition to these physical factors, a number of biological conditions alter the radiation response of tissue. Some of these factors have to do with the inherent state of the tissue, such as age and metabolic rate. Other factors are related to artificially introduced modifiers of the biologic system.

Oxygen Effect

Tissue is more sensitive to radiation when irradiated in the oxygenated, or aerobic, state than when irradiated under anoxic (without oxygen) or hypoxic (low-oxygen) conditions. This characteristic of tissue is called the *oxygen effect* and is described numerically by the **oxygen enhancement ratio (OER),** as follows:

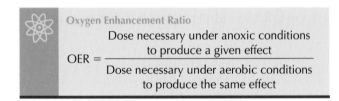

Oxygen Enhancement Ratio

$$OER = \frac{\text{Dose necessary under anoxic conditions to produce a given effect}}{\text{Dose necessary under aerobic conditions to produce the same effect}}$$

Generally, the irradiation of tissue is conducted under conditions of full oxygenation. Hyperbaric (high-pressure) oxygen has been used in radiation oncology in an attempt to increase the radiosensitivity of nodular, avascular tumors, which are less radiosensitive than tumors with an adequate blood supply.

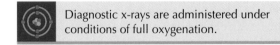 Diagnostic x-rays are administered under conditions of full oxygenation.

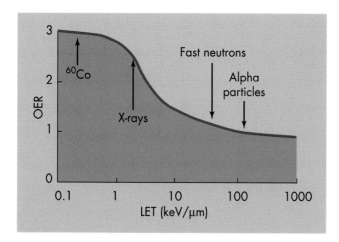

FIGURE 34-2 The OER is high for low-LET radiation and decreases in value as the LET increases.

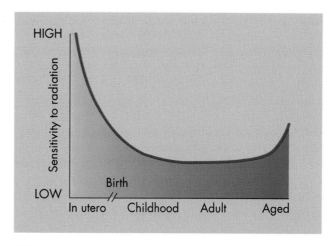

FIGURE 34-3 Radiosensitivity varies with age. Experiments with animals have shown that the very young and the very old are more sensitive to radiation.

Question: When experimental mouse mammary carcinomas are clamped and irradiated under hypoxic conditions, the tumor control dose is 10,600 rad (106 Gy$_t$). When the tumors are not clamped and are irradiated under aerobic conditions, the tumor control dose is 4050 rad (40.5 Gy$_t$). What is the OER for this system?

Answer: $OER = \dfrac{10,600}{4050}$

$= 2.6$

The OER is LET dependent (Figure 34-2). The OER is highest for low-LET radiation, having a maximum of approximately 3, and decreases to approximately 1 for high-LET radiation.

Age

The age of a biologic structure affects its radiosensitivity. The response of humans is characteristic of this age-related radiosensitivity (Figure 34-3). Humans are most sensitive before birth. The sensitivity then decreases until maturity, which is when humans are most resistant to radiation effects. In old age, humans again become somewhat more radiosensitive. Many theories have been developed to explain this pattern of response, but none is universally accepted.

Recovery

In vitro experiments show that human cells are capable of recovering from radiation damage. If the radiation dose is sufficient to kill the cell before its next division, interphase death will occur. If the radiation dose is not sufficient to kill the cell before its next division, the cell will recover from the sublethal radiation damage it has sustained.

  Interphase death occurs when the cell dies before replicating.

This intracellular recovery is due to a repair mechanism inherent in the biochemistry of the cell. Some types of cells have greater capacity for the repair of sublethal damage than others.

At the whole-body level, this recovery from radiation damage is assisted through **repopulation** by the surviving cells. If a tissue or organ receives a sufficient radiation dose, it will respond by shrinking in size. This is called **atrophy** and occurs because some cells die, disintegrate, and are carried away as waste products. If a sufficient number of cells sustain only sublethal damage and survive, they may proliferate and repopulate the irradiated tissue or organ. The combined processes of repair and repopulation contribute to recovery from radiation damage.

Recovery = Repair + Repopulation

Chemical Agents

Some chemicals can modify the radiation response of cells, tissues, and organs. For the chemical agents to be effective, they must be present at the time of irradiation. Application after irradiation does not usually alter the degree of radiation response.

Radiosensitizers. Agents that enhance the effect of radiation are called **sensitizing agents.** Some examples are halogenated pyrimidines, methotrexate, actinomycin D, hydroxyurea, and vitamin K. The halogenated pyrimidines become incorporated into the deoxyribonucleic acid (DNA) of the cell and cause the radiation effects on that molecule to be amplified. All the radiosensitizers have an effectiveness ratio of approximately 2; that is, if 90% of a cell culture is killed by 200 rad (2 Gy$_t$), then in the presence of a sensitizing agent, only 100 rad (1 Gy$_t$) will be required for the same percentage of lethality.

Radioprotectors. The radioprotective compounds include molecules containing a sulfhydryl group (sulfur and hydrogen bound together), such as cysteine and cysteamine. Hundreds of others compounds have been tested and found effective by a factor of approximately 2. For example, if 600 rad (6 Gy$_t$) is a lethal dose to a mouse, then in the presence of a radioprotective agent, 1200 rad (12 Gy$_t$) would be required to produce death. Radioprotective agents have not found human application because to be effective, they must be administered in toxic levels. The protective agent can be worse than the radiation.

Hormesis

Some evidence suggests that a little radiation actually produces a helpful effect. Several animal studies have shown that those receiving low-radiation doses live longer than controls. The prevailing explanation is that a little radiation stimulates hormonal and immune responses to other toxic environmental agents. There are many nonradiation examples of hormesis. In large quantities, fluoride is deadly; in small quantities, it is a known tooth preservative.

RADIATION DOSE-RESPONSE RELATIONSHIPS

Radiobiology is a relatively new science. Although some scientists were working with animals to observe the effects of radiation, within a few years after the discovery of x-rays, these studies were not experimentally sound. Interest in radiobiology increased enormously, however, with the advent of the atomic age during the 1940s.

The object of nearly all radiobiologic research is the establishment of radiation dose-response relationships. A **radiation dose-response relationship** is a mathematic relationship between various radiation dose levels and the magnitude of the observed response.

Radiation dose-response relationships have two important applications in radiology. First, these experimentally determined relationships are used to design therapeutic treatment routines for patients with cancer. Second, radiobiologic studies have been designed to provide information on the effects of low-dose irradiation. These studies and the dose-response relationships obtained are the basis for radiation-control activities and are of particular significance to diagnostic radiology.

Every radiation dose-response relationship has two characteristics: it is either linear or nonlinear and it is either threshold or nonthreshold. These characteristics can be described mathematically or graphically. This discussion avoids the math.

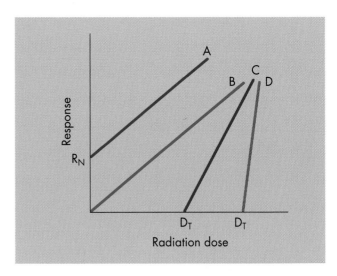

FIGURE 34-4 Linear dose-response relationships *A* and *B* are nonthreshold types; *C* and *D* are threshold types.

Linear Dose-Response Relationships

Figure 34-4 shows examples of a linear dose-response relationship, so called because the response is directly proportional to the dose. When the radiation dose is doubled, the response to radiation is likewise doubled.

Dose-response relationships *A* and *B* intersect the dose axis at zero or below in Figure 34-4. These relationships are therefore the linear, nonthreshold type. In a nonthreshold dose-response relationship, any dose, regardless of its size, is expected to produce a response. At zero dose, relationship *A* exhibits a measurable response, R$_N$. The level R$_N$ is called the natural response level and indicates that even without a radiation exposure, that type of response (cancer, for example) occurs.

 Radiation-induced cancer and genetic effects follow a linear, nonthreshold dose-response relationship.

Dose-response relationships *C* and *D* in Figure 34-4 are linear, threshold type because they intercept the dose axis at some value greater than zero. The threshold doses for *C* and *D* is D$_T$. At doses below these values, no response would be expected. Relationship *D* has a steeper slope than *C*, and therefore above the threshold dose, any increment of dose will produce a larger response if that response follows relationship *D* rather than *C*.

Nonlinear Dose-Response Relationships

All other radiation dose-response relationships are defined as nonlinear (Figure 34-5). Curves *A* and *B* are nonlinear, nonthreshold. Curve *A* shows that a large response results from very little radiation dose. At high-dose levels the radiation is not as efficient, since an in-

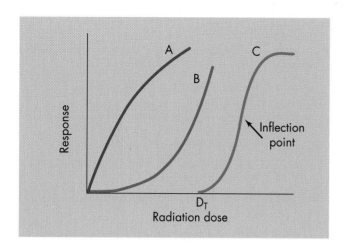

FIGURE 34-5 Nonlinear dose-response relationships can assume several shapes. Curves *A* and *B* are nonthreshold. Curve *C* is threshold.

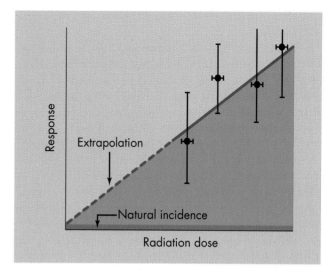

FIGURE 34-6 A dose-response relationship is produced by extrapolating high-dose experimental data to low doses.

cremental dose at high levels results in less relative damage than the same incremental dose at low levels.

The dose-response relationship represented by curve *B* in Figure 34-5 is just the opposite. Incremental doses in the low-dose range result in very little response. At high doses, however, the same increment of dose produces a much larger response.

Curve *C* in Figure 34-5 is a nonlinear, threshold relationship. At doses below D_T, no response is measured. As the dose is increased above the D_T for *C*, it becomes increasingly effective per increment of dose until it reaches the dose corresponding to the inflection point of the curve. The inflection point occurs when the curve stops bending up and begins bending down. Above this level, incremental doses become less effective. Relationship *C* is sometimes called an *S-type*, or *sigmoid-type, radiation dose-response relationship*.

 Radiation death and the skin effects of high-dose fluoroscopy follow a sigmoid-type dose-response relationship.

We refer to these general types of radiation dose-response relationships in discussing the type and degree of human radiation injury. Diagnostic radiology is almost exclusively concerned with the late effects of radiation exposure and therefore with linear, nonthreshold dose-response relationships. For completeness, however, Chapter 36 contains a brief discussion of early radiation damage.

Constructing a Dose-Response Relationship

Determining the radiation dose-response relationship for the whole body is tricky. It is very difficult to determine the degree of response, even that of early effects, because the number of experimental animals that can be used is

usually small. It is nearly impossible to measure low-dose, late effects, and that is the area of greatest interest to diagnostic imaging.

Therefore we resort to irradiating a limited number of animals to very large doses of radiation in hopes of observing a statistically significant response. Figure 34-6 shows the results of such an experiment in which four groups of animals were irradiated to a different dose. The observations on each group results in an ordered pair of data: a dose and the associated biologic response.

The error bars in each ordered pair indicate the confidence associated with each data point. The error bars on the dose measurements are very narrow; the radiation dose can be measured very accurately. The error bars on the response, however, are very wide because of biologic variability and the limited number of observations at each dose.

The principal interest in diagnostic imaging is to estimate the response at very low doses. Since this cannot be done directly, the dose-response relationship is extrapolated from the high-dose, known region into the low-dose, unknown region. This invariably results in a linear, nonthreshold dose-response relationship. Such an extrapolation, however, may not be correct because of the many qualifying conditions on the experiment.

SUMMARY

In 1906, two French scientists first theorized that radiosensitivity was a function of the metabolic state of tissue being irradiated. Their theory is known as *the law of Bergonie and Tribondeau* and state the following: (1) stem cells are radiosensitive, and mature cells are less so; (2) young tissue is more radiosensitive than older tissue; (3) high metabolic activity is radiosensitive, and low metabolic rate is radioresistant; and (4) increases in the proliferation and growth rates of cells makes them more radiosensitive.

Physical and biologic factors affect tissue radiosensitivity. The physical factors are the LET (rate at which energy is transferred from radiation to soft tissue), RBE (as LET increases, the damage to tissue increases), fractionation (dose delivered over a long time), and protraction (a lower dose delivered continuously). The biologic factors affecting radiosensitivity are the oxygen effect (the aerobic state of tissue is more radiosensitive), the age-related effect (the human fetus is most sensitive to radiation than an adult), and the recovery effect (intracellular recovery is due to intrinsic repair mechanisms and the progression of the cell through the cell cycle). Some chemicals can modify the response of cells. They are called *radiosensitizers* and *radioprotectors*.

Radiobiology research concentrates on radiation dose-response relationships. A radiation dose-response relationship is the relationship between different radiation doses and the magnitude of the observed response. In linear dose-response relationships the response is directly proportional to the dose. In nonlinear dose-response relationships, varied responses are produced from varied doses. The threshold dose-response is the level below which there is no response. The nonthreshold dose-response relationship means that any dose is expected to produce a response. For establishing radiation-protection guidelines for diagnostic imaging, the linear, nonthreshold dose-response model is used.

CHALLENGE QUESTIONS

1. Define or otherwise identify:
   a. Linear energy transfer
   b. Standard radiation
   c. Oxygen enhancement ratio
   d. Repopulation
   e. Interphase death
   f. Dose protraction
   g. Tissue weighting factor
2. Write the formula for relative biologic effectiveness.
3. Give an example of fractionated radiation.
4. When is high-pressure (hyperbaric) oxygen used in radiation oncology?
5. Write the formula for the oxygen enhancement ratio.
6. How does age affect the radiosensitivity of tissue?
7. Name three agents that enhance the effect of radiation.
8. Name three radioprotective agents.
9. Are radioprotective agents used for human application? Why or why not?
10. Explain the meaning of a radiation dose-response relationship.
11. What occurs in a nonlinear radiation dose-response relationship?
12. Explain why the linear, nonthreshold dose-response relationship is used as the model for radiation-protection guides for diagnostic imaging.
13. State two of the corollaries to the law of Bergonie and Tribondeau.
14. Approximately 800 rad of 220-kVp x-rays are necessary to produce death in the armadillo. ^{60}Co gamma rays have a lower LET than 220-kVp x-rays, and therefore 940 rad is required for death. What is the RBE of ^{60}Co compared with 220-kVp x-rays?
15. Under fully oxygenated conditions, 90% of human cells in culture are killed by 150-rad. If the cells are made anoxic, the dose required for 90% lethality is 400 rad. What is the OER?
16. What are the units of LET?
17. Describe how RBE and LET are related.
18. How do you receive your occupational radiation exposure: fractionated, protracted, or continuous? Explain.
19. Describe how OER and LET are related.

Molecular and Cellular Radiobiology

OBJECTIVES

At the completion of this chapter, the student should be able to:

1. Discuss the three principal effects of in vitro irradiation of macromolecules
2. Explain the effects of radiation on DNA macromolecules
3. Identify the chemical reactions involved in the radiolysis of water
4. Describe the effects of in vivo irradiation
5. Describe the principles of the target theory of radiobiology
6. Discuss the kinetics of human cell survival after irradiation

OUTLINE

Even though the initial interaction between radiation and tissue occurs at the electron level, observable human radiation injury results from change at the molecular level. The occurrence of molecular lesions is categorized into effects on macromolecules and effects on water. The irradiation of macromolecules and the radiolysis of water are discussed in this chapter. Since the human body is an aqueous solution containing 80% water molecules, radiation interaction with water is the principal radiation interaction in the body. However, the ultimate damage is to the target molecule deoxyribonucleic acid (DNA), which controls cellular metabolism and reproduction.

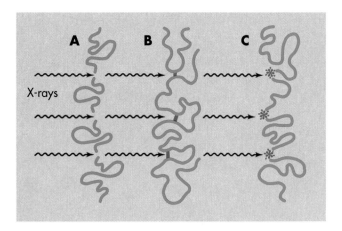

FIGURE 35-1 Results of the irradiation of macromolecules. **A,** Main-chain scission. **B,** Cross-linking. **C,** Point lesions.

IRRADIATION OF MACROMOLECULES

Although the initial interaction between radiation and tissue occurs at the electron level, the observed human radiation injury results from molecular change. Such molecular changes can be conveniently separated into either effects on macromolecules or effects on water. The results of irradiation of macromolecules are quite different from those of irradiation of water.

A **solution** is a suspension of particles or molecules in a fluid such as water. A solution can also be a mixture of fluids, such as water and alcohol. When macromolecules are irradiated in a solution **in vitro** (outside the body or outside the cell), a considerable radiation dose is required to produce a measurable effect. **In vivo** irradiation (irradiation of macromolecules in the living cell) demonstrates that molecules are considerably more radiosensitive in their natural state.

In Vitro Irradiation
Macromolecules are irradiated outside the body or outside the cell.

In Vivo Irradiation
Macromolecules are irradiated inside a living cell.

When macromolecules are irradiated in solution in vitro, the following major effects occur (Figure 35-1): (1) main-chain scission, (2) cross-linking, and (3) point lesions. Laboratory experiments have shown that all these types of radiation effects on macromolecules are reversible through intracellular repair and recovery.

Main-Chain Scission

Scission is the act of cutting or dividing or the state of being cut or divided. **Main-chain scission** is the breakage in the long-chain molecule that divides a long, single

molecule into many molecules. Each of these smaller molecules may still be macromolecular in nature. Main-chain scission not only reduces the size of the macromolecule but also changes the viscosity of the solution in which irradiation occurs. A **viscous** solution is one that is very thick and slow to flow, such as cold maple syrup. Tap water, on the other hand, has a low viscosity. Measurement of viscosity determines the degree of main-chain scission. The more scission that has occurred, the less viscous the solution.

Cross-Linking

Some macromolecules have small, spurlike side structures that extend from the main chain. Others produce these spurs as a consequence of irradiation. If these side spurs are created by irradiation, they will attach to a neighboring molecule or to another segment of the same molecule. This process is called **cross-linking.** Radiation-induced molecular cross-linking increases the viscosity of a macromolecular solution.

Point Lesions

The irradiation of macromolecules can also result in disruption of single chemical bonds, producing **point lesions** in a molecule. A *lesion* can be defined as any change that results in impairment or loss of function. Point lesions occur at the point of a single chemical bond. Such lesions are not detectable by current analytic techniques, but they can result in a minor modification of the molecule, which can in turn cause it to malfunction in the cell.

At low radiation doses, point lesions are considered to be the cellular radiation damage resulting in the late radiation effects observed at the whole-body level.

Macromolecular Synthesis

Modern molecular biology has developed a generalized scheme for the function of a normal human cell. This scheme involves the processes of catabolism, anabolism, and synthesis. Recall from Chapter 33 that **catabolism** is a process that creates energy for a cell by breaking down molecular nutrients brought to and diffused through the cell membrane. An important use of this energy is the construction, or synthesis, of macromolecules from smaller molecules. The process of synthesizing smaller molecules into a larger macromolecule is called *anabolism.* Anabolism is the constructive phase of metabolism, in which smaller molecules are converted to larger molecules; catabolism is the destructive phase of metabolism, in which larger molecules are converted to smaller molecules.

Catabolism
Catabolism is the breaking down of nutrient molecules into energy for the cell.

Anabolism
Anabolism is the production of large molecules for form and function.

The synthesis of proteins and nucleic acids is critical to the survival of the cell and to cell reproduction. Proteins depend on nucleic acids for synthesis. Chapter 33 discusses protein synthesis and its dependence on nucleic acids. Figure 35-2 provides a schematic review of how proteins are manufactured: messenger ribonucleic acid (mRNA) transcribes the genetic code, which is brought to transfer RNA (tRNA), which then translates it into a protein.

Radiation damage to any of these macromolecules may result in cell death or late effects. Proteins are less radiosensitive than nucleic acids. Proteins occurring abundantly are continuously synthesized throughout the cell cycle, and multiple copies of specific protein molecules are always present in the cell. Likewise, multiple copies of both types of RNA molecules are present in the cell, although RNA molecules are not as abundant as protein molecules. The DNA molecule, on the other hand, with its unique assembly of bases, is not so abundant.

DNA is the most radiosensitive macromolecule.

DNA is synthesized somewhat differently than proteins. During the G_1 portion of interphase, the deoxyribose, phosphate, and base molecules accumulate in the nucleus. These molecules combine to form one large molecule that during the S portion of interphase, is attached to an existing single chain of DNA (Figure 35-3).

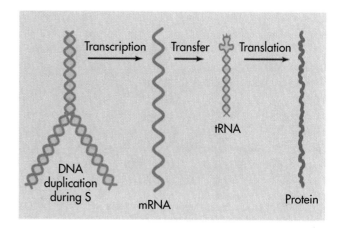

FIGURE 35-2 The genetic code of DNA is transcribed by mRNA and transferred to tRNA, which translates it into a protein.

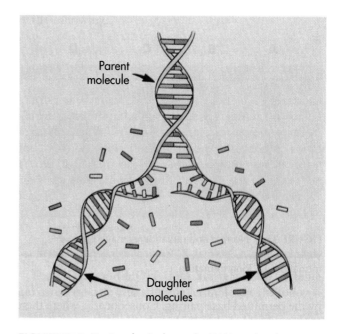

FIGURE 35-3 During the S phase, the DNA molecule separates like a zipper, and two daughter DNA molecules are formed, each alike and each a replicate of the parent molecule.

During G_1, the molecular DNA is in the familiar double-helix form.

In G_1, there is half as much DNA as in G_2.

As the cell moves in S phase, the ladder begins to open up in the middle of each rung, much like a zipper. Now, the DNA consists of only a single chain, and there is no pairing of bases. This state does not last long, however, because the combined base-sugar-phosphate molecule attaches to the single-strand DNA sequence as determined

The free radicals are another story. Because of their single, unpaired electron in the outermost shell, free radicals are highly reactive. They are so unstable that they exist with a lifetime of less than 1 ms. During that time, however, they are capable of diffusion through the cell and interaction at a distant site. Free radicals contain excess energy that can be transferred to other molecules to disrupt bonds and produce point lesions at some distance from the initial ionizing event. Free radicals can also produce other products that are poisonous to the cell and act as toxic agents.

The OH* free radical can join with a similar molecule to form hydrogen peroxide, as follows:

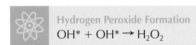

Hydrogen Peroxide Formation
$$OH^* + OH^* \rightarrow H_2O_2$$

The H* free radical can interact with molecular oxygen to form the hydroperoxyl radical, as follows:

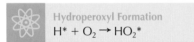

Hydroperoxyl Formation
$$H^* + O_2 \rightarrow HO_2^*$$

The hydroperoxyl radical, along with hydrogen peroxide, is considered to be the principal damaging product after the radiolysis of water. Hydrogen peroxide can also be formed by interaction of two hydroperoxyl free radicals, as follows:

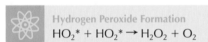

Hydrogen Peroxide Formation
$$HO_2^* + HO_2^* \rightarrow H_2O_2 + O_2$$

Two other species of free radicals can be created. Some organic molecules, symbolized as *RH*, can become reactive free radicals, as follows:

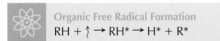

Organic Free Radical Formation
$$RH + \gamma \rightarrow RH^* \rightarrow H^* + R^*$$

When oxygen is present, yet another species of free radical is possible, as follows:

Organic Free Radical Formation
$$R^* + O_2 \rightarrow RO_2^*$$

Free radicals are energetic molecules because of their unique structure. This excess energy can be transferred to DNA and result in bond breaks.

DIRECT AND INDIRECT EFFECT

The harmful effects on biologic material irradiated in vivo can be direct or indirect. A **direct effect** occurs when the ionizing radiation interacts directly with a particularly radiosensitive molecule, such as DNA. An **indirect effect** results from the production of free radicals after the radiolysis of water. For example, a water molecule far from the DNA molecule may be the initial site of ionization. When the water molecule is irradiated, a free radical is formed and can migrate to the DNA molecule. The excess energy of the free radical is transferred to the DNA molecule and creates a point lesion.

Direct Effect
If the initial ionizing event occurs on the most radiosensitive molecule, DNA, the effect of radiation is direct.

Indirect Effect
If the initial ionizing event occurs on any other molecule, usually water, which then transfers energy to the DNA, the effect of radiation is indirect.

It is impossible to know for certain whether the damage to the DNA molecule results from direct or indirect effect. However, since the human body is 80% water and less than 1% DNA, it is generally concluded that most of the effects of irradiation in vivo result from indirect effect. When oxygen is present, as in living tissue, the indirect effects are amplified because of the additional types of free radicals that are formed.

The principal effect of radiation on humans is indirect.

TARGET THEORY

The cell contains many species of molecules, most of which exist in abundance. Radiation damage to such molecules probably would not result in noticeable injury to the cell because similar molecules would be available to continue to support the cell. On the other hand, some molecules in the cell are considered to be particularly necessary for normal cell function. These molecules are not in abundant supply, and in fact, there may be only one such molecule. Radiation damage to such a molecule could affect the cell severely, since there would be no similar molecules available as substitutes to carry on normal cell function.

This concept of a sensitive key molecule is the basis for the **target theory**. According to target theory, for a cell to die after radiation exposure, its so-called target molecule must be inactivated (Figure 35-9). There is considerable experimental evidence in support of the target theory, which suggests that the key molecular target is the DNA.

DNA is the target molecule.

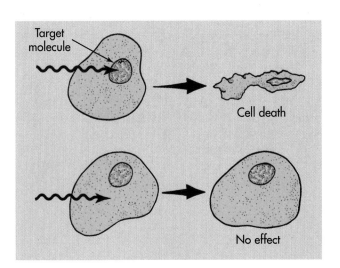

FIGURE 35-9 According to target theory, cell death will occur only if the target molecule is inactivated. DNA, the target molecule, is located in the cell nucleus.

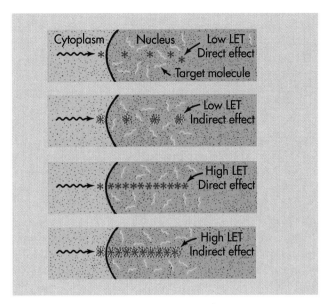

FIGURE 35-10 In the presence of oxygen, the indirect effect is amplified, and the volume of action for low-LET radiation is enlarged. The effective volume of action for high-LET radiation remains unchanged, since maximal injury will have been inflicted by direct effect.

Originally, target theory was used to represent cell lethality. It can be used equally well, however, to describe nonlethal radiation-induced cell abnormalities.

In target theory, the target is considered to be an area of the cell occupied by the target molecule or by a sensitive site on the target molecule. This area changes position with time because of intracellular molecular movement.

The interaction between radiation and cellular components is random, and therefore, when an interaction does occur with a target, it occurs randomly. Radiation does not seek the target molecule. The target molecule's sensitivity to radiation occurs simply because of its vital function in the cell.

When a radiation interaction does occur with the target, a **hit** is said to have occurred. Radiation interaction with molecules other than the target molecule can also result in a hit. It is not possible to distinguish between a direct and an indirect hit.

 Hits occur through both the direct and the indirect effects.

When a hit occurs through indirect effect, the size of the target appears considerably larger because of the mobility of the free radicals. This increased target size contributes to the importance of the indirect effect of radiation.

Figure 35-10 illustrates some of the consequences of using target theory to explain the relationships among linear energy transfer (LET), the oxygen effect, and di-

rect vs. indirect effect. With low-LET radiation, in the absence of oxygen, the probability of a hit on the target molecule is low because of the relatively large distances between ionizing events. If oxygen is present, free radicals are formed, and the volume of effectiveness surrounding each ionization is enlarged. Consequently, the probability of a hit is increased.

When high-LET radiation is used, the distance between ionizations is so close that the probability of a hit by direct effect is high, possibly higher than that for the low-LET, indirect effect. When oxygen is added to the system and high-LET radiation is used, the effect of the radiation may not be increased. The added sphere of influence for each ionizing event, although somewhat larger, will not result in additional hits, since the maximum number of hits has already been produced by direct effect with the high-LET radiation.

 A hit is not simply an ionizing event but rather an ionization that inactivates the target molecule.

CELL SURVIVAL KINETICS

Early radiation experiments at the cell level were conducted with simple cells, such as bacteria. It was not until the middle of the 1950s that laboratory techniques were developed to allow the growth and manipulation of human cells in vitro. These techniques required the development of an artificial growth medium that would nourish a human cell. Now cells can be grown in tubes,

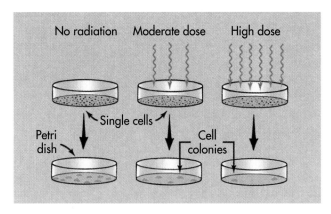

FIGURE 35-11 When single cells are planted in a Petri dish, they grow into visible colonies. Fewer colonies develop if the cells are irradiated.

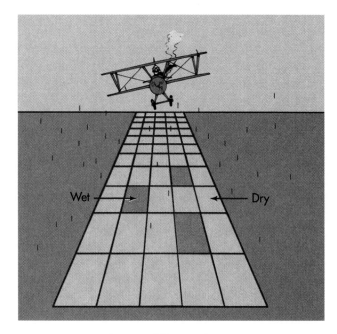

FIGURE 35-12 When rain falls on a dry pavement consisting of a large number of squares, the number of squares that remains dry decreases exponentially as the number of raindrops increases.

flasks, Petri dishes, or nearly any type of laboratory container.

One technique for measuring the lethal effects of radiation on cells is shown in Figure 35-11. If normal cells are planted individually in a Petri dish and incubated for 10 to 14 days, they will divide many times and produce a visible colony consisting of as many as 1000 cells. This is **cell cloning.** After the irradiation of such single cells, some will not survive, and therefore fewer colonies will be formed. The higher the radiation dose, the fewer the colonies formed.

 The lethal effects of radiation are determined by observing cell survival, not cell death.

When a mathematic extension of target theory is used, two models of cell survival result. The models are the radiation dose-response relationships for the cell. The **single-target, single-hit model** applies to biologic targets, such as enzymes, viruses, and simple cells such as bacteria. The **multitarget, single-hit model** applies to more complicated biologic systems, such as human cells.

The following discussion concerns the equation of these models. The mathematics of these models is relatively unimportant but is given here for the interested student.

Single-Target, Single-Hit Model
Consider for a moment, the situation illustrated in Figure 35-12. A large concrete runway containing 100 squares is shown, and it is raining. A square is considered wet when one or more raindrops have fallen on it.

When the first drop falls on the pavement, 1 of the 100 squares will be wet. When the second drop falls, it will probably fall on a dry square and not the one already wet. Consequently, 2 of 100 squares will be wet.

When the third raindrop falls, there will probably be 3 wet and 97 dry squares. As the number of raindrops increases, however, it will become more probable that a given square will be hit by two or more drops.

Because the raindrops are falling randomly, the probability that a square will become wet is governed by a statistical law called the *Poisson distribution*. According to this law, when the number of raindrops is equal to the number of squares (100 in this case), 63% of the squares will be wet, and 37% of the squares will be dry. If the raindrops had fallen uniformly, all 100 squares would become wet with 100 raindrops.

 Radiation interacts randomly with matter.

Obviously, many of the 63 squares in this example have been hit twice and even more. When the number of raindrops equals twice the number of squares, then 0.37 × 0.37, or 14, squares will be dry. After 300 raindrops, only 5 squares will remain dry. A graph of the number of dry squares as a function of the number of raindrops is shown in Figure 35-13. If the number of squares exposed to the rain were large or unknown, the scale on the right, expressed in percentages, would be used.

The wet-squares analogy can be extended to the irradiation of a large number of biologic specimens (for example, 1000 bacteria). Each bacterium presumably contains a single sensitive site or target that must be

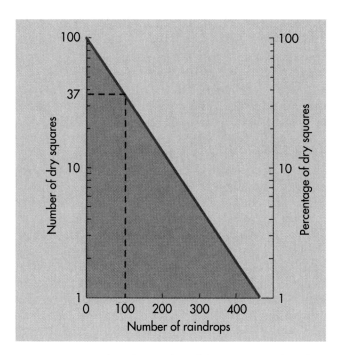

FIGURE 35-13 When the number of dry squares is plotted on semilogarithmic paper as a function of the number of raindrops, a straight line results because after a few drops, some squares will be hit more than once.

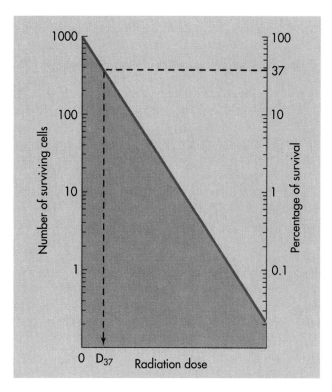

FIGURE 35-14 After the irradiation of 1000 cells, the dose-response relationship is exponential. The D_{37} is that dose that results in 37% survival.

inactivated for the cell to die. As the 1000 bacteria are irradiated with increasing increments of dose, more will be killed (Figure 35-14). Just as with the wet squares, however, as the dose increases, some cells will suffer two or more hits. All hits per target in excess of one represent wasted radiation dose, since the bacteria had already been killed by the first hit. Remember, a hit is not simply an ionizing event, but rather an ionization that inactivates the target molecule.

When the radiation dose reaches a level sufficient to kill 63% of the cells (37% survival), it is called D_{37}. After a dose equal to $2 \times D_{37}$, 14% of the cells would survive, and so on. D_{37} is a measure of the radiosensitivity of the biologic specimen. A low D_{37} represents a highly radiosensitive specimen, and a high D_{37} represents radioresistance.

 If there were no wasted hits (uniform interaction), D_{37} is the dose that would be sufficient to kill 100% of the cells.

The equation that describes the dose-response relationship represented by the graph in Figure 35-14 is the single-target, single-hit model of radiation-induced lethality, as follows:

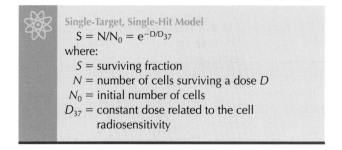

Single-Target, Single-Hit Model
$$S = N/N_0 = e^{-D/D_{37}}$$
where:
S = surviving fraction
N = number of cells surviving a dose D
N_0 = initial number of cells
D_{37} = constant dose related to the cell radiosensitivity

Multitarget, Single-Hit Model

Returning to the wet-squares analogy, suppose that each pavement square were divided into two equal parts (Figure 35-15). By definition, each half must now be hit with a raindrop for the square to be considered wet. The first few raindrops will probably hit only one half of any given square, and therefore, after a very light rain, no squares may be wet. Many raindrops must fall before any single square suffers a hit in both halves so that it can be considered wet. This represents a threshold, since according to our definition, many raindrops can fall and all squares will remain dry.

As the number of raindrops increases, eventually some squares will have both halves hit and therefore will

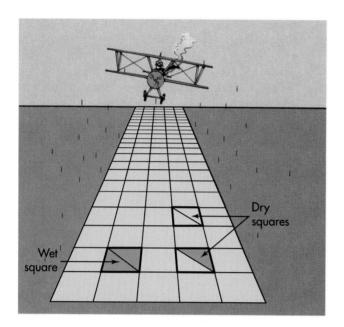

FIGURE 35-15 If each pavement square has two equal parts, each part must be hit for the square to be considered wet.

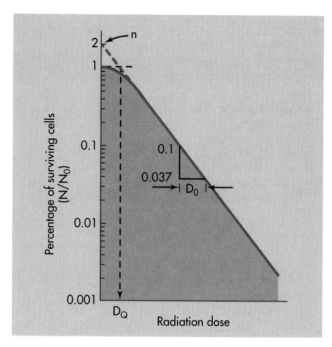

FIGURE 35-17 The multitarget, single-hit model of cell survival is characteristic of human cells containing two targets.

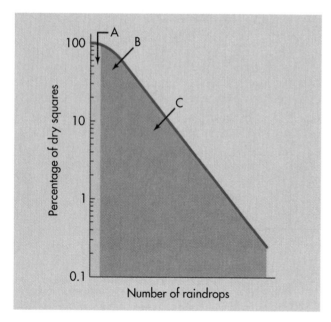

FIGURE 35-16 When a square contains two equal parts and both have to be hit to be considered wet, three regions of the dry-square vs. raindrops relationship can be identified.

by the single-target, single-hit model. The intermediate region *B* is the region of accumulation of hits.

Complex biologic specimens, such as human cells are thought to have more than a single critical target. Suppose that the human cell has two targets, each of which has to be inactivated for the cell to die. This would be analogous to the square having two halves, each of which had to be hit by rain for it to be considered wet. Figure 35-17 is a graph of single-cell survival for human cells having two targets.

At very low radiation doses, there will be nearly 100% cell survival. As the radiation dose increases, fewer cells will survive because more will have sustained a hit in both target molecules. At some higher radiation dose, all cells will have sustained at least one hit in one of its two targets. All cells that survive this dose will have one target hit, and therefore at all higher doses, the dose-response relationship would appear as the single-target, single-hit model.

The model of cell survival just described is the multitarget, single-hit model, as follows:

be considered wet. This portion of the curve is represented by region *A* in Figure 35-16. When many raindrops have fallen, region *C* will be reached, and every square will have at least one half wet. When this occurs, each additional raindrop will produce a wet square. In region *C* the relationship between the number of raindrops and the number of wet squares is that described

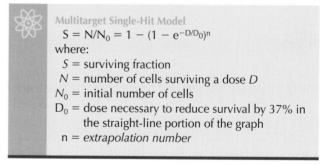

Multitarget Single-Hit Model

$$S = N/N_0 = 1 - (1 - e^{-D/D_0})^n$$

where:

S = surviving fraction

N = number of cells surviving a dose D

N_0 = initial number of cells

D_0 = dose necessary to reduce survival by 37% in the straight-line portion of the graph

n = *extrapolation number*

TABLE 35-1	D_0 and D_Q for Experimental Mammalian Cell Lines	
Cell Type	D_0 (rad)	D_Q (rad)
Mouse occytes	91	62
Mouse skin	135	350
Human bone marrow	137	100
Human fibroblasts	150	160
Mouse spermatogonia	180	270
Chinese hamster ovary	200	210
Human lymphocytes	400	100

The D_0 is called the **mean lethal dose,** and it is a constant related to the radiosensitivity of the cell. It is equal to D_{37} in the linear portion of the graph and therefore represents the dose that would result in one hit per target in the straight-line portion of the graph if no radiation were wasted.

 A large D_0 indicates a radioresistant cell line, and a small D_0 is characteristic of radiosensitive cells.

The extrapolation number is also called the *target number.* The extrapolation number represents the number of targets that must be hit to cause cell death. This number is determined by extrapolating the linear portion of the curve back to its intersection with the y-axis. When this type of experiment was first conducted with human cells, the observed extrapolation number was 2. That result agreed with the hypothesis that similar regions on two homologous chromosomes (an identical pair) had to be inactivated to produce cell death. Since chromosomes come in pairs, the experimental results confirmed the hypothesis. Subsequent experiments, however, have resulted in extrapolation numbers ranging from 2 to 12, and therefore the precise meaning of *n* is unknown.

The D_Q is called the **threshold dose.** It is a measure of the width of the shoulder of the multitarget, single-hit model and is related to the capacity of the cell to recover from sublethal damage. Table 35-1 lists reported values for D_0 and D_Q for experimental cell lines.

 A large D_Q indicates that the cell can readily recover from sublethal damage.

Recovery
The shoulder of the graph of the multitarget, single-hit model shows that for mammalian cells, some damage must be accumulated before the cell dies. This accumulated damage is termed **sublethal damage.** The wider the shoulder, the more sublethal damage that can be sustained and the higher the value of D_Q.

Figure 35-18 demonstrates the results of a split-dose irradiation designed to describe the capacity of a cell to

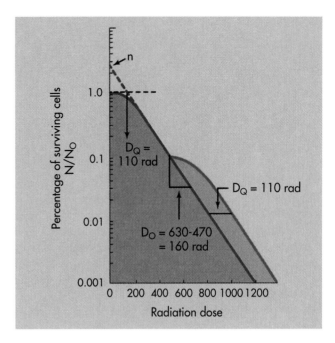

FIGURE 35-18 Split-dose irradiation results in a second cell survival curve, with the precise characteristics of the first displaced along the dose axis by a dose equal to D_Q.

recover from sublethal damage. This illustration shows a rather typical human cell survival curve with $D_0 = 160$ rad (1.6 Gy$_t$), $D_Q = 110$ rad (1.1. Gy$_t$), and $n = 2$. If the cells that survive any large dose (for example, 470 rad [4.7 Gy$_t$]) are reincubated in a growth medium, they will grow into another large population.

This new population of cells can then be used to perform a second cell-survival experiment. When the cells that survived the first dose are subsequently subjected to additional incremental radiation doses, a second dose-response curve will be generated that has precisely the same shape as the first. The extrapolation number is the same, the D_0 is the same, and it is separated along the dose axis from the first dose-response curve by D_Q. The time between such split doses must be at least as long as the cell generation time for full recovery to occur.

Such experiments show that cells that survive an initial radiation insult exhibit precisely the same characteristics as nonirradiated cells, and therefore they have fully recovered from the sublethal damage produced by the initial irradiation.

 D_Q is not only a measure of the capacity to accumulate sublethal damage but is also a measure of the ability of the cell to recover from sublethal damage.

Question: Using Figure 35-18, estimate the overall surviving fraction for a cell receiving a split-dose of 400 rad followed by 400 rad (4 Gy$_t$).

Answer: At a dose of 400 rad, approximately 0.15 of the cells survive. Therefore at a split-dose of 400 rad and 400 rad, the surviving fraction should equal $0.15 \times 0.15 = 0.023$. The total dose is 800 rad ($8\ Gy_t$), and the surviving fraction on the split-dose curve at 800 rad should equal 0.023, and it does. Had the 800 rad been delivered at one time, the surviving fraction would have been 0.012, as shown by the single-dose curve of Figure 35-18.

Cell Cycle Effects

When human cells replicate by mitosis, the average time from one mitosis to another is called the **cell cycle time** or the **generation time**. Most human cells that are in a state of normal proliferation have generation times of 10 to 20 hours. Some specialized cells have generation times extending to hundreds of hours, and some cells, such as neurons (nerve cells), do not normally replicate. Longer generation times primarily result from a lengthening of the G_1 phase of the cell cycle.

 The length of the G_1 phase is the most variable of cell phases.

Techniques are now available for taking a randomly growing population of cells that are uniformly distributed in position throughout the cell cycle and synchronizing them. A population of synchronized cells can then be subdivided into smaller populations and irradiated sequentially as they pass through the phases of the cell cycle.

Figure 35-19 is representative of results obtained from human fibroblasts. The fraction of cells surviving a given dose can vary by a factor of 10 from the most sensitive to the most resistant phase of the cell cycle. This pattern of change in radiosensitivity as a function of phase in the cell cycle is known as the **age-response function**. It varies from cell type to cell type, but the results illustrated in Figure 35-19 are characteristic of most human cells. Cells in mitosis are always most sensitive. The fraction of surviving cells is the lowest in this phase. The next most sensitive phase of the cell cycle occurs at the G_1-S transition. The most resistant portion of the cell cycle occurs late in the S phase.

 Human cells are most radiosensitive in the M phase and most radioresistant late in the S phase.

LET, RBE, and OER

Mammalian cell survival experiments have been used extensively to measure the effects of various types of radiation and to determine the magnitude of various dose-modifying factors, such as oxygen. Since the D_0 is related to radiosensitivity, the ratio of D_0 for one condition of irradiation compared with another will be a measure of

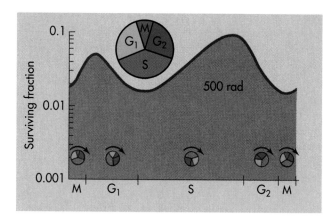

FIGURE 35-19 Age-response function of human fibroblasts after irradiation. There is minimal survival during the M phase and maximal survival during the late S phase. Such cells are most radiosensitive during mitosis and most radioresistant during the late S phase.

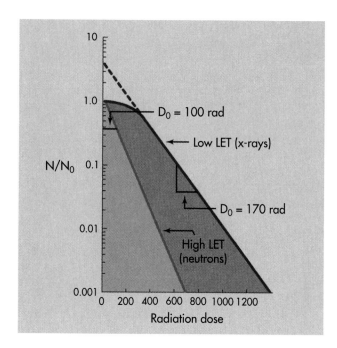

FIGURE 35-20 Representative cell survival curves for human fibroblasts after exposure to 200-kVp x-rays and 14-MeV neutrons.

the effectiveness of the dose modifier, whether it is physical or biologic.

Recall from Chapter 34 that as electrons pass through tissue, they create a track of ionized molecules. The way in which energy is distributed along this track is called the *linear energy transfer (LET)* of radiation. X-rays in the diagnostic range have a low LET.

If the same cell type is irradiated by two different radiations under identical physical and biologic conditions, the possible results may be those that appear in Figure 35-20. At the very high LET values (as with alpha particles and neutrons), even with mammalian cells, the cell survival kinetics follow the single-target, single-hit model. With low-LET radiation (x-rays) the multitarget, single-hit model is representative. The mean lethal dose after low-LET irradiation is always greater than that after high-LET irradiation. If the low-LET D_0 is representative of x-rays, then the ratio of one D_0 to another will equal the relative biologic effectiveness (RBE) for the high-LET radiation, as follows:

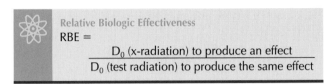

Relative Biologic Effectiveness

$$RBE = \frac{D_0 \text{ (x-radiation) to produce an effect}}{D_0 \text{ (test radiation) to produce the same effect}}$$

To review Chapter 34, the RBE measures the relative effect of ionizing radiation at a given dose compared with the potential of another type of radiation (for example the potential of x-rays to create biologic damage relative to the potential toxicity of alpha particles at the same dose). The RBE is most often expressed as the ratio of the energy required to produce a given biologic effect using 200 keV of x-ray over the amount of energy of one kind of radiation required to produce that same biologic effect. Thus the REB can be expressed alternatively as follows:

Relative Biologic Effectiveness

$$RBE = \frac{\text{Dose at 200 keV}}{\text{Dose unknown}}$$

Question: Figure 35-20 shows the radiation dose-response relationship of human fibroblasts exposed to x-rays and to 14-MeV neutrons. The D_0 after x-radiation is 170 rad (1.7 Gy_t); the D_0 for neutron irradiation is 100 rad (1 Gy_t). What is the RBE of 14-MeV neutrons relative to x-ray?

Answer: $RBE = \dfrac{170 \text{ rad}}{100 \text{ rad}}$

$= 1.7$

The most completely studied dose modifier is oxygen. In the presence of oxygen, the effect of low-LET radiation is maximal because of the increased number of free radicals produced during radiolysis. When hypoxic or anoxic cells are exposed, a considerably higher dose is required to produce a given effect. When high-LET radiation is used, there is little difference between the response of oxygenated cells and that of anoxic cells. Figure 35-21 shows typical cell survival curves for each of these combinations of LET and oxygen.

Such experiments are designed to measure the magnitude of the oxygen effect. The oxygen enhancement ratio

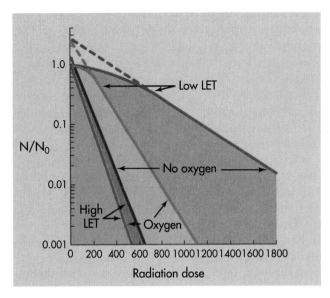

FIGURE 35-21 Cell survival cures for human cells irradiated in the presence and absence of oxygen with high- and low-LET radiation.

determined from single-cell survival experiments is defined as follows:

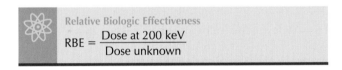

Oxygen Enhancement Ratio

$$OER = \frac{D_0 \text{ (anoxic) to produce an effect}}{D_0 \text{ (oxygenated) to produce the same effect}}$$

Question: What is the estimated OER for human cells exposed to low- and high-LET radiation? (Refer to Figure 35-21.)

Answer: Low LET, no oxygen $D_0 = 340$ rad
Low LET, oxygen $D_0 = 140$ rad

$$OER = \frac{340 \text{ rad}}{140 \text{ rad}} = 2.4$$

High LET, no oxygen, $D_0 = 90$ rad
High LET, oxygen, $D_0 = 70$ rad

$$OER = \frac{90 \text{ rad}}{70 \text{ rad}} = 1.3$$

The interrelationships among LET, RBE, and OER are complex. However, it is LET that determines the magnitude of RBE and OER.

SUMMARY

When macromolecules are irradiated in vitro, the following effects occur: (1) main-chain scission, the breakage of the backbone of a long-chain macromolecule; (2)

cross-linking, the attachment of side sections of the macromolecule to a neighboring macromolecule; and (3) point lesions, the disruption of single chemical bonds in a macromolecule. Each type is reversible through intercellular repair and recovery.

Because DNA is not abundant in the cell, it is the most radiosensitive of all macromolecules. Chromosome aberrations or abnormal metabolic activity can result from DNA damage. The three observable effects of DNA irradiation are cell death, malignant disease, and genetic damage.

Because the human body is 80% water, the irradiation of water is the principal interaction in the body. Water dissociates into free radicals that are highly reactive and are capable of diffusion through the cell to cause point lesions at some distance. The initial ionizing event is said to be a *direct effect* if the interaction was with a DNA molecule. If the ionizing event occurs with water and transfers that energy to DNA, an indirect effect has occurred.

The concept of a sensitive key molecule in a cell is the basis for the target theory. For a cell to die after radiation exposure, the target molecule, DNA, must be inactivated.

Two models describe cell survival after radiation exposure. The single-target, single-hit model is used mostly for simple cells such as bacteria. The multitarget, single-hit model states that at low radiation doses, there is 100% cell survival. However, at higher doses, the relationship becomes a single-hit, single-target (lethal dose) model. Experiments in cell recovery show that cells have the ability to recover from sublethal radiation damage.

CHALLENGE QUESTIONS

1. Define or otherwise identify:
   a. In vitro
   b. Relative biologic effectiveness
   c. Point mutation
   d. Free radical
   e. Target theory
   f. D_{37}
   g. Mean lethal dose
   h. Radiation hit
   i. Extrapolation number
   j. D_Q

2. List the effects of irradiation of macromolecules in solution in vitro.

3. How is solution viscosity used to determine the degree of macromolecular radiation damage?

4. What is the difference between catabolism and anabolism?

5. In what phase of the cell cycle does the DNA ladder open up in the middle of each rung and consist of only a single chain?

6. Name the three principal observable effects of DNA irradiation.

7. Diagram the point mutations of DNA that transfer the incorrect genetic code to one of the two daughter cells.

8. Write the formula for the radiolysis of water in which the atom of water is ionized and dissociates into two ions.

9. What happens to radiation-induced free radicals within the cell?

10. Explain the target theory of radiobiology.

11. Does radiation interact with tissue uniformly or randomly? Explain.

12. Write the equation for the single-target, single-hit model of dose-response relationships.

13. Write the equation for the multitarget, single-hit model of dose-response relationships.

14. Complete the following chemical equations:
    a. H_2O + Radiation $\rightarrow$
    b. HOH^+ (dissociation) $\rightarrow$
    c. HOH^- (dissociation) $\rightarrow$

15. The D_{37} of a cellular species that follows the single-target, single-hit model is 150 rad. What percentage of cells will survive 450 rad?

16. What is the REB of alpha radiation if the D_0 is 40 rad, compared with 180 rad for x-rays?

17. What is the difference between direct effect and indirect effect?

18. How does the radiosensitivity of human cells vary with stages of the cell cycle?

19. What is the difference between in vitro and in vivo?

Early Effects of Radiation

OBJECTIVES

At the completion of this chapter, the student should be able to:

1. Describe the three acute radiation syndromes
2. Identify the two stages leading to acute radiation lethality
3. Define $LD_{50/60}$
4. Discuss local tissue damage after high-dose irradiation
5. Explain the early radiation effects on the hemopoietic system
6. Review the cytogenetic effects of radiation exposure

OUTLINE

If the radiation injury is sufficiently severe, the reduction in the number of blood cells continues unchecked until the body no longer has any defense against infection. Just before death, hemorrhage and dehydration may be pronounced. Death occurs because of generalized infection, electrolyte imbalance, and dehydration.

Gastrointestinal syndrome. After radiation doses extending from approximately 1000 to 5000 rad (10 to 50 Gy_t), the GI syndrome occurs. The prodromal symptoms of vomiting and diarrhea occur within hours of exposure and persist for hours to as long as a day. A latent period of 3 to 5 days follows, during which time no symptoms are present.

The manifest illness period begins with a second wave of nausea and vomiting, followed by diarrhea. The individual experiences a loss of appetite (anorexia) and may become lethargic. The diarrhea persists and increases in severity, leading to loose and then watery and bloody stools. Supportive therapy is unable to prevent the rapid progression of symptoms that ultimately leads to death within 4 to 10 days of exposure.

 Death in the GI syndrome occurs principally because of severe damage to the cells lining the intestines.

Intestinal cells are normally in a rapid state of proliferation and are continuously being replaced by new cells. The turnover time for this cell-renewal system in a normal individual is 3 to 5 days. However, radiation exposure kills the most sensitive cells—the stem cells—and this factor controls the length of time until death. When the intestinal lining is completely denuded of functional cells, there is uncontrolled passage of fluids across the intestinal membrane, a severe destruction of electrolyte balance, and conditions promoting infection.

At doses consistent with the GI syndrome, damage to the hematologic system also occurs. It takes a longer time for the cell-renewal system of the blood to effect the development of stem cells into mature cells, and therefore, sufficient time is not provided for maximal hematologic effects to occur. Measurable and even severe hematologic changes accompany GI death.

Central nervous system syndrome. **CNS syndrome** occurs after a radiation dose in excess of approximately 5000 rad (50 Gy_t). A series of signs and symptoms occur that lead to death within a matter of hours to 3 days. First, there is an onset of severe nausea and vomiting, usually within a few minutes of exposure. During this time, the individual may become extremely nervous and confused, complain of a burning sensation in the skin, lose vision, and even lose consciousness within the first hour. This may be followed by a latent period lasting up to 12 hours, during which time the earlier symptoms subside or disappear.

After the latent period is the period of manifest illness, during which time the symptoms of the prodromal stage return but more severely. The person becomes disoriented; loses muscle coordination; has difficulty breathing; may go into convulsive seizures; experiences loss of equilibrium, ataxia, and lethargy; lapses into a coma; and dies.

Regardless of the medical attention given the patient, the symptoms of manifest illness appear rather suddenly and always with extreme severity. At radiation doses sufficiently high to produce CNS effects, the outcome is always death within a few days of exposure.

 The ultimate cause of death in CNS syndrome is apparently an elevated fluid content of the brain.

The CNS syndrome is characterized by increased intracranial pressure, inflammatory changes in the blood vessels of the brain (vasculitis), and inflammation of the meninges (meningitis). At doses sufficient to produce CNS damage, damage to all other organs of the body would be equally severe. The classic radiation-induced changes in the GI tract and the hematologic system cannot occur because there is insufficient time between exposure and death for them to appear.

$LD_{50/60}$

 The $LD_{50/60}$ is the dose of radiation to the whole body that will result in death within 60 days to 50% of irradiated subjects.

If experimental animals are irradiated with varying doses of radiation (for example, 100 to 1000 rad [1 to 10 Gy_t]), a plot of the percentage dying as a function of radiation dose would appear as in Figure 36-1. This figure illustrates the radiation dose-response relationship for acute human lethality. At the lower dose of approximately 100 rad (1 Gy_t), no one is expected to die. Above approximately 600 rad (6 Gy_t), all those irradiated would die unless vigorous medical support was available. Above 1000 rad (10 Gy_t), even vigorous medical support would not prevent death.

 Acute radiation lethality follows a nonlinear, threshold dose-response relationship.

If death is to occur, it usually happens within 60 days of exposure. Acute radiation lethality is measured quantitatively by the $LD_{50/60}$. The $LD_{50/60}$ for humans is estimated to be approximately 350 rad (3.5 Gy_t). With clinical support, humans can tolerate much higher doses, the maximum reported to be 850 rad (8.5 Gy_t). Table 36-3 lists values of $LD_{50/60}$ for various experimental species and humans.

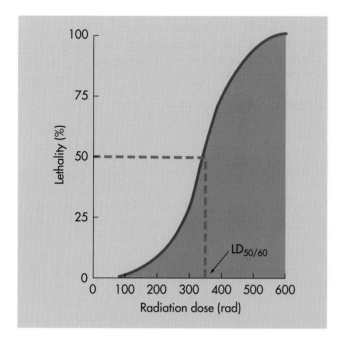

FIGURE 36-1 Radiation-induced death in humans follows a nonlinear, threshold dose-respoonse relationship.

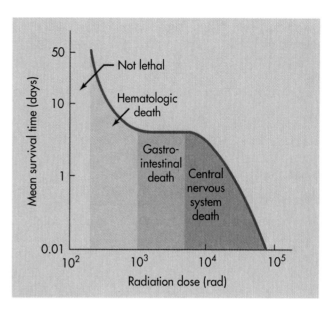

FIGURE 36-2 Mean survival time after radiation exposure shows three distinct regions. If death is due to hematologic or CNS effects, the mean survival time varies with the dose. If GI effects cause death, it occurs in approximately 4 days.

TABLE 36-3	Approximate LD$_{50/60}$ for Various Species after Whole-Body Radiation Exposure
Species	**LD$_{50/60}$ (rad)**
Pig	250
Dog	275
Human	350
Guinea pig	425
Monkey	475
Opossum	510
Mouse	620
Goldfish	700
Hamster	700
Rat	710
Rabbit	725
Gerbil	1050
Turtle	1500
Armadillo	2000
Newt	3000
Cockroach	10,000

Sometimes, additional measures of acute lethality are identified. LD$_{10/60}$ and LD$_{90/60}$ would indicate a dose resulting in 10% lethality or 90% lethality within 60 days, respectively. LD$_{50/30}$ is the lethal dose to 50% when the observed survival time is shortened to 30 days. Normally, this is not much different from the LD$_{50/60}$.

Question: Using Figure 36-1, estimate the radiation dose that will produce 25% lethality in humans within 60 days.

Answer: First, draw a horizontal line from the 25% level on the y-axis until it intersects the S curve. Now, drop a vertical line from this point to the x-axis. This intersection with the x-axis occurs at the LD$_{25/60}$, which is approximately 250 rad (2.5 Gy$_t$).

Mean Survival Time

As the whole-body radiation dose increases, the average time between exposure and death decreases. This time is known as the **mean survival time.** A graph of radiation dose vs. mean survival time is shown in Figure 36-2. There are three distinct regions to this graph, and they are associated with the three radiation syndromes.

As the radiation dose increases from 200 to 1000 rad (2 to 10 Gy$_t$), the mean survival time decreases from approximately 60 to 4 days, and this region is consistent with death resulting from the hematologic syndrome. Mean survival time is dose dependent with the hematologic syndrome.

In the dose range associated with the GI syndrome, however, the mean survival time remains relatively constant, at 4 to 6 days. With larger doses (those associated with the CNS syndrome), the mean survival time is again dose dependent, varying from approximately 3 days to a matter of hours.

LOCAL TISSUE IRRADIATION

When only part of the body is irradiated, compared with whole-body irradiation, a higher dose is required to produce a response. Every organ and tissue of the body can

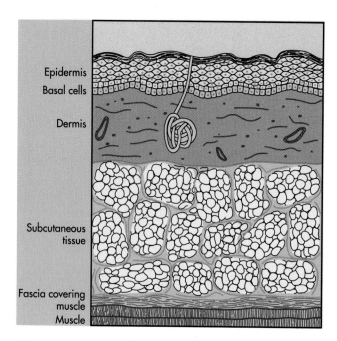

FIGURE 36-3 Sectional view of the anatomic structures of the skin. The basal cell layer is most radiosensitive.

be affected by partial-body irradiation. The effect is cell death, resulting in a shrinkage or reduction in size of the organ or tissue. This can lead to a total nonfunction of that organ or tissue, or it can be followed by recovery.

> Atrophy is the shrinkage of an organ or tissue caused by cell death.

There are many examples of local tissue damage immediately after radiation exposure. In fact, if the dose is high enough, any local tissue will respond. The manner in which local tissues respond depends on their intrinsic radiosensitivity and the kinetics of cell proliferation and maturation. Examples of local tissues that can be affected immediately are the skin, gonads, and bone marrow.

Effects on Skin

The tissue with which we have most experience is the skin. Normal skin consists of three layers: an outer layer (the epidermis), an intermediate layer of connective tissue (the dermis), and a subcutaneous layer of fat and connective tissue. There are additional accessory structures in the skin, such as hair follicles, sweat glands, and sensory receptors (Figure 36-3). All the cell layers and the accessory structures participate in the response to radiation exposure.

The skin, like the lining of the intestine, represents a continuing cell renewal system, only at a much slower rate than that experienced by intestinal cells. Almost 50% of the cells lining the intestine are replaced every day, whereas skin cells are replaced at the rate of only approximately 2% per day.

The outer skin layer, the epidermis, consists of several layers of cells, the innermost layer being the basal cells.

The **basal cells** are the **stem cells** that mature as they migrate to the surface of the epidermis. Once these cells arrive on the surface as mature cells, they slowly die, are shed, and must be replaced by new cells from the basal layer.

 Damage to basal cells results in the earliest manifestation of radiation injury to the skin.

Before the advent of cobalt and linear accelerator teletherapy, the limitations of radiation therapy with orthovoltage x-rays (200- to 300-kVp x-rays) were determined by the tolerance of the patient's skin. The object of x-ray therapy is to deposit x-ray energy in the tumor while sparing the surrounding normal tissue.

Since the x-rays must pass through the skin to reach the tumor, the skin was often necessarily subjected to higher radiation doses than the tumor. The resultant skin damage was **erythema** (a sunburn-like reddening of the skin), followed by **desquamation** (ulceration and denudation of the skin), which often required that the therapy be interrupted.

After a single dose of 300 to 1000 rad (3 to 10 Gy_t), an initial mild erythema may occur within the first or second day. This first wave of erythema then subsides, only to be followed by a second wave that reaches maximal intensity in about 2 weeks. At higher doses, this second wave of erythema is followed by a moist desquamation, which in turn, may lead to a dry desquamation. Moist desquamation is known as **clinical tolerance** for radiation therapy.

During radiation therapy, the skin is exposed in a fractionated scheme, usually approximately 200 rad/day (2 Gy_t/day) 5 days a week. The radiation oncologist plans patient treatments using isoeffect curves that have been generated to accurately project the dose necessary to produce skin erythema or clinical tolerance after a prescribed treatment routine (Figure 36-4).

Erythema was perhaps the first observed biologic response to radiation exposure. Many of the early x-ray pioneers, including Roentgen, suffered x-ray–induced skin burns. One of the hazards to the patient during the early years of radiology was x-ray–induced erythema. During those years, x-ray tube potentials were so low that it was usually necessary to position the tube very close to the patient's skin, and 10- to 30-minute exposures were commonly required to obtain a suitable radiograph. Often the patient would return several days later suffering from an x-ray burn.

These skin effects follow a nonlinear, threshold dose-response relationship similar to that described for radiation-induced lethality. Small doses of x-radiation do not cause erythema. Extremely high doses of x-radiation cause erythema in all people so irradiated. Whether intermediate doses produce erythema depends on the individual's radiosensitivity, the dose rate, and the size of the skin field irradiated. An analysis of people irradiated therapeutically with superficial x-rays has shown that the

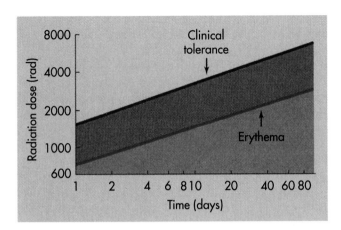

FIGURE 36-4 These isoeffect curves show the relationship between the number of daily fractions and the total radiation dose that produces erythema or moist desquamation. As the fractionation of the dose increases, so does the total dose required.

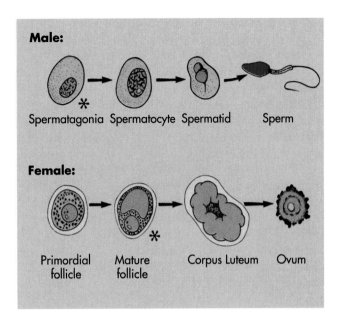

FIGURE 36-5 Progression of germ cells from the stem cell phase to the mature cell. Asterisk indicates the most radiosensitive cell.

skin erythema dose required to affect 50% of those irradiated (**SED50**) is about 600 rad (6 Gy$_t$).

Before the definition of the roentgen and the development of accurate radiation-measuring apparatus, the skin was observed and its response to radiation used in formulating radiation-protection practices. The unit used was the SED$_{50}$, and permissible radiation exposures were specified in fractions of SED$_{50}$.

Another response of the skin to radiation exposure is **epilation,** or loss of hair. For many years, soft x-rays (10 to 20 kVp), called **grenz rays,** were used as the treatment of choice for skin diseases such as tinea (ringworm). Tinea capitis (ringworm of the scalp), common in children, was successfully treated by grenz radiation, but unfortunately the patient's hair would fall out for weeks or even months. In instances in which unnecessarily high doses of grenz rays were used, the epilation was permanent.

The response of the skin to x-rays is currently receiving more attention because of high-dose fluoroscopy. The longer fluoroscopy times required for cardiovascular and interventional procedures, coupled with allowed exposure rates exceeding 20 R/min, are of great concern. Injuries to patients have been reported, and steps are being taken to better control such exposures. Table 36-4 summarizes the potential effects of high-dose fluoroscopy.

Effects on Gonads

The human gonads are critically important target organs. As an example of local tissue effects, they are particularly sensitive to radiation. Responses to doses as low as 10 rad have been observed. Since these organs pro-

TABLE 36-4	Potential Radiation Responses of Skin from High-Dose Fluoroscopy	
Potential Radiation Response	**Approximate Threshold Dose (rad)**	**Approximate Time of Onset**
Early transient erythema	200	Hours
Main erythema	600	10 days
Temporary epilation	300	3 weeks
Permanent epilation	700	3 weeks
Moist desquamation	1500	4 weeks

duce the germ cells that control fertility and heredity, their response to radiation has been studied extensively.

Much of what is known about the type of radiation response and dose-response relationships is derived from numerous animal experiments. Some significant data are also available, however, from human populations. Radiotherapy patients, radiation accident victims, and volunteer convicts have all provided data to allow a rather complete description of the response of the gonads to radiation.

The cells of the testes, the male gonads, and the ovaries, the female gonads, respond differently to radiation because of differences in progression from the stem cell phase to the mature cell. Figure 36-5 illustrates this progression, indicating the most radiosensitive phase of cell maturation.

 Ovaries and testes produce oogonia and spermatogmia, which mature into ova and sperm, respectively.

Germ cells are produced by both ovaries and testes, but they develop from the stem cell phase to the mature cell phase at different rates and at different times. This process of development is called **gametogenesis.** The stem cells of the ovaries are the **oogonia,** and they multiply in number only during fetal life. The oogonia reach a maximum number of about 7 million during midfetal development and then begin to decline because of spontaneous degeneration.

During late fetal life many primordial follicles grow to encapsulate the oogonia, which become **oocytes.** These follicle-containing oocytes remain in a suspended state of growth until puberty. In prepuberty the number of oocytes is reduced to only several hundred thousand. Commencing at puberty, the follicles rupture with regularity, ejecting a mature germ cell, the **ovum.** There will be only 400 to 500 such ova available for fertilization during approximately 30 to 40 years of menstruating an average of 13 times per year.

The germ cells of the testes are continually being produced from stem cells progressively through a number of stages to maturity, and like the ovaries, the testes provide a sustaining cell-renewal system. The male stem cell is the **spermatogonia,** which matures into the **spermatocyte.** The spermatocyte in turn multiplies and develops into a spermatid, which finally differentiates into the functionally mature germ cell, the **spermatozoa,** or **sperm.** The maturation process from stem cell to spermatozoa requires 3 to 5 weeks.

Ovaries. Irradiation of the ovaries early in life reduces their size (atrophy) by germ cell death. After puberty, such irradiation also suppresses and delays menstruation.

 The most radiosensitive cell during female germ cell development is the oocyte in the mature follicle.

Radiation effects on the ovaries are somewhat age dependent. During fetal life and into early childhood, the ovaries are especially radiosensitive. They decline in sensitivity, reaching a minimum in the 20- to 30-year age range and then increase continually with age. Doses as low as 10 rad (100 mGy$_t$) in the mature female may result in the delay or suppression of menstruation. A dose of approximately 200 rad (2 Gy$_t$) produces a pronounced temporary infertility; approximately 500 rad (5 Gy$_t$) to the ovaries is necessary to produce permanent sterility.

In addition to the destruction of fertility, irradiation of the ovaries of experimental animals produces genetic mutations. Even moderate doses, such as 25 to 50 rad (250 to 500 mGy$_t$), are associated with measurable increases in genetic mutations. There is also some evidence to indicate that oocytes surviving such a modest dose are

capable of repairing some genetic damage as they mature into ova.

Testes. The testes, like the ovaries, atrophy after high doses of radiation. Many data on testicular damage have been gathered from observations of volunteer convicts and radiotherapy patients treated for carcinoma in one testis while the other was shielded. Many investigators have recorded normal births to the partners of patients whose remaining, functioning testis received a radiation dose between 50 and 300 rad (0.5 and 3 Gy$_t$). Nevertheless, procreation for a period of months after testicular irradiation is ill advised.

The spermatogonial stem cells are the most sensitive phase in the gametogenesis of the spermatozoa. After irradiation of the testes, the maturing cells, spermatocytes, and spermatids are relatively radioresistant and continue to mature. Consequently, there is no significant reduction in spermatozoa until several weeks after exposure, and therefore fertility continues during this time. At this time, the irradiated spermatogonia would have developed into mature spermatozoa had they survived.

Radiation doses as low as 10 rad (100 mGy$_t$) can result in a reduction in the number of spermatozoa (Table 36-5), which is similar to the radiation response of the ovaries. With increasing dose, the depletion of spermatozoa becomes greater and extends over a longer period of time. A total of 200 rad (2 Gy$_t$) produces temporary infertility, which commences approximately 2 months after irradiation and persists for up to 12 months. A total of 500 rad (5 Gy$_t$) produces permanent sterility. Even after doses sufficient to produce permanent sterility, the male normally retains his potency and ability to engage in sexual intercourse.

Since male gametogenesis is a self-renewing system, there is some evidence to suggest that the genetic mutations induced in surviving postspermatogonial cells represent the most hazardous mutations. Consequently, after testicular irradiation of doses above approximately 10 rad (100 mGy$_t$), the male should refrain from procreation for 2 to 4 months until all cells in the spermatogonial and postspermatogonial stages at the time of irradiation have matured and disappeared. This will reduce, but probably not eliminate, any increase in genetic mutations because of the persistence of the stem cell. Evidence from animal experiments suggests that there is

TABLE 36-5	Response of the Ovaries and Testes to Radiation
Approximate Dose (rad)	**Response**
10	Minimally detectable response
200	Temporary infertility
500	Sterility

some repair of genetic mutations even when the stem cell is irradiated.

HEMATOLOGIC EFFECTS

As pointed out in the chapter introduction, x-ray workers in the 1920s and 1930s were often required to submit to a blood test each week to check the level of white blood cells (leukocytes). If the leukocyte level was depressed by more than 25% of the normal, the employee was either given time off or assigned to nonradiation activities until the count returned to normal. What was not really understood at the time, however, is that the minimum whole-body dose necessary to produce a measurable hematologic depression is approximately 25 rad (250 mGy$_t$). These workers were being heavily irradiated by today's standards.

Hemopoietic System

The hemopoietic system consists of bone marrow, circulating blood, and lymphoid tissue. Lymphoid tissues are the lymph nodes, spleen, and thymus. The principal effect of radiation on this system is the depression of the number of blood cells in the peripheral circulation. The time- and dose-related effects on the various types of circulating blood cells are determined by the normal growth and maturation of these cells.

All cells of the hemopoietic system apparently develop from a single type of stem cell (Figure 36-6). This stem cell is called a **pluripotential stem cell** because it has the ability to develop into several different types of mature cells.

Although the spleen and thymus manufacture one type of leukocyte, the lymphocyte, most circulating blood cells, including lymphocytes, are manufactured in the bone marrow. In a child, the bone marrow is rather uniformly distributed throughout the skeleton. In an adult, the active bone marrow responsible for producing circulating cells is restricted to flat bones, such as the ribs, sternum, and skull, and the ends of long bones.

From the single pluripotential stem cell, a number of cell types are produced. Principally these are the **lymphocytes** (those involved in the immune response), the **granulocytes** (scavenger type of cells used to fight bacteria), **thrombocytes** (cells also called *platelets* and involved in the clotting of blood to prevent hemorrhage), and **erythrocytes** (red blood cells that are the transportation agents for oxygen). These cell lines develop at different rates in the bone marrow and are released to the peripheral blood as mature cells.

While in the bone marrow, the cells proliferate in number, differentiate in function, and mature. The developing granulocytes and erythrocytes spend about 8 to 10 days in the bone marrow. Thrombocytes have a lifetime of approximately 5 days in the bone marrow. Lymphocytes are produced over varying times and have varying lifetimes in the peripheral blood. Some are thought to have lives measured in terms of hours and others in terms of years. In the peripheral blood, the granulocytes have a lifetime of only a couple of days. Thrombocytes have a lifetime of approximately 1 week and erythrocytes a lifetime of nearly 4 months.

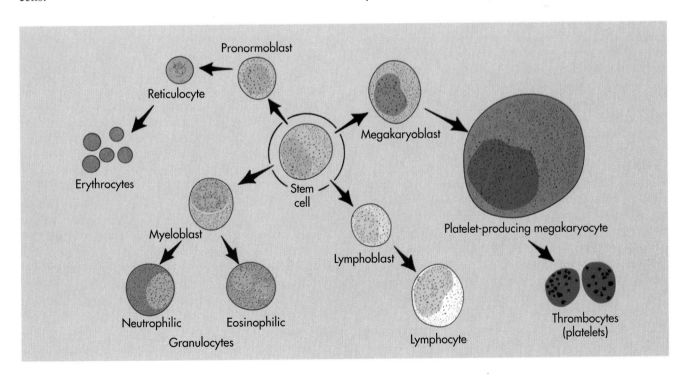

FIGURE 36-6 The four principal types of blood cells—lymphocytes, granulocytes, erythrocytes, and thrombocytes—develop and mature from a single pluripotential stem cell.

The hemopoietic system is therefore another example of a cell-renewal system. The effect of radiation on this system is determined by normal cell growth and development.

Hemopoietic Cell Survival

The principal response of the hemopoietic system to radiation exposure is a decrease in the number of all types of blood cells in the circulating peripheral blood. Lethal injury to the stem cells and other precursor cells causes the depletion of the mature circulating cells.

Figure 36-7 shows the radiation response of three circulating cell types. Examples are given for low, moderate, and high radiation doses, showing that the degree of cell depletion increases with increasing dose. These figures are the results of observations on experimental animals, radiotherapy patients, and the few radiation accident victims.

After exposure, the first cells to become affected are the lymphocytes. Within minutes or hours after exposure, these cells are reduced in number (lymphopenia), and they are very slow to recover. Because their response is so immediate, the radiation effect is apparently a direct one on the lymphocytes themselves, rather than on the precursor cells.

 The lymphocytes and the spermatogonia are the most radiosensitive cells in the body.

Granulocytes experience a rapid rise in number (granulocytosis), followed first by a rapid decrease and then a slower decrease in number (granulocytopenia). If the radiation dose is moderate, then approximately 15 to 20 days after irradiation, an abortive rise in the granulocyte count may occur. Minimum granulocyte levels are reached approximately 30 days after irradiation. If recovery is to occur, return to normal will take approximately 2 months.

The depletion of platelets (thrombocytopenia) after irradiation develops more slowly, again because of the longer time required for the more sensitive precursor cells to reach maturity. Thrombocytes reach a minimum number in about 30 days and recover in approximately 2 months, similar to the response of granulocytes.

The erythrocytes are less sensitive than the other blood cells. This occurs apparently because of their very long lifetime in the peripheral blood. Injury of these cells is not apparent for a matter of weeks. Total recovery may take 6 months to a year.

CYTOGENETIC EFFECTS

A technique developed in the early 1950s contributed enormously to human genetic analysis and radiation genetics. The technique calls for a culture of human cells to be prepared and treated so that the chromosomes of each cell can be easily observed and studied. This has resulted in many observations on radiation-induced chromosome damage.

 Cytogenetics is the study of the genetics of cells and in particular, cell chromosomes.

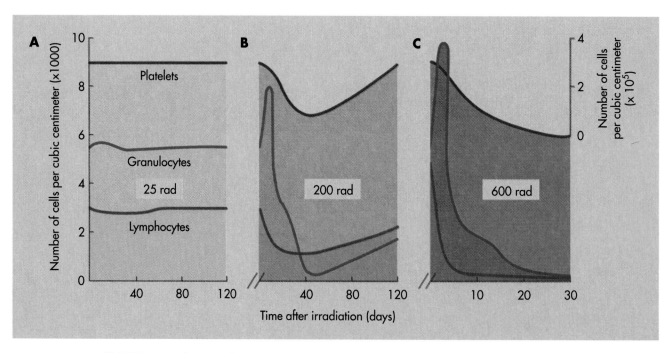

FIGURE 36-7 These graphs show the radiation response of the major circulating blood cells. **A,** 25 rad. **B,** 200 rad. **C,** 600 rad.

The chromosomes of a human cancer cell after radiation therapy are shown in the photomicrograph in Figure 36-8. The many chromosome aberrations seen represent a high degree of damage. Radiation cytogenetic studies have shown that nearly every type of chromosome aberration can be induced by radiation and that some may be specific to radiation. The induction rate of chromosome aberrations is related in a complex way to the radiation dose and differs among the various types of aberrations.

 Radiation-induced chromosome aberrations follow a nonthreshold dose-response relationship.

Attempts to measure chromosome aberrations in patients after diagnostic x-ray examination have been largely unsuccessful. However, some studies involving high-dose fluoroscopy have shown the presence of radiation-induced chromosome aberrations soon after the examination.

High doses of radiation, without question, cause chromosome aberrations. Low doses, no doubt, do also, but it is difficult technically to observe aberrations at doses that are less than approximately 5 rad (50 mGy$_t$). An even more difficult task is the identification of the link between radiation-induced chromosome aberrations and latent illness or disease.

When the body is irradiated, all cells can suffer cytogenetic damage. Such damage is an early response to radiation because if the cell survives, the damage will be manifested during the next mitosis after the radiation exposure.

Human peripheral lymphocytes are most often used for cytogenetic analysis, and these lymphocytes do not move into mitosis until stimulated in vitro by an appropriate laboratory technique. Cytogenetic damage to the stem cells is sustained immediately but may not be manifested for the considerable time required for the stem cells to reach maturity as circulating lymphocytes.

Although chromosome damage is produced at the time of irradiation, it can be months and even years before the damage is measured. Some workers who were irradiated in industrial accidents 20 years ago continue to show chromosome abnormalities in their circulating lymphocytes.

Normal Karyotype

The human chromosome consists of many long strings of deoxyribonucleic acid (DNA) mixed with a protein and folded back on itself many times. A normal chromosome is shown in Figure 33-11 as it would appear in the G$_1$ phase of the cell cycle, when only two chromatids are present, and in the G$_2$ phase of the cell cycle after

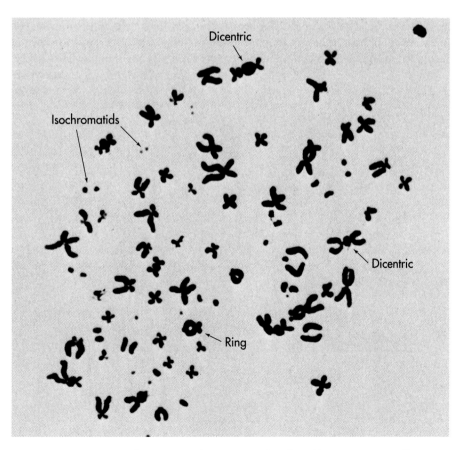

FIGURE 36-8 Chromosome damage in an irradiated human cancer cell.

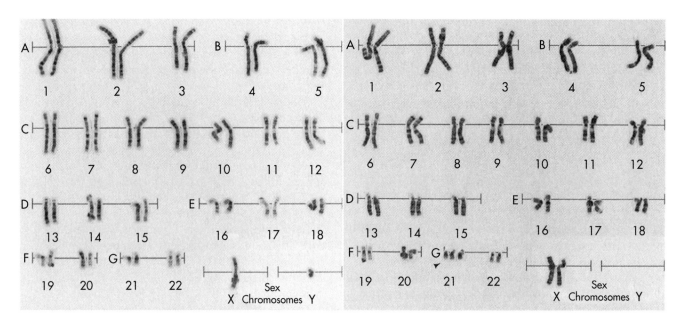

FIGURE 36-9 A photomicrograph of the human cell nucleus at metaphase shows each chromosome distinctly. The karyotype is made by cutting and pasting each chromosome like paper dolls and aligning them largest to smallest. The left karyotype is male, the right female. *(Courtesy Carolyn Caskey.)*

DNA replication. The chromosome structure of four chromatids represented for the G_2 phase is the same as that visualized in the metaphase portion of mitosis. For certain types of cytogenetic analyses of chromosomes, photographs are taken and enlarged so that each individual chromosome can be cut out like a paper doll and paired with its sister into a chromosome map, which is called a **karyotype** (Figure 36-9).

 Each cell has 22 pairs of autosomes and a pair of sex chromosomes, the X chromosome from the female and the Y chromosome from the male.

Structural radiation damage to individual chromosomes can be visualized without constructing a karyotype. These are the single- and double-hit chromosome aberrations. Reciprocal translocations require a karyotype for detection. Point genetic mutations are undetectable even with karyotype construction.

Single-Hit Chromosome Aberrations

When radiation interacts with chromosomes, the interaction can occur through a direct or an indirect effect. In either mode, these interactions result in a hit. The hit, however, is somewhat different from that described previously in radiation interaction with DNA, in which the hit results in an invisible disruption of the molecular structure of the DNA. A chromosome hit, on the other hand, produces a visible derangement of the chromosome. Since the chromosomes contain DNA, the hit has disrupted many molecular bonds and has severed many chains of DNA.

 A chromosome hit represents severe damage to the DNA.

Single-hit effects produced by radiation during the G_1 phase of the cell cycle are shown in Figure 36-10. The breakage of a chromatid is called **chromatid deletion**. During the S phase, both the remaining chromosome and the deletion are replicated. The chromosome aberration visualized at metaphase consists of a chromosome with material missing from the ends of two sister chromatids and two acentric fragments (without a centromere). These fragments are called **isochromatids**.

Chromosome aberrations could also be produced by single-hit events during the G_2 phase of the cell cycle (Figure 36-10). The probability of ionizing radiation passing through sister chromatids to produce isochromatids as low. Usually the radiation produces a chromatid deletion in only one arm of the chromosome. The result is a chromosome with an arm that is obviously missing genetic material and a chromatid fragment.

Multihit Chromosome Aberrations

A single chromosome can sustain more than one hit, resulting in a multihit aberration (Figure 36-11). In the G_1 phase of the cell cycle, ring chromosomes are produced if two hits occur on the same chromosome. Dicentrics are produced when adjacent chromosomes each suffer one hit and recombine as shown. The mechanism for the joining of chromatids depends on a condition termed *stickiness* that is radiation-induced and appears at the site of the severed chromosome.

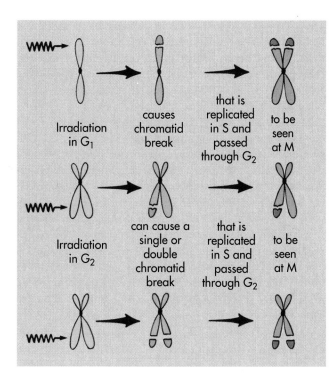

FIGURE 36-10 Single-hit chromosome aberrations after irradiation in the G₁ and G₂ phases. The aberrations are visualized and recorded during the M phase.

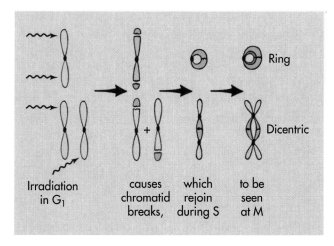

FIGURE 36-11 Multihit chromosome aberrations after irradiation in the G₁ phase result in ring and dicentric chromosomes in addition to chromatid fragments. Similar aberrations can be produced by irradiation during the G₂ phase, but they are rarer.

In the G₂ phase of the cell cycle, similar aberrations can be produced; however, such aberrations again require that (1) either the same chromosome be hit at least twice or (2) adjacent chromosomes be hit and joined together. However, these effects are rare.

Reciprocal translocations. The multihit chromosome aberrations previously described represent rather severe

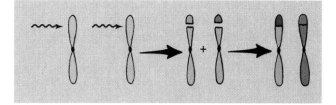

FIGURE 36-12 Radiation-induced reciprocal translocations are multihit chromosome aberrations that require karyotypic analysis for detection.

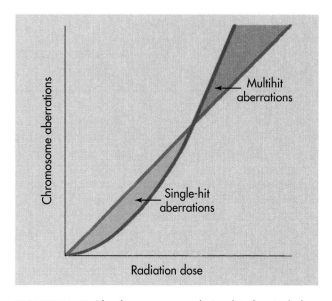

FIGURE 36-13 The dose-response relationship for single-hit aberrations is linear and nonthreshold, whereas that for multihit aberrations is nonlinear and nonthreshold.

damage to the cell. At mitosis, the acentric fragments are either lost or are attracted to only one of the daughter cells, since they are unattached to a spindle fiber. Consequently, one or both of the daughter cells can be missing considerable genetic material.

Reciprocal translocations are multihit chromosome aberrations that require karyotypic analysis for detection (Figure 36-12). Radiation-induced reciprocal translocations result in no loss of genetic material, simply a rearrangement of the genes. Consequently, all or nearly all genetic codes are available; they simply may be organized in an incorrect sequence.

Kinetics of Chromosome Aberration
At very low doses of radiation, only single-hit types of aberrations are observed. When the radiation dose exceeds perhaps 100 rad (1 Gy₁), the frequency of multihit aberrations increases more rapidly.

The general dose-response relationship for the production of single-hit and multihit aberrations is shown in Figure 36-13. Single-hit aberrations are produced with a linear, nonthreshold dose-response relationship. Multihit aberrations are produced with a nonlinear, non-threshold relationship. These relationships have been determined experimentally by a number of investigators.

Radiation Dose-Response Relationships for Cytogenetic Damage

Single Hit: $Y = a + bD$

Multihit: $Y = a + bD + cD^2$

where:

Y = number of single-hit or multihit chromosome aberrations

a = naturally occurring frequency of chromosome aberrations

b and c = radiation dose (D) coefficients of damage for single-hit and multihit aberrations, respectively

Some laboratories use cytogenetic analysis as a biologic radiation dosimeter. The multihit aberrations are considered to be the most significant in terms of latent human damage. If the radiation dose is unknown yet not life threatening, the approximate chromosome aberration frequency will be two single-hit aberrations per rad per 1000 cells and one multihit aberration per 10 rad per 1000 cells. This approximation holds through a total dose of perhaps 200 rad.

SUMMARY

After exposure to a high radiation dose (approximately 25 rad and up), there can be a response in humans within a few days to a few weeks. This immediate response is called an *early effect of radiation exposure.* Such early effects are usually deterministic: the severity of response is dose related, and there is a dose threshold.

The sequence of events after high-dose radiation exposure leading to death within days or weeks is called the *acute radiation syndrome.* The sequence of events are hematologic syndrome, GI syndrome, CNS syndrome. The syndromes are dose related.

$LD_{50/60}$ is the dose of radiation to the whole body in which 50% of the subjects will die within 60 days. For humans, this dose is estimated at approximately 300 rad. As radiation doses increase, the time between exposure and death decreases. This time between exposure and death is termed the *mean survival time.*

When tissue is irradiated locally, higher doses are tolerated. Examples of local tissue damage are the effects on the skin, gonads, and bone marrow. The first manifestation of radiation injury to the skin is damage to the basal cells. Resulting skin damage is erythema, desquamation, or epilation. Analysis of superficial x-ray therapy has shown that the skin erythema dose, or SED_{50}, is approximately 600 rad.

Radiation of the male testes can result in a reduction in the number of spermatozoa. A dose of 200 rad produces temporary infertility. A dose of 500 rad to the testes produces permanent sterility. In the male, as in the female, stem cell development is the most radiosensitive phase.

The hemopoietic system consists of bone marrow, circulating blood, and lymphoid tissue. The principal effect of radiation on this system is a depression of the number of blood cells in the peripheral circulation. Radiation exposure decreases the number of all precursor cells, which reduces the number of mature cells in the circulating blood. Lymphocytes and spermatogonia are considered the most radiosensitive cells in the body.

The study of chromosome damage from radiation exposure is called *cytogenetics.* Chromosome damage takes on the following different forms: (1) chromatid deletion, (2) dicentric chromosome aberration, and (3) reciprocal translocations.

CHALLENGE QUESTIONS

1. Define or otherwise identify:
   a. GI syndrome
   b. Latent period
   c. $LD_{50/60}$
   d. Erythema
   e. Clinical tolerance
   f. Acute radiation syndrome
   g. Erythrocyte
   h. Karyotype
   i. Epilation
   j. Multihit aberration
2. What is the minimum dose that results in reddening of the skin?
3. Explain the prodromal syndrome.
4. The clinical signs and symptoms of the manifest illness stage of acute radiation lethality are classified into what three groups?
5. Which stage of acute radiation syndrome simulates recovery?
6. What dose of radiation results in the GI syndrome?
7. What is the reason for death in the GI syndrome?
8. Identify the cause of death in the CNS syndrome.
9. Describe the stages of gametogenesis in the female. Identify the most radiosensitive phases.
10. What cells arise from pluripotential stem cells?
11. Discuss the maturation of basal cells in the epidermis.
12. What two cells are the most radiosensitive cells in the human body?
13. Describe the changes in mean survival time with increasing dose.

14. What are the approximate values of $LD_{50/60}$ and SED_{50} in humans?

15. What are the four principal blood cell lines and the function of each?

16. Diagram the mechanism for the production of a reciprocal translocation.

17. List the clinical signs and symptoms of the hematologic syndrome.

18. What is cytogenetics?

19. If the ambient incidence of single hit–type chromosome aberrations is 0.15 per 100 cells and the dose coefficient is 0.0094, how many such aberrations would be expected after a dose of 38 rad?

20. If the ambient incidence of multihittype chromosome aberrations is 0.082 and the dose coefficient is 0.0047, how many dicentrics per 100 cells would be expected after a whole-body dose of 160 rad?

Late Effects of Radiation

OBJECTIVES

At the completion of this chapter, the student should be able to:

1. Define the late effects of radiation exposure
2. Identify the radiation dose needed to produce late effects
3. Discuss the results of epidemiologic studies of people exposed to radiation
4. List the local tissue effects of low-dose radiation to the skin, chromosomes, and cornea
5. Explain the estimates of radiation risk
6. Analyze radiation-induced leukemia and cancer
7. Review the risks of low-dose radiation to fertility and pregnancy

OUTLINE

The early effects of radiation exposure are produced by high radiation doses. The late effects of radiation exposure are the result of low doses delivered over a long time. The radiation exposures experienced by personnel in diagnostic imaging are low dose and low linear energy transfer (LET). In addition, the exposures in diagnostic imaging are delivered intermittently over long periods.

The principal late effects of low-dose radiation over long periods are radiation-induced malignancy and genetic effects. Most late effects are also known as *stochastic effects*. Stochastic effects exhibit an increasing incidence, not severity, of response with increasing dose. Life-span shortening and effects on local tissues have also been reported as late effects but are not considered significant. Radiation-protection guides are based on the suspected or observed effects of radiation and on an assumed linear, nonthreshold dose-response relationship.

This chapter reviews these late effects and introduces the subject of risk estimation. Radiation effects during pregnancy are of considerable importance in diagnostic x-ray imaging, and such effects are covered here.

TABLE 37-1	Minimum Population Sample Required to Show that the Given Radiation Dose Significantly Elevated the Incidence of Leukemia	
Dose (rad)	Required Sample Size (No. of People)	
5	6,000,000	
10	1,600,000	
15	750,000	
20	500,000	
50	100,000	

EPIDEMIOLOGIC STUDIES

Epidemiology is the study of the occurrence, distribution, and causes of disease in humans. Epidemiologic studies of people exposed to radiation are difficult because (1) the dose is usually not known but presumed to be low and (2) the frequency of response is very low. Consequently, the results of radiation epidemiologic studies do not carry the statistical accuracy that the observations of early radiation effects do.

Table 37-1 illustrates the difficulty of the problem. It shows the minimum number of people who must be observed as a function of radiation dose to definitely link an increase in the incidence of leukemia with the radiation dose in question.

LOCAL TISSUE EFFECTS
Skin

In addition to the acute early effects of erythema and desquamation, late effects can occur. One such late effect is skin cancer. Chronic irradiation of the skin can also result in severe nonmalignant changes. The skin of the hands and forearms of early radiologists who performed fluoroscopic examinations without protective gloves developed a very callused, discolored, and weathered appearance. The skin was also very tight and brittle and sometimes severely cracked or flaked. This late effect was called *radiodermatitis*. The dose necessary to produce such an effect is very high, and it is extremely unlikely to occur in the current practice of radiology.

Chromosomes

Irradiation of blood-forming organs can produce hematologic depression as an early response or leukemia as a late response. Chromosome damage in the circulating lymphocytes can be produced as both an early and a late response. An early response would be a reduced white blood cell count. An example of a more serious late response is leukemia. A low dose of radiation can produce chromosome aberrations that may not be apparent until many years after the radiation exposure. Chromosome abnormalities in the peripheral lymphocytes of individuals irradiated accidentally with rather high radiation dose continue to show as long as 20 years, presumably as a result of radiation damage to the lymphocytic stem cells. These stem cells may not have been stimulated into replication and maturation for many years. Specific chromosome damage is now linked to specific malignancies, such as ovarian cancer and neuroblastoma.

Cataracts

In 1932, E.O. Lawrence of the University of California developed the first **cyclotron**, a 5-inch-diameter machine capable of accelerating charged particles to very high energies. These charged particles were used as "bullets" shot at the nuclei of target atoms in the study of nuclear structure. By 1940, every university physics department of any worth had built its own cyclotron and was engaged in what has become high-energy physics.

The modern cyclotron is used principally to produce radionuclides for use in nuclear medicine (Figure 37-1). The largest particle accelerators in the world are located at Argonne National Laboratory in the United States and at Conseil Européen pour la Recherche Nucléaire (CERN) in Geneva. These accelerators are used to discover the ultimate fine structure of matter and to describe exactly what happened at the moment of the creation of the universe.

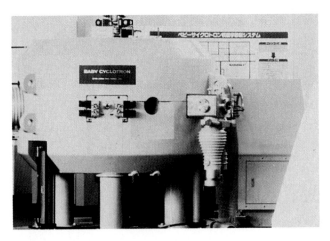

FIGURE 37-1 Cyclotron used to produce radionuclides for nuclear medicine. *(Courtesy Positron Corporation.)*

Early machines might be located in one room and a beam of high-energy particles would be extracted through a tube and steered and focused by electromagnets onto the target material in the adjacent room. At that time, sophisticated electronic equipment was not available for controlling this high-energy beam. The cyclotron physicists used a tool of the radiologist, the fluorescent screen, to aid in locating the high-energy beam. Unfortunately, in so doing, these physicists would receive high radiation doses to the lens of the eye because they had to look directly into the beam. In 1949, the first paper reporting cataracts in cyclotron physicists appeared. By 1960, several hundred such cases had been reported. (This was particularly tragic, since there were few high-energy physicists.)

On the basis of these observations and animal experimentation, the following conclusions can be drawn regarding radiation-induced cataracts:

1. The radiosensitivity of the lens of the eye is age dependent.
2. The older the individual, the greater the radiation effect and the shorter the latent period.
3. Latent periods varying from 5 to 30 years have been observed in humans, but the average is approximately 15 years.
4. High-LET radiation, such as neutron and proton, has a high relative biologic effectiveness (RBE) for the production of cataracts.
5. Radiation-induced cataracts occur on the posterior pole of the lens.

 The dose-response relationship for radiation-induced cataracts is nonlinear and threshold.

If the lens dose is high enough, in excess of approximately 1000 rad (10 Gy$_t$), nearly 100% of those who are irradiated develop cataracts. Although the precise level of the threshold dose is difficult to assess, most investi-

gators would suggest that the threshold after an acute x-ray exposure is approximately 200 rad (2 Gy$_t$). The threshold after fractionated exposure, such as that received in radiology, is probably in excess of 1000 rad (10 Gy$_t$). Occupational exposures to the lens of the eye are too low to require protective lens shields for radiologic technologists. It is nearly impossible for a medical radiation worker to reach the threshold dose.

Radiation administered to patients undergoing head and neck examination by either fluoroscopy or computed tomography can be significant. In computed tomography, the lens dose can be 5 rad per slice. In this situation, usually no more than one or two slices intersect the lens. In computed tomography it is common to modify examinations to reduce the dose to the eyes.

LIFE-SPAN SHORTENING
Risks to Radiographers

Many experiments conducted with animals after both acute and chronic exposure show that irradiated animals die young. Figure 37-2 graphs the results of several such representative experiments and shows that the relationship between life-span shortening and dose is apparently linear and nonthreshold. When all the animal data are considered collectively, it is difficult to attempt a meaningful extrapolation to humans. At worst, humans can expect a reduced life span of approximately 10 days for every rad.

The data presented in Table 37-2 was compiled by Bernard L. Cohen of the University of Pittsburgh and extrapolated from various statistical sources of mortality. The expected loss of life in days is given as a function of occupation, disease, or another factor (for example, gender). Whereas the average life-span shortening caused by occupational accidents is 74 days, that for radiation workers is only 12 days.

 Radiologic technology is considered a safe occupation.

One investigator has evaluated the death records of radiologic technologists who operated field x-ray equipment during World War II. These imaging units were poorly designed and inadequately shielded, so the technologists received higher-than-normal exposures. A total of 7000 such technologists have been studied, and no radiation effects have been observed.

An investigation of health effects from radiation exposure of American radiologic technologists is underway. This is a mail survey covering many work-related conditions of approximately 150,000 subjects and will take many years to complete. Early reports show no effects.

Radiation-induced life-span shortening is nonspecific; that is, there are no characteristic disease entities associated with it, and it does not include late

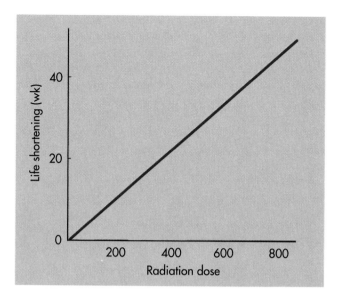

FIGURE 37-2 In chronically irradiated animals, the extent of life-span shortening appears linear and nonthreshold. This graph shows the representative results of several such experiments with mice.

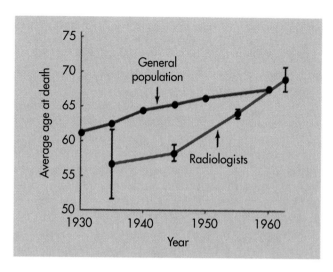

FIGURE 37-3 Radiation-induced life-span shortening is shown for American radiologists. The age at death in the radiologists was lower than that of the general population, but this difference has disappeared.

TABLE 37-2	Risk of Life-Span Shortening as a Result of Occupation, Disease, or Another Factor	
Risk Factor		**Expected Days of Life Lost**
Male rather than female		2800
Heart disease		2100
Unmarried status		2000
Smoking (one pack of cigarettes a day)		1600
Coal miner		1100
Cancer		980
Obesity: 30 pounds overweight		900
Stroke		520
All accidents		435
Service in Vietnam		400
Motor vehicle accidents		200
Average occupational accidents		74
Speed limit increase from 55 to 65 mph		40
Radiation worker		12
Airplane crashes		1

TABLE 37-3	Death Statistics for Three Groups of Physicians	
	Median Age at Death	**Deaths per 1000 Age-Adjusted**
1935 to 1944		
RSNA	71.4	18.4
ACP	73.4	15.4
AAOO	76.2	13.0
1945 to 1954		
RSNA	72.0	16.4
ACP	74.8	13.7
AAOO	76.0	11.9
1955 to 1958		
RSNA	73.5	13.6
ACP	76.0	11.4
AAOO	76.4	10.6

malignant effects. Radiation-induced life-span shortening simply means accelerated premature aging and death.

Observations on human populations have not yielded convincing evidence of life-span shortening. No life-span shortening has been observed in atomic bomb survivors, and some received rather substantial radiation doses. Life-span shortening in watch-dial painters, x-ray patients, and other human populations exposed to radiation has not been reported.

Risks to Radiologists

American radiologists are one population that has been rather extensively studied. Such studies have many shortcomings, not the least of which is the fact that they are retrospective in nature. Figure 37-3 shows the results obtained when the age at death for radiologists was compared with the age at death for the general population. Radiologists dying in the early 1930s were approximately 5 years younger than the average age at death of the general population. However, this difference in age at death had shrunk to zero by 1965.

A more thorough study used two other physician groups as controls rather than the general population. Table 37-3 summarizes the results of this investigation.

The physician groups observed in this study were members of the Radiological Society of North America (RSNA) as the high-risk group and members of the American Academy of Ophthalmology and Otolaryngology (AAOO) as the low-risk group. Members of the American College of Physicians (ACP) represented an intermediate risk group.

A comparison of the median age at death and age-adjusted death rates for these physician specialties demonstrates a significant difference in age at death during the early years of radiology. This difference has disappeared in the contemporary practice of diagnostic imaging, presumably because of better attention to radiation protection through proper procedures and equipment design.

When these differences in mortality were first described, British investigators began looking for similar effects in British radiologists. None were found, which raises some questions about the validity and significance of the findings in American radiologists.

RISK ESTIMATES

The early effects of high-dose radiation exposure are usually easy to observe and measure. The late effects are also easy to observe, but it is nearly impossible to associate a particular late response with a previous radiation exposure. Consequently, precise dose-response relationships are often not possible, and therefore **risk estimates** are used. There are three types of risk estimates; relative, excess, and absolute. Each represents different statements of risk and has different dimensions.

Relative Risk

Relative risk involves estimating late radiation effects in large populations without having any precise knowledge of their radiation dose. Relative risk is computed by comparing the number of people in the exposed population showing a given late effect with the number who developed the same late effect in an unexposed population. For instance, a relative risk of 1 would indicate no risk at all. A relative risk of 1.5 indicates that the frequency of a late response is 50% higher in the irradiated population compared with the nonirradiated population.

> **Relative Risk**
>
> $$\text{Relative risk} = \frac{\text{Observed cases}}{\text{Expected cases}}$$

Of particular importance are the relative risk factors for radiation-induced late effects observed in the range of 1 to 2 in human populations.

Occasionally, an investigation results in a relative risk of less than 1. This would indicate that the exposed population receives some protective benefit, which is consistent with the theory of radiation hormesis. However, the usual interpretation of such studies is that the results are

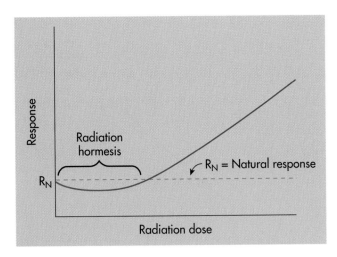

FIGURE 37-4 Radiation hormesis is indicated when the relative risk is less than 1.

not statistically significant either because of the small number of observations or because of inadequate identification of irradiated and control populations.

Radiation hormesis. The theory of **radiation hormesis** suggests that a little radiation, less than approximately 10 rad (100 mGy$_t$), may be good for you. Like a vaccine, such low doses may provide a protective effect by stimulating molecular repair and immunologic response mechanisms. An example of a reported dose-response relationship indicating radiation hormesis is shown in Figure 37-4. The low-dose region where the response is less than the natural level is the hormetic region. The crossover to a positive response is usually in the range between 5 and 20 rad (50 and 200 mGy$_t$). Nevertheless, radiation hormesis remains a theory, and until it is proved, ALARA (as low as reasonably achievable) is practiced (see Chapter 1).

Question: In a study of radiation-induced leukemia after diagnostic levels of radiation, 227 cases were observed in 100,000 persons so irradiated. The normal incidence of leukemia in the United States is 150 cases per 100,000. Based on this data, what is the relative risk of radiation-induced leukemia?

Answer:
$$\text{Relative risk} = \frac{\text{Observed cases}}{\text{Expected cases}}$$
$$\frac{227}{100,000} \div \frac{150}{100,000} = \frac{0.00227}{0.00150} = 1.51$$

Excess Risk

Often when an investigation of human radiation response indicates the induction of some late effect, the magnitude of the effect will be reflected by the excess cases induced. Leukemia, for instance, is known to occur spontaneously in nonirradiated populations. If the leukemia incidence in an irradiated population exceeds that which is expected, the difference between the observed number of cases and the expected number would be **excess risk**.

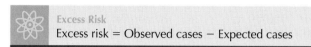

Excess Risk

Excess risk = Observed cases − Expected cases

The excess cases in this instance are assumed to be radiation induced. Determining the number of excess cases requires a comparison of the observed number of cases in the irradiated population with the number of cases that would have been expected on the basis of known population levels.

Question: A total of 23 cases of skin cancer were observed in a population of 1000 radiologists. The incidence in the general population is 0.5/100,000. How many excess skin cancers were produced in the population of radiologists?

Answer: Excess cases = Observed cases − Expected cases

$$= \frac{23}{1000} - \frac{0.5}{100,000}$$

$$= \frac{23}{1000} - \frac{0.005}{1000}$$

$$\simeq 23$$

Since none would be expected, all 23 cases represent radiation risk.

Absolute Risk

If at least two different dose levels are known, it may be possible to determine an absolute risk factor. Unlike the relative risk, which is a dimensionless ratio, the **absolute risk** has units of number of cases/10^6 persons/rad/yr. The absolute risk of radiation-induced malignant disease is approximately 10 cases/10^6 persons/rad/yr. This value is a considerable simplification of the results of many studies.

A linear dose-response relationship must be assumed if the absolute risk is to be determined. If the dose-response relationship is assumed to be nonthreshold, then only one dose level is required. The value of the absolute radiation risk is equal to the slope of the dose-response relationship (Figure 37-5). The error bars on each data point indicate the precision of the observation of response.

Question: The absolute risk for radiation-induced breast cancer is approximately 6 cases/10^6 persons/rad/yr for a 20-year at-risk period. If 100,000 women receive 100 mrad during mammography, how many radiation-induced cancers would be expected?

Answer: (6 cases/10^6 persons/rad/yr)(10^5 persons)(0.1 rad) (20 yr) = 1.2 cases

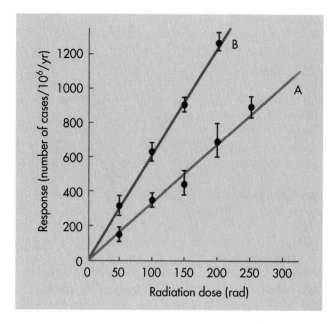

FIGURE 37-5 The slope of the linear, nonthreshold dose-response relationship is equal to the absolute risk. *A* and *B* show absolute risks of 3.4 and 6.2 cases 10^6 persons/rad/yr, respectively.

Question: There are approximately 300,000 American radiologic technologists, and they receive an annual effective dose of 10 mrem. What is the expected number of annual deaths because of this occupational exposure?

Answer: (10 cases/10^6 persons/rad/yr)(0.3×10^6)(0.01 rad)
= (10 cases)(0.003)
= 0.03 cases/yr

Death from malignant disease occurs in approximately 20% of the population.

RADIATION-INDUCED MALIGNANCY

All the late effects, including radiation-induced malignancy, have been observed in experimental animals, and from these animal experiments, dose-response relationships have been developed. At the human level, these late effects have been observed, but often there are insufficient data to precisely identify the dose-response relationship. Consequently, some of the conclusions drawn regarding human responses are based in part on animal data.

Leukemia

Considering the incidence of radiation-induced leukemia in laboratory animals, there is no question that this response is real and that the incidence increases with increasing radiation dose. The form of the dose-response relationship is apparently linear and nonthreshold. A number of human population groups have exhibited an elevated incidence of leukemia after radiation exposure: A-bomb survivors, American radiologists, radiotherapy patients, and children irradiated in utero, to name a few.

A-bomb survivors. Probably the greatest wealth of information that we have on radiation-induced leukemia in humans results from observations of the survivors of the atomic bombings of Hiroshima and Nagasaki, Japan. At the time of the bomb (**ATB**), approximately 300,000 people lived in those two cities. Nearly 100,000 were killed from the blast and early effects of radiation. Another 100,000 people received significant doses of radiation and survived. The remainder were unaffected, since their radiation exposure was less than 10 rad (100 mGy$_t$).

After World War II, scientists of the Atomic Bomb Casualty Commission (ABCC), now known as the *Radiation Effects Research Foundation (RERF)*, attempted to determine the radiation dose received by each of the A-bomb survivors in both cities. They first established the position of each person ATB and estimated the dose to that survivor by considering not only distance from the explosion but also terrain, type of bomb, type of construction if the survivor were inside, and other factors that might influence dose.

A summary of the data obtained by these investigations is given in Table 37-4, and the data analysis is shown graphically in Figure 37-6. The natural incidence of leukemia in the Japanese ATB was approximately 25 cases/10⁶ persons/yr. After high doses, the leukemia incidence is as much as 100 times that in the nonirradiated population. Even though there are large error bars at each dose increment, it is clear that the response appears linear and nonthreshold.

If, however, the data in the low-dose region (for example, below 200 rad) are expanded, it could be concluded that a threshold exists in the neighborhood of 50 rad. Nevertheless, neither this information nor other available information is interpreted to support a threshold response.

 Radiation-induced leukemia follows a linear, nonthreshold dose-response relationship.

Figure 37-7 demonstrates the temporal distribution of the onset of leukemia in the A-bomb survivors for the 40 years after the bombs. The data are presented as cases per 100,000 and include for comparison the leukemia rate in the population at large and in the nonexposed populations of the bombed cities. There was a rather rapid rise in leukemia incidence that reached a plateau after approximately 5 years. The incidence declined slowly for approximately 20 years when it reached the natural level experienced by the nonexposed. The at-risk period is that time after irradiation during which the radiation effect might be expected to occur. It is interesting to note that the at-risk period for radiation-induced cancer is a lifetime.

 Radiation-induced leukemia is considered to have a latent period of 4 to 7 years and an at-risk period of approximately 20 years.

The data from the A-bomb survivors show without a doubt that the radiation exposure to those survivors caused the later development of leukemia. It is interesting, however, to reflect on some additional aspects of these events. The first A-bomb was dropped on Hiroshima; it was fueled with uranium, so the radiation dose was about equally distributed between gamma rays and neutrons. The Nagasaki bomb was a plutonium bomb. A total of 90% of its radiation was caused by gamma rays and only 10% by neutrons. Neutron radiation has a higher RBE than gamma rays, and this difference contributes to the difficulties in assessing the dose for each survivor. Acute leukemia and chronic myelocytic leukemia were observed most often in the atomic bomb survivors.

TABLE 37-4	Incidence of Leukemia in A-Bomb Survivors		
	Hiroshima	**Nagasaki**	**Total**
Total number of survivors in study	74,356	25,037	99,393
Observed cases of leukemia	102	42	144
Expected cases of leukemia	39	13	52

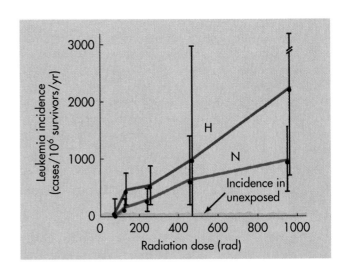

FIGURE 37-6 Data from the A-bomb survivors of Hiroshima *(H)* and Nagasaki *(N)* suggest a linear, nonthreshold dose-response relationship.

Chronic lymphocytic leukemia is rare and therefore is not considered to be a form of radiation-induced leukemia.

Taken to the final analysis, the data from the A-bomb survivors pointed to an absolute risk of 1.5 cases/10^6 persons/rad/yr. The overall relative risk based on the total number of observed leukemia deaths (144) vs. the number of expected leukemia deaths (52) is approximately 2.8:1.

Radiologists. By the second decade of radiology, reports of pernicious anemia and leukemia in radiologists began to appear. In the early 1940s, several investigators had reviewed the incidence of leukemia in American radiologists and found it alarmingly high. These early radiologists functioned without the benefit of modern radiation-protection devices and procedures, and many served as both radiation oncologists and diagnostic radiologists. In radiotherapeutic activities, they received substantial radiation exposures from radium applications. It has been estimated that some of these early radiologists received doses exceeding 100 rad/year (1 Gy$_t$/yr).

One report of the death records of medical specialists dying between 1929 and 1943 showed that 8 of 175 deaths in radiologists were caused by leukemia. In non-radiologist physicians, there were 221 leukemia deaths from a total of 55,160. These data indicate a relative risk of 10.3:1. Another study covering the years 1948 to 1963 was based on a total of 12 leukemia cases in 425 radiology-related deaths. A relative risk of 4:1 was observed. Currently, American radiologists do not exhibit an elevated incidence of leukemia when compared with other physician specialists.

On the other hand, a rather exhaustive study of mortality in radiologists in Great Britain covering the period from the turn of the century to 1960 did not show such an elevated risk of leukemia. The reasons for such a different experience between American and British radiologists is unknown. Some suggest that it is because the radiation-therapy activities in Great Britain have always been attended by medical physicists, who presumably were more conscious of radiation safety.

Studies of radiation-induced leukemia in American radiologic technologists have been conducted, and they consistently show no evidence of such an effect.

Patients with ankylosing spondylitis. In the 1940s and 1950s, in Great Britain particularly, it was common practice to use radiation to treat patients with ankylosing spondylitis. Ankylosing spondylitis is an arthritis-like condition of the vertebral column. Such patients cannot walk upright or move except with great difficulty. For relief they would be given rather high doses of radiation to the spinal column, and the treatment was quite successful. Patients who previously had to walk hunched over were able to stand erect. Radiation therapy was a permanent cure and remained the treatment of choice for approximately 20 years, until it was discovered that

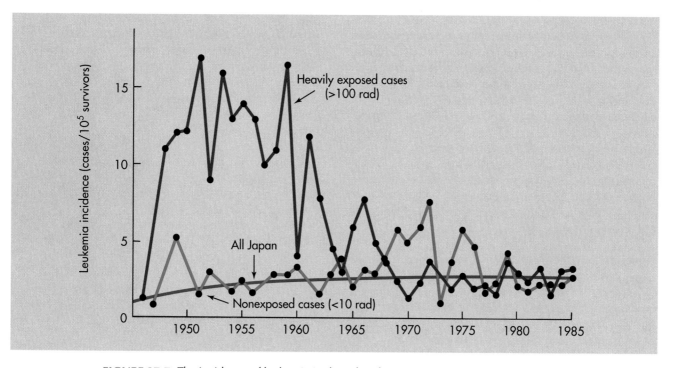

FIGURE 37-7 The incidence of leukemia in the A-bomb survivors increased rapidly for the first few years and then declined to natural incidence by about 1975.

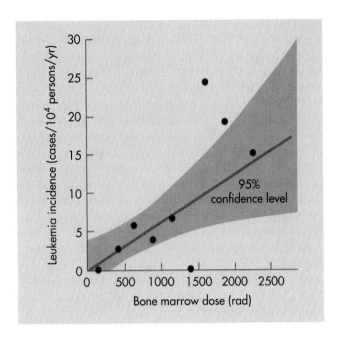

FIGURE 37-8 The results of observations of leukemia in patients with ankylosing spondylitis treated with x-ray therapy suggest a linear, nonthreshold dose-response relationship.

some who had been cured by radiation were dying from leukemia. The graphic results on the observations of these patients are shown in Figure 37-8.

From 1935 to 1955, 14,554 male patients were treated at 81 different radiation-therapy centers in Great Britain. Review of the treatment records showed the dose to the bone marrow of the spinal column to range from 100 to 4000 rad (1 to 40 Gy$_t$). A total of 52 cases of leukemia occurred in this population.

The rate of leukemia in patients receiving more than 2000 rad was 17 cases/10,000 persons; in Great Britain the normal incidence of leukemia was 0.5 cases/10,000. The relative risk therefore is approximately 34:1. When one considers all 52 cases and compares the incidence of leukemia with that of the general population, the relative risk is 9.5:1.

The absolute risk can be obtained from these data by determining the slope of the best-fit line through the data points (Figure 37-8). Such an analysis results in approximately 0.8 cases/10^6 persons/rad/yr. If 95% confidence limits are placed on the data, the possibility of a threshold dose at approximately 300 rad cannot be ruled out.

Leukemia in other populations. A number of studies have been designed to link leukemia incidence with environmental radiation. Natural background radiation levels increase in general with altitude and with latitude, but the range of levels observed is not sufficient to demonstrate a relationship with leukemia.

Other population groups that have provided evidence, both positive and negative, regarding the leukemia-inducing action of radiation are radium watch-dial painters, children receiving superficial x-ray treatment, and some additional adult radiotherapy groups.

Cancer

Although the human data linking cancer and radiation are not as significant as that linking leukemia and radiation, it may be said that radiation can cause cancer. Nearly all types of human cancer can be radiation induced.

The relative and absolute risks for cancer are similar to those reported for leukemia. Many types of cancer have been implicated as radiation induced, and a discussion of the more important ones is in order.

It is not possible to link any case of cancer to a previous radiation exposure, regardless of its magnitude, because cancer is so common. Approximately 20% of all deaths are caused by cancer, therefore any radiation-induced cancers are obscured. Leukemia, on the other hand, is a relatively rare disease. That makes analysis of radiation-induced leukemia easier.

Thyroid cancer. Thyroid cancer has developed in three groups of patients whose thyroid glands were irradiated in childhood. The first two groups, called the Ann Arbor series and the Rochester series, consist of individuals who, in the 1940s and early 1950s, were treated shortly after birth for thymic enlargement. The thymus is a gland lying just below the thyroid gland that can enlarge in response to infection.

At these facilities, radiation was often the treatment of choice. After a dose of up to 500 rad (5 Gy$_t$), the thymus gland would shrink so that all enlargement disappeared. No further problems were evident until up to 20 years later, when some of these patients began to develop thyroid nodules and some cases of thyroid cancer.

In the Ann Arbor series, several thousand children were involved. The dose to the thyroid gland was estimated to be 20 to 30 rad (200 to 300 mGy$_t$) and was received mainly from scatter radiation from the adjacent useful beam to the thymus gland. Reasonable beam collimation was practiced.

In the Rochester series, there were a smaller number of cases, but the practice was to irradiate a rather large area so that the thymus gland and thyroid gland were equally irradiated. The estimated thyroid dose was approximately 300 rad (3 Gy$_t$).

The final group included 21 children who were natives of the Rongelap Atoll in 1954; they were subjected to high levels of fallout during an A-bomb test. The winds shifted during the test, carrying the fallout over an adjacent inhabited island rather than one that had been evacuated. These children received radiation doses to the thyroid gland from both external exposure and internal ingestion of approximately 1200 rad (12 Gy$_t$).

If the incidence of thyroid nodularity, considered preneoplastic, in these three groups, is computed and the incidence plotted as a function of estimated dose, the result

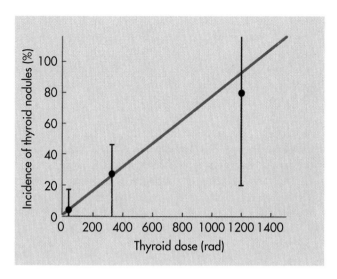

FIGURE 37-9 Radiation-induced preneoplastic thyroid nodularity in three groups whose thyroid glands were irradiated in childhood follows a linear, nonthreshold dose-response relationship.

is that shown in Figure 37-9. Admittedly, the error bars on both the dose data and the incidence levels are large. Still, the implication of a linear, nonthreshold dose-response relationship is clear.

In a similar population of children irradiated for thymic enlargement, 24 thyroid carcinomas were reported in nearly 3000 irradiated patients; none was reported in 5000 nonirradiated siblings. The absolute risk factor was reported as 2.5 cases/10^6 persons/rad/yr.

Bone cancer. Two population groups have contributed an enormous amount of data showing that radiation causes bone cancer. The first group consists of the radium watch-dial painters.

In the 1920s and 1930s, there were various small laboratories whose employees, mostly female, worked at benches painting watch dials with paint laden with radium sulfate. To prepare a fine point on the paintbrushes, the employees would touch the tip of the brush to the tongue. In this manner, substantial quantities of radium were ingested.

Radium salts were used because the emitted radiation, principally alpha and beta particles, would continuously excite the luminous compounds so that the watch dial would glow in the dark. Current technology uses harmlessly low levels of tritium (^{3}H) and promethium (^{147}Pm) for this purpose.

When ingested, the radium would behave metabolically like calcium and deposit in bone. Because of radium's long half-life (1620 yr) and alpha emission, these employees received radiation doses up to 50,000 rad (500 Gy$_t$) to bone.

A total of 72 bone cancers in about 800 people have been observed during a follow-up period in excess of 50

years. Analysis of these data has resulted in an overall relative risk of 122:1. The absolute risk is equal to 0.11 cases/10^6 persons/rad/yr.

Another population to develop excess bone cancer is patients treated with radium salts for a variety of diseases from arthritis to tuberculosis. Such treatments were common practice in many parts of the world until about 1950.

Skin cancer. Skin cancer usually begins with the development of a radiodermatitis. Significant data have been developed from several reports of skin cancer induced in radiotherapy patients treated with orthovoltage (200 to 300 kVp) or superficial x-rays (50 to 150 kVp).

 Radiation-induced skin cancer follows a threshold dose-response relationship.

From these data it can be concluded that the latent period is approximately 5 to 10 years, but there are not enough data to develop absolute risk values. When the dose delivered to the skin was in the range of 500 to 2000 rad (5 to 20 Gy$_t$), the relative risk of developing skin cancer was 4:1. If the dose were 4000 to 6000 rad (40 to 60 Gy$_t$) or 6000 to 10,000 rad (60 to 100 Gy$_t$), the relative risks were 14:1 and 27:1, respectively.

Breast cancer. Some of the radiographic techniques used in mammography are discussed in Chapter 23. The radiation dose to mammography patients is considered in Chapter 40. At this time, a discussion of the risk of radiation-induced breast cancer is considered.

A continuing controversy exists regarding the risk of radiation-induced breast cancer, and the implications of this controversy carry to breast cancer detection by x-ray mammography. The concern of such risk first surfaced in the middle 1960s after the published reports of breast cancer developing in patients with tuberculosis.

For many years tuberculosis was treated by isolation in a sanitarium. During the patient's stay, one mode of therapy was to induce a pneumothorax in the affected lung under nonimage-intensified fluoroscopy. Many patients received multiple treatments and up to several hundred fluoroscopic examinations. Precise dose determinations are not possible, but levels of several hundred rad would have been common. In some of these patient populations the relative risk for radiation-induced breast cancer was as high as 10:1.

One such population exhibited no excess risk. This finding, however, was explained as a consequence of fluoroscopic technique. In the positive studies, the patient faced away from the radiologist, toward the fluoroscopic x-ray tube, during exposure. In the study that reported negative findings, the patients were fluoroscoped facing the radiologist so that the radiation beam entered posteriorly. The breast tissue was exposed only to the low-intensity beam exiting the patient.

Additional studies have produced results suggesting radiation-induced breast cancer in patients treated with x-rays for acute postpartum mastitis. The dose to these patients ranged from 75 to 1000 rad (0.75 to 10 Gy_t). The relative risk factor in this population was approximately 2.5:1.

Radiation-induced breast cancer has also been observed in the A-bomb survivors. Through 1980, observations on nearly 12,000 women who received radiation doses of 10 rad or more to the breasts exhibited a relative risk of 4:1.

In some of these studies, only one breast was irradiated. In nearly every such case, breast cancer developed only in the irradiated breast. These patients have now been followed for up to 25 years. On the basis of all available data regarding radiation-induced breast cancer, the best estimate for absolute risk is 6 cases/10^6 persons/rad/yr.

Lung cancer. Early in this century, it was observed that approximately 50% of the workers in the Bohemian pitchblende mines of Germany died of lung cancer. Lung cancer incidence in the general population was negligible by comparison. The dusty mine environment was considered to be the cause of this lung cancer. Now it is known that radiation exposure from radon in the mines contributed to the incidence of lung cancer in these miners.

Recently, observations of the American uranium miners active in the Colorado plateau in the 1950s and 1960s have also shown elevated levels of lung cancer. The peak of this activity occurred in the early 1960s when there were approximately 5000 miners active in nearly 500 underground mines and 150 open-pit mines. Most of the mines were worked by fewer than 10 men; therefore for such a small operation, a lack of proper ventilation could be expected.

The radiation exposure in these mines occurred because of the high concentration of uranium ore. Uranium, which is radioactive with a very long half-life of 10^9 years, decays through a series of radioactive nuclides by successive alpha and beta emissions, each accompanied by gamma radiation.

One of the decay products of uranium is **radon** (^{222}Rn). This radionuclide is a gas that emanates through the rock to produce a high concentration in the air. When breathed, the radon can be deposited in the lung, where it undergoes additional successive series decay to a stable isotope of lead. During these subsequent decay actions, several alpha particles are released, resulting in a rather high local dose. Also, alpha particles are high-LET radiation and therefore have a high RBE.

To date, more than 4000 uranium miners have been observed, and they have received estimated doses to lung tissue as high as 3000 rad (30 Gy_t); on this basis the relative risk was approximately 8:1. Smoking uranium miners have a relative risk of approximately 20:1.

The available data indicate a dose-response relationship that is linear and nonthreshold with an absolute risk of 1.3 cases/10^6 persons/rad/yr.

Liver cancer. Thorium dioxide (ThO_2) in a colloidal suspension known as *Thorotrast* was widely used in diagnostic radiology between 1925 and 1945 as a contrast agent for angiography. Thorotrast was approximately 25% by weight ThO_2, and it contained several radioactive isotopes of thorium and its decay products. Radiation that was emitted produced a dose in the ratio of approximately 100:10:1 of alpha, beta, and gamma radiation, respectively.

The use of Thorotrast is responsible for several types of carcinoma after a latent period of approximately 15 to 20 years. After extravascular injection, it is carcinogenic at the site of the injection. After intravascular injection, ThO_2 particles are deposited in phagocytic cells of the reticuloendothelial system and are concentrated in the liver and spleen. The half-life and high alpha radiation dose of ThO_2 have resulted in many cases of cancer in these organs.

TOTAL RISK OF MALIGNANCY

From the basis of many of these observations on human population groups after exposure to low-level radiation and with all the risk estimates taken collectively for leukemia and cancer, some simplified conclusions can be made. The overall absolute risk for induction of malignancy is approximately 4 cases/10,000-rad and 10 cases/10^6 persons/rad/yr, with the at-risk period extending 20 to 25 years after exposure. This is approximately 400 deaths from radiation-induced malignancy after an exposure of 1 rad to 1,000,000 persons when all such cases occurring within 25 years of exposure are counted.

Three Mile Island

To make these values somewhat more meaningful, we can consider the Three Mile Island incident in 1979. Approximately 2,000,000 people reside within a 80-km (50-mile) radius of this island. On the basis of population statistics alone, approximately 330,000 cancer deaths would be expected. During the total period of the radiation incident, the average dose to persons living within a 160-km (100-mile) radius was 1.5 mrad (15 μGy_t); to those within the 80-km (50-mile) radius, it was 8 mrad (80 μGy_t). When 8 mrad is applied as an upper limit, it can be predicted that this incident will result in no more than one additional malignant death as a result of this population radiation exposure. Clearly, this response is not detectable in the face of approximately 400,000 natural cancer deaths in that population.

Predicted Deaths at Three Mile Island
2×10^6 people $\times$ 2 deaths/10^4 people-rad $\times$
0.0015 rad = 0.6 deaths

BEIR Committee/NCRP

The 1990 report of the Committee on the Biologic Effects of Ionizing Radiation (BEIR), an arm of the National Academy of Sciences, reviewed the data on late effects of low-dose, low-LET radiation. After the BEIR report and several others issued by the National Council on Radiation Protection and Measurements (NCRP), it became possible to make several generalizations are possible. Table 37-5 shows such generalizations, and they are considered authoritative.

The BEIR committee examined three situations. First, they estimated the excess mortality from malignant disease after a one-time accidental exposure to 10 rad; such a situation is highly unlikely in radiology. Second, they considered the response to a dose of 1 rad/yr for life; this situation is possible in diagnostic radiology but is certainly rare. Finally, they considered excess radiation-induced cancer mortality after a continuous dose of 100 mrad/yr. This is still considerably higher than the experience of most radiologic technologists but can serve as a good upper limit of occupational radiation risk.

The dose-response relationship is the linear, non-threshold model. These analyses showed an additional 800 cases of malignant-disease death in a population of 100,000 after 10 rad and an additional 550 after 100 mrad/yr. These cases are in addition to the normal incidence of cancer death, which is approximately 19,000 per 100,000 persons.

The BEIR Committee has further stated that because of the uncertainty in their analysis, less than 1 rad/yr may not be harmful.

TABLE 37-5	BEIR Committee Estimated Excess Mortality from Malignant Disease in 100,000 People	
	Male	**Female**
Normal expectation	20,560	16,680
Excess cases		
Single exposure to 10 rad (100 mGy$_t$)	770	810
Continuous exposure (10 mGy$_t$/yr)	2880	3070
Continuous exposure to 100 mrad/yr (1 mGy$_t$/yr)	520	600

The BEIR Committee and the NCRP have also analyzed the available human data with regard to the age at exposure with a limited time of expression and whether the response was absolute or relative. If a person is irradiated at an early age and the response is limited in time, the radiation-induced excess will appear as a bulge on the age-response relationship (Figure 37-10). Childhood leukemia is a good example.

An **absolute age-response relationship** is shown in Figure 37-11. There, the increased incidence of cancer is a constant number of cases after a minimal latent period. Most subscribe to a **relative age-response relationship,** in which the increased incidence of cancer is proportional to the natural incidence (Figure 37-12).

Perhaps the best way to present these radiation risk data is to compare them with other known causes of death. As might be imagined, there are many tables that analyze risk. This information is presented in simplified

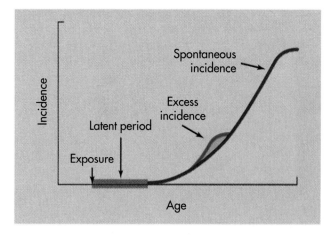

FIGURE 37-10 Exposure at an early age can result in an excess bulge of cancer after a latent period.

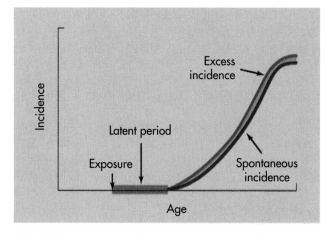

FIGURE 37-11 The absolute-risk model predicts that the excess radiation-induced cancer is constant for life.

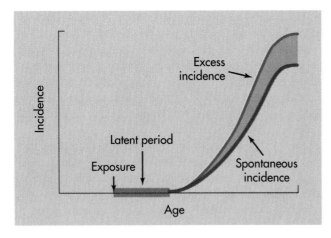

FIGURE 37-12 The relative-risk model predicts that the excess radiation-induced cancer is proportional to the natural incidence.

TABLE 37-6	Average Annual Risk of Death from Various Causes
Cause	Your Chance of Dying This Year
All causes (all ages)	1 in 100
Smoking of 20 cigarettes per day	1 in 280
Heart disease	1 in 300
Cancer	1 in 520
All causes (25-year old)	1 in 700
Stroke	1 in 1200
Motor vehicle accident	1 in 4000
Drowning	1 in 30,000
Alcohol (light drinker)	1 in 50,000
Air travel	1 in 100,000
Radiation, 100 mrad	**1 in 100,000**
Texas Gulf Coast hurricane	1 in 4,500,000
Occupation as a rodeo cowboy	1 in 6,200,000

form in Table 37-6. Note that in these common situations, risk from radiation exposure is near the bottom of the list. Our actual occupational risk is even less, since we use protective apparel during fluoroscopy and the radiation-risk estimate assumes whole-body exposure.

RADIATION AND PREGNANCY

Since the first medical applications of x-rays, there has been concern and apprehension regarding the effects of radiation before, during, and after pregnancy. Before pregnancy, the concern is interrupted fertility. During pregnancy, concern is directed to possible congenital effects in newborns. The postpregnancy concerns are related to suspected genetic effects. All these effects have been demonstrated in animals, and some have been observed in humans.

Effects on Fertility

The early effect of high-level radiation on fertility in males and females is discussed in Chapter 36. There is ample evidence to show that such an effect does exist and is dose related. The effects of low-dose, long-term irradiation on fertility, however, are less well defined.

Animal data indicate that even when radiation is delivered at the rate of 100 rad per year, there is no noticeable depression in the fertility rate.

There have been two national surveys of American radiologists, one reported in 1927 and the other in 1955. In each case, a finding of depressed fertility rate and increased rate of congenital abnormalities in the offspring of radiologists was reported. Both studies have been questioned because of their experimental methods. The conclusions reported are not generally accepted.

The health effects analysis of 150,000 American radiologic technologists mentioned earlier has indicated no effect on fertility. The number of births during a 12-year sampling period equaled the number expected.

 Low-dose, chronic irradiation does not impair fertility.

Irradiation In Utero

Irradiation in utero concerns the following two types of exposures: that of the radiation worker and that of the patient. The recommended techniques and radiation-control procedures associated with these exposed persons are considered fully in Chapter 40. At this time, the biologic effects of such irradiation is considered.

Substantial animal data are available to describe rather completely the effects of relatively high doses of radiation delivered during various periods of gestation. Because the embryo is a rapidly developing cell system, it is particularly sensitive to radiation. With age, the embryo (and then the fetus) becomes less sensitive to the effects of radiation, and this pattern continues into adulthood. After maturity, however, radiosensitivity increases with age. Figure 37-13 is a summary of the observed $LD_{50/60}$ in mice exposed at various times, showing this aggregated radiosensitivity. The scale of human age is included to describe the suspected age-related radiosensitivity in humans.

 All observations point to the first trimester of pregnancy as the most radiosensitive period.

Such findings are of particular concern because an x-ray exposure often occurs when pregnancy is unknown.

The effects of irradiation in utero are time and dose related. They include prenatal death, neonatal death, congenital abnormalities, malignancy induction, general impairment of growth, genetic effects, and mental re-

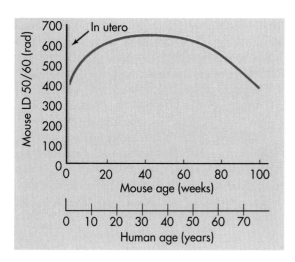

FIGURE 37-13 LD$_{50/60}$ of mice in relation to age at the time of irradiation.

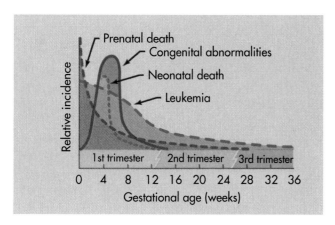

FIGURE 37-14 Following 200 rad delivered at various times in utero, a number of effects can be observed.

tardation. Figure 37-14 is redrawn from studies designed to observe the effects of a 200-rad (2-Gy$_t$) dose delivered at various stages in utero in mice. The scale along the x-axis indicates the approximate comparable time in humans.

Within 2 weeks of fertilization, the most pronounced effect of a high radiation dose is prenatal death, which is manifested as a spontaneous abortion. Observations in radiotherapy patients have confirmed this effect but only after rather high doses.

On the basis of animal experimentation, it would appear that this response is very rare. The best estimate is that a 10-rad (100-mGy$_t$) dose during the first 2 weeks induces perhaps 0.1% spontaneous abortions. This is in addition to the 25% to 50% normal incidence of spontaneous abortions.

Fortunately, this response is of the all-or-none variety. Either there is a radiation-induced abortion, or the pregnancy will carry to term with no ill effect.

TABLE 37-7	Relative Risk of Childhood Leukemia after Irradiation In Utero by Trimester
Time of X-Ray Examination	**Relative Risk**
First trimester	8.3
Second trimester	1.5
Third trimester	1.4
TOTAL	1.5

 The first 2 weeks of pregnancy may be of least concern for radiation exposure because the response is all or nothing.

During the period of major organogenesis, from the second through the tenth week, two effects are likely to occur. Early in this period, skeletal and organ abnormalities can be induced. As major organogenesis continues, congenital abnormalities of the central nervous system can be observed if the pregnancy is carried to term.

If the radiation-induced congenital abnormalities are severe enough, the result will be neonatal death. After a dose of 200 rad (2 Gy$_t$) to the mouse, nearly 100% of the fetuses suffered significant abnormalities. In 80%, it was sufficient to cause neonatal death.

Such effects are rare after diagnostic levels of exposure and are essentially undetectable after radiation doses lower than 10 rad (100 mGy$_t$). A dose of 10 rad (100 mGy$_t$) during organogenesis is expected to increase the incidence of congenital abnormalities by 1% above the natural incidence. To complicate matters, there is approximately a 5% incidence of naturally occurring congenital abnormalities in the unexposed population.

Irradiation in utero at the human level has been associated with childhood malignancy by a number of investigators. Perhaps the most complete study of this effect was conducted by Alice Stewart and her co-workers in a project known as the *Oxford Survey*, a study of childhood malignancy, in England, Scotland, and Wales. Nearly every case of such childhood malignancy in these countries since 1946 has been investigated. The nationalization of health care resulted in well-maintained health records. Each case was first identified and then investigated through an interview with the mother, a review of hospital charts, and a review of physician records. Each case of childhood malignancy was matched with a control for age, gender, place of birth, socioeconomic status, and other demographic factors. The control was a child who matched with the case in all respects except the control did not have cancer or leukemia. The Oxford Survey is being continued at this time and has now considered more than 10,000 cases and a like number of matched controls.

Although the Oxford Survey has reviewed all malignancies, it is the findings of radiation-induced leukemia that have been of particular importance. Table 37-7 shows the results of this survey in terms of relative risk. A relative risk of the development of childhood leukemia after irradiation in utero of 1.5 is significant. This indicates an increase of 50% over the nonirradiated rate. The number of cases involved, however, is small.

 The relative risk of childhood leukemia after irradiation in utero is 1.5.

The incidence of childhood leukemia in the population at large is approximately 9 cases per 100,000 live births. According to the Oxford Survey, if all 100,000 had been irradiated in utero, perhaps 14 cases of leukemia would have resulted. Although these findings have been substantiated in several American populations, there is no consensus among radiation scientists that this effect after receiving such low doses is indeed real.

Other effects after irradiation in utero have been studied rather fully in animals and have been observed in some human populations. An unexpected finding in offspring of the A-bomb survivors is mental retardation. Children of exposed mothers have performed poorly on IQ tests and have demonstrated poor scholastic performance in comparison with unexposed Japanese children. These differences are marginal, yet significant. When assessed by test scores, measurable mental retardation is apparent in approximately 6% of all children. A 10-rad dose in utero is expected to increase this incidence by an additional 0.5%.

Radiation exposure in utero does retard the growth and development of the newborn. Irradiation in utero, principally during the period of major organogenesis, has been associated with microcephaly (small head) and, as just discussed, mental retardation.

The human data bearing on these effects are obtained from patients irradiated medically, the A-bomb survivors, and the residents of the Marshall Islands who were exposed to radioactive fallout in 1954 during weapons testing. For instance, the heavily irradiated children at Hiroshima are, on average, 2.25 cm (0.9 in) shorter, 3 kg (6.6 lb) lighter, and 1.1 cm (0.4 in) smaller in head circumference than members of the nonirradiated control groups.

These effects, as well as mental retardation, have been observed principally in those receiving doses in excess of 100 rad (1 Gy_t) in utero. The lack of appropriate and sensitive tests of mental function make it impossible to draw similar conclusions at doses below 100 rad (1 Gy_t).

A summary of the effects of irradiation in utero is shown in Table 37-8. There are four responses of concern to radiology: spontaneous abortion, congenital abnormalities, mental retardation, and childhood malignancy. Spontaneous abortion causes the least concern of the four, since it is an all-or-none effect. Congenital abnormalities, mental retardation, and childhood malignancy are of real concern, but the probability of such a response after a fetal dose of 10 rad (100 mGy_t) is nil. Furthermore, 10 rad (100 mGy_t) to the fetus is very rarely experienced in radiology.

The form of the dose-response relationship for each of these effects is unknown. They do, however, appear to be linear and nonthreshold when based on doses higher than 100 rad (1 Gy_t). When large experimental animal populations were acutely exposed, the minimum reported dose for observing such effects as statistically significant was approximately 10 rad (100 mGy_t).

No evidence in either humans or animals indicate that the levels of radiation exposure currently experienced occupationally and medically are responsible for any such effects on growth and development.

Although efforts for protecting the unborn from the harmful effects of radiation are principally directed at diagnostic x-ray exposures, radiologic technologists must also be aware of similar hazards from radioisotope examinations. For example, radioiodine is known to concentrate principally in the thyroid gland. After an administration of radioactive iodine, the dose to thyroid tissue is several orders of magnitude higher than the whole-body dose because of this organ concentration effect.

The thyroid gland begins to function at approximately 10 weeks of gestation, and since radioiodine readily crosses the placental barrier from the mother's blood to the fetal circulation, radioiodine should be administered during pregnancy only in trace doses and before the tenth week of gestation. At any time thereafter, the hazard of such an administration increases.

TABLE 37-8	Summary of Effects After 10 Rad in Utero		
Time of Exposure	**Type of Response**	**Natural Occurrence**	**Radiation Response**
Up to 2 weeks	Spontaneous abortion	25%	0.1%
2-10 weeks	Congenital abnormalities	5%	1%
2-15 weeks	Mental retardation	6%	0.5%
Up to 9 months	Malignant disease	8/10,000	12/10,000
Up to 9 months	Impaired growth and development	1%	Nil
Up to 9 months	Genetic mutation	10%	Nil

Genetic Effects

Unfortunately, the weakest area of knowledge in radiation biology is the area of radiation genetics. Essentially all the data indicating that radiation causes genetic effects have come from rather large-scale experiments with either flies or mice. There are no substantive data on humans.

Observations of the A-bomb survivors have shown no radiation-induced genetic effects, and survivors are now into the third generation. Other human populations have likewise provided only negative results. Consequently, in the absence of accurate human data, there is no choice but to rely on information from experimental laboratory studies.

In 1927, the Nobel prize-winning geneticist H.J. Muller from the University of Texas reported the results of his irradiation of *Drosophila*, the fruit fly. He irradiated mature flies before procreation and then measured the frequency of lethal mutations in the offspring. The radiation doses used were thousands of rad, but as the data in Figure 37-15 show, the dose-response relationship for radiation-induced genetic damage is unmistakably linear and nonthreshold.

From Muller's studies, other conclusions were drawn. Radiation does not alter the quality of mutations but rather increases the frequency of the spontaneous mutations that are observed. Muller's data showed no dose rate or dose fractionation effects. Hence, he concluded that such mutations were single-hit phenomena.

It was principally on the basis of Muller's work that the National Council on Radiation Protection in 1932 lowered the recommended dose limit and acknowledged officially for the first time the existence of nonthreshold radiation effects. Since that time, all radiation-protection guides have assumed a linear, nonthreshold dose-response relationship and have been based on the suspected genetic, as well as somatic, effects of radiation.

The only other experimental work of any significance is that of William Russell. Beginning in 1946, he commenced to irradiate a rather large mouse colony with radiation dose rates that varied from 0.001 to 90 rad/min (0.01 to 900 mGy$_t$/min) and total doses up to 1000 rad (10 Gy$_t$). These studies are continuing, and observations have now been made on over 8 million mice! The experiment requires the observation of seven specific genes that control readily recognizable characteristics, such as ear shape, coat color, and eye color.

Russell's data show that a dose-rate effect does exist, which would indicate that the mouse has the capacity to repair genetic damage. He has confirmed the linear, nonthreshold form of the dose-response relationship and has not detected any types of mutations that did not occur naturally.

The average mutation rate per unit dose in the mouse is approximately 15 times that observed in the fruit fly. Whether an increased sensitivity exists in humans relative to the mouse is unknown.

From these experimental studies has developed the concept of **doubling dose**. The doubling dose in humans is estimated to lie in the range between 50 and 250 rad (0.5 and 2.5 Gy$_t$).

The doubling dose is that dose of radiation that will produce twice the frequency of genetic mutations as would have been observed without the radiation.

So, what is the significance of all this in our daily practice? What is the significance to either patients or radiation workers? First, it can be said with certainty that radiation-induced genetic mutations after the levels of exposure experienced in diagnostic radiology are essentially zero. The probability of such an effect is extremely low.

Under nearly all such exposures, no action is required; however, if a high radiation dose (for example, that in excess of 10 rad) is experienced, some protective action may be required. The prefertilized egg, in its various stages, exhibits a constant sensitivity to radiation; however, it also demonstrates some capacity for repair of genetic damage. If repair occurs, it is rapid, and therefore a delay in procreation of only a few days may be appropriate. In the male, on the other hand, it might be prudent to refrain from procreation for a period of 60 days to allow cells that were in a resistant stage of development at the time of exposure to mature to functioning spermatids. Box 37-1 summarizes some additional conclusions regarding radiation genetics.

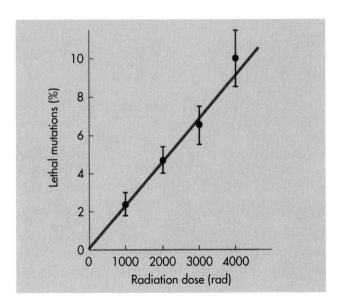

FIGURE 37-15 The irradiation of flies by H.J. Muller shows the genetic effects to be linear and nonthreshold. Note that the doses were exceedingly high.

BOX 37-1 Additional Conclusions Regarding Radiation Genetics

- Radiation-induced mutations are usually harmful.
- Any dose of radiation, however small, to a germ cell, results in some genetic risk.
- The frequency of radiation-induced mutations is directly proportional to dose, so a linear extrapolation of data obtained at high doses provides a valid estimate for low-dose effects.
- The effect depends on the rate at which the radiation is delivered (protraction) and on the time between exposures (fractionation).
- For most prereproductive life, the female is less sensitive to the genetic effects of radiation than the male.
- Most radiation-induced mutations are *recessive*. These require that the mutant genes be present in both the male and the female to produce the trait. Consequently, such mutations may not be expressed for many generations.
- The frequency of radiation-induced genetic mutations is extremely low. It is approximately 10^{-7} mutation/rad/gene.

SUMMARY

The late effects of radiation exposure occur a long period of time after an exposure incident. Late effects can develop from high-dose, short-term exposure, but the concern in diagnostic imaging is low-dose exposures over time. Many epidemiologic studies have reported positive results; however, there are problems: (1) the exact dose is usually not known, and (2) the frequency of observable response is low. Most late effects are stochastic: the incidence of response is dose related, and there is no dose threshold.

Local tissues can be affected by low-dose radiation. The late effects appear as nonmalignant changes in the skin. The skin develops a weathered, calloused, and discolored appearance. Chromosome damage in circulating lymphocytes and cataracts in the cornea of the eye have been observed as late effects of radiation exposure.

Because dose-response relationships are not precise when the late effects of radiation exposure are observed, risk estimates are used to predict radiation response in a population. Relative risk is calculated when the population's radiation dose is not known. Relative risk is computed by comparing the number of people in the exposed population with late effects to the number in an unexposed population who developed the

same condition. Excess risk determines the magnitude of the late effect as the difference between cases and controls.

The effects of low-dose, long-term irradiation in utero can include the following effects: prenatal death, neonatal death, congenital abnormalities, malignancy, impairment of growth, genetic effects, and mental retardation. However, these abnormalities are based on doses greater than 100 rad, with the minimum reported doses in animal experiments at approximately 10 rad. No evidence at either the human or animal level indicate that the levels of radiation exposure currently experienced occupationally or medically are responsible for any such effects on fetal growth or development.

CHALLENGE QUESTIONS

1. Define or otherwise identify:
   a. Epidemiology
   b. In utero
   c. ABCC or RERF
   d. Stochastic effect
   e. Oxford Survey
   f. H.J. Muller
   g. Doubling dose
   h. Radon (^{222}Rn)

2. What population group experienced the radiation-induced cataracts that were reported in 1960?

3. What is the risk of life-span shortening for radiation workers?

4. What is the significance of the change in death statistics of American radiologists from 1935 to 1944 and from 1955 to 1958?

5. Write the formula for relative risk.

6. What is the absolute risk of three cases of leukemia developing per year in 100,000 people after an average dose of 2 rad?

7. When should excess risk be used as the preferable risk index?

8. A total of 20 million people in Scandinavia were exposed to an average of 0.7 mrad as a result of the accident at Chernobyl. Assuming an absolute risk of 10 cases/10^6/rad/yr over a 30-year period, how many malignancies will be induced?

9. What is the suspected reason that British radiologists did not have an elevated risk of leukemia compared with American radiologists?

10. Discuss the experience of radiation-induced leukemia in patients with ankylosing spondylitis.

11. Why was the thymus gland irradiated in the Ann Arbor and Rochester series? What were the late effects of this irradiation?

12. Discuss how bone cancer developed in watch-dial painters in the 1920s and 1930s.

13. Explain the risk of radon gas to uranium miners.

14. Explain the relative age-response relationship.

15. What are the effects of low-dose, long-term irradiation on fertility?

16. Are radiation-induced mutations dominant or recessive? Explain.

17. In a population of 30,367 irradiated people, 13 cases of leukemia developed; in a control population of 86,672 people, 31 cases of leukemia developed. What was the relative risk?

18. What is the absolute risk if 32 cases of leukemia develop per year in 100,000 persons after an average dose of 2 rad?

19. How many cases of radiation-induced leukemia are suspected to have occurred in the A-bomb survivors?

20. What is the difference between relative risk and excess risk?

Health Physics

OBJECTIVES

At the completion of this chapter, the student should be able to:

1. Define *health physics*
2. List the cardinal principles of radiation protection and discuss the ALARA concept
3. Explain the purpose of the National Council on Radiation Protection and Measurements
4. Name the recommended dose limits observed for radiation workers and the public.
5. Discuss the radiosensitivity of the stages of pregnancy
6. Describe the recommended management procedures for pregnant radiation workers and for the pregnant patient

OUTLINE

Immediately after their discovery, x-rays were applied to the healing arts. It was recognized within months, however, that radiation could cause harmful effects. The first American fatality from radiation exposure was Thomas Edison's assistant, Clarence Dally. Since that time, a great deal of effort has been devoted to developing equipment, techniques, and procedures to control radiation levels and reduce unnecessary radiation exposure to radiation workers and to the public.

The cardinal principles for radiation protection are simplified rules to provide safety in radiation areas for occupational workers. In 1931, the first dose-limiting recommendations were made. Today the National Council on Radiation Protection and Measurements (NCRP) continuously reviews the recommended dose limits.

DEFINITION OF *Health Physics*

Providing radiation protection for workers and public is the practice of **health physics**. The term *health physics* was coined during the early days of the Manhattan Project, the secret effort during World War II to develop the atomic bomb. The health physicist can be a radiation scientist, an engineer, or a physician concerned with the research, teaching, or operational aspects of radiation safety. Health physicists design equipment, calculate and construct barriers, and develop administrative protocols to maintain radiation exposure as low as reasonably achievable (ALARA).

Health physics is concerned with providing occupational radiation protection and minimizing radiation dose to workers and the public.

CARDINAL PRINCIPLES OF RADIATION PROTECTION

All health physics activity in radiology is designed to minimize radiation exposure of patients and personnel. Three cardinal principles of radiation protection developed for nuclear activities—time, distance, and shielding—find equally useful application in diagnostic radiology. When these cardinal principles are observed, radiation exposure can be minimized (Box 38-1).

Minimize Time

The dose to an individual is directly related to the duration of exposure. If the time during which one is exposed to radiation is doubled, the exposure will be doubled, as follows:

BOX 38-1 Cardinal Principles of Radiation Protection

1. Keep the time of exposure to radiation as short as possible.
2. Maintain as large a distance as possible between the source of radiation and the exposed person.
3. Insert shielding material between the radiation source and the exposed person.

Time

Exposure = Exposure rate × Exposure time

Question: A radiation source has an exposure rate of 230 mR/hr (2.3 mGy$_a$/hr) at a position occupied by a radiation worker. If the worker remains at that position for 36 minutes, what will be the total occupational exposure?

Answer: Occupational exposure = 230 mR/hr $\dfrac{36 \text{ min}}{60 \text{ min/hr}}$

               = 138 mR

Question: The parent of a patient is asked to remain next to the patient during fluoroscopy in which the radiation exposure level is 600 mR/hr (6 mGy$_a$/hr). If the allowable daily exposure is 50 mR, how long may the parent remain?

Answer: Time = Exposure ÷ Exposure rate

               = 50 mR ÷ 600 mR/hr

               = $^1/_{12}$ hr

               = 8 min

During radiography, the time of exposure is kept to a minimum to reduce motion blur. During fluoroscopy, the time of exposure should also be kept to a minimum to reduce patient and personnel exposure. This is an area of radiation protection not directly controlled by the radiologic technologist.

Radiologists are trained to depress the fluoroscopic foot switch in an alternating fashion, sequencing on-off, rather than continuous on during the course of the examination. A repeated up-and-down motion on the fluoroscopic foot switch permits a high-quality examination to be made with a considerably reduced exposure to the patient. The use of pulsed progressive fluoroscopy can reduce patient dose to a factor of 0.1 or less.

The 5-minute reset timer on all fluoroscopes reminds the radiologist that a considerable fluoroscopic time has elapsed. The timer records the amount of on-time for the x-ray beam. Most fluoroscopic examinations take less than 5 minutes. Only during difficult cardiovascular and interventional procedures should it be necessary to exceed 5 minutes of exposure time.

Question: A fluoroscope emits 4.2 R/min (42 mGy$_a$/min) at the tabletop for every milliampere of operation (4.2 R/mAmin). What is the patient exposure in a barium enema examination that is conducted at 1.8 mA and requires 2.5 minutes of fluoroscopic time?

Answer: Patient exposure $= \left(\dfrac{4.2 \text{ R}}{\text{mAmin}}\right)(1.8 \text{ mA})(2.5 \text{ min})$
$= 18.9 \text{ R}$

Maximize Distance

As the distance between the source of radiation and a person increases, the radiation exposure decreases rapidly. The decrease in exposure is calculated using the inverse square law (see Chapter 5) if the source of radiation can be considered a point source.

Most radiation sources are point sources. The x-ray tube target, for example, is a point source of radiation. The scattered radiation generated within a patient appears, however, to come not from a point source but rather from an extended area source. As a rule of thumb, even an extended source can be considered a point source at sufficient distance.

If the distance from the source exceeds five times the source diameter, it can be assumed to be a point source.

Distance and Exposure
To calculate the decrease in exposure gained by distance, assume a point source and apply the inverse square law.

Question: An x-ray tube has an output intensity of 2.6 mR/mAs at 100 cm source-to-image receptor distance when operated at 70 kVp. What would be the radiation exposure 350 cm from the target?

Answer: $\dfrac{I_1}{I_2} = \dfrac{d_2{}^2}{d_1{}^2}$

$I_1 = I_2 \dfrac{d_2{}^2}{d_1{}^2}$

$= (2.6 \text{ mR/mAs})\left(\dfrac{100 \text{ cm}}{350 \text{ cm}}\right)^2$

$= (2.6 \text{ mR/mAs})(0.082)$

$= 0.21 \text{ mR/mAs}$

In radiography, the distance from the radiation source to the patient is generally fixed by the type of examination, and the radiologic technologist is positioned behind a protective barrier.

During fluoroscopy, the radiologic technologist can exercise good radiation-protection procedures. Figure 38-1 shows the approximate radiation exposure levels at waist height during a fluoroscopic examination. The lines on the plot plan are called *isoexposure lines* and represent positions of equal exposure in the fluoroscopy room. At the normal position for a radiologist or a radiologic technologist, the exposure rate is approximately 300 mR/hr (3 mGy$_a$/hr).

During portions of the examination when it is not necessary for the radiologic technologist to remain close to the patient, the technologist should back away from the patient. Two steps back, the exposure rate is only approximately 5 mR/hr (500 μGy$_a$/hr). This reduction in exposure does not follow the inverse square law, since during fluoroscopy, the patient is an extended source of radiation because of scattered x-rays generated within the body.

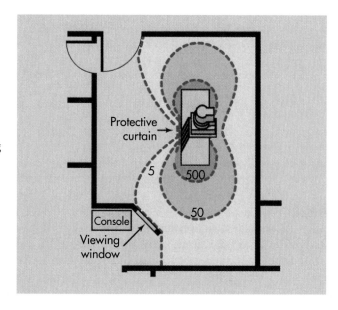

FIGURE 38-1 Typical isoexposure contours during fluoroscopic examination (mR/hr).

During fluoroscopy, the radiologic technologist should remain as far from the patient as possible.

Question: What is the approximate occupational exposure of a radiologic technologist at a position where the exposure level is 300 mR/hr, and at a position two steps farther back, where the exposure level is 20 mR/hr, during a fluoroscopic examination lasting 4 minutes, 15 seconds?

Answer: Occupational exposure equals
Position *A:* (300 mR/hr)(4.25 min)(1 hr/60 min)
= 21.25 mR
Position *A′:* (20 mR/hr)(4.25 min)(1 hr/60 min)
= 1.4 mR

Maximize Shielding

Positioning shielding between the radiation source and exposed people greatly reduces the level of radiation exposure. Shielding used in diagnostic radiology usually consists of lead, although conventional building materials are often used. The amount that a protective barrier reduces radiation intensity can be estimated if the half-value layer (HVL) or the tenth-value layer (TVL) of the barrier material is known. The HVL is defined and discussed in Chapter 12. The TVL is similarly defined as follows:

One TVL is the thickness of absorber that will reduce the radiation intensity to one tenth of its original value.

Table 38-1 shows approximate HVLs and TVLs for lead and concrete for diagnostic x-ray beams between 40 and 150 kVp.

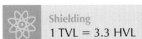
Shielding
1 TVL = 3.3 HVL

Question: When operated at 80 kVp, an x-ray imager emits 3.6 mR/mAs at a distance of 100 cm. How much shielding (concrete or lead) would be required to reduce the intensity to less than 0.25 mR/mAs?

Answer: The amount of shielding in the first or second column of the following chart will reduce the beam intensity to the value in the third column. The last row is the answer.

Lead (mm)	Concrete (in)	Beam intensity (mR/mAs)
0	0	3.60
0.19	0.42	1.80
0.38	0.84	0.60
0.57	1.26	0.45
0.76	1.68	0.23

For the next question, remember that workload is the radiation output during the week that the imaging system delivers radiation.

Question: An x-ray imaging system is used strictly for chest radiography at 125 kVp. The useful beam is always pointed to a wall containing 0.8-mm lead shielding. How much additional shielding will be required if the workload doubles?

Answer: When the workload doubles, so will the exposure on the other side of the wall. From Table 38-1, it is seen that one HVL, or 0.27 mm of lead, will be necessary to reduce that exposure to its original level.

Another example of the application of shielding in radiology is the use of protective apparel. It is recommended that protective aprons contain 0.5 mm of lead. This is approximately equivalent to two HVLs, which should reduce occupational exposure to 25%. Actual measurements show that such protective aprons reduce exposure to approximately 10% because scattered x-rays are often incident on the apron at an oblique angle.

Usually, applications of the cardinal principles of radiation protection involve a consideration of all three.

TABLE 38-1	Approximate HVLs and TVLs of Lead and Concrete at Various Tube Potentials				
	HVL			TVL	
Tube Potential (kVp)	Lead (mm)	Concrete (in)		Lead (mm)	Concrete (in)
40	0.03	0.13		0.06	0.40
60	0.11	0.25		0.34	0.87
80	0.19	0.42		0.64	1.4
100	0.24	0.60		0.80	2.0
125	0.27	0.76		0.90	2.5
150	0.28	0.86		0.95	2.8

The typical problem involves a known radiation level at a given distance from the source. The level of exposure at any other distance, behind any shielding, for any length of time can be calculated. The order in which these calculations are made makes no difference.

Question: The operating kVp of a radiographic imaging system rarely exceeds 100 kVp. The output intensity is 4.6 mR/mAs at 100-cm SID. The distance to the desk of the administrative assistant on the other side of the wall to which the x-ray beam is directed is 200 cm. The wall contains 0.96 mm of lead, and 300 mAs is anticipated daily. If exposure is to be restricted to 2 mR/wk, how long each day may the assistant remain at the desk?

Answer: Daily x-ray output at 100 cm =
$$(4.6 \text{ mR/mAs})(300 \text{ mAs}) = 1380 \text{ mR}$$
Daily output at 200 cm =
$$(1380)(100/200)^2 = 345 \text{ mR}$$
Daily output behind 0.96 mm of lead, or four
$$\text{HVLs} = 22 \text{ mR}$$
$$= 110 \text{ mR/wk}$$
$$\text{Time allowed} = \frac{2 \text{ mR}}{110 \text{ mR/wk}} =$$
$$0.018 \text{ week} = 43 \text{ minutes}$$
However, this analysis does not take into account the x-ray beam attenuation by the patient, which is approximately two TVLs, or 0.01.

Therefore:

Daily output behind 0.96 mm of lead
and the patient = (110 mR)(0.01) = 1.1 mR
$$\text{Time allowed} = \frac{2 \text{ mR}}{1.1 \text{ mR/wk}} =$$
$$1.8 \text{ wk (unlimited)}$$

Question: Suppose an analysis shows that if an administrative assistant remains at his desk for more than 24 minutes each week, his dose limit will be exceeded. How much additional protective lead would be required?

Answer: Full occupancy is 40 hr × 60 min/hr = 2400 min
$$\frac{2400 \text{ min}}{24 \text{ min}} = 100$$
The additional shielding should reduce exposure to 1/100 the present level: That is two TVLs, or an additional 1.6 mm of lead.

DOSE LIMITS

A continuing effort of health physicists has been the description and identification of occupational dose limits. For many years a **maximum permissible dose**

(MPD) was specified. The MPD was the dose of radiation that, in light of current knowledge, would be expected to produce no significant radiation effects. Therefore at radiation doses below the MPD, no responses should occur. At the level of the MPD, the risk is not zero but it is small: lower than the risk associated with other occupations and reasonable in light of the benefits derived. The concept of MPD is now obsolete and has been replaced by dose limits.

Whole-Body Effective Dose Limits

The self-stated goal of the **National Council on Radiation Protection and Measurements (NCRP)** is to formulate and widely disseminate information, guidance, and recommendations on radiation protection and measurements that represent the consensus of leading scientific thinking. The NCRP has also assessed risk based on data from the reports of the National Academy of Sciences (Committee on the Biologic Effects of Ionizing Radiation) and the National Safety Council (Table 38-2) to arrive at occupational dose limits.

Current DLs are prescribed for various organs as well as the whole body and for various working conditions. If the DL were received by a radiation worker each year, the lifetime risk will not exceed 10^{-4} yr^{-1}. The value 10^{-4} yr^{-1} is the approximate risk of death to those working in safe industries. The DLs set by the NCRP ensure that radiation workers have the same risk as those in safe industries.

 DLs imply that if received annually, the risk of death would be approximately 1 in 10,000.

Question: Suppose all 300,000 American radiologic technologists receive the DL (5000 mrem) this year. How many would be expected to die prematurely?

TABLE 38-2	Fatal Accident Rates in Various Industries	
Industry	**Rate (× 10^{-4} yr^{-1})**	
Trade	0.4	
Manufacturing	0.4	
Service	0.4	
Government	0.9	
Radiation workers	0.9	
All Groups	**0.9**	
Transport	2.2	
Public utilities	2.2	
Construction	3.1	
Mining	4.3	
Agriculture	4.4	

Answer: $(300,000)(10^{-4}) = 30$

Of course, they actually receive approximately 50 mrem/yr; therefore the expected mortality is as follows:

$$30\left(\frac{50}{5000}\right) = 0.3;\ \text{less than 1!}$$

Particular care is taken to make certain that no radiation worker receives a radiation dose in excess of the DL. The DL is specified only for occupational exposure. It should not be confused with medical x-ray exposure received as a patient. Although patient dose should be kept low, there is no patient DL.

The first dose limit, 50,000 mrem/wk (500 mSv/wk), was recommended in 1902. The current DL is 100 mrem/wk (1 mSv/wk). Through the years, there has been a downward revision of the DL. The history of these recommendations is given in Table 38-3 and is shown graphically in Figure 38-2.

In the early years of radiology, the DL consisted of a single value considered the safe working level for whole-body exposure. It was based primarily on the known acute response to radiation exposure and presumed that

a threshold dose existed. The **threshold dose** is that below which a person has a negligible chance of sustaining specific biologic damage.

Today the DL is specified not only for whole-body exposure but also for partial-body exposure, organ exposure, and exposure of the general population, again excluding medical exposure as a patient and exposure from natural sources (Table 38-4).

The DLs included in Table 38-4 were first published by the NCRP in 1987 and further refined in 1993. They replace the previous MPDs, which had been in effect since 1959. These DLs have been adopted by state and federal regulatory agencies and are now the law of the United States. Notice that SI units are preferred.

The basic annual DL remains the same: 50 mSv/yr (5000 mrem/yr). Substantial changes were made in other specified DL values. The DL for the lens of the eye was raised to 150 mSv/yr (15 rem/yr) and that for other organs to 500 mSv/yr (50 rem/yr). The cumulative whole-body DL is now 10 mSv (1000 mrem) times one's age in years. The DL during pregnancy remains fixed at 5 mSv (500 mrem); once pregnancy is declared, the monthly effective dose shall not exceed 0.5 mSv (50 mrem).

TABLE 38-3	Historical Review of Dose Limits for Occupational Exposure		
Year	Recommendation	Approximate Daily Dose Limit (mrem)	Source
1902	Dose limited by fogging of a photographic plate after 7-minute contact exposure	10,000	Rollins
1915	Lead shielding of tube needed (no numerical exposure levels given)		British Roentgen Society
1921	General methods to reduce exposure		British X-Ray and Radium Protection Committee
1925	"It is entirely safe if an operator does not receive every thirty days a dose exceeding 1/100 of an erythema dose."	200	Mutscheller
1925	10% of an SED per year	200	Sievert
1926	1 SED per 90,000 working hours	40	Dutch Board of Health
1928	0.000028 of an SED per day	175	Barclay and Cox
1928	0.001 of an SED per month 5 R/day permissible for the hands	150	Kaye
1931	Limit exposure to 0.2 R/day	200	Advisory Committee on X-Ray and Radium Protection of the U.S.
1932	0.001 of an SED per month	30	Failla
1934	5 R/day permissible for the hands	5000	Advisory Committee on X-Ray and Radium Protection of the U.S.
1936	0.1 R/day	100	Advisory Committee on X-Ray and Radium Protection of the U.S.
1941	0.02 R/day	20	Taylor
1943	200 mR/day is acceptable	200	Patterson
1959	5 rem/yr, 5 (N-18) rem accumulated	20	NCRP
1987	50 mSv/yr, 10 × N mSv cumulative	20	NCRP
1991	20 mSv/yr	8	IRCP

SED, Skin erythema dose.

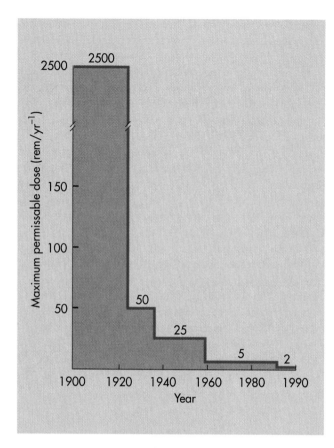

FIGURE 38-2 Dose limits over the past century.

Current DLs are based on a *linear, nonthreshold dose-response relationship*. They are considered the level of radiation exposure acceptable as an occupational hazard.

In practice, at least in diagnostic radiology, it is seldom necessary to exceed even one tenth of the appropriate DL. However, since the basis for the DL assumes a linear, nonthreshold dose-response relationship, all unnecessary radiation exposure should be avoided.

Occupational exposure is described as dose equivalent in units of millisieverts (mrem). This scheme has been adopted to be more precise in radiation-protection practices.

The effective dose (E) concept accounts for different types of radiation because of their varying relative biologic effectiveness. Effective dose also considers the relative radiosensitivity of various tissues and organs. This is a particularly important consideration when a protective apron is worn. Wearing a protective apron reduces radiation dose to many tissues and organs to near zero. Therefore effective dose is much less than that recorded by a collar-positioned radiation monitor.

Effective Dose

Effective dose (E) = Radiation weighting factor (W_r) × Tissue weighting factor (W_t) × Absorbed dose

TABLE 38-4	DLs Recommended by the NCRP
Exposure	**Dose**
Occupational exposures	
Effective dose	Annual: 50 mSv (5000 mrem)
	Cumulative: 10 mSv × age (1000 mrem × age)
Equivalent annual dose for tissues and organs	
Lens of eye	150 mSv (15 rem)
Skin, hands, and feet	500 mSv (50 rem)
Public exposures (annual)	
Effective dose for continuous or frequent exposure	1 mSv (100 mrem)
Effective dose for infrequent exposure	5 mSv (500 mrem)
Equivalent dose for tissues and organs	
Lens of eye	15 mSv (1500 mrem)
Skin, hands, and feet	50 mSv (5000 mrem)
Child (under 18 years of age) exposures (annual)	
Effective dose	1 mSv (100 mrem)
Equivalent dose for tissues and organs	
Lens of eye	15 mSv (1500 mrem)
Skin, hands, and feet	50 mSv (5000 mrem)
Embryo-fetus exposures	
Total effective dose	5 mSv (500 mrem)
Effective dose in a month	0.5 mSv (50 mrem)
Negligible individual dose (annual)	0.01 mSv (10 mrem)

Adoption of this scheme is progressing. For our purposes, effective dose is the quantity of importance. It is expressed in millisieverts (mSv) (millirems [mrem]) and is the basis for our DLs. As seen in Table 38-5, the radiation weighting factor (W_r) is equal to one for the types of radiation we use in medicine. The value of W_r for other types of radiation depends on the LET of that radiation.

The tissue weighting factor (W_t) accounts for the relative radiosensitivity of various tissues and organs. Tissues with higher values are more radiosensitive (Table 38-6). Practical implementation of these factors does not change the previous approach. The dose limit is high enough that it is rarely exceeded in diagnostic radiology.

With a collar-positioned radiation monitor, a change in procedure is necessary to estimate effective dose. Since essentially all a radiologic technologist's radiation exposure occurs during fluoroscopy and the trunk is shielded by a protective apron, the response of the monitor overestimates the effective dose to the whole body or trunk.

A conversion factor of 0.3 should be applied to the collar-monitor value to estimate effective dose. If a protective apron is not worn (for example, a radiographer who does no fluoroscopy), then the monitor response may be considered the effective dose.

Effective Dose Limits for Tissues and Organs

The whole-body DL of 50 mSv/yr (5000 mrem/yr) is an effective dose, which takes into account the weighted average to various tissues and organs. The NCRP also identifies several specific tissues and organs with specific recommended dose limits.

Skin. Some organs have a DL higher than that for the whole body. The skin DL is 500 mSv/yr (50 rem/yr); this is an increase from the earlier recommendation of 150 mSv/yr (15 rem/yr). This limit is not normally of concern in diagnostic radiology, since it applies to nonpenetrating radiation such as alpha and beta radiation and very soft x-rays. Radiologic technologists exclusively engaged in soft tissue radiography or nuclear medicine are very unlikely to sustain radiation exposures to the skin in excess of 10 mSv/yr (1000 mrem/yr).

Extremities. Radiologists often have their hands near the primary radiation beam, and therefore extremity exposure may be of concern. The DL for the extremities is the same as that for the skin, 500 mSv/yr (50 rem/yr).

These radiation levels are quite high and under normal circumstances should not even be approached. For certain occupational groups, such as cardiovascular and interventional radiologists and nuclear medicine technologists, extremity personnel monitors should be provided. Such devices are worn on the wrist or the finger.

Public Exposure

The general population is limited to 5 mSv/yr (500 mrem/yr) if the exposure is infrequent. If the exposure is frequent, such as in hospital workers who regularly visit x-ray rooms, the DL is 1 mSv/yr (100 mrem/yr).

The DL for nonoccupationally exposed persons is one tenth of that for the radiation worker.

This 1 mSv/yr is the DL that medical physicists use when computing the thickness of protective barriers. If a barrier separates an x-ray examining room from an area occupied by the general public, then the shielding is designed so that the annual exposure in the adjacent area cannot exceed 1 mSv/yr (100 mrem/yr).

If the adjacent area is occupied by radiation workers, then the shielding must be sufficient to maintain an annual exposure level less than 10 mSv/yr (1000 mrem/yr). This approach to shielding derives from the 10 mSv × N cumulative DL.

Radiation exposure of the general public or individuals in the population is rarely measured because it is not necessary. Most radiology personnel do not even receive this level of exposure.

Educational Considerations

There are several special situations associated with the whole-body occupational DL. Students under the age of 18 may not receive more than 1 mSv/yr (100 mrem/yr) during the course of their educational activities. This is

TABLE 38-5	W_r for Various Types of Radiation	
Type of Energy Range		**W_r**
X-rays and gamma rays, electrons		1
Neutrons, energy		
<10 keV		5
10 keV to 100 keV		10
>100 keV to 2 MeV		20
>2 MeV to 20 MeV		10
>20 MeV		5
Protons		2
Alpha particles		20

TABLE 38-6	W_t for Various Tissues
Tissue	**W_t**
Gonad	0.20
Active bone marrow	0.12
Colon	0.12
Lung	0.12
Stomach	0.12
Bladder	0.05
Breast	0.05
Esophagus	0.05
Liver	0.05
Thyroid	0.05
Bone surface	0.01
Skin	0.01

included in, not in addition to, the 1 mSv (100 mrem) permitted each year as a nonoccupational exposure.

Consequently, student radiologic technologists under the age of 18 may be engaged in x-ray imaging, but their exposure must be monitored and must remain below 1 mSv/yr (100 mrem/yr). Because of this, it is general practice not to accept underaged students into schools of radiologic technology unless their eighteenth birthday is within sight.

Even more changes in the DL are on the way. The changes are not made because of fear that current limits are dangerous or even harmful; they are made in keeping with ALARA; that is, they maintain radiation exposures *as low as reasonably achievable*.

The changes also acknowledge that radiologic technologists can function efficiently even with these more restrictive dose-limiting recommendations. In 1991, the ICRP issued a number of recommendations that includes an annual whole-body DL of 20 mSv (2000 mrem). Such a reduction is currently under consideration in the United States.

X-RAYS AND PREGNANCY

Two situations in diagnostic radiology require particular care and action. Both are associated with pregnancy. Their importance is obvious from both a physical and an emotional standpoint.

Radiobiologic Considerations

The severity of the potential response to radiation exposure in utero is both time and dose related. (see Chapter 37). Unquestionably, the most sensitive period to radiation exposure occurs before birth. Furthermore, the fetus is more sensitive early than late in pregnancy. As a general rule, the higher the radiation dose, the more severe the radiation response.

Time dependence. A grave misconception is that the most critical time for irradiation is during the first 2 weeks when it is most unlikely that a woman knows of her pregnancy. In fact, this is the time during pregnancy when irradiation is least hazardous.

The most likely biologic response to irradiation during the first 2 weeks of pregnancy is resorption of the embryo and termination of pregnancy. No other response is likely. The induction of congenital abnormalities during the first 2 weeks of pregnancy has not been demonstrated in humans or experimental animals after any level of radiation dose.

The time from approximately the second week to the tenth week of pregnancy is called the *period of major organogenesis*. During this time, the major organ systems of the body are developing. If the radiation dose is sufficient, congenital abnormalities may result. Early in this interval, the most likely congenital abnormalities are associated with skeletal deformities. Later in this period, neurologic deficiencies are more likely to occur.

During the second and third trimesters, the responses previously noted are unlikely. The results of numerous investigations strongly suggest that if a response occurs after diagnostic irradiation during the last two trimesters, the principal response would be the appearance of malignant disease during childhood. Malignant disease induction in childhood is also a possible response to irradiation during the first trimester.

These responses require a very high radiation dose before there is significant risk of occurrence. No such responses would occur at less than 25 rad (250 mGy). Such dose levels are remote, yet possible with patients who receive multiple x-ray studies of the abdomen or pelvis. They are essentially impossible with radiologic technologists because their exposures are so low. There are no other significant responses after irradiation in utero.

Dose dependence. There is virtually no information available for low doses of radiation that occur in diagnostic radiology to construct dose-response relationships for irradiation in utero. There is, however, a large body of data from animal irradiation, particularly rats and mice, from which such relationships can be estimated. The statements that follow, although attributed to human exposure, represent estimates based on extrapolation from animal studies.

After an in utero radiation dose of 200 rad (2 Gy_t), it is nearly certain that each of the effects noted previously will occur. There is little likelihood, however, that an exposure of this magnitude would be experienced in diagnostic radiology.

Spontaneous abortion after irradiation during the first 2 weeks of pregnancy is unlikely at radiation doses less than 25 rad (250 mGy_t). The precise nature of the dose-response relationship is unknown, but a reasonable estimate of risk suggests that 0.1% of all conceptions would be resorbed after a dose of 10 rad (100 mGy_t). The response at lower doses would be proportionately lower. It should be kept in mind, however, that the expected incidence of spontaneous abortion in the absence of radiation exposure is estimated to be 25% to 50%.

In the absence of radiation exposure, approximately 5% of all live births exhibit a manifest congenital abnormality. A 1% increase in congenital abnormalities is estimated to follow a 10-rad (100-mGy_t) fetal dose, and there is a proportionately lower increase at lower doses.

The induction of a childhood malignancy after irradiation in utero is difficult to assess. Risk estimates are even lower than those reported for spontaneous abortion and congenital abnormalities. The best approach to assessing risk of childhood malignancy is to use a relative risk estimate.

During the first trimester, the relative risk of radiation-induced childhood malignancy is in the range of 5 to 10; it drops to approximately 1.4 during the third trimester. The overall relative risk is accepted to be 1.5, a 50% increase over the naturally occurring incidence.

Pregnant Technologist

When a radiologic technologist becomes pregnant, she should notify her supervisor. The pregnancy then becomes declared, and the DL becomes 0.5 mSv/mo (50 mrem/mo). The supervisor should then review her previous radiation-exposure history, since this will aid in deciding what protective actions are necessary.

The DL for the fetus is 5 mSv (500 mrem) for the period of pregnancy, a dose level that most radiologic technologists do not reach regardless of pregnancy. Although some may receive doses that exceed 5 mSv/yr (500 mrem/yr), most receive less than 1 mSv/yr (100 mrem/yr).

This is usually indicated with the personnel monitoring device positioned at the collar above the protective apron. The exposure at the waist under the protective apron will not normally exceed 10% of these values, and therefore, under normal conditions, specific protective action is not necessary.

It is recommended that protective aprons be 0.25-mm lead equivalent but most are 0.5-mm lead equivalent. The 0.5-mm lead equivalent aprons provide approximately 90% attenuation at 75 kVp, which is sufficient. A 1-mm lead equivalent apron is available, but such a thickness is not necessary, particularly in view of the additional weight of the apron. Back problems during pregnancy constitute a greater hazard than radiation exposure. The length of the apron need not extend below the knees, but wraparound aprons are preferred during pregnancy. If necessary, a special effort should be made to provide an apron of proper size because of its weight.

It is reasonable to provide the pregnant radiographer with a second radiation monitor, which is positioned under the protective apron at waist level. The exposure reported on this second monitor should be maintained on a separate record and identified as exposure to the fetus. The monitors should never be switched and the record confused. Color-coding the monitors may help: red for the collar badge—red neck; yellow for the waist badge—yellow belly! Additional or thicker lead aprons are normally not necessary.

The use of an additional monitor shows consistently that exposures to the fetus are insignificant. Suppose, for instance, that a pregnant radiologic technologist wearing a single radiation monitor at collar level receives 10 mSv (1000 mrem) during the 9-month period. The dose at waist level under a protective apron would be less than 10% of the collar dose or 1 mSv (100 mrem). Because of attenuation by the maternal tissues overlying the fetus, the dose to the fetus would be approximately 30% of the abdominal skin dose or 300 μSv (30 mrem). Consequently, when normal protective measures are taken, it is nearly impossible for the fetal DL to even approach 5 mSv (500 mrem).

When pregnancy is declared, regardless of the nature of the x-ray facilities or the technologist's work experience, the supervisor should review acceptable practices of radiation protection. This review should emphasize the cardinal principles of radiation protection: minimize time, maximize distance, and use available shielding.

Management Principles

A biologic response to occupational radiation exposure in radiologic personnel is not expected. Nevertheless, it is essential for the director of radiology to incorporate three steps into the radiation protection program: (1) new employee training, (2) periodic in-service training, and (3) counseling during pregnancy.

New employee training. The initial step for any administrative protocol dealing with pregnant employees involves orientation and training. During these orientation discussions, all female employees should be instructed as to their responsibility regarding pregnancy and radiation.

Each radiologic technologist should be provided with a copy of the facility radiation protection manual and other appropriate materials. This material might include a 1-page summary of doses, responses (Box 38-2), and proper radiation-control working habits.

The new employee should then read and sign a form, indicating that she has been instructed in this area of radiation protection. A female radiologic technologist must notify her supervisor when she is pregnant or suspects she is pregnant.

BOX 38-2   Pregnancy in Diagnostic Radiology

Human responses to low-level x-ray exposure

Life-span shortening: 10 days/rad
Cataracts: none below 200 rad
Leukemia:10 cases/10^6/rad/yr
Cancer: 4 cases/10^4/rad
Genetic effects: doubling dose = 50 rad
Death from all causes: 4 deaths/10^4/rad

Effects of irradiation in utero

Up to 14 days
   Spontaneous abortion: 25% natural incidence; 0.1% increase/10 rad
2-10 weeks
   Congenital abnormalities: 5% natural incidence; 1% increase/10 rad
Second and third trimester
   Cell depletion: no effect at less than 50 rad
   Latent malignancy: 4:10,000 natural incidence; 6:10,000/rad
Entire pregnancy
   Genetic effects: 10% natural incidence; 5×10^{-7} mutations/rad

Protective measures for the pregnant radiologic technologist

Two occupational radiation monitors: collar and waist
Dose limit: 5 mSv/9mo, 0.5 mSv/mo

In-service training. Every well-run radiology service maintains a regular schedule of in-service training. Usually, this training is conducted at monthly intervals but sometimes more often. At least twice each year such training should be devoted to radiation protection, and a portion of these sessions should be directed at the potentially pregnant employee.

The material to be covered in such sessions is outlined in Figure 38-3. Although it is good to review doses and responses, it is probably more appropriate to emphasize radiation-control procedures. These, of course, affect the radiation safety of all radiologic technologists, not just the pregnant technologist.

BOX 38-3 Important Facts to Emphasize During Training

- The effective DL is 50 mSv/yr (5000 mrem/yr).
- Environmental background radiation is approximately 1 mSv/yr (100 mrem/yr).
- Occupational exposures are closer to environmental background radiation than to effective dose limits.

A review of personnel monitoring records is particularly important. A helpful procedure is to post the most recent radiation monitoring report for all to see. The year-end report should be initialed by each radiologic technologist, and the director of radiology should be sure that they understand the nature and magnitude of their annual exposure.

Through such training, radiologic personnel will realize that their occupational exposure is minimal, usually much less than 10% of the DL. The material listed in Box 38-3 should be emphasized during training.

Counseling during pregnancy. The director of radiology takes the next action when the radiologic technologist declares her pregnancy. First, the director should counsel the employee, including a review of her radiation-exposure history and any appropriate modifications to her schedule that she requests.

 Under no circumstance should termination or an involuntary leave of absence occur as a consequence of pregnancy.

New Employee Notification

This is to certify that _____ , a new employee of this radiologic facility, has received instructions regarding mutual responsibilities should she become pregnant during this employment.

In addition to personal counseling by _____ , she has been given to read several documents dealing with pregnancy in diagnostic radiology. Furthermore, the additional reading material that follows is available in the departmental office:

1. *Review of NCRP radiation dose limit for embryo and fetus in occupationally-exposed women,* NCRP Report No 53, Washington, DC, 1977, National Council on Radiation Protection and Measures.
2. *Medical radiation exposure of pregnant and potentially pregnant women,* NCRP Report No 54, Washington, DC, 1977, National Council on Radiation Protection and Measures.
3. Wagner, LK et al: *Exposure of the pregnant patient to diagnostic radiation,* Philadelphia, 1985, JB Lippincott.
4. *The effects on populations of exposure to low levels of ionizing radiation,* Washington, DC, 1990, National Academy of Sciences.

I understand that should I become pregnant and I decide to declare my pregnancy, it is my responsibility to inform my supervisor of my condition so that additional protective measures can be taken.

_____   _____
Supervisor   Employee

_____
Date

FIGURE 38-3 Form for new employee notification.

In all likelihood, a review of the employee's radiation exposure history will show a low-exposure profile. Those who wear the radiation monitor positioned at the collar, as recommended, and who are also heavily involved in fluoroscopy may receive an exposure greater than 5 mSv/yr (500 mrem/yr). Such employees, however, are protected by lead aprons so that exposure to the trunk of the body would not normally exceed 500 μSv/yr (50 mrem/yr).

This review of occupational radiation exposure is the appropriate time to emphasize that the DL during pregnancy is 5 mSv (500 mrem) and 0.5 mSv/mo (50 mrem/mo). Furthermore, it should be shown that this DL refers to the fetus and not to the radiologic technologist. This level of 5 mSv (500 mrem) to the fetus during gestation is considered an absolutely safe. In view of this discussion, the director of radiology should point out to the radiologic technologist that an alteration in her work schedule is not normally requested.

For radiologic technologists involved in radiation oncology, nuclear medicine, or ultrasound, a similar consultation and level of modification as previously discussed is appropriate. In radiation oncology, the pregnant technologist may continue her normal workload but should be advised not to participate in brachytherapy applications.

In nuclear medicine, the pregnant technologist should handle only small quantities of radioactive material. She should not elute radioisotope generators or inject millicurie quantities of radioactive material.

Ultrasound technologists are not normally classified as radiation workers. A sizable portion of ultrasound patients, however, have previously been nuclear medicine patients and therefore become a potential source of exposure to the ultrasonographer. This possibility is remote, since the quantity of radioactivity used is so low. It may be advisable during the pregnancy to provide the ultrasonographer with a radiation monitor.

Finally, the pregnant technologist should be required to read and sign a form (Figure 38-4), attesting to the fact that she has been given proper attention and that she understands that the level of risk associated with her employment is much less than that experienced by nearly all occupational groups.

Pregnant Patient

Safeguards against accidental irradiation early in pregnancy are complex administrative problems. This situa-

---

Acknowledgment of Radiation Risk During Pregnancy

I, _____ , do acknowledge that I have received counseling from _____ regarding my employment responsibilities during my pregnancy.

It is clear to me that there is a vanishly small probability that my employment will in any way adversely affect my pregnancy. The reading material listed below has been made available to me to demonstrate that the additional risk during my pregnancy is much less than that for most occupational groups. I further understand that, although I may be assigned to low-exposure duties and provided with a second radiation monitor, these are simply added precautions and do not in any way convey that any assignment in this department is especially hazardous during pregnancy.

1. *Review of NCRP radiation dose limit for embryo and fetus in occupational-exposed women,* NCRP Report No 53, Washington, DC, 1977, National Council on Radiation Protection and Measures.
2. *Medical radiation exposure of pregnant and potentially pregnant women,* NCRP Report No 54, Washington, DC, 1977, National Council on Radiation Protection and Measures.
3. Wagner, LK et al: *Exposure of the pregnant patient to diagnostic radiation,* Philadelphia, 1985, JB Lippincott.
4. *The effects of populations of exposure to low levels of ionizing radiation,* Washington, DC, 1990, National Academy of Sciences.

_____   _____
Supervisor   Employee

_____
Date

FIGURE 38-4 Form for acknowledgment of radiation risk during pregnancy.

X-Ray Consent for Women of Childbearing Age

X-ray examinations of abdomen and pelvis exposing the uterus to radiation are:

Abdomen (KUB)	Colon (barium enema)	Pyelograms (IVP and retrograde)
Stomach (UGI)	Gallbladder	Cystograms
Small Intestine (SI)	Hips, sacrum, coccyx	Lumbar spine and pelvis
All nuclear medicine studies		

The 10 days after onset of menstural period are generally considered safe for x-ray examinations.

Onset of last menstural period   Date _____   Date today _____

I am pregnant	Yes _____	No _____	Don't know _____
I have had a hysterectomy	Yes _____	No _____	Don't know _____
I use an IUD	Yes _____	No _____	Don't know _____

I recognize that if I am pregnant and have radiation to the abdomen, there is a possibility of injury to the fetus. However, I understand that the likelihood of such injury is slight and that my physician feels that the information to be gained from this examination is important to my health. I therefore wish to have this x-ray examination performed now.

_____
Name of examination

_____
Signature of patient

_____
Witness

FIGURE 38-5 X-ray consent for women of childbearing age.

tion is particularly critical during the first 2 months of pregnancy, when such a condition may not be suspected and when the fetus is particularly sensitive to radiation exposure. After a couple of months, the risk of irradiating an unknown pregnancy becomes small because the patient is generally aware of her condition.

If the state of pregnancy is known, then under some circumstances the radiologic examination should not be conducted. A pregnant patient should never knowingly be examined with x-rays unless a documented decision to do so has been made. When such an examination does proceed, it should be conducted with all of the previously discussed techniques for minimizing patient dose.

For many years, radiologists subscribed to the **10-day rule.** This rule was first stated in 1970 by the ICRP. Because it was less likely that a woman would be pregnant during the first 10 days after the onset of menstruation, this rule recommended that examinations of the abdomen or pelvis of fertile women be performed only during the 10 days after the onset of menstruation. Because of a better understanding of the radiobiology of radiation and pregnancy, the 10-day rule is considered obso-

lete today and has been abandoned by many practitioners. The risk of injury after irradiation in utero is small and the usual benefit so great that if the examination is clinically indicated, it should be performed.

When a pregnant patient must be examined, the examination should be done with precisely collimated beams and carefully positioned protective shields. The use of a high-kVp technique is most appropriate in such situations.

Elective booking. The most direct way to ensure against the irradiation of an unsuspected pregnancy is to institute **elective booking.** This requires that the clinician, radiologist, or radiologic technologist determine the start of the patient's previous menstrual cycle. X-ray examinations in which the fetus is not in or near the primary beam may be allowed, but they should be accompanied by pelvic shielding.

Ideally, the referring physician should be responsible for determining the menstrual cycle and for withholding the examination request if there is any question about the necessity of the examination. This may require a radiologist-sponsored educational program that can be easily conducted at regularly scheduled medical staff meetings.

Patient questionnaire. An alternative procedure is to have the patient herself indicate her menstrual cycle. In many radiology departments, the patient must complete an information form before examination. These forms often include questions such as, "Are you or could you be pregnant?" and "What was the start date of your last menstrual period?" Figure 38-5 is an example of such a simple, yet effective questionnaire for protecting against irradiation of a pregnant patient.

Posting. If neither elective booking nor the request form seems appropriate to a radiology service, an equally successful method is to post signs of caution in the radiology waiting room. Such signs could read, "Are you pregnant or could you be? If so, inform the radiologic technologist, "Warning: special precautions are necessary if you are pregnant," or "Caution: if there is any possibility that you are pregnant, it is very important that you inform the radiologic technologist before you have an x-ray examination." Such posting satisfies our responsibility to the patient and to the health care facility. However, it remains the ethical and professional responsibility of the radiologic technologist to verbally screen for pregnancy.

It has been estimated that fewer than 1% of all women referred for x-ray examination are potentially pregnant. If a pregnant patient escapes detection and is irradiated, however, what is the subsequent responsibility of the radiology service to the patient and what should be done?

The first step is to estimate the fetal dose. The medical physicist should be consulted immediately and requested to estimate the fetal dose. If a preliminary review of the examination techniques used (for example, type of examination, kVp, and mAs) determines that the dose may have exceeded 1 rad (10 mGy$_t$), a more complete dosimetric evaluation should be conducted.

Table 38-7 presents representative radiation levels for many examinations. With a knowledge of the types of examinations performed and the techniques and apparatus used, the medical physicist can accurately determine the fetal dose. Phantoms and dosimetry materials are available to ensure that this determination can be made with confidence.

Once the fetal dose is known, the referring physician and radiologist should determine the stage of gestation at which the x-ray exposure occurred. With this information, there are only two alternatives: allow the patient to continue to term or to terminate the pregnancy. Recommendations for abortion after diagnostic x-ray exposures have not been made by consulting or regulatory authorities. Since the natural incidence of congenital anomalies is approximately 5%, no such effects can rea-

TABLE 38-7	Representative Entrance Exposures and Fetal Doses for Frequently Performed Radiographic Examinations with a 400-Speed Image Receptor	
Examination	**Entrance Skin Exposure (mR)**	**Fetal Dose (mrad)**
Skull (lateral)	40	0
Cervical spine (AP)	60	0
Shoulder	50	0
Chest (PA)	50	0
Thoracic spine (AP)	90	1
Cholecystogram (PA)	80	1
Lumbosacral spine (AP)*	130	40
Abdomen or kidneys, ureters, and bladder (AP)*	110	30
Intravenous pyelogram*	110	30
Hip*	120	30
Wrist or foot	5	0

AP, Anterior-posterior; *PA,* posterior-anterior.
*Gonadal shields should be used if possible.

sonably be considered a consequence of diagnostic x-ray doses. Manifest damage to the newborn is unlikely at fetal doses below 25 rad (250 mGy$_t$), although some suggest that lower doses may cause mental developmental abnormalities.

In view of the available evidence, a reasonable approach is to apply a 10- to 25-rad rule. Below 10 rad (100 mGy$_t$) a therapeutic abortion is not indicated unless additional risk factors are involved. Above 25 rad (250 mGy$_t$) the risk of latent injury may justify a therapeutic abortion. Between 10 and 25 rad, the precise time of irradiation, the emotional state of the patient, the effect an additional child would have on the family, and other social and economic factors must be carefully considered.

Fortunately, experience with such situations has shown that fetal doses have been consistently low. The fetal dose rarely exceeds 5 rad (50 mGy$_t$) after a series of x-ray examinations.

SUMMARY

Health physics is concerned with the research, teaching, and operational aspects of radiation protection. The three cardinal principles developed for radiation workers are as follows: minimize the time of radiation exposure, maximize the distance from the radiation source, and use shielding to reduce radiation exposure. ALARA (as low as reasonably achievable) defines the principal concept of radiation protection.

Dose limits are prescribed for various organs, the whole body, and various working conditions so that the life-time risk of each year's occupational exposure does not exceed 10^{-4} per year^{-1}. The NCRP recommends a cumulative whole-body DL of 10 mSv multiplied by one's age in years. The DL during pregnancy is 5 mSv. In diagnostic imaging, however, it is seldom necessary to exceed one tenth the appropriate DL.

Occupational radiation exposure is measured in millisieverts (millirems) and the description of such exposure is effective dose (E). The effective dose accounts for the type of radiation and the relative radiosensitivity of tissues and organs.

The radiobiology of pregnancy requires particular attention for the pregnant radiologic technologist and the pregnant patient. The pregnant radiologic technologist should be provided with a second radiation-monitoring device to be worn under the protective apron at waist level. Posting the waiting room and examination room with education signs meets the ethical responsibility to the pregnant patient.

CHALLENGE QUESTIONS

1. Define or otherwise identify:
   a. Health physics
   b. TVL
   c. NCRP
   d. Effective dose
   e. ALARA
   f. Tissue weighting factor (W_t)
   g. Fetal DL
   h. Extremity monitor
   i. Elective booking

2. Write the equation for the radiation dose as a function of time of exposure.

3. What is the function of the 5-minute reset timer on a fluoroscopy imaging system?

4. A fluoroscope emits 3.5 R/min at the tabletop for every mA of operation. What is the approximate patient entrance skin exposure after a 3.2-minute fluoroscopic examination at 1.5 mA?

5. What are the three cardinal principles of radiation protection?

6. What does the value 10^{-4} yr^{-1} mean in regards to the NCRP-recommended dose limits?

7. How do some radiation occupational groups such as nuclear medicine technologists monitor their extremity doses?

8. What is the whole-body occupational DL for radiography students under 18 years of age?

9. What is the embryo's response to irradiation above 25 rad during the first 2 weeks after conception?

10. During the fetal period of major organogenesis, what radiation responses are possible?

11. State the management protocol for the pregnant radiologic technologist.

12. What information regarding radiation protection should be covered in regularly scheduled in-service training classes?

13. A nuclear power plant worker is assigned to an area where the radiation exposure level is 500 mR/hr. If the allowable daily exposure is 50 mR, how long may the worker remain?

14. The output intensity of a radiographic unit is 4.2 mR/mAs. What is the total output after a 200-ms exposure at 300 mA?

15. What is the approximate entrance skin exposure (ESE) after a 3.2-minute fluoroscopic examination at 1.5 mA? The fluoroscope emits 4.2 R/min for every milliampere of operation.

16. List five procedures that could result in a measurable fetal dose.

17. How can the three cardinal principles of radiation protection be best applied in diagnostic radiology?

18. What exposure will a radiologic technologist receive when exposed for 10 minutes at 4 m from a source with intensity of 100 mR/hr at 1 m while wearing a protective apron equivalent to 2 HVLs?

19. What wartime effort introduced the term *health physicist?*

Designing for Radiation Protection

OBJECTIVES

At the completion of this chapter, the student should be able to:

1. Name the leakage radiation limit for x-ray tubes
2. List the radiation-protection features of a radiographic imaging system
3. List the radiation-protection features of a fluoroscopic imaging system
4. Discuss the design of primary and secondary radiation barriers
5. Describe the types of radiation dosimeters used in diagnostic imaging

OUTLINE

A number of features of modern x-ray equipment designed to improve radiographic quality are discussed in previous chapters. Many are also designed to reduce patient dose during x-ray studies. For instance, proper beam collimation contributes to improved image contrast and is also effective in reducing patient dose. Filtration, on the other hand, is added to the x-ray beam only to reduce the patient dose.

More than 100 individual radiation-protection devices and accessories are associated with modern x-ray equipment. Some are characteristic of either radiographic or fluoroscopic assemblies, and some are determined by federal regulation for all diagnostic x-ray equipment. The list of devices required for all diagnostic x-ray imaging systems follow.

RADIOGRAPHIC PROTECTION FEATURES

Many radiation-protection devices and accessories are incorporated into modern x-ray imaging systems. Some are characteristic of either radiographic or fluoroscopic assemblies, and some are required for all diagnostic x-ray equipment. Two of those appropriate for all diagnostic x-ray equipment relate to the protective housing of the x-ray tube and to the control panel. Other radiation-protection features include the source-to-image receptor distance (SID) indicator, collimation, positive beam limiting (PBL), beam alignment, filtration, reproducibility, linearity, and operator shield.

Protective X-Ray Tube Housing

Every x-ray tube must be contained within a protective housing that reduces radiation leakage to less than 100 mR/hr (1 mGy$_a$/hr) at a distance of 1 m from the housing.

Control Panel

The control panel must indicate the conditions of exposure and positively indicate when the x-ray tube is energized. These requirements are usually satisfied with kVp and mA indicators. Sometimes visible or audible signals indicate when the x-ray beam is energized.

 X-ray beam-on must be positively and clearly indicated to the operator.

Source-to-Image Receptor Distance Indicator

An SID indicator must be provided. It can be as simple as a tape measure attached to the tube housing or as advanced as laser lights, but it must be accurate to within 2% of the indicated SID.

Collimation

Light-localized variable-aperture rectangular collimators should be provided. The x-ray beam and light beam must coincide to within 2% of the SID. Cones and diaphragms may replace the collimator for special examinations. The attenuation of the useful beam by the collimator shutters must be equivalent to that attenuated by the protective housing.

Question: Most radiographs are taken at an SID of 100 cm. How much difference is allowed between the projection of the light field and the x-ray beam at the image receptor?

Answer: 2% of 100 cm = 2 cm

Positive Beam Limitation

Automatic light-localized variable-aperture collimators were required on all but special x-ray imaging systems manufactured in the United States between 1974 and 1994. These PBL devices are no longer required but continue to be a part of most new radiographic systems. They must be adjusted so that with any film size in use and at all standard SIDs the collimator shutters automatically provide an x-ray beam equal to the image receptor. The PBL must be accurate to within 2% of the SID.

Beam Alignment

In addition to proper collimation, each radiographic tube should be provided with a mechanism to ensure proper alignment of the x-ray beam and the image receptor. It does no good to align the light field and the x-ray beam and not have the image receptor also aligned.

Filtration

All general-purpose diagnostic x-ray beams must have a total filtration (inherent plus added) of at least 2.5 mm Al when operated above 70 kVp. Radiographic tubes operated between 50 and 70 kVp must have at least 1.5 mm Al. Below 50 kVp, a minimum of 0.5 mm Al total filtration is required. X-ray tubes designed for mammography usually have 30 μm Mo or 60 μm Rh filtration.

As discussed in Chapter 31, it is not normally possible to physically examine and measure the thickness of each component of total filtration. An accurate measurement of half-value layer (HVL) is sufficient. If the HVL is equal to or greater than the value given in Table 31-3 at the various kVps, total filtration is adequate.

Question: The following data are obtained on a three-phase radiographic imaging system operating at 70 kVp, 100 mA, and 100 ms. Is the filtration adequate?

Added filtration (mm Al)	0	0.5	1.0	1.5	2.0	3.0	4.0	5.0
Exposure (mR)	87	74	65	56	49	39	31	25

Answer: A plot of this data indicates an HVL of 2.5 mm Al. Table 31-3 shows that of 70 kVp a HVL of 2.2 mm Al or greater is sufficient. The filtration is adequate.

Reproducibility

For any given radiographic technique, the output radiation intensity should be constant from one exposure to another. This is checked by making repeated exposures at the same technique and observing the average variation in radiation intensity. Reproducibility of x-ray exposure should not exceed 5% intensity change.

Linearity

When adjacent mA stations are used (for example, 100 and 200 mA) and exposure time is adjusted for constant mAs, the output radiation intensity should remain constant. Alternately, and perhaps better, the exposure time should remain constant, causing the mAs to increase in proportion to the increase in mA. This takes any inaccuracy in the exposure timer out of the analysis. The radiation intensity is expressed in the following units: mR/mAs (mGy$_a$/mAs). The maximum acceptable variation in linearity is 10% change in intensity from one mA station to the adjacent mA station.

Operator Shield

It must not be possible to expose an image receptor while the radiologic technologist stands outside a fixed protective barrier, usually the operating console booth. The exposure control should be fixed to the operating console and not to a long cord. The radiologic technologist may be in the examination room during exposure but only if protective apparel is worn.

Mobile X-Ray Imaging System

A protective lead apron should be assigned to each mobile x-ray imaging system. The exposure switch of such a system must allow the operator to remain at least 2 m from the x-ray tube during exposure. Of course, the use-ful beam must be directed away from the radiologic technologist while positioned at this minimum distance.

FLUOROSCOPIC PROTECTION FEATURES

The features of fluoroscopic imaging systems that follow are designed primarily to reduce patient and personnel exposure.

Source-to-Skin Distance

It might be thought that increasing the distance between any x-ray tube and the patient would result in reduced patient dose because of the increased distance. This is true, but maintaining the exposure to the image intensifier requires the mA to be increased to compensate for the increased distance. Because of the divergence of the x-ray beam, the entrance skin exposure (ESE) is less for the required exit exposure as the source-to-skin distance (SSD) is increased. The SSD must be not less than 38 cm on stationary fluoroscopes and not less than 30 cm on mobile fluoroscopes.

In Figure 39-1, a 20-cm abdomen is five HVLs thick. If the fluoroscopic x-ray tube is moved from a 40-cm (**A**) to a 20-cm (**B**) SSD, there is a great increase in the ESE. The exposure required at the image intensifier is 1 mR. In situations A and B the ESE will be 2.25 mR and 4.0 mR, respectively, solely because of the divergence of the x-ray beam: the inverse square law. When the x-ray attenuation of five HVLs are added for each geometry, the ESEs become 72 and 128 mR, respectively.

Primary Protective Barrier

The image-intensifier assembly serves as a primary protective barrier and must be 2 mm Pb equivalent. It must be coupled with the x-ray tube and interlocked so that the fluoroscopic x-ray tube cannot be energized when the image intensifier is in the parked position.

Filtration

The total filtration of the fluoroscopic x-ray beam must be at least 2.5 mm Al equivalent. The tabletop, patient

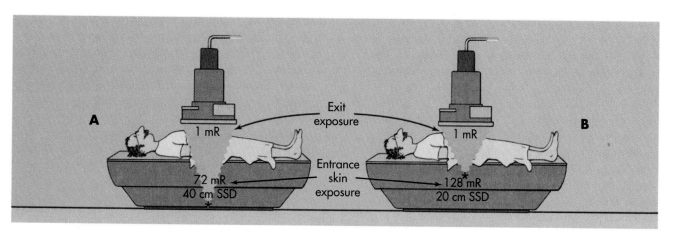

FIGURE 39-1 The patient ESE is higher and magnification greater when the fluoroscopic x-ray tube is too close to the tabletop. See text for explanation.

cradle, or other material positioned between the x-ray tube and the tabletop are included as part of the total filtration. When the filtration is unknown, the HVL should be measured. The minimum HVL reported in Table 33-3 must be met so that adequate filtration may be assumed.

Collimation

The fluoroscopic x-ray beam collimators must be adjusted so that an unexposed border is visible on the television monitor when the input phosphor of the image intensifier is positioned 35 cm above the tabletop and the collimators are fully open. For automatic collimating devices, such an unexposed border should be visible at all heights above the tabletop. The collimator shutters should track with height above the tabletop.

Exposure Control

The fluoroscopic exposure control should be the deadman type; that is, if the operator drops dead, the exposure is terminated unless he or she falls on the switch! The conventional foot pedal or pressure switch on the image-intensifier tower satisfies this condition.

Bucky Slot Cover

During fluoroscopy, the Bucky tray is moved to the end of the examining table, leaving an opening in the side of the table approximately 5 cm wide at gonadal level. This opening should automatically be covered with at least 0.25 mm Pb equivalent.

Protective Curtain

A protective curtain or panel of at least 0.25 mm Pb equivalent should be positioned between the fluoroscopist and the patient. Figure 39-2 shows the typical isoexposure distribution for a fluoroscope. Without the curtain and Bucky slot cover, the exposure of radiology personnel is many times higher.

Cumulative Timer

A cumulative timer that produces an audible signal when the fluoroscopic time has exceeded 5 minutes must be provided. This device is designed to make sure the radiologist is aware of the relative beam-on time during each procedure. The assisting radiologic technologist should record total fluoroscopy beam-on time for each examination.

X-Ray Intensity

The intensity of the x-ray beam at the tabletop of a fluoroscope should not exceed 2.1 R/min (21 mGy$_a$/min) for each mA of operation at 80 kVp. If there is no optional high-level control, the total intensity must not exceed 10 R/min (100 mGy$_a$/min) during fluoroscopy. If an optional *high-level control* is provided, the maximum tabletop intensity allowed is 20 R/min (200 mGy$_a$/min). There is no limit on x-ray intensity when the image is recorded as in cineradiography or videography.

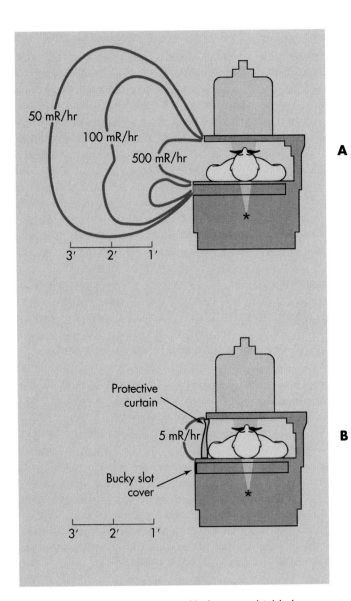

FIGURE 39-2 A, Isoexposure profile for an unshielded fluoroscope demonstrates need for protective curtains and Bucky slot covers. **B,** Exposure profile with these protective devices.

DESIGN OF PROTECTIVE BARRIERS

When one is designing a radiology department or an individual x-ray examination room, it is not sufficient to consider only general architectural characteristics. Great attention must be given to the location of the x-ray imaging system within the examination room. The use of adjoining rooms is also of great importance when designing for radiation safety. It is often necessary to insert protective barriers, usually sheets of lead, in the walls of x-ray examination rooms. If the radiology facility is located on an upper floor, it may be necessary to shield the floor as well.

A great number of factors are considered when designing a protective barrier. This discussion touches on only the fundamentals and some basic definitions. Any

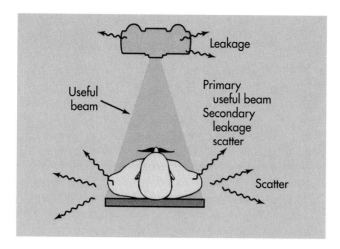

FIGURE 39-3 Three types of radiation—the useful beam, leakage radiation, and scatter radiation—must be considered in designing the protective barriers of an x-ray room.

TABLE 39-1	**Lead and Concrete Equivalents for Primary Protective Barriers**			
LEAD			**CONCRETE**	
(mm)	(in)	(lb/ft²)	(cm)	(in)
0.4	1/64	1	2.4	1 3/8
0.8	1/32	2	4.8	1 7/8
1.2	3/64	3	7.2	2 7/8
1.6	1/16	4	9.6	3 3/4

when the useful beam intercepts any object, causing some x-rays to be scattered. For the purpose of protective shielding calculations, the scattering object can be considered as a new source of radiation. During both radiography and fluoroscopy, the patient is the most important scattering object.

 The intensity of scatter radiation 1 m from the patient is approximately 0.1% of the intensity of the useful beam at the patient.

Question: The patient ESE is 410 mR (4.1 mGy$_a$) for a kidney, ureter, and bladder (KUB) examination. What will be the approximate radiation exposure at 1 m from the patient? At 3 m from the patient?

Answer: At 1 m: 410 mR × 0.1% = 410 mR × 0.001
  = 0.41 mR = 410 μR
  At 3 m: = 0.41 mR = (1/3)²
  = 0.41 mR (1/9)
  = 0.036 mR = 36 μR

Leakage radiation is that radiation emitted from the x-ray tube housing in all directions other than that of the useful beam. If the tube housing is properly designed, the leakage radiation will never exceed the regulatory limit of 100 mR/hr (1 mGy$_a$/hr) at 1 m. Although in practice, leakage radiation levels are much less than this limit, 100 mR/hr at 1 m is used for barrier calculations.

Barriers designed to shield areas from secondary radiation are called **secondary protective barriers.** Secondary protective barriers are always less thick than primary protective barriers.

Often, lead is not required for secondary protective barriers because the computation usually results in less than 0.4 mm Pb. In such cases, conventional gypsum board, glass, or lead acrylic is adequate.

Many walls that are secondary protective barriers can be adequately protected with four thicknesses of 5/8-in gypsum board. Operating console booth barriers are secondary protective barriers—the useful beam is never directed at the operating console booth. Four thicknesses of gypsum board and ½-in plate glass may be all that is necessary. Sometimes glass walls ½- to 1-in thick can be

time new x-ray facilities are being designed or old ones renovated, a medical physicist must be consulted for assistance in designing proper radiation shielding.

Type of Radiation

For the purpose of protective barrier design, two types of radiation are considered, primary and secondary radiation (Figure 39-3). Primary radiation, the useful beam, is the most intense, and therefore, the most hazardous and the most difficult to protect against. When a chest board is positioned on a given wall, it can be assumed that it will intercept the useful beam frequently. Therefore, it is sometimes necessary to provide shielding directly behind the chest board in addition to that specified for the rest of the wall.

 Any wall to which the useful beam can be directed is designated a **primary protective barrier.**

Lead bonded to sheet rock or wood paneling is most often used as a primary protective barrier. Such lead shielding is available in various thicknesses, and it is specified for architects and contractors in units of pounds per square foot (lb/ft²). Rarely is it necessary to use in excess of 4 lb/ft² in a diagnostic room.

Concrete, concrete block, or brick may be used instead of lead. As a rule of thumb, 4 inches of masonry is equivalent to ¹/₁₆ inch of lead. Table 39-1 shows available lead thicknesses and equivalent thicknesses of concrete. The thinnest available shielding is 1 lb/ft², but because of some difficulties in fabrication, 2 lb/ft² lead is often no more costly.

There are two types of secondary radiation: scatter radiation and leakage radiation. Scatter radiation results

TABLE 39-2	Equivalent Material Thicknesses for Secondary Barriers				
		SUBSTITUTES			
Computed Lead Required	Steel (mm)	Glass (mm)	Gypsum (mm)	Wood (mm)	
0.1	0.5	1.2	2.8	19	
0.2	1.2	2.5	5.9	33	
0.3	1.8	3.7	8.8	44	
0.4	2.5	4.8	12	53	

TABLE 39-3	Levels of Occupancy of Areas Adjacent to X-Ray Rooms*
Occupancy	Area
Full	Work areas (for example, offices, laboratories, shops, wards, nurses' stations), living quarters, children's play areas, occupied space in nearby buildings
Frequent	Corridors, restrooms, elevators using operators, unattended parking lots
Occasional	Waiting rooms, stairways, unattended elevators, janitors' closets, outside area

*As suggested by the NCRP.

used for operating console booth barriers. Table 39-2 contains equivalent thicknesses for material for secondary protective barriers.

Question: What percentage of the recommended dose limit (100 mrem/wk) will be incident on an operating console booth barrier located 3 m from the x-ray tube and patient? Assume that the x-ray output is 3 mR/mAs and that the weekly beam-on time is 5 min at an average 100 mA, a generous assumption.

Answer: *From scatter radiation, the barrier will receive:*
Total primary beam = 3 mR/mAs × 100 mA ×
$$5 \text{ min} \times 60 \text{ s/min}$$
$$= 90,000 \text{ mR}$$
Scatter radiation = 90,000 mR × 1/1000
$$\times (1/3)^2$$
$$= 10 \text{ mR}$$
From leakage radiation, the barrier will receive:
Leakage radiation at 1 m = 100 mR/hr ×
$$5/60 \text{ hr} = 8.3 \text{ mR}$$
Leakage radiation = 8.3 mR $(1/3)^2$
$$= 0.9 \text{ mR}$$
Total secondary radiation = 10 mR + 0.9 mR
$$= 10.9 \text{ mR, or } 11\% \text{ of}$$
the recommended
dose limit

This analysis is representative of the clinical environment. The estimated exposure is to the operating console booth barrier, not to the radiologic technologist. The composition of the barrier and the additional distance reduce technologist exposure even more. This is why personnel radiation exposure during radiography is very low. Radiologic technologists get most of their occupational radiation exposure during fluoroscopy.

Factors Affecting Barrier Thickness

Many factors must be taken into consideration when calculating the required protective barrier thickness. A thorough discussion of these factors is beyond the scope of this book; however, a definition of each is useful for understanding the problems involved.

Distance. The thickness of a barrier naturally depends on the distance between the source of radiation and the barrier. The distance is that to the adjacent occupied area, not to the inside of the wall of the x-ray room. A wall along which an x-ray imaging system is positioned probably requires more shielding than the other walls of the room. In such a case, the leakage radiation may be more hazardous than the scatter radiation or even the useful beam. It may be desirable to position the x-ray imaging system in the middle of the room because then no single wall is subjected to especially intense radiation exposure.

Occupancy. The use of the area being protected is of principal importance. If the area were a rarely occupied closet or storeroom, the required shielding would be less than if it were an office or laboratory occupied 40 hours a week. This reflects the **time of occupancy factor (T)**. Table 39-3 reports the occupancy levels of various areas as suggested by the National Council on Radiation Protection and Measurements (NCRP).

Control. An area occupied primarily by radiology personnel and patients is called a **controlled area**. Radiology personnel and patients who may be exposed in excess of population recommended dose limits are monitored for radiation exposure. The design limits for a controlled area are based on the proportionate weekly exposure and therefore require that the barrier reduce the exposure rate in the area to less than 100 mrem/wk (1 mSv/wk). Design limits for a controlled area are based on the cumulative recommended dose limit of 5000 mrem/yr (50 mSv/yr).

An **uncontrolled area** can be occupied by anyone, and therefore the maximum exposure rate allowed is based on the recommended dose limit for the public of 100 mrem/yr (1 mSv/yr). This is equivalent to 2 mrem/wk (20 μSv/wk), which is the design limit for an uncontrolled area. Furthermore, the protective barrier should ensure that no individual receives more than 2 mrem (20 μSv) in any 1 hour.

Workload. The shielding required for an x-ray examining room depends on the level of radiation activity in that room. The greater the number of examinations performed each week, the thicker the shielding required. This characteristic is called workload (W) and has units of milliampere-minutes per week (mAmin/wk). A busy, general purpose x-ray room may have a workload of 500 mAmin/wk. Rooms in private offices have workloads of less than 100 mAmin/wk.

Question: The plans for a community hospital call for two x-ray examination rooms. The estimated patient load for each room is 15 patients per day, and each patient will average three films taken at 80 kVp, 70 mAs. What is the projected workload of each room?

Answer:

$$15 \text{ pts/day} \times 5 \text{ days/wk} = 75 \text{ pts/wk}$$
$$75 \text{ pts/wk} \times 3 \text{ films/pt} = 225 \text{ films/wk}$$
$$225 \text{ films/wk} \times 70 \text{ mAs/film} = 15,750 \text{ mAs/wk}$$
$$15,750 \text{ mAs/wk} \times \frac{1 \text{ min}}{60 \text{ s}} = 262.5 \text{ mAmin/wk}$$

For combination radiographic/fluoroscopic rooms, usually only the radiographic workload need be considered for barrier calculations. When the fluoroscopic x-ray tube is energized, a primary protective barrier in the form of the fluoroscopic screen always intercepts the useful x-ray beam. Consequently, the primary barrier requirements are always much less for fluoroscopic beams than for radiographic beams.

Use factor. The percentage of time during which the x-ray beam is on and directed toward a particular barrier is called the **use factor** (U) for that barrier. The NCRP recommends that walls be assigned a use factor of ¼ and the floor a use factor of 1. Studies have shown these recommendations to be high and therefore very conservative. Many medical physicists suggest that primary barriers in fact do not exist, that all barriers are secondary, since the useful beam is always intercepted by the patient and the image receptor.

If an x-ray room has a special design, other use factors may be assigned. A room designed strictly for chest radiography has one wall with a use factor of 1. All others have a use factor of zero for primary radiation and thus would be considered secondary radiation barriers. The ceiling is nearly always considered a secondary protective barrier. The use factor for secondary barriers is always 1, since leakage and scatter radiation are present 100% of the time that the tube is energized.

 The use factor for secondary barriers is always 1.

Kilovolt peak. The final consideration in the design of an x-ray protective barrier is the penetrability of the x-ray beam. For protective barrier calculations, kilovolt peak (kVp) is used as the measure of penetrability. Most modern x-ray imaging systems are designed to operate at up to 150 kVp. Most examinations, however, are conducted at an average of 75 kVp. Usually constant operation is assumed to be at a kVp greater than that actually used, 100 kVp for general radiography, 30 kVp for mammography. Therefore it is more likely for the protective barrier to be too thick than too thin.

Alternatively, a workload distribution such as that shown in Figure 39-4 may be used. Workload distribution results in a more precise determination of required barrier thickness, but it is a considerably more difficult computation.

Measurements of radiation exposure outside the x-ray examination room always result in radiation levels far less than those anticipated by calculation. The total beam-on time is always less than that assumed. The av-

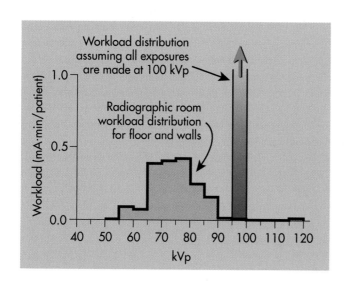

FIGURE 39-4 Workload distribution.

erage kVp is usually closer to 75 kVp than to 100 kVp. The calculations do not account for the fact that the patient and image receptor always intercept the useful beam. Therefore, although the calculations are intended to result in a dose limit of 100 mrem/wk or 2 mrem/wk outside the x-ray room, the actual exposure rarely exceeds one tenth of those dose limits. To confirm this for yourself, keep records for 1 week of kVp, mAs, and beam direction.

RADIATION DETECTION AND MEASUREMENT

Instruments are designed either to detect radiation, measure radiation, or perform both measurements. Those designed for detection generally operate in the **pulse** or **rate mode** and are used to indicate the presence of radiation. If the instrument is in the pulse mode, the presence of radiation is indicated by a ticking, chirping, or beeping sound. In the rate mode, the instrument response is in milliroentgens or roentgens per hour.

Instruments designed to measure the intensity of radiation usually operate in the **integrate mode.** They accumulate the signal and respond with a total exposure

in milliroentgens or roentgens. Such application is called **dosimetry,** and the radiation-measuring devices are called **dosimeters.**

The earliest radiation-detection device was the photographic emulsion, and it is still a primary means of radiation detection and measurement. However, other devices have been developed that have more favorable characteristics than the photographic emulsion for some applications. Table 39-4 lists most of the currently available radiation-detection and radiation-measurement devices along with some of their principal characteristics and uses.

The use of film as a radiation monitor (film badges) is covered in Chapter 40. Other types of radiation-detection devices that are of particular importance in diagnostic radiology include (1) the gas-filled radiation detector, which is used widely as a device to measure radiation intensity and to detect radioactive contamination; (2) thermoluminescence dosimetry (TLD), which is used for both patient and personnel radiation monitoring; and (3) scintillation detection, which is the basis for the gamma camera (an imaging device used in nuclear medicine) and which is also used in most computed tomography (CT) imagers.

Gas-Filled Detectors

Three types of gas-filled radiation detectors exist: ionization chambers, proportional counters, and Geiger-Muller (G-M) detectors. Although they are different in response characteristics, each is based on the same principle of operation. As radiation passes through gas, it ionizes atoms of the gas. The electrons released in ionization are detected as an electrical signal proportional to radiation intensity.

 The ionization of gas is the basis for gas-filled radiation detectors.

Consider an ideal gas-filled detector as shown schematically in Figure 39-5. It consists of a cylinder filled with air or any of a number of other gases. Xenon under pressure, for instance, is used to measure x-rays in some CT scanners.

Along the central axis of the cylinder is positioned a rigid wire called the *central electrode*. If a voltage difference occurs between the central electrode and the wall such that the wire is positive and the wall negative, then any electrons liberated in the chamber by ionization will be attracted to the central electrode. These electrons form an electric signal either as a pulse of electrons or as a continuous current. This electric signal is then amplified and measured. Its intensity is proportional to the radiation intensity that caused it.

In general, the larger the chamber, the more gas molecules there are for ionization and therefore the more

TABLE 39-4	Characteristics and Uses of Radiation-Detection and Radiation-Measuring Device
Device	**Characteristics and Uses**
Photographic emulsion	Has a limited range, is sensitive, is energy dependent—can be used for personnel monitoring, imaging
Ionization chamber	Has a wide range, is accurate and portable—can be used to survey for radiation levels >1 mR/hr
Proportional counter	Is a laboratory instrument, is accurate and sensitive—can be used to assay small quantities of radionuclides
Geiger-Muller counter	Is limited to <100 mR/hr, is portable—can be used to survey for low radiation levels and radioactive contamination
Thermoluminescence dosimetry	Has a wide range, is accurate and sensitive—can be used for personnel monitoring, stationary area monitoring
Scintillation detection	Has a limited range, is very sensitive, is a stationary or a portable instrument—photon spectroscopy, imaging

sensitive the instrument. Similarly, if the chamber is pressurized, then more molecules will be available for ionization, and an even higher sensitivity will result. A high sensitivity means that an instrument can detect very low radiation intensities.

Sensitivity is not the same as accuracy. A high accuracy means that an instrument can detect and precisely measure the intensity of a radiation field. Instrument accuracy is controlled by the overall electronic design of the device.

Region of recombination. If the voltage across the chamber of the ideal gas-filled detector is slowly increased from zero to a high level, the resulting electric signal will increase in stages (Figure 39-6). In the first stage, when the voltage is very low, no electrons are attracted to the central electrode. The ion pairs produced in the chamber recombine. This is known as the *region of recombination,* shown as stage R in Figure 39-6.

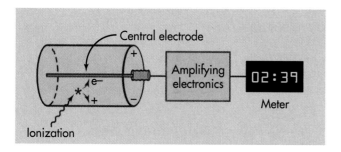

FIGURE 39-5 Ideal gas-filled detector consists of a cylinder of gas and a central collecting electrode. When a voltage is maintained between the central electrode and the wall of the chamber, electrons produced in ionization can be collected and measured.

Ion-chamber region. As the chamber voltage is increased, a condition will be reached in which every electron released by ionization will be attracted to the central electrode and collected. The voltage at which this occurs varies according to the design of the chamber, but for most conventional instruments it is in the range of 100 to 300 V. This portion of the gas-filled detector performance curve is known as the *ionization region,* indicated by *I* in the Figure 39-6. Ion chambers are operated in this region.

A number of different types of ion chambers are used in radiology, the most familiar being the portable survey instrument. This instrument is used principally for area radiation surveys. It can measure a wide range of radiation intensities, from 1 mR/hr (10 μGy_a/hr) to several thousand R/hr (Gy_a/hr). The **ion chamber** is the instrument of choice for measuring the radiation intensity in areas around a fluoroscope, around radionuclide generators and syringes, in the vicinity of patients containing therapeutic quantities of radioactive materials, and outside protective barriers.

Other, more accurate, ion chambers are used for the precise calibration of the output intensity of diagnostic x-ray imaging systems and external-beam radiation therapy units (Figure 39-7). Another application of a precision ion chamber is the dose calibrator (Figure 39-8). These devices find daily use in nuclear medicine laboratories for the assay of quantities of radioactive material.

Proportional region. As the chamber voltage of the ideal gas-filled detector is increased still farther above the ionization region, electrons of the filling gas released by primary ionization are accelerated more rapidly to the central electrode. The faster these electrons travel, the higher the probability that they will cause secondary ionization on their way to the central electrode. A secondary ionization occurs when an electron is released from an

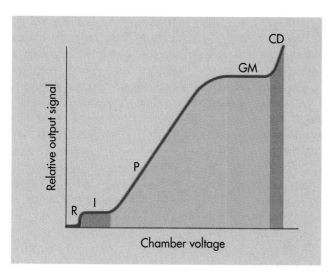

FIGURE 39-6 The amplitude of the signal from a gas-filled detector increases in stages as the voltage across the chamber is increased.

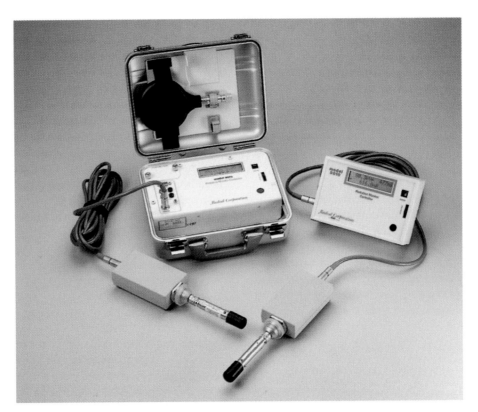

FIGURE 39-7 This ion chamber dosimeter is used for the accurate measurement of diagnostic x-ray beams. *(Courtesy Radcal Corp.)*

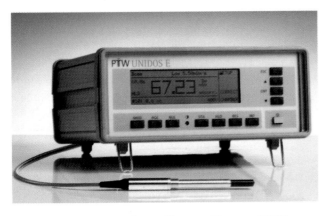

FIGURE 39-8 A dose calibrator. *(Courtesy PTW.)*

initial ionizing event and knocks out another electron in its path, thereby ionizing a second atom.

These secondary electrons will also be attracted to the central electrode and collected. The total number of electrons collected in this fashion increases with increasing chamber voltage. The result is a rather large electron pulse for each primary ionization. This stage of the voltage response curve is known as the *proportional region.*

Proportional counters are sensitive instruments used primarily as stationary laboratory instruments for the assay of small quantities of radioactivity. Some portable survey instruments operate in the proportional region, but they are generally used to detect only alpha and beta radiation.

One characteristic of proportional counters that makes them particularly useful is their ability to distinguish between alpha and beta radiation. Nevertheless, proportional counters find little applications in clinical radiology.

Geiger-Muller region. The fourth region of the voltage response curve for the ideal gas-filled chamber is the G-M region. This is the region in which Geiger counters operate. In the G-M region, the voltage across the ionization chamber is sufficiently high that when a single ionizing event occurs, a cascade of secondary electrons is produced in a fashion similar to a very brief, yet violent chain reaction. The effect is that nearly all the molecules of the gas are ionized, liberating a large number of electrons. This results in a large electron pulse.

When sequential ionizing events occur soon after one another, the detector may not be capable of responding to a second event if the filling gas has not been restored to its initial condition. Therefore a quenching agent is added to the filling gas of the G-M counter to enable the chamber to return to its original condition; subsequent ionizing events can then be detected. The minimum time between ionizations that can be detected is known as the *resolving time.*

G-M counters are used for contamination control in nuclear medicine laboratories. As portable survey instruments, they are used to detect the presence of radioactive contamination on work surfaces and laboratory apparatus. They are not particularly useful as dosimeters because they are difficult to calibrate for varying conditions of radiation. G-M counters are sensitive instruments capable of detecting and indicating single ionizing events. If they are equipped with an audio amplifier and speaker, the crackle of individual ionizations can be heard. The G-M counter does not have a very wide range. Most instruments are limited to less than 100 mR/hr (1 mGy$_a$/hr).

Region of continuous charge. If the voltage across the gas-filled chamber is increased still further, a condition will be reached whereby a single ionizing event will completely discharge the chamber, as in operation in the G-M region. Because of the high voltage, however, electrons will continue to be stripped from atoms of the filling gas, producing a continuous current or signal from the chamber. In this condition, the instrument is useless for detecting radiation, and continued operation in this region results in damage. The region is known as the *region of continuous discharge* and is indicated as *CD* in Figure 39-5.

Scintillation Detectors

Scintillation detectors are used in several areas of radiologic science. The scintillation detector is the basis for the gamma camera in nuclear medicine and is used in the detector arrays of many CT scanners.

Scintillation process. Certain types of material scintillate when irradiated; that is, they emit a flash of light immediately in response to the absorption of ionizing radiation. The amount of light emitted is proportional to the amount of energy absorbed by the material. Consider for example, the two gamma-ray interactions in Figure 39-9. If a 50-keV gamma ray interacts photoelectrically in the crystal, all the energy (50 keV) would reappear as light. If, however, that same gamma ray interacts by a Compton scattering event in which only 20 keV of energy was absorbed, then a proportionately lower quantity of light would be emitted in the scintillation.

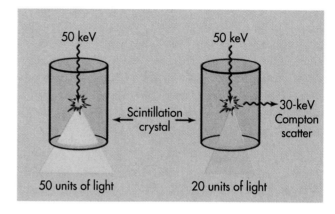

FIGURE 39-9 During scintillation, the intensity of the light emitted is proportional to the amount of the energy absorbed in the crystal.

Only materials with a particular crystalline structure scintillate. At the atomic level, the process involves the rearrangement of valence electrons into traps. The return of the electron from the trap to its normal position is immediate in scintillation and delayed in luminescence. This property was considered under an earlier discussion of luminescence (see Chapter 16).

Types of scintillation phosphors. Many different types of liquids, gases, and solids can respond to ionizing radiation by scintillation. Scintillation detectors are most often used to indicate individual ionizing events and are incorporated into either fixed or portable radiation-detection devices. They can be used to measure radiation either in the rate or the integrate mode.

Nearly all the noble gases can be made to respond to radiation by scintillation. Such applications are rare, however, because the detection efficiency is very low and therefore the probability of interaction is small.

Liquid scintillation detectors are frequently used in the research laboratory to detect the low-energy beta emissions from carbon-14 (^{14}C) and tritium (^{3}H). Because they present a relatively harmless radiation hazard and are easily incorporated into biologic molecules, ^{14}C and ^{3}H are useful research radionuclides.

These radionuclides emit low-energy beta particles with no associated gamma rays. This makes them hard to detect. With liquid scintillation counting, however, the biologic molecules can be mixed with a liquid scintillation phosphor so that the beta emission interacts directly with the phosphor, causing a flash of light to be emitted. Liquid scintillation counters have nearly 100% detection efficiency for beta radiation.

By far the most widely used scintillation phosphors are the inorganic crystals: thallium-activated sodium iodide (NaI:T1) or thallium-activated cesium iodide (CsI:T1). The activator atoms of thallium are impurities grown into the crystal to control the spectrum of the light emitted and to enhance its intensity. The NaI:T1 crystals are incorporated into gamma cameras; CsI:T1 is the phosphor incorporated into image-intensifier tubes as the input phosphor. Both types of crystals have been incorporated into CT detector arrays. Many of today's CT scanners, however, use cadmium tungstate ($CdWO_4$) or a ceramic as the scintillation detector.

Scintillation detector assembly. Light produced during scintillation is emitted isotropically (that is, with equal intensity in all directions). Consequently, when used as radiation detectors, scintillation crystals are enclosed in aluminum that has a polished inner surface in contact with the crystal. This allows the light flash to be reflected internally to the one face of a crystal that is not enclosed, called the *window.*

The aluminum containment is also necessary to hermetically seal the crystal. A hermetic seal is one that prevents the crystal from coming into contact with air or moisture. This is necessary because many scintillation crystals are hygroscopic; that is, they absorb moisture. When moisture is absorbed, the crystals swell and crack. Cracked crystals are not useful because the crack produces an interface that reflects and attenuates the scintillation.

Figure 39-10 shows the basic components of a single crystal–photomultiplier (PM) tube assembly representative of the type used in a portable survey instrument. The detector portion of the assembly is the NaI:T1 crystal contained in the aluminum hermetic seal. Coupled to the window of the crystal is a PM tube that converts the light flashes from the scintillator into an electric signal of pulses.

The PM tube is an electron vacuum tube that contains a number of elements. The tube consists of a glass envelope, which provides structural support for the internal elements and maintains the vacuum inside the tube. The portion of the glass envelope that is coupled to the scintillation crystal is called the *window of the tube.* The crystal window and the PM tube window are sandwiched together with a silicone grease, which provides optical coupling so that the light emitted by the scintillator is transmitted to the interior of the PM tube with minimal loss.

As the light passes from the crystal into the PM tube, it is incident on a thin metal coating called a *photocathode,* which consists of a compound of cesium, antimony, and bismuth. Electrons are emitted by a process called *photoemission* that is similar to thermionic emission in the filament of an x-ray tube except that the stimulus is light rather than heat.

 A photocathode is a device that emits electrons when illuminated.

The flash of light from the scintillation crystal therefore hits the photocathode, and electrons are released by photoemission. The number of electrons emitted is directly proportional to the intensity of the light.

These photoelectrons are accelerated to the first of a series of platelike elements called *dynodes.* Each dynode serves to amplify the electron pulse by secondary electron emission. For each electron incident on the dynode, several secondary electrons are emitted and directed to the next stage. Consequently, there is an electron gain for each dynode in the PM tube. The dynode gain is the ratio of secondary electrons to incident electrons.

The number of dynodes and the gain of each dynode determine the overall electron gain of the PM tube. Photomultiplier tube gain is the dynode gain raised to the power of the number of dynodes.

 Photomultiplier Tube Gain
PM tube gain = g^n
where g is dynode gain, and n is the number of dynodes.

Question: An eight-stage PM tube (eight dynodes) has a dynode gain of three (three electrons emitted for each incident electron). What is the PM tube gain?

Answer: PM tube gain = 3^8
= 6561

The last platelike element of the PM tube is called the *collecting electrode* or *collector.* The collector absorbs the electron pulse from the last dynode and conducts it to the preamplifier. The preamplifier provides an initial state of pulse amplification. It is attached to the base of the PM tube, a structure that provides support for the glass envelope and internal structures.

The overall result of scintillation detection is that a single photon interaction produces a burst of light; this in turn produces photoelectron emission, which is then amplified to produce a relatively large electron pulse. The size of the electron pulse is proportional to the energy absorbed by the crystal from the incident photon.

It is this property of scintillation detection that promotes its use as an energy-sensitive device for gamma spectrometry using pulse height analysis. Through such

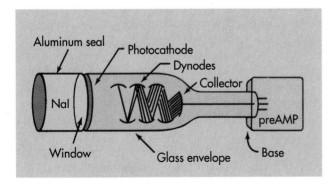

FIGURE 39-10 Scintillation detector assembly characteristics of the type used in a portable survey instrument.

application, unknown gamma emitters can be identified, and more sensitive radioisotope imaging can be accomplished by counting only pulses having energy representing a total gamma-ray absorption.

Scintillation detectors are sensitive devices for x-rays and gamma rays. They can measure radiation intensities as low as single-photon interactions. This property of scintillation detectors results in their use as portable radiation devices in much the same manner as G-M counters.

A portable scintillation detector is more sensitive than a G-M counter because it has much higher detection efficiency. For this application, the scintillation detector would be used to monitor the presence of contamination and perhaps low levels of radiation. It is not normally used as a dosimeter because of difficulties involved in calibration.

Thermoluminescence Dosimetry

Some materials glow when heated. This is a thermally stimulated emission of visible light called *thermoluminescence*. In the early 1960s, Cameron and co-workers at the University of Wisconsin experimented with some thermoluminescent materials and were able to show that exposure to ionizing radiation caused some materials to glow particularly brightly when subsequently heated. **Thermoluminescence dosimetry** (TLD) is the emission of light by a thermally stimulated crystal after irradiation.

This radiation-induced thermoluminescence has been developed into a sensitive and accurate method of radiation dosimetry for monitoring personnel radiation and for measuring patient dose during diagnostic and therapeutic radiation procedures. Thermoluminescence is also used in experimental radiation science, especially in cases when a small detector size is important and when low-level environmental monitoring is performed. Personnel and patient radiation monitoring are discussed in Chapter 40; however, at this time it is important to know some of the basic principles of TLD (Figure 39-11).

After irradiation, the TLD phosphor is placed on a special dish, or planchet, for analysis in an instrument called a *TLD analyzer*. The temperature of the planchet

can be carefully controlled. Directly viewing the planchet is a PM tube. The PM tube is the same type of light-sensitive and light-measuring vacuum tube described previously as a major component of scintillation detectors.

The PM tube–planchet assembly is in a chamber with a light tight seal. The output signal from the PM tube is amplified and displayed either on a meter or chart reorder. Figure 39-12 is a cutaway drawing of a commercially available TLD analyzer.

Glow curve. As the temperature of the planchet is increased, the amount of light emitted by the TLD increases in an irregular manner. Figure 39-13 shows the

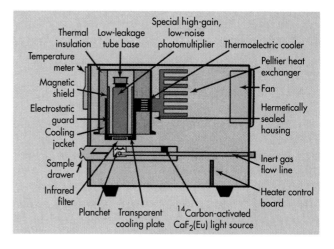

FIGURE 39-12 Cutaway schematic of a representative TLD analyzer. *(Courtesy Harshaw Chemical Company.)*

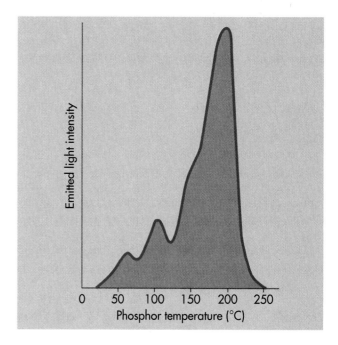

FIGURE 39-13 Thermoluminescence glow curve for LiF.

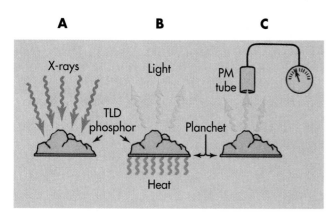

FIGURE 39-11 TLD is a multistep process. **A,** Exposure to ionizing radiation. **B,** Subsequent heating. **C,** Measurement of the intensity of the emitted light.

TABLE 39-5	Some Thermoluminescent Phosphors and Their Characteristics and Uses			
		Phosphor		
	Lithium Fluoride	Lithium Borate	Calcium Fluoride	Calcium Sulfate
Composition	LiF	$Li_2B_4O_7$:Mn	CaF_2:Mn	$CaSO_4$:Dy
Density $\times 10^3$ (kg/m³)	2.64	2.5	3.18	2.61
Effective atomic number	8.2	7.4	16.3	15.3
Temperature of main peak (°C)	195	200	260	220
Principal use	Patient and personnel dose	Research	Environmental monitoring	Environmental monitoring

light output from lithium fluoride (LiF) as the temperature increases. There are several prominent peaks in the graph, and each occurs because of a specific electron transition in the TL crystals. Such a graph is known as a **glow curve,** and each TL material has a characteristic glow curve. Both the height of the highest temperature peak and the total area under the curve are directly proportional to the energy deposited in the TLD by ionizing radiation. The TLD analyzers are electronic instruments designed to measure the height of the glow curve or the area under the curve and relate this to exposure or dose through a conversion factor.

Types of TLD material. Many materials, including some body tissues, exhibit the property of radiation-induced thermoluminescence. Materials that are used for TLD, however, are somewhat limited in number and are principally types of inorganic crystals. Lithium fluoride (LiF) is the most widely used TLD material. It has an atomic number of 8.2 and therefore has x-ray absorption properties similar to that of soft tissue. LiF is relatively sensitive. It can measure doses as low as 5 mrem (0.1 mSv) with modest accuracy, and at doses exceeding 10 rad (100 mGy_t), accuracy is better an ±5%.

 LiF is a nearly tissue equivalent radiation dosimeter.

Calcium fluoride (CaF) that is activated with manganese (CaF_2:Mn) has a higher effective atomic number (Z = 16.3) than LiF, making it considerably more sensitive to ionizing radiation. CaF_2:Mn can measure radiation doses less than 1 mrad (10 μGy_t) with moderate accuracy. Other types of TLDs are available, and Table 39-5 lists some thermoluminescent phosphors and their principal characteristics and applications.

Properties of TLD. A particular advantage of TLD is size. The TLD can be obtained in several solid crystal shapes and sizes. Rectangular rods measuring 1 × 1 × 6 mm long and flat chips measuring 3 × 3 × 1 mm thick

are the most popular sizes. The TLD can also be obtained in powder form, which allows for its irradiation in nearly any configuration. TLDs are also available with the phosphor matrixed with Teflon or plated onto a wire and sealed in glass.

The TLD is reusable. When irradiated, the energy absorbed by the TLD remains stored until released as visible light by heat during analysis. The heating restores the crystal to its original condition and makes it ready for another exposure.

The TLD responds proportionately to dose. If the dose is doubled, the TLD response will also be doubled. The TLD is rugged, and its small size makes it useful for monitoring dose in small areas, such as body cavities. The TLD does not respond to individual ionizing events, and therefore it cannot be used as a rate meter. The TLD is suitable only for integral dose measurements, but it does not give immediate results. It must be analyzed after irradiation for dosimetry results.

Optically Stimulated Luminescence

An additional radiation dosimeter especially adapted for personnel monitoring was developed by Landauer in the late 1990s (Figure 39-14). Optically stimulated luminescence (OSL) uses aluminum oxide (Al_2O_3) to detect radiation.

Irradiation of Al_2O_3 stimulates some electrons into an excited state. During processing, laser light stimulates these electrons, causing them to return to their ground state with the emission of visible light. The intensity of the visible light emission is proportional to the radiation dose received by the Al_2O_3.

The OSL process is not unlike TLD. Both are based on stimulated luminescence. However, OSL has several advantages over TLD, especially as applied to occupational radiation monitoring. With a minimum reportable dose of 1 mrem, OSL is more sensitive than TLD. OSL has a precision of ±1 mrem, which beats TLD. Other features of OSL include (1) reanalysis for confirmation of dose, (2) qualitative information about exposure conditions, (3) a wide dynamic range, and (4) excellent long-term stability.

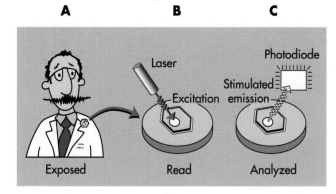

FIGURE 39-14 OSL is a multistep process. **A,** Exposure to ionizing radiation. **B,** Laser illumination. **C,** Measurement of the intensity of the emitted light.

SUMMARY

There are many radiation protection devices, accessories, and protocols associated with modern x-ray imaging systems. This chapter discusses the radiation-protection devices that are common for all radiographic and fluoroscopic imaging systems. Many of the devices are federally mandated; others are features added by manufacturers.

Leakage radiation emitted by the x-ray tube during exposure must be contained by a protective tube housing. The limit of leakage must be no more than 100 mR/hr at a distance of 1 m from the housing. The operating console must indicate exposure by either kVp and mA meters or visible and audible signals.

Great attention is given to the design of x-ray examination rooms, placement of x-ray imaging systems, and use of adjoining rooms. There are two types of protective barriers: the primary and secondary. Primary barriers intercept the useful beam and require the most lead. Secondary barriers protect personnel from scatter and leakage radiation and are often constructed of materials other than lead.

Dosimeters are instruments designed to detect and measure radiation. Other than photographic emulsion, there are four types of highly accurate devices for measuring radiation. The gas-filled detectors are the ionization chamber, the proportional counter, and the G-M counter. The scintillation detector is a very sensitive device used in nuclear medicine. Two other radiation-detection devices used especially for occupational radiation monitoring are TLD and OSL.

CHALLENGE QUESTIONS

1. Define or otherwise identify:
   a. TLD
   b. Use factor
   c. Pulse mode/rate mode
   d. Glow curve
   e. Primary protective barrier, secondary protective barrier
   f. Occupancy factor
   g. Scintillation detector
   h. Dosimetry
2. What do audible and visible signals indicate on the radiographic operating console?
3. List as many devices used for radiation protection on radiographic equipment as you can.
4. What happens if the x-ray beam and the film are not properly aligned?
5. What filtration is used for mammographic equipment operated below 30 kVp?
6. How are reproducibility and linearity different when measuring the intensity of the x-ray beam?
7. What characteristics of fluoroscopic equipment are designed for radiation protection?
8. How can filtration be measured if the amount of inherent and added filtration is unknown?
9. Name the two types of radiation exposure that are of concern when protective barriers are being designed.
10. List four factors that are taken into consideration when designing a protective barrier for a radiographic room.
11. What is the difference between a controlled area and uncontrolled area?
12. What are the units of workload for an x-ray examination room?
13. Explain the use factor (U) as it relates to a protective barrier in an x-ray examination room.
14. Why is the use factor for secondary barriers always 1?
15. Name the three gas-filled dosimeters.
16. Discuss the properties of TLD that make it suitable for personnel monitoring.
17. Which modality of diagnostic imaging uses scintillation detection as a radiation-detection process?
18. Discuss the advantage of OSL over TLD.
19. A photomultiplier has nine dynodes, each of which has a gain of 2.2. What is the overall tube gain?
20. Given the following conditions of operation, compute the weekly workload: (a) 20 patients per day, (b) 3.2 films per patient, and (c) 80 mAs per view on average.

CHAPTER

40

Radiation-Protection Procedures

OBJECTIVES

At the completion of this chapter, the student will be able to:

1. Discuss the units and concepts of occupational radiation exposure
2. Indicate three ways that patient dose can be reported
3. Describe the intensity and distribution of radiation dose in mammography and computed tomography
4. Discuss ways to reduce occupational radiation exposure
5. Explain occupational radiation monitors and the places where they should be positioned
6. Discuss personnel radiation-monitoring reports
7. List the available thicknesses of protective apparel
8. Discuss the principles of "as low as reasonably achievable" that are applied to patient radiation safety
9. Identify screening x-ray examinations that are no longer routinely performed
10. Discuss the various technical factors affecting patient radiation dose
11. Explain when to use gonadal shields

OUTLINE

All medical health physics activity is directed in some way to minimizing the radiation exposure of radiologic personnel and the radiation dose to patients during x-ray examination. Radiation exposure of radiologists and radiologic technologists is measured with occupational radiation-monitoring devices. Patient dose is usually estimated by conducting simulated x-ray examinations with human phantoms.

If radiation-control procedures are adopted, occupational radiation exposure and patient dose can be kept acceptably low. Health physicists subscribe to ALARA: keep all radiation exposure *as low as reasonably achievable*. Radiologic technologists should follow this guide as well.

TABLE 40-1	Occupational Radiation Exposure of Radiologic Personnel	
Exposure Category		**Value**
Average whole-body dose		70 mrem/yr
Those receiving less than minimum detectable dose		53%
Those receiving less than 100 mrem/yr		88%
Those receiving more than 5000 mrem/yr		0.05%

OCCUPATIONAL RADIATION EXPOSURE

Radiation dose is measured in units of rad (Gy_t). Radiation exposure is measured in roentgen (Gy_a). When the exposure is to radiologic technologists and radiologists, the proper unit is the rem (Sv). The rem is the unit of effective dose and is used for radiation-protection purposes. Although *exposure, dose,* and *effective dose* have precise and different meanings, they are often used interchangeably in radiology because they have approximately the same numerical value.

When properly used, *exposure* (R, Gy_a) refers to radiation intensity in air. *Dose* (rad, Gy_t) measures the radiation energy absorbed as a result of radiation exposure and is used to identify irradiation of patients. *Effective dose* (rem, Sv) identifies the biologic effectiveness of the radiation energy absorbed. This unit is usually applied to occupationally exposed persons and to population exposure.

Although the recommended dose limit for radiologic personnel is 50 mSv/yr (5000 mrem/yr), experience has shown that considerably lower exposures are routine. The occupational radiation exposure of radiologic personnel engaged in general x-ray activity should not normally exceed approximately 1 mSv/yr (100 mrem/yr).

Radiologists generally receive slightly higher exposures than radiologic technologists because of their frequency of exposure to fluoroscopy and because the radiologist is usually closer to the radiation source and the patient during such procedures. Table 40-1 reports the results of an analysis of the annual occupational radiation exposure of radiologic personnel. Clearly, the radiation exposures are low.

Fluoroscopy

Unquestionably, the highest occupational exposure of diagnostic x-ray personnel occurs during fluoroscopy.

During radiographic exposure, the radiologist is rarely present, and the radiologic technologist is behind the operating console protective barrier.

During fluoroscopy, both radiologist and radiologic technologist are exposed to relatively high levels of radiation. Personnel exposure, however, is directly related to the x-ray beam-on time. With care, personnel exposures can be maintained ALARA.

Question: A barium enema examination requires 2.5 min of fluoroscopic x-ray beam-on time. If the radiographer is exposed to 250 mR/hr, what will be the occupational radiation exposure?

Answer: Exposure = Exposure rate × Time
= 250 mR/hr × 2.5 min
= 250 mR/hr × 0.0417 hr
= 10.4 mR

Remote fluoroscopy results in low personnel exposures because personnel are usually not in the examination room with the patient. Some fluoroscopes have the x-ray tube over the table and the image receptor under the table. This geometry offers some advantage to image quality, but personnel exposures are higher because the secondary radiation (scatter plus leakage) levels are higher. This condition should be kept in mind during mobile and C-arm fluoroscopy, in which it is best to position the x-ray tube under the patient (Figure 40-1).

Cardiovascular and Interventional Procedures

Personnel engaged in cardiovascular and interventional procedures often receive higher exposures than those in general radiologic practices because of the longer fluoroscopic x-ray beam-on time. The frequent absence of a protective curtain on the image-intensifier tower and the extensive use of cineradiography also contribute to higher personnel exposure.

Extremity exposure for fluoroscopists may be significant. Even with protective gloves, exposure of the forearm can approach the recommended dose limit of 500 mSv/yr (50 rem/yr) if care is not taken. Without protective gloves, excessive hand exposures are possible.

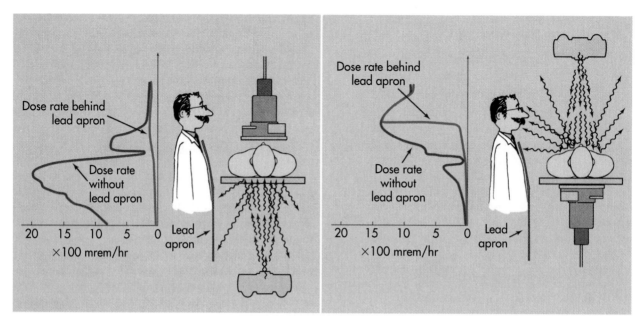

FIGURE 40-1 Scatter radiation during portable fluoroscopy is more intense with the x-ray tube over the patient. *(Courtesy Stephen Balter.)*

 Extremity monitoring must be provided for cardiovascular and interventional fluoroscopists.

Mammography

Personnel exposures associated with mammography are low because the low kVp of operation results in less scatter radiation. Usually, a conventional wall or window wall is sufficient to provide adequate protection. Rarely does a room used strictly for mammography require protective lead shielding. Lead glass, lead acrylic, and even plate glass are integral components of personnel protective barriers made for dedicated mammographic systems. Usually, such barriers are entirely adequate.

Computed Tomography

Personnel exposures in computed tomography (CT) facilities are low. Since the CT x-ray beam is finely collimated and only secondary radiation is present in the examination room, the radiation levels are low compared with those experienced in fluoroscopy. Figure 40-2 shows the isoexposure profiles for both the horizontal and vertical planes of a multislice spiral CT scanner. These data are given as milliroentgen per 360 degrees and show that personnel can be permitted to remain in the room during scanning. However, protective apparel should always be worn in such situations.

Question: It is necessary for a radiologic technologist to remain in the CT room at the midtable position during a 20-scan examination. What would be the occupational exposure if no protective apron were worn?

Answer: From Figure 40-2, we may assume an exposure of 0.47 mR/scan.

Occupational exposure = 0.47 mR/scan × 20 = 8 mR

Of course, with a protective apron, the trunk of the body would receive essentially zero.

Surgery

Nursing personnel and others working in the operating room and in intensive care units are sometimes exposed to radiation from mobile x-ray imaging systems and C-arm fluoroscopes. Although these personnel are often anxious about such exposures, many studies have shown that their occupational exposure is near zero. It is usually not necessary to provide occupational radiation monitors for such personnel.

Mobile Radiography

When fixed protective barriers are not available, such as during mobile examination, the mobile x-ray imaging system is equipped with an exposure cord long enough to allow the technologist to leave the immediate examination area. The radiologic technologist should wear a protective apron for each such mobile examination.

Occupational radiation monitors are not necessary during mobile radiography except for the radiologic technologist and anyone *routinely* required to restrain or hold patients. Personnel that regularly operate or are in the immediate vicinity of a C-arm fluoroscope should wear an occupational radiation monitor in addition to protective apparel. During C-arm fluoroscopy, the x-ray

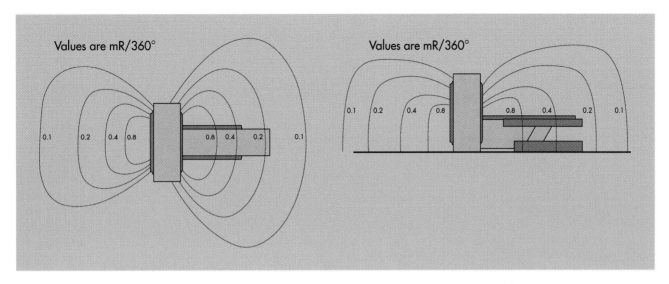

FIGURE 40-2 Isoexposure profiles in both the horizontal and the vertical planes for multislice spiral CT.

beam may be on for a relatively long time, and the beam can be pointed in virtually any direction.

It should *never* be necessary for radiologic personnel to exceed 50 mSv/yr (5000 mrem/yr). In smaller hospitals, emergency centers, and private clinics, occupational exposures rarely exceed 5 mSv/yr (500 mrem/yr). As Table 40-1 reports, average exposures in most facilities are less than 1 mSv/yr (100 mrem/yr).

PATIENT DOSE

The exposure of patients to medical x-rays is commanding increased attention in society for two reasons. First, the frequency of x-ray examination is increasing among all age groups: at a rate of approximately 10% per year in the United States. This rate of increase is exceeded in many other countries. This indicates that physicians are relying more and more on x-ray diagnosis to assist them in patient care even when accounting for the newer imaging modalities. This is to be expected. X-ray diagnosis is considered much more accurate today than in the past. The more rigorous training programs required of radiologists and radiologic tecnologists and the improvements in diagnostic x-ray equipment allow for more difficult, but more substantive, x-ray examinations. Efficacy and diagnostic accuracy are much improved.

Second, there is increasing concern among public health officials and radiation scientists regarding the risk associated with medical x-ray exposure. Acute effects on superficial tissues after cardiovascular and interventional procedures are being reported with increasing frequency.

The possible late effects of diagnostic x-ray exposure are of concern, and therefore attention must be given to good radiation-control practices. The same level of diagnostic information can be obtained with lower radia-

tion dose and therefore with reduced risk. This is in keeping with **ALARA.**

Estimation of Patient Dose

Patient dose from diagnostic x-rays is generally reported in one of three ways. The exposure to the entrance surface, or **entrance skin exposure (ESE)**, is most often reported because it is easy to measure. The **gonadal dose,** the exposure to the reproductive organs, is important because of the possible genetic responses to medical x-ray exposure. The dose to the gonads is not difficult to measure or estimate. The dose to the bone marrow, or **mean marrow dose,** is important because bone marrow is the target organ believed responsible for radiation-induced leukemia. Bone marrow dose cannot be measured directly; it is estimated from the ESE.

Table 40-2 presents some representative values of ESE and gonadal dose for various x-ray examinations. The mean marrow dose for each procedure is also presented. Note that these are only approximate values and should not be used to estimate patient dose at any facility. In any given x-ray facility, actual doses delivered may be considerably different. The efficiency of x-ray production and image-receptor speed are the most important variables.

The values in Table 40-2 provide for relative dose comparisons among radiologic examinations. Doses during fluoroscopy are too dependent on technique, equipment, and beam-on time to be easily estimated. Usually, such doses must be measured.

Entrance Skin Exposure (ESE). ESE is most often referred to as the *patient dose.* It is widely used because it is easy to measure and because reasonably accurate estimates can be made in the absence of measurements.

TABLE 40-2	Representative Radiation Quantities from Diagnostic X-Ray Procedures			
Examination	Technique (kVp/mAs)	ESE (mR)	Mean Marrow Dose (mrad)	Gonadal Dose (mrad)
Skull	76/50	200	10	<1
Chest	110/3	10	2	<1
Cervical spine	70/40	150	10	<1
Lumbar spine	72/60	300	60	225
Abdomen	74/60	400	30	125
Pelvis	70/50	150	20	150
Extremity	60/5	50	2	<1
CT (head)	125/300	3000	20	50
CT (pelvis)	124/400	4000	100	3000

The measurement technique often employed uses thermoluminescence dosimeters (TLDs). The size, sensitivity, and accuracy of TLDs make them very satisfactory patient-radiation monitors. A small grouping or pack of 3 to 10 TLDs can easily be taped to the patient's skin in the center of the x-ray field. Since the response of the TLD is proportional to exposure and dose, the TLD can be used to measure all levels experienced in diagnostic radiology. With proper laboratory technique, the results of such measurements are accurate to within 5%

Two rather straightforward methods for estimating ESE are available in the absence of patient measurements. The first requires the use of a nomogram such as that shown in Figure 40-3. This figure contains a family of curves from which the output intensity of a radiographic unit can be estimated if the technique is known or assumed. The output intensity of different x-ray imaging systems varies widely, so the use of this nomogram method is only good to perhaps ±50%.

Using this nomogram first requires knowledge of the total filtration in the x-ray beam. This is usually available from the medical physics report, but if not, 3 mm Al is a good estimate. Next, the kVp and mAs of the intended examination must be identified. A vertical line is drawn that rises from the value of total filtration until it intersects with the kVp of the examination. From this intersection, a horizontal line is drawn to the left until it intersects the mR/mAs axis. The resulting mR/mAs value is the approximate output intensity of the radiographic unit. This value is multiplied by the examination mAs to obtain the approximate patient exposure.

Question: Referring to Figure 40-3, estimate the ESE from a lateral skull film taken at 66 kVp and 150 mAs with a radiographic unit having 2.5 mm Al total filtration.

Answer: Estimate the intersection between a vertical line rising from 2.5 mm Al and a horizontal line through 66 kVp. Extend the horizontal line to the y-axis and read 3.8 mR/mAs.
3.8 mR/mAs × 150 = 570 mR

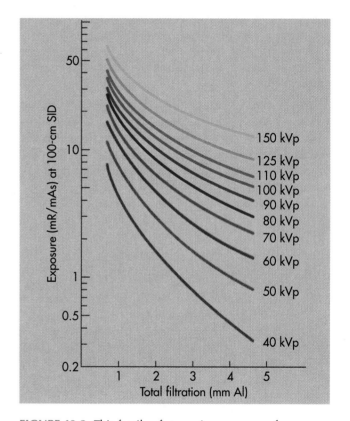

FIGURE 40-3 This family of curves is a nonogram for estimating output x-ray intensity from a single-phase radiographic unit. *(Courtesy John R. Cameron.)*

A better approach requires that a medical physicist construct a nomogram such as that shown in Figure 40-4 for each radiographic unit. A straight edge between any kVp and mAs crosses the ESE scale at the correct mR value.

Question: Using the nomogram of Figure 40-4, find the ESE for a radiographic exposure made at 66 kVp and 150 mAs?

Answer: When the prescribed line is drawn, it crosses the ESE scale at approximately 1000 mR.

A third method for estimating ESE requires knowledge of the output intensity for at least one operating condition. During the annual or special radiation-control survey and calibration of an x-ray facility, the medical physicist measures this output intensity, usually in units of milliroentgens per milliampere-second, at 80 cm, the approximate source-to-skin distance (SSD), or at 100 cm, the source-to-image receptor distance (SID). At 70 kVp, the radiographic output intensity varies from about 2 to 10 mR/mAs at 80-cm SSD.

Knowledge of this calibration value would allow an adjustment for a different SSD via application of the inverse square law.

Question: The output intensity of a radiographic unit is reported as 3.7 mR/mAs (37 μGy_a/mAs) at 100-cm SID. What is the intensity at 75-cm SSD?

Answer: At 75-cm SSD the intensity is greater by $(100/75)^2$
$$= (1.33)^2$$
$$= 1.78$$
3.7 mR/mAs $\times$ 1.78 = 6.6 mR/mAs

The known ESE is scaled according to the kVp and mAs of the examination. Output intensity varies according to the square of the ratio in the change in kVp. (See Chapter 12 to review this relationship.)

Question: The output intensity at 70 kVp and 75-cm SSD is 6.6 mR/mAs (66 μGy_a/mAs). What is the output intensity at 76 kVp?

Answer: At a higher kVp, the output intensity is greater by the square of the ratio of the kVp or change.
$$(76/70)^2 = (1.09)^2 = 1.18$$
6.6 mR/mAs $\times$ 1.19 = 7.8 mR/mAs

The final step in estimating ESE is to multiply the output intensity in mR/mAs by the examination mAs since they are proportional.

Question: If the radiographic technique for intravenous pyelography calls for 80 mAs, what is the ESE when the output intensity is 7.8 mR/mAs (78 μGy_a/mAs)?

Answer: 7.8 mR/mAs $\times$ 80 mAs = 624 mR

These steps can be combined into a single calculation as illustrated in the following example.

Question: The output intensity for a radiographic unit is 4.5 mR/mAs (4.5 μGy_a/mAs) at 70 kVp and 80 cm. If a lateral skull film is taken at 66 kVp and 150 mAs, what will be the ESE at an 80-cm SSD? What would be the skin dose at a 90-cm SSD?

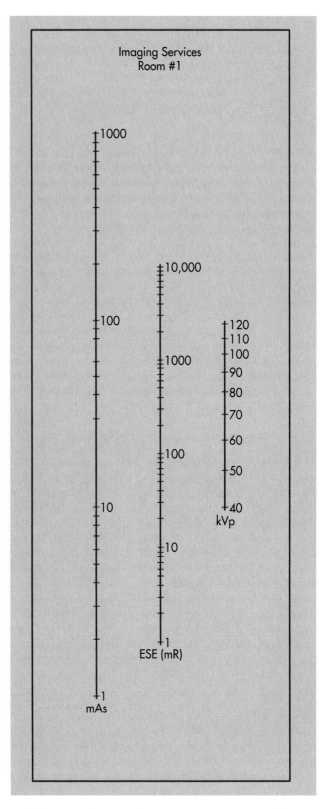

FIGURE 40-4 This type of nomogram is very accurate but must be fashioned individually for each radiographic unit. *(Courtesy Michael D. Harpen.)*

Answer: *At 80-cm SSD:*

$$\text{Dose} = (4.5 \text{ mR/mAs})\left(\frac{66 \text{ kVp}}{70 \text{ kVp}}\right)^2 (150 \text{ mAs})$$

$$= 600 \text{ mR}$$

At 90-cm SSD:

$$\text{Dose} = (600 \text{ mR})\left(\frac{80}{90}\right)^2$$

$$= 474 \text{ mR}$$

The ESE in fluoroscopy is more difficult to estimate because the x-ray field moves and sometimes varies in size. If the field were of one size and stationary, the ESE would be directly related to exposure time. In the absence of measurements, the fluoroscopic ESE can be estimated at 4 R/mAs.

 For the average fluoroscopic examination, an ESE of 4 R/min can be assumed.

Question: A fluoroscopic procedure requires 2.5 min at 90 kVp and 2 mA. What is the approximate ESE?

Answer: $\text{ESE} = (4 \text{ R/min})(2.5 \text{ min})$
$= 10 \text{ R}$

Mean marrow dose. The hematologic effects of radiation are rarely, if ever, experienced in diagnostic radiology. It is appropriate, however, to understand the mean marrow dose, which is one measure of patient dose during diagnostic procedures. The mean marrow dose is the average radiation dose to the entire active bone marrow. For instance, if during a particular examination, 50% of the active bone marrow were in the primary beam and received an average dose of 25 mrad (250 μGy_t), the mean marrow dose would be 12.5 mrad (125 μGy_t).

Table 40-2 includes the approximate mean marrow dose in adults for various radiographic examinations. In children, these levels would generally be less because the radiographic techniques used are considerably less. Table 40-3 shows the distribution of active bone marrow in the adult and provides some clues as to which diagnostic x-ray procedures involve exposure to large amounts of bone marrow.

In the United States the mean marrow dose from diagnostic x-ray examinations averaged over the entire population is approximately 100 mrad/yr (1 mGy$_t$/yr). Such a dose never results in the hematologic responses described in Chapter 36. It is a dose concept, however, used by some to estimate, on a population basis, the risk of one late effect of radiation: leukemia.

Genetically significant dose. Measurements and estimates of gonadal dose are important because of the suspected genetic effects of radiation. Although the gonadal dose from diagnostic x-rays is low for each individual, it may have some significance in terms of population effects.

TABLE 40-3	Distribution of Active Bone Marrow in Adults	
Anatomic Site		**Percentage of Bone Marrow**
Head		10
Upper limb girdle		8
Sternum		3
Ribs		11
Cervical vertebrae		4
Thoracic vertebrae		13
Lumbar vertebrae		11
Sacrum		11
Lower limb girdle		29
TOTAL		100

The population gonadal dose of importance is the **genetically significant dose (GSD)**, the radiation dose to the population gene pool. **The GSD is the gonad dose which, if received by every member of the population, would produce the total genetic effect on the population as the sum of the individual doses actually received.** Thus it is a weighted-average gonadal dose. It takes into account people who are and who are not irradiated and averages the results. The GSD can be estimated only through large-scale epidemiologic studies.

Genetically Significant Dose

$$\text{GSD} = \frac{\Sigma DN_X P}{\Sigma N_T P}$$

where:
Σ = mathematical symbol meaning to sum or add values
D = average gonadal dose per examination
N_X = number of people receiving x-ray examinations
N_T = total number of people in the population
P = expected future number of children per person (progeny)

For computational purposes therefore, the GSD considers the age, gender, and expected number of children for each person examined with x-rays. It also acknowledges the various types of examinations and the gonadal dose per examination type.

Estimates for GSD have been conducted in many countries (Table 40-4). The estimate reported by the U.S. Public Health Service is 20 mrad/yr (200 μGy_t/yr). Thus this is a genetic radiation burden over and above the existing natural background radiation level of approximately 100 mrad/yr (1 mGy$_t$/yr). The genetic effects of this total GSD, 120 mrad/yr (1.2 mGy$_t$/yr), are not detectable.

Patient Dose in Special Examinations

Mammography. Because of the considerable application of x-rays for examination of the female breast and the

TABLE 40-4	Estimated GSD from Diagnostic X-Ray Examination	
Population	**GSD (mrad)**	
Denmark	22	
Great Britain	12	
Japan	27	
New Zealand	12	
Sweden	72	
United States	20	

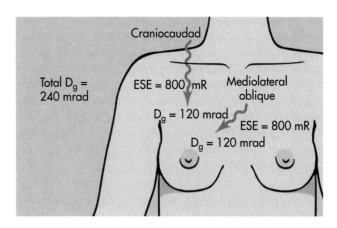

FIGURE 40-5 Two mammographic exposures result in a total glandular dose that is the sum of the individual glandular doses.

concern for the induction of breast cancer by radiation, it is imperative that radiologic technologists have some understanding of the radiation doses involved in such examinations.

Screen-film and digital mammography currently are the only acceptable techniques. Direct-exposure film and xeromammography are history. An ESE of approximately 800 mR/view (8 mGy$_a$/view) is normal. Increasing the x-ray tube potential much beyond 26 kVp degrades the image unacceptably, so further dose reduction by technique manipulation is unlikely. Faster image receptors may make even lower-dose mammography possible.

Radiographic grids are used in most screen-film mammography examinations. Grid ratios of 4:1 and 5:1 are most popular. The contrast enhancement produced by using such grids is significant, but so is the increase in patient dose. Patient dose is increased by approximately two times with the use of such grids when compared with nongrid technique.

The values stated for patient dose in mammography can be misleading. Because of the low x-ray energies used in mammography, the dose falls off very rapidly as the beam penetrates the breast. If the ESE for a craniocaudad view is 800 mR (8 mGy$_a$), the dose to the midline of the breast may be only 100 mrad (1.0 mGy$_t$). The biologic effect of such an examination is presumed to be more closely associated with the total energy absorbed by glandular tissue.

Fortunately, it is known that the risk of an adverse biologic response from mammography is small. Certainly, it is nothing about which a patient should be concerned. Any possible response, however, is related to the average radiation dose to glandular tissue, the **glandular dose (Dg)** and not the skin exposure. The D$_g$ varies in a complicated way with variations in x-ray beam quality and quantity. For screen-film mammography, the D$_g$ is approximately 15% of the ESE.

Specification of an ESE can also be misleading when evaluating a two-view examination, such as that used for screening (Figure 40-5). In an examination consisting of craniocaudad and mediolateral oblique views, the views produce an ESE of 800 mR (8 mGy$_a$) each. It would be incorrect to describe this total examination procedure as

resulting in an ESE of 1.6 R (16 mGy$_a$). Skin exposures from different projections cannot be added. Either the skin exposure for each view must be specified, or there must be an attempt to estimate the total D$_g$.

The total D$_g$ can be estimated by approximating that the contribution from each view will be 15% of the ESE. Consequently, the total D$_g$ would be the sum of contribution from each of the craniocaudad and mediolateral oblique views: 0.15 × 800 = 120 mrad (1.2 mGy$_t$). The total D$_g$ would therefore be 240 mrad (2.4 mGy$_t$).

 Glandular dose should not exceed 100 mrad/view with nongrid screen-film mammography or 300 mrad/view with a grid.

From this discussion, it would seem that patient dose in mammography can be considerably reduced if the number of views is restricted. For screening programs, no more than two views per breast are advisable.

CT scanning. An important consideration in CT scanning, as with any x-ray procedure, is not only the skin dose but also the distribution of dose to internal organs and tissues. On the basis of skin dose, CT is somewhat higher than most other diagnostic x-ray procedures. The skin dose delivered by a series of contiguous CT slices is much higher than that delivered by a single radiographic view; however, a typical radiographic head or body examination often involves several views. Furthermore, for many CT examinations, considerably less tissue volume is irradiated than in conventional radiography.

However, because of increasing use of spiral CT and multislice imaging, CT is now a high-dose procedure. U.S. Public Health Service data suggest that 5% of all x-ray examinations are CT; yet CT accounts for 35% of total patient dose. The CT dose is approximately equal to average fluoroscopic procedures.

As was pointed out in Chapters 29 and 30, CT differs in many important ways from other x-ray examinations. A regular x-ray film can be likened to a photograph taken with a flash: the patient is "floodlighted" with x-rays to directly expose the image receptor, whether it is film or an image intensifier. On the other hand, CT incorporates a fine, collimated beam of x-rays. This difference in radiation delivery also means that the dose distribution from CT is different that from radiographic procedures.

 CT dose is nearly uniform throughout the imaging volume; radiographic and fluoroscopic doses are high at the entrance surface and very low at the exit surface.

Part of the dose efficiency of CT is because of the precise collimation of the x-ray beam. Scatter radiation increases patient dose and reduces radiographic contrast. Because CT uses narrow, well-collimated x-ray beams, scatter radiation is significantly reduced and contrast resolution significantly improved. Thus a larger percentage of the x-rays contribute usefully to the image.

The precise collimation used in CT means that only a well-defined volume of tissue is irradiated during each scan. The ideal x-ray beam for CT would have sharp boundaries. There would be no overlap between adjacent scans. Thus the dose delivered to a patient from a series of ideal adjacent CT scans should be the same as that from a single slice.

Figure 40-6 illustrates how this ideal situation cannot be attained in practice. The size of the focal spot of the x-ray tube blurs the sharp boundaries of the section.

Also, the x-ray beam is not precisely parallel, so some spreading occurs as the beam traverses the image field.

If a series of adjacent images is performed with an automatically indexed patient couch, the couch movement must be precise. If the couch moves too much between scans, some tissue will be missed. If it moves too little, some tissue in each scan will be double exposed.

 It is essential that CT collimators be periodically monitored for proper adjustment.

Finally, and perhaps most important, if the prepatient collimators are too wide, tissues near the interface of each image may receive twice the dose that they otherwise should. Thus in practice, a series of adjacent images delivers a slightly higher dose than a single image because of the overlapping dose profiles.

Typical CT doses range from 3000 to 5000 mrad (30 to 50 mGy_t) during head imaging and 4000 to 6000 mrad (40 to 60 mGy_t), during body imaging. These values are only approximate and vary widely depending on the type of CT scanner and the examination technique. Because the CT x-ray beam is well collimated, the area of irradiation can be precisely controlled. Thus radiosensitive organs such as the eyes can be selectively avoided.

Shields as protection from the primary x-ray beam in CT are of little use. Not only does the metal from these shields produce terrible artifacts in the image, but the rotational scheme of the x-ray source also greatly reduces their effectiveness. The patient, however, can effectively be shielded from the low levels of scatter radiation as long as the direct x-ray beam does not intersect the shield.

Patient dose during multislice spiral CT is somewhat

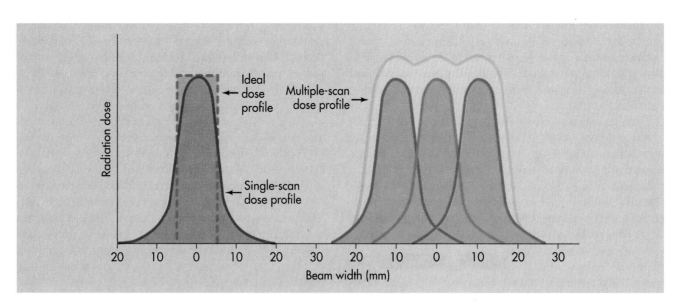

FIGURE 40-6 Patient dose distribution in CT is complicated because the profile of the x-ray beam cannot be made sharp.

more difficult to assess than the dose during conventional CT. At a pitch of 1.0:1, the patient dose is about the same. At a higher beam pitch, the dose is reduced compared with conventional CT. At a lower beam pitch, patient dose is increased. (see Chapter 30 for a discussion of beam pitch.)

As with any radiographic procedure, many factors influence patient dose. For CT scanning a generalization is possible.

CT Patient Dose

$$\text{Patient dose} = k\frac{IE}{\sigma^2 w^3 h}$$

where k = conversion factor

I = beam intensity in milliampere-seconds

E = average beam energy in kiloelectron volts (approximately $\frac{1}{2}$ kVp)

σ = a system noise

w = pixel size

h = slice thickness

Note that, as with radiography, patient dose is proportional to the x-ray beam intensity. It is also directly proportional to the average beam energy. Other factors are variables unique to CT scanning. Sigma *(σ)* is the noise. This is equivalent to quantum mottle in screen-film radiography and represents random statistical variations in the CT numbers. The *w* stands for the pixel size, one of the determinants of spatial resolution. The last factor, *h*, is the slice thickness. A decrease in either the noise, pixel size, or slice thickness while the other factors remain constant results in increased patient dose.

All other factors being equal, a low-noise, high-resolution CT image results in a higher patient dose. The challenge in CT, as indeed with all x-ray imaging, is not so much to deliver fantastically good resolution and low noise (since this could be achieved at the cost of very high patient dose) but to use the x-ray beam efficiently, producing the best possible image at a reasonable dose to the patient.

REDUCTION OF OCCUPATIONAL EXPOSURE

The radiologic technologist can do much to minimize occupational radiation exposure. Most exposure-control procedures require not sophisticated equipment or especially vigorous training but simply a conscientious attitude in the performance of assigned duties. Most equipment characteristics, technique changes, and administrative procedures designed to minimize patient dose also reduce occupational exposure.

In diagnostic radiology, at least 95% of the radiologic technologist's occupational radiation exposure come from fluoroscopy and mobile radiography. Attention to the cardinal principles of radiation protection (time, dis-

tance, and shielding) and ALARA is the most important aspect of occupational radiation control.

During fluoroscopy, the radiologist should minimize x-ray beam-on time. This can be done by careful technique, which includes intermittent activation of the fluoroscopic beam rather than one long period of x-ray beam-on time. It is a common radiation-protection practice to maintain a log of fluoroscopy time by recording the x-ray beam-on time, using the 5-minute reset timer.

During fluoroscopy, the radiologic technologist should step back from the table when his or her immediate presence and assistance is not required. The radiologic technologist should also take maximal advantage of all protective shielding, including the apron, curtain, Bucky slot cover, and radiologist.

Each mobile x-ray unit should have a protective apron assigned to it. The radiologic technologist should wear a protective apron during all mobile studies and maintain maximum distance from the source. The exposure cord on a portable x-ray unit must be at least 2 m long. The primary beam should never be pointed at the radiologic technologist or other nearby personnel.

During radiography, the radiologic technologist is positioned behind an operating console barrier. These barriers are usually considered secondary barriers because they intercept leakage and scatter radiation. Thus leaded glass and leaded gypsum board are often unnecessary for such barriers. The useful beam should never be directed toward the operating console barrier.

Other work assignments in diagnostic imaging, such as scheduling, darkroom duties, and filing, result in essentially no occupational radiation exposure.

Occupational Radiation Monitoring

Radiologists and radiologic technologists are routinely exposed to ionizing radiation. The level of exposure depends on the type and frequency of activity in which these professionals are engaged. Determining the quantity of radiation received requires a program of occupational radiation monitoring. *Occupational radiation monitoring* refers to procedures instituted to estimate the amount of radiation received by individuals who work in a radiation environment.

Occupational radiation monitoring is required when there is any likelihood that an individual will receive more than one tenth of the recommended dose limit. Most clinical diagnostic imaging personnel must be monitored; however, it is usually not necessary to monitor diagnostic radiology secretaries and file clerks. Furthermore, it is usually not necessary to monitor operating room personnel, except perhaps those routinely involved in cystoscopy and C-arm fluoroscopy.

The occupational radiation monitor offers no protection against radiation exposure. This monitor simply measures the quantity of radiation to which the monitor was exposed and therefore is used as an indicator of the exposure of the wearer. There are basically four types of personnel monitors in use in diagnostic radiology: film badges, TLDs, optically stimulated luminescence dosimeters, and pocket ionization chambers.

Regardless of the type of monitor, it is essential that it be obtained from a certified laboratory. In-house processing of radiation monitors should not be atttempted.

Film badges. Film badges came into general use during the 1940s and have been widely used in diagnostic radiology ever since. Film badges are specially designed devices in which a small piece of film similar to dental radiographic film is sandwiched between metal filters inside a plastic holder. Figure 40-7 is a view of two typical film badge monitors.

The film incorporated into a film badge is special radiation dosimetry film that is particularly sensitive to x-rays. The optical density on the exposed and processed film is proportional to the exposure received by the film badge.

Carefully controlled calibration, processing, and analyzing conditions are necessary for the film badge to accurately measure occupational radiation exposure. Usu-ally, exposures less than 10 mR (100 μGy_a) are not measured by film badge monitors, and the film badge vendor reports only that a minimum exposure was received. When higher exposures are received, they can be accurately reported.

The metal filters, along with the window in the plastic film holder, allows estimation of the x-ray energy. The usual filters are made of aluminum and copper. If the radiation exposure is a result of penetrating x-rays, the image of the filters on the processed film will be faint, and there may be no image at all of the window in the plastic holder. If the badge is exposed to soft x-rays, the filters will be well imaged, and the optical densities under the filters will allow estimation of the x-ray energy.

Often, the filters to the front of the badge differ in shape from the filters to the back of the badge. Radiation that had entered through the back of the badge would normally indicate that the person wearing the badge received considerably higher exposure than indicated, since the x-rays would have penetrated through the body before interacting with the film badge. For this reason, film badges must be worn with their proper side facing the front.

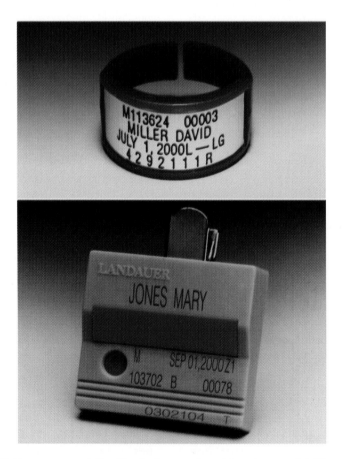

FIGURE 40-7 Some representative film badge monitors. Many have metal filters incorporated to help identify the type of radiation and its energy. *(Courtesy Landauer, Inc.)*

Film badges must be worn with their proper side to the front.

Several advantages of film badge occupational radiation monitors continue to make them popular. They are inexpensive, easy to handle, easy to process, and reasonably accurate, and they have been in use for several decades.

Film badge monitors also have disadvantages. They cannot be reused, and since they incorporate film as the sensing device, they cannot be worn for long periods because of fogging caused by temperature and humidity.

Film badge monitors should never be left in an enclosed car or other area where excessive temperatures may occur. The fogging produced by elevated temperature and humidity results in a falsely high evaluation of exposure. Film badge monitors should not be worn for longer than 1 month.

Thermoluminescence dosimeters. The sensitive material of the TLD monitor (Figure 40-8) is lithium fluoride (LiF) in crystalline form, either as a powder or more often as a small chip approximately 3 mm square and 1 mm thick. When exposed to x-rays, the TLD absorbs energy and stores it in the form of excited electrons in the crystalline lattice.

When heated, these excited electrons fall back to their normal orbital state with the emission of visible light. The intensity of visible light is measured with a photomultiplier tube and is proportional to the radiation dose received by the crystal. This sequence was described in Chapter 39.

The TLD occupational radiation monitor has several advantages over film. It is more sensitive and more accurate. Properly calibrated TLD monitors can measure exposure as low as 5 mR (50 μGy_a). The TLD monitor does not suffer from loss of information after exposure to excessive heat or humidity. Consequently, TLDs can be worn for up to 1 year.

The primary disadvantage of TLD personnel monitoring is cost. The price of a typical TLD monitoring service is perhaps twice that of film badge monitoring. If the frequency of monitoring is quarterly, however, the cost is about the same.

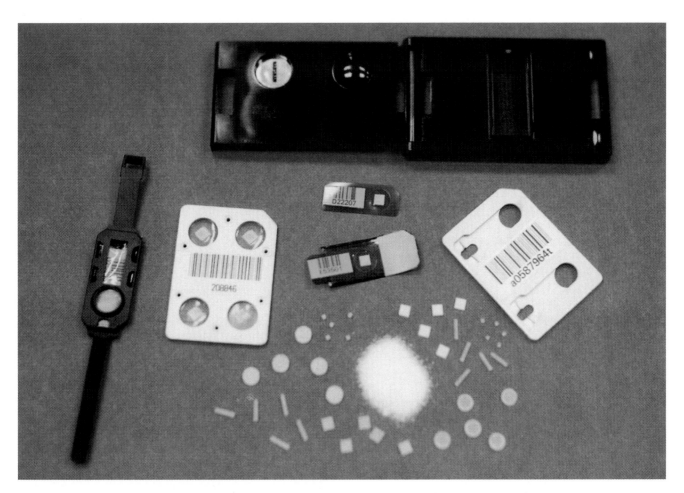

FIGURE 40-8 TLDs are available as chips, disks, rods, and powder. They are used for area and environmental radiation monitoring and especially for occupational radiation monitoring. *(Courtesy Bicron.)*

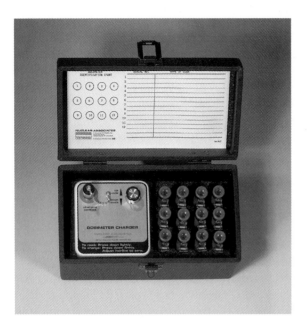

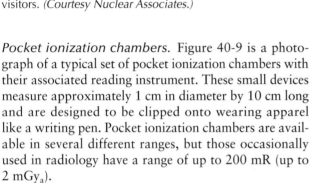

FIGURE 40-9 Pocket ionization chambers may be used in diagnostic radiology for employees exposed occasionally and visitors. *(Courtesy Nuclear Associates.)*

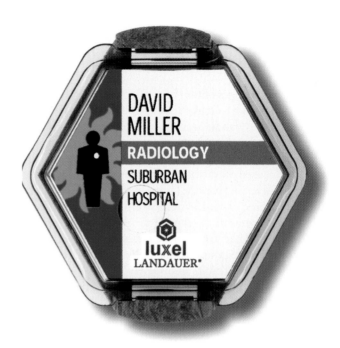

FIGURE 40-10   OSL dosimeter. *(Courtesy Landauer.)*

Pocket ionization chambers. Figure 40-9 is a photograph of a typical set of pocket ionization chambers with their associated reading instrument. These small devices measure approximately 1 cm in diameter by 10 cm long and are designed to be clipped onto wearing apparel like a writing pen. Pocket ionization chambers are available in several different ranges, but those occasionally used in radiology have a range of up to 200 mR (up to 2 mGy$_a$).

The use of a pocket ionization chamber can be somewhat time consuming because it is an electroscope. The chamber must be charged to a predetermined voltage before use so that the scale indicates zero. As the chamber is exposed to radiation, the charge is neutralized so that a subsequent analysis of the chamber voltage indicates the total radiation exposure.

Pocket ionization chambers are not normally used in diagnostic radiology. Their use requires daily identification of personnel exposures. Manipulation of the charging and reading mechanism is required daily. They may be used for a day or so to monitor nonradiologic personnel such as nurses.

Pocket ionization chambers are reasonably accurate and sensitive, but they do have a limited range. If exposure exceeds the range of the dosimeter, the precise level of exposure would never be known. Pocket ionization chambers are fairly expensive and can be easily damaged.

Optically stimulated luminescence. Optically stimulated luminescence (OSL) dosimeters have come into use the past few years (Figure 40-10). They are worn and

handled just as film badges and TLD are and are about the same size. The OSL dosimeters have some advantages to all of the previous dosimeters (see Chapter 39). They are sensitive and more accurate and can be used for a year.

Placement of the occupational radiation monitor. Much discussion and research in health physics have gone into providing precise recommendations about where a radiologic technologist should wear the occupational radiation monitor. The official publications of the National Council on Radiation Protection and Measurements (NCRP) offer suggestions that have been adopted as regulations in most states.

Many radiologic technologists wear their personnel monitors in front at the waist or chest level because it is convenient to clip the badge over a belt or a shirt pocket. If the technologist is not involved in fluoroscopic procedures, these locations are acceptable.

If the radiologic technologist participates in fluoroscopy, then the occupational radiation monitor should be positioned on the collar above the protective apron. The recommended dose limit of 5000 mrem/yr (50 mSv/yr) refers to the effective dose. When a protective apron is worn during fluoroscopy, exposure to the collar region is approximately 20 times greater than that to the trunk of the body beneath the protective apron. Thus, if the occupational radiation monitor is worn beneath the protective apron, it will record a falsely low exposure and will not indicate what could be a hazardous exposure to unprotected body parts.

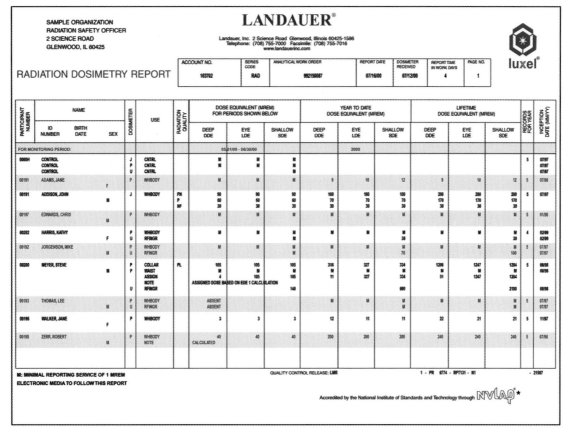

FIGURE 40-11 The occupational radiation monitoring report must include the items of information shown here. *(Courtesy Landauer, Inc.)*

Nearly all state radiation-control programs recommend or require that the occupational radiation monitor be worn at collar level. This is the official recommendation of the Council of Radiation Control Program Directors (CRCPD).

In some clinical situations, it may be advisable to wear more than one radiation monitor; however, this is not normally necessary for radiologist technologists. Two exceptions exist: during pregnancy and extremity exposure. The abdomen should be monitored during pregnancy. The extremities should be monitored during cardiovascular and interventional procedures during which the radiologist's hands are in close proximity to the useful beam. Nuclear medicine technologists should wear extremity monitors when handling radioactive material.

Occupational Radiation Monitoring Report

State and federal regulations require that the results of the occupational radiation monitoring program be recorded in a precise fashion and maintained for review. Annual, quarterly, monthly, or weekly monitoring periods are acceptable.

The occupational radiation monitoring report must contain a number of specific items of information (Figure 40-11). The first column is an identification number assigned to the radiation worker and monitor. The second column identifies the date of birth. The third column lists the employee sex and is followed by other columns containing information about use and radiation dose equivalent. Additional personal data required include birthdate and gender.

The exposure data that must be included on the form are the current exposure, cumulative annual exposure, and cumulative lifetime exposure. Separate monitors (for example, extremity monitors or fetal monitors) would be identified separately from the whole-body monitor.

Occasionally, if occupational exposure involves low-energy radiation, a dose to the skin might occur that is greater than the dose of penetrating radiation. In such case, the skin dose is separately identified. There are areas on the report for neutron radiation exposure to accommodate nuclear reactor and particle accelerator workers.

When a radiologic technologist changes employment, the total radiation exposure history must be transferred to the records of the new employer. Consequently, when leaving a job, he or she should automatically receive a report of the total radiation-exposure history at that facility. Such a report should be given automatically; if it is not, it must be requested.

When establishing an occupational radiation monitoring program, the supplier of the monitor should be informed of the type of radiation facility involved. That information influences the method of calibration of the monitors and the control monitors. After processing, the response of the control monitor is subtracted from each individual monitor. That way, the report for each individual monitor represents only occupational radiation exposure. The control monitor is used to measure the background exposure during transportation, handling and storage of all film badges and serves as a comparison badge. The control monitor should never be stored in or adjacent to a radiation area. It should be kept in a distant room or office.

All monitors should be returned to the supplier together and in a timely fashion so that they can be processed together. Lost or inadvertently exposed monitors must be evaluated, and an estimate of the true exposure should be made by the medical physicist. Unless there are unusual circumstances, the estimate can be made by averaging the exposures from the previous 6 months.

Protective Apparel

The operating console is usually positioned behind fixed protective barriers during diagnostic radiographic procedures. During fluoroscopy or mobile radiography, radiologic personnel are in the examination room and near the x-ray source.

 Protective apparel must be worn during fluoroscopy and mobile radiology.

Protective gloves and aprons are available in many sizes and shapes. They are usually constructed of lead-impregnated vinyl. Some protective garments are impregnated with tin or other metals because other metals have some advantages over lead as a shielding material in the diagnostic x-ray energy range.

The normal thicknesses for protective apparel are 0.25, 0.5, and 1 mm Pb equivalent. The garments themselves are much thicker than these dimensions, but they provide shielding equivalent to that thickness of lead (Table 40-5). Protection of at least 0.25 mm Pb is required.

Of course, maximum exposure reduction is obtained with the 1-mm lead equivalent garment but an apron of this material can weigh as much as 10 kg (22 lb). The wearer could be exhausted by end of the fluoroscopy schedule just from having to carry the protective apron.

The x-ray attenuation at 75 kVp for 0.25-mm lead equivalent and 1-mm lead equivalent is 66% and 99%, respectively. Most radiology departments find 0.5-mm lead equivalent protective garments a workable compromise between unnecessary weight and desired protection.

Protective aprons for cardiovascular and interventional radiographic suites should be the wrap-around type. During these procedures, there can be a lot of personnel movement, and some professionals, such as an anesthesiologist, may even have their back to the radiation source.

 Protective aprons and gloves should be fluoroscoped at least once a year to check for cracks.

When not in use, protective apparel must be stored on properly designed racks. If they are continuously folded or heaped in the corner, cracks can develop. At least once a year, aprons and gloves should be fluoroscoped to be sure that no such cracks have appeared. If fluoroscopy is not available, high-kVp radiography (for example, 120 kVp/10 mAs) may be used.

Position

During fluoroscopy, all personnel should remain as far from the patient as possible, keeping the front of the apron facing the radiation source at all times. After loading spot films, the radiologic technologist should take a step or two backward from the table when his or her presence is not required. The radiologist should be trained to use the deadman's foot switch sparingly. Naturally, when x-ray beam-on time is high, the radiation exposure to patient and personnel is proportionately high.

Patient Holding

Many patients referred for x-ray examination are not physically able to support themselves (for example, infants, the elderly, and the incapacitated). Mechanical restraining devices should be available for such patients. Otherwise, a relative or friend accompanying the patient should be asked to help. As a last resort, other hospital employees, such as nurses and orderlies (but never diagnostic imaging employees) may be used *occasionally* to hold patients. In some states, such as New York, it is illegal for radiologic technologists to hold patients, and it is illegal to hire someone for this purpose.

TABLE 40-5	Some Physical Characteristics of Protective Lead Aprons			
		PERCENTAGE OF X-RAY ATTENUATION		
Equivalent Thickness (mm Pb)	**Weight (lb)**	**50 kVp**	**75 kVp**	**100 kVp**
0.25	3-10	97	66	51
0.50	6-15	99.9	88	75
1.00	12-25	99.9	99	94

Radiology staff should never hold patients.

When it is necessary to have another person hold the patient, protective apparel must be provided to that person. An apron and gloves are necessary, and the holder should be carefully positioned and instructed so that he or she is not exposed to the useful beam. Because a child's holder is often the mother, the radiologic technologist should be sure to ask if she could be pregnant.

REDUCTION OF UNNECESSARY PATIENT DOSE

There are many sources of unnecessary patient dose over which the radiologic technologist has considerable control. *Unnecessary patient dose* is defined as any radiation dose that is not required for the patient's well-being or proper management and care.

Unnecessary Examinations

The radiologic technologist has practically no control over what some consider the largest source of unnecessary patient dose: the unnecessary x-ray examination. This is almost exclusively the radiologist's or clinician's responsibility. Radiologic technologists can help by inquiring whether the patient has had a previous x-ray examination. If so, perhaps those films should be obtained for review before continuing.

Unfortunately, this source of unnecessary patient dose presents a serious dilemma for the radiologist and the clinician. Many x-ray examinations are knowingly requested when the yield of helpful information may be extremely low or nonexistent. When such an examination is performed, the benefit to the patient in no way compensates for the radiation dose.

If the examination is not performed, the clinician and radiologist may be severely criticized if the patient's ultimate management results in failure, even though the examination in question would have contributed little, if anything, to effective patient management; the radiologist may even be sued. In such situations, the radiologist is caught between the proverbial "rock and a hard place."

Routine x-ray examinations should not be performed when there is no precise medical indication. Substantial evidence shows that such examinations are of little benefit because they are not cost-effective and the disease detection rate is very low. Examples of such cases follow:

1. **Mass screening for tuberculosis.** General screening has not been found effective. Better methods of tuberculosis testing are now available. Some x-ray screening may be appropriate in high-risk groups (for example, medical and paramedical personnel), in service personnel posing a potential community hazard (for example, food handlers or teachers), and in special occupational groups (for example, miners and workers having contact with beryllium, asbestos, glass, or silica).

2. **Hospital admission.** Chest x-ray examinations for routine hospital admission when there is no clinical indication of chest disease should not be performed. Among patients who might be candidates for such examination are those admitted to the pulmonary service.

3. **Preemployment physicals.** Chest and lower back x-ray examinations are not justified because little knowledge can be gained about previous injury or disease.

4. **Periodic health examinations.** Many physicians and health care organizations promote annual or biannual physical examinations. Certainly, when such an examination is conducted on an asymptomatic patient, it should not include x-ray examination, especially fluoroscopic examination.

5. **Whole-body multislice spiral CT screening.** Some facilities now advertise this procedure to the public for self-referral. Until there is evidence of a significant disease-detection rate, this should not be done. The radiation dose is too high.

Repeat Examinations

One area of unnecessary radiation exposure that the radiologic technologist can influence is that of repeat examinations. The frequency of repeat examinations has been variously estimated to range as high as 10% of all examinations. In the typical busy hospital facility, repeat examinations do not normally exceed 5%. Examinations with the highest repeat rates are those of lumbar spine, thoracic spine, and abdomen.

Some repeat examinations are caused by equipment malfunctions. However, most are caused by error by the radiologic technologist. Studies of causes of repeat examinations have shown that improper positioning and poor radiographic technique resulting in overexposure or underexposure are primarily responsible for repeats. Motion and improper collimation are responsible for some repeats. Infrequent errors that also contribute to repeat examinations are dirty screens, use of improperly loaded cassettes, light leaks, chemical fog, artifacts caused by a dirty processor, wrong projection, improper patient preparation, grid errors, and multiple exposure.

Radiographic Technique

In general, the use of a high-kVp technique results in reduced patient dose. Increases in kVp are always associated with a reduced mAs to obtain an acceptable radiographic optical density, and this in turn results in reduced patient dose. This occurs because the patient dose is linearly related to the mAs, but it is related to approximately the square of the kVp. An area of radiography where high-kVp technique is widely accepted is examination of the chest.

CHALLENGE QUESTIONS

1. Define or otherwise identify:
   a. GSD
   b. Entrance skin exposure
   c. Shadow shield
   d. Mean marrow dose
   e. Glandular dose
   f. Contact shield

2. What is the dose limit for diagnostic imaging personnel?

3. During what two examination procedures is occupational radiation exposure usually the highest?

4. Why is diagnostic medical radiation exposure to patients commanding increased attention?

5. List the three ways that patient dose is reported.

6. What is the estimated GSD caused by diagnostic x-ray examination?

7. Why are measurements of gonadal dose important?

8. Why is the ESE not used in values stated for patient dose in mammography?

9. What is the difference between ESE in CT vs. ESE in routine radiography?

10. What is the required length of the exposure cord on the mobile radiographic unit?

11. When must personnel radiation monitoring be provided?

12. Describe the design of film badges. How are they worn and where are they placed on the body?

13. List the exposure data that must be included in the personnel monitoring report.

14. What is an appropriate thickness of protective apparel?

15. What is the procedure for holding patients during an x-ray examination?

16. What types of screening x-rays are not recommended?

17. Describe the features of optically stimulated dosimetry that make it particularly effective for occupational radiation monitoring.

Answers to Challenge Questions

CHAPTER 1

1. a. The ability to do work or physical influence surroundings because of position or chemical state or nuclear state.
   b. $E = mc^2$, where E is energy expressed in joule, m is mass expressed in kilograms, and c is the speed of light expressed in meters per second.
   c. Any electromagnet or particulate radiation that has sufficient energy to remove an electron from an atom.
   d. 2/1000 of a rad where the rad (radiation absorbed dose) is the definition of 100 ergs of energy per gram of absorbing material.
   e. Approximately 300 mrad.
   f. The first heated filament x-ray tube was developed by a physicist, William Coolidge, in 1913.
   g. The production of continuous x-ray images in real time using a specialized x-ray imaging system, the fluoroscope, with low continuous mA. The fluoroscope was first demonstrated by Thomas Edison in 1898.
   h. The procedure of confining the x-rayed beam to the area of anatomic interest to limit patient radiation dose.
   i. Biochemistry
   j. A phosphor that glows when excited with x-rays. This is the phosphor that Roentgen was experimenting with when he discovered x-rays.
3. Weight is determined by the force of gravity. Weight changes in value with position from a gravitational mass such as the Earth or moon. Mass is constant. It is independent of position and is determined by its energy equivalence.

5. X-rays interact at the electron level or nuclear level, ionizing an atom or ejecting a nuclear particle respectively. Lower-energy electromagnetic radiation interacts with molecule cells and larger objects in a way that usually will not always elevate the temperature of the object.

7. An x-ray, for instance, interacts with an orbital electron of an atom of tissue. The electron absorbs some energy from the x-ray and is released from the atom. The electron (negative ion) and resulting atom (positive ion) are called an *ion pair*.

9. It was a casual and unexpected finding; in fact, others had produced x-rays before Roentgen, but because they were focused on a known area of physics, the x-ray findings were discarded.

11. As low as reasonably achievable.

13. In Roentgen's time, glass plates were used. Leonard cut exposure time in half by exposing two glass plates with emulsion sides together, leading to the development of double-emulsion film. During World War I, radiologists began to use film, substituting cellulose nitrate for glass.

15. Radon 222, a gas.

17. Electrons emitted from the filament of an electronic vacuum tube, an x-ray tube for instance.

19. See Box 1-3.

CHAPTER 2

1. a. Equal lengths have equal value.
   b. The last numeral to the right that is meaningful to the answer. A figure is significant if it is followed by a number greater than zero.
   c. A special unit to express radiation exposure, radiation absorbed dose, effective dose equivalent, and radioactivity.
   d. Coordinate values on a two-dimensional graph (x, y).
   e. Joule-second (J s).
   f. The mathematical relationship between similar quantities such as feet to the mile or pounds to the kilogram.
   g. Equal length varied by an order of magnitude.
   h. The denominator.
   i. Method of describing a wide range of values using exponents to the base 10 (e.g., a (10^b).

3. 2^3.

5. a. 0.7.
   b. 0.081.
   c. 0.467.

7. a. 4.2×10^{-3}.
   b. 1.067×10^{-2}.

9. a. 7.
   b. 2.14.

11. 0.003.

13. Find a common denominator.

15. As one factor increases or decreases, the accompanying factor increases or decreases by the same amount.

17. 6.59.

19. 6.56 km/L.

CHAPTER 3

1. a. The three fundamental units of measurements: length (meter, m), mass (kilogram, kg), and time (seconds, s).
   b. Secondary quantities that are derived from a combination of one or more of the three base quantities (for example, volume, density, and velocity).
   c. Quantities derived from the base quantities that are used only in specialty areas of science such as the radiological units used in radiologic science.
   d. The property of matter that acts to resist change in its state of motion. Described in Newton's first law: the state of a mass will remain constant until acted on by an outside force.
   e. The rate of change of velocity with time.
   f. The transfer of thermal energy from one position to another by the transfer of molecules or particles physically.
   g. The force applied to an object multiplied by the distance over which it is applied.
   h. The rate of change of position with time, sometimes called *speed*.
   i. The scaler quantity has only magnitude. A vector quantity has magnitude and direction.
   j. The force on an object is equal to its mass multiplied by its acceleration.

3. 250 in³.

5. Approximately 0.7 m/s.

7. 0.1 ft/sec.

9. 770 N.

11. 735 N (on Earth), 120 N (on moon).

13. 3.0 kgm²/s³ or 3 W.

15. 88.2 J.

17. 25° C.

19. Exposure, dose, effective dose, and radioactivity.

CHAPTER 4

1. a. Form of electromagnetic radiation that has no mass and no charge.
   b. The first description of an atom having a nucleus.
   c. Electromagnetic and particulate radiation.
   d. Neutrons and protons.
   e. An arrangement of all known elements into rows and columns. The rows relate to the number of electron shells present; the columns relate to the number of electrons in the outermost shell.
   f. Time required to reduce radioactivity to half its original value.

g. Tungsten.

h. The nucleus of the helium atom, two neutrons and two protons.

i. Innermost electron shell.

j. New substance that is formed when two or more atoms of different elements combine.

3. 8, 9, 8, 17; 13, 14, 13, 27; 27, 33, 27, 60; 88, 138, 88, 226.

5. K = 2, L = 8, M = 8, N = 2.

7. a. 57.43 keV.
   b. 66.71 keV.
   c. 69.53 keV.

9. Approximately 2.5 curies.

11. Periodic table of the elements.

13. Electron, proton, and neutron.

15. No, positive charges do not move but are confined to the nucleus.

17. The arrangements of electron in the outermost shells.

19. Size and charge on the particle. An alpha particle has four units of mass and two units of charge. A beta particle has essentially no mass and one unit of charge.

CHAPTER 5

1. a. The smallest quantity of any type of electromagnet radiation; it may be pictured as a small bundle of energy, sometimes called a *quantum*.

   b. Characteristic of materials that allow x-rays to penetrate with a minimum of absorption. Radiolucent structures are nearly invisible to x-rays.

   c. A mathematical relationship describing the reduction in radiation intensity with distance from a point source. This decrease in intensity is inversely proportional to the square of the distance of the object to the source.

   d. The number of wavelengths passing a point per second.

   e. Energy can be transmuted, but it cannot be created or destroyed.

   f. A form of ionizing electromagnet radiation emitted from the nuclei of radioactive atoms.

   g. The wide range of electromagnet radiation described by its frequency wavelength or energy.

   h. The mathematical or graphical description of a simple harmonic motion.

   i. A single unit of electromagnet radiation.

   j. A narrow region in the middle electromagnet spectrum extending from approximately 400 nm (blue) to 700 nm (red).

3. 400 m/s; 2400 m or about 1½ mi.

5. 2.88 m.

7. 2.6×10^{19} Hz, 1.15×10^{-11} m.

9. 0.75 mR/mAs.

11. Velocity = frequency × wavelength ($v = f \times \lambda$).

13. $I_1 / I_2 = d_2^2 / d_1^2$ or $I_1 / I_2 = (d_2 / d_1)^2$, where I_1 is the intensity at distance d_1 from the source and I_2 is the intensity at distance d_2 from the source. The reduction in intensity with distance from a point source of radiation.

15. Radiofrequency (hertz), visible light (meters), and x-radiation (electron volts).

17. Origin. X-rays are emitted from the electron cloud. Gamma rays are emitted from the nucleus.

19. Partial absorption of energy; the combination of absorption and scatter.

CHAPTER 6

1. a. Electric charge is a fundamental property of matter. It comes in discrete units that are either positive or negative particles: the proton and the electron. These units are too small to be useful, so the fundamental unit of electric charge is the coulomb (C).

   b. The study of electric charges in motion; measured in amperes (A).

   c. Electric potential is equal to electric current multiplied by the resistance of the conductor: V = IR.

   d. Energy produced or consumed per unit time. The product of electric current and electric potential; the time rate at which work can be done.

   e. The form of electricity provided by your local power company. Current in which electrons oscillate back and forth.

   f. An ordered assembly of electric components and wiring. An electric circuit results when resistance is controlled and the conductor is made into a closed path.

   g. Material that impedes the movement of electrons opposite of conductor.

   h. The study of stationary electric charges.

   i. Material that exhibits no resistance below a critical temperature. Allows an electric current to flow in a supercooled conductor without supplying an electric potential.

   j. A devise to measure the intensity of electric current.

3. 1.57×10^{20} electrons.

5. a. 2.2 amp.
   b. 45.8 amp.

7. a. 242 watts.
   b. 5038 watts.

9. The coulomb (C). One C = 6.3×10^{18} electron charges.

11. Contact, friction, and induction.

13. 1. Unlike charges attract; like charges repel. 2. Coulomb's law 3. Electric-charge distribution 4. Electric-charge concentration.

15. Water (water vapor, moisture). The moisture in Houston allows electrified objects to be drained of electrons spontaneously or easily.

17. A material such as silicon or germanium that will conduct electrons under some conditions and will impede electron flow under other conditions. The development of semiconductors led first to the transistor, then to integrated circuits, and finally to microchips, which are responsible for the present explosion in computer technology.
19. The watt.

CHAPTER 7

1. a. Two poles.
   b. Intensified magnetic field at the end of a magnetized object measured in ampere meter.
   c. The ability to transfer energy from one object to another without touching.
   d. Magnetic force is proportional to the product of the magnetic pole strength divided by the square of the distance between them.
   e. An accumulation of many atomic magnets with their dipoles aligned.
   f. The degree to which materials can be magnetized.
   g. Ability of certain materials to be strongly attracted by a magnet and (usually) permanently magnetized.
   h. Both are units of magnetic intensity. 10,000 gauss = 1 tesla.
   i. A naturally occurring magnet.
3. 0.5 mt.
5. Lodestone was discovered in Asia Minor (currently western Turkey) and was used to locate water.
7. Natural magnets, artificially induced permanent magnets, and electromagnets.
9. Diamagnetic.
11. Transformer design; magnetic resonance imaging.
13. The magnetic field of the domain can be transferred to the object.
15. It loses its magnetic properties.
17. Yes.
19. From approximately 50 to 100 microtesla.

CHAPTER 8

1. a. Material that inhibits or stops the flow of electrons.
   b. Force applied to move electrons in a conductor; also called *electromotor force*.
   c. A coil of wire that can induce a magnetic field.
   d. Induction of a magnetic field in one object by the magnetic field of a nearby object.
   e. A device that allows alternating current to power a direct-current power motor.
   f. A transformer having a single iron core with only one winding of wire.
   g. A device to measure electric current.
   h. A multicore transformer used in the high-voltage generator of an x-ray imaging system. Because it traps even more of the magnetic field lines of the primary wiring, it is more efficient than a closed-core transformer.
   i. An electron tube whose components are fixed in a vacuum created inside a glass or metal envelope.
3. By supplying current to a group of wires, which creates a magnetic field, making the wire act like a tiny electromagnet.
5. 27 milliamps.
7. 1000:1.
9. A material that either conducts or insulates depending on an applied electric field. The basis for modern microelectronics.
11. 44 ohms.
13. A helix coil of current-carrying wire that produces a magnetic field along the axis of the helix.
15. The process of inducing a current flow through a secondary coil by passing a varying current through the primary coil.
17. Mechanical energy, such as steam or falling water, is used to turn a loop of wire in the presence of a magnetic field.

CHAPTER 9

1. a. An electronic device designed to terminate x-ray exposure after properly exposing an image receptor.
   b. A method of adjusting the voltage to the x-ray imaging system through a constant value in response to changes in voltage supplied by the power company.
   c. An electrical circuit device that stores charge.
   d. Placed in the tube circuit; connected at the center of the secondary winding of the high-voltage step-up transformer.
   e. An electrical device that contains two electrodes.
   f. The magnitude of change in the voltage potential applied to the x-ray tube.
   g. A single-core transformer designed to supply a precise voltage to the filament circuit and to the high-voltage circuit of the x-ray imaging system.
   h. The process of changing alternating-current voltage to direct-current voltage.
3. 71.7 volt peak.
5. 6 amps.
7. Answers vary.
9. Extremity x-rays.
11. On/off control, kVp selection, mA selection, time (mAs) selection, and automatic-exposure controls.
13. Primary voltage and secondary voltage are in direct relation to the number of turns of the transformer.
15. 3.3 mAs.
17. The high-voltage transformer is just one component of a high-voltage generator.
19. Single phase, 100%; three phase, twelve pulse, 4%; three phase, six pulse, 14%; high frequency, 1%.

CHAPTER 10

1. a. The graph of the rate at which the housing of an x-ray tube will cool.
   b. X-rays that escape through the protective housing; they contribute nothing in the way of diagnostic information.
   c. A measure of thermal energy. HU = kVp × mA × s.
   d. Component of an x-ray tube cathode designed to confine the electron beam to a small area of the anode.
   e. Most anodes revolve at 3400 rpm; anodes of high-capacity tubes rotate at 10,000 rpm.
   f. Material used to make filament of the cathode. Addition of 1% to 2% thorium to the tungsten increases efficiency and prolongs tube life.
   g. The electric current flowing from cathode to anode, measured in milliamperes.
   h. A specially designed x-ray tube allowing rapid serial exposure.
   i. A form of heat dissipation. Transfer of heat by movement of heated molecules from one place to another.
   j. The electron cloud that surrounds the heated filament of an x-ray tube.
   k. X-rays emitted through the window.
3. Source-to-image receptor distance.
5. Computer control.
7. Filament failure. Thorium.
9. The large focal spot provides for high-capacity imaging. The small focal spot improves spatial resolution.
11. Stationary anodes serve low tube current and low-power uses. Rotating anodes are needed in most cases when high-intensity beams are required.
13. High atomic number results in increased efficiency of x-ray production. High thermal conductivity and melting point allow for longer, more intense x-ray examination.
15. Via an electromagnet induction motor.
17. Radiation intensity on the cathode side of the x-ray beam is higher than that on the anode side, allowing the radiographer to position the cathode side of the x-ray tube over the thicker part of the anatomic structure.
19. Space-charge-limited tubes are those under conditions of low kVp and high mA.

CHAPTER 11

1. a. Electrons emitted by the filament and directed to the target (traveling from the cathode to the anode).
   b. The intensity with which electrons are bound to the nucleus.
   c. X-rays produced by transitions of orbital electrons from outer to inner shells.

   d. X-rays produced by interaction of a projectile electron with a target nucleus.
   e. X-ray intensity, measured in milliroentgen (mR).
   f. Effective energy of the x-ray.
   g. The monoenergetic equivalent of an x-ray beam.
   h. Overall result is an increase in the effective energy of the x-ray beam (higher quality) and an accompanying reduction in x-ray quantity.
   i. The measure of x-ray energy of all x-rays.
   j. The x-ray tube target material principally used for mammography.
3. 0.6.
5. See Figure 11-10.
7. X-ray intensity and effective energy are increased.
9. By increasing the kVp.
11. Only approximately 1% of projectile electron energy is converted to x-rays.
13. Significantly helpful above the K absorption edge of 70 keV.
15. 0.014 nm.
17. A 15% increase in kVp is equivalent to doubling the mAs.
19. Characteristic x-rays.

CHAPTER 12

1. a. The filtration provided by the window of the x-ray tube.
   b. Milliroentgens (mR).
   c. Addition of a filter shifts the x-ray emission spectrum to the high-energy side, resulting in an x-ray beam with higher effective energy, greater penetrability, and higher quality.
   d. 15%.
   e. The thickness of filter or other absorbing material that will reduce intensity to half its original value.
   f. A compensating filter designed to shape the useful x-ray beam to the anatomic structure under examination so that the optical density of the finished radiograph will be more uniform.
   g. Identified numerically by half-value layer; also influenced by kVp and the added filtration in the useful beam.
   h. Method of reducing patient dose and increasing x-ray beam quality by selectively removing low-energy x-rays that have no chance of getting to the image receptor. Usually totals 2 to 3 mm of aluminum equivalent.
   i. Another term for x-ray quantity, measured in mR.
3. 1083 mR.
5. 38.9 mR.
7. 3.2 mm Al.
9. 3.12 (10^{17} electrons.
11. $I_1/I_2 = (d_2/d_1)^2$.

13. Double the mAs.
15. The square law involves compensating for a change in SID by changing the mAs by the factor SID². When the SID is increased, the mAs must be increased by SID² to maintain constant OD.
17. Because it is efficient at removing low-energy x-rays and because it is readily available, inexpensive, and easily shaped into filters.
19. Yes, the quantity is reduced with an increase in filtration.

CHAPTER 13

1. a. The relationship among transmitted x-rays, photoelectrically absorbed x-rays, and Compton's scattered x-rays resulting in the x-ray image.
   b. Scattering of very-low-energy x-rays with no loss of energy; also called *coherent* or *Thompson scattering*.
   c. The quantity of matter per unit volume, usually specified in kilograms per cubic meter (kg/m³). Sometimes reported in grams per cubic centimeter (gm/cm³).
   d. The threshold energy required by a photon to undergo pair production.
   e. A high-atomic-number material (for example, iodine and barium) administered in liquid form to improve the contrast resolution of an x-ray examination.
   f. X-ray ionization resulting in x-ray scattering.
   g. The result of absorption and scattering.
   h. Having a single energy. Characteristic x-rays are monoenergetic and the effective x-ray energy of an x-ray beam is the monoenergetic equivalent of the actual beam.
   i. Electrons released in ionization as the result of photoelectric interaction and Compton scattering.
   j. An x-ray absorption interaction in which the x-rays are not scattered but are totally absorbed. An electron or photoelectron is then removed from the atom.
3. 23.9 keV.
5. High atomic number; Z = 53. High mass density (4930 kg/m³) and relatively nontoxic.
7. Compton-scattered x-rays leave the target atom in the approximate direction of the incident x-ray beam.
9. Classic scattering, pair production, and photo disintegration. The x-ray energies involved are outside of the diagnostic imaging range.
11. The energy of the incident x-ray and the energy of the ejected electron.
13. When kVp is increased the probability of any interaction is reduced, but since the probability of photoelectric interaction is reduced much more rapidly than the probability of Compton interaction, the relative number of Compton interactions increases.

15. The relative frequency of photoelectric interaction compared with Compton interaction decreases with increasing x-ray energy.
17. Differential absorption resulting from photoelectric effect is proportional to the third power of the atomic number. Compton effect is unrelated to atomic number.
19. 1809:1.

CHAPTER 14

1. a. The material of which the base of modern x-ray film is made.
   b. The region of the silver halide crystal containing an impurity at which the latent image begins to form.
   c. The invisible image on an unprocessed radiograph.
   d. The ability to intercept more x-rays with fewer silver halide crystals.
   e. Film that is sensitive to the blue and green visible light spectrum.
   f. Silver bromide and silver iodide crystals.
   g. Using a film emulsion that has the same absorption properties as the color of light emitted under a radiographic intensifying screen.
   h. Marks, spurious objects, or unwanted optical density on the image that does not represent the anatomic structure.
   i. A reduction in image contrast resulting from x-ray exposure of unprocessed film by other than the useful beam; usually occurs during storage.
   j. The length of time radiographic film can be stored without objectionable increased fog. From top to bottom, one should label overcoat emulsion, adhesive layer base, adhesive layer emulsion overcoat. See Figure 14-1.
3. The base maintains its size and shape during use and processing so that no dimension of the film is changed.
5. $AgNO_3 + KBr \rightarrow AgBr \downarrow + KNO_3$.
7. Panchromatic film is sensitive to the entire visible light spectrum. Orthochromatic film is sensitive to only blue and green light.
9. In addition to precautions for other film handling and storage, the emulsion side must be loaded into the cassette against the radiographic intensifying screen.
11. The emulsion has not changed significantly in composition, but the manner in which silver halide crystals are grown, sized, and shaped has changed. Film base has evolved from glass to cellulose to polyester.
13. The amount of silver bromide in the emulsion and its covering power.
15. The sensitivity center attracts a few interstitially mobile electrons to form atomic silver. This process is amplified during processing.

17. At exposure times that are very short, as in angiography, or very long, as in mammography, with the use of the screen film image receptor, resulting optical density may be considerably lower than that expected.

19. Conventional screen film radiography uses two screens and film with double emulsion. Mammography uses a single screen and film having a single emulsion.

CHAPTER 15

1. a. A liquid into which other liquids or powder can be easily dissolved.
   b. The hardener in a developer that controls the swelling and softening of the emulsion.
   c. A chemical that supplies electrons to the positive silver ion, converting it to a silver atom.
   d. The action of two different chemicals combined is greater than the sum of the action of the individual chemicals.
   e. Maintenance of image quality with time; the image does not deteriorate with age. Absence of archival quality results in a loss of image contrast resulting from fog and an increasing brownish tint.
   f. Component of the turnaround assembly that with the master roller and guide shoes, controls the movement of film during processing.
   g. Another component of the turnaround assembly; a curved metal lip with smooth grooves to guide the film around the bend.
   h. Total processing time of 3 min rather than 90 s to improve image contrast and reduce patient dose.
   i. Light-emitting diode.
   j. Total processing time, from start to finish; normally 90 s. Development, 22 s. Fixing, 22 s. Washing, 20 s. Drying, 26 s.

3. Hydroquinone is rather slow acting but is responsible for the very blackest shades. Phenidone acts quickly and influences the lightest shades of gray. Phenidone controls the toe of the characteristic curve, and hydroquinone, the shoulder.

5. The cassette is automatically loaded from a supply rack and automatically unloaded into the processor.

7. Reduction and oxidation of a chemical compound. Think EUROPE: electrons are used in reduction/ oxidation produces electrons.

9. The Eastman Kodak Company.

11. Water.

13. $AG^+ + E^- = AG$.

15. They are toxic and can cause skin burns and eye irritation or injury.

17. Probably lack of glutaraldehyde in the developer.

19. This represents lack of archival quality, inadequate fixing, and retention of the fixing agent; it may also be caused by inadequate washing.

CHAPTER 16

1. a. The undesirable continuing emission of light after exposure of the phosphor to x-rays.
   b. With equal intensity in all directions.
   c. The ability to produce an accurate and clear image; also called *image blur*.
   d. The proper marriage of the sensitivity of a film emulsion to the light spectrum emitted by the radiographic intensifying screen.
   e. Loss of spatial resolution created by the size and distribution of the grains of phosphor in a radiographic intensifying screen.
   f. Appears on a radiograph as a speckled background; occurs most often when fast screens and high-kVp techniques are used.
   g. The active ingredient of a radiographic intensifying screen that converts the x-ray beam into light.
   h. Any device used to maintain close screen-film contact when the cassette is closed and latched. The result is improved contrast resolution and spatial resolution.
   i. The visible light.

3. Base followed by a reflective layer, followed by the phosphor, covered by a protection coating (see Figure 16-1).

5. Fine-detail screens with a speed of 50 to 100, par 50 to 80. Par-speed screens with a speed of 100. High-speed screens with speeds of 200 to 1200.

7. By radiographing a wire-mesh test tool.

9. A low-Z front contact material, base, phosphor, emulsion, film base, emulsion, phosphor, intensifying screen base, contact material, and a high-Z back.

11. Approximately 5% to 20%.

13. It can be a source of image blur and can reduce spatial resolution.

15. DQE represents the probability that an x-ray will be absorbed by a radiographic intensifying screen. CE represents the amount of light emitted by each absorbing event.

17. Intensification factor represents the speed of a radiographic intensifying screen. It is the ratio of the exposures required to produce the same optical density with and without the use of screens. IF = Exposure required without screens ÷ Exposure required with screens.

19. The splotchy appearance of a radiograph that has been exposed by a limited number of x-ray photons.

21. Handle very carefully; handle screens only when they are new and being installed in cassettes and when they are being cleaned. Clean them periodically. Check screen-film contact by radiographing a wire mesh; correct or replace cassettes.

CHAPTER 17

1. a. kVp, field size, and patient thickness.
   b. 1.0 mm of aluminum equivalent.
   c. Opening in a radiation-opaque material to allow only the useful beam to be emitted.
   d. When the image receptor and radiographic cone are not properly aligned so that part of the useful beam is attenuated in the column.
   e. Characteristic of any device that confines the useful x-ray beam to the anatomic structure under examination.
   f. X-rays produced from an area of the anode other than the focal spot.
   g. Positive beam–limiting device; an automatic, variable-aperture, light-localizing collimator.
   h. Reduced patient dose, improved image contrast.
   i. The x-rays transmitted through the patient and scattered in the patient that intersect the image receptor and contribute to the image formation.
   j. Reducing the thickness of tissue to improve both spatial and contrast resolution.
3. 1.83×2.28 cm.
5. 3.75×4.5 cm.
7. Image-forming x-rays are those transmitted to the patient and those scattered in the patient that interact with the image receptor. Remnant radiation includes image-forming x-rays plus the x-rays scattered in the patient but away from the image receptor.
9. Upper two diaphragms.
11. Mammography.
13. An opening in a radiopaque barrier of size just sufficient to allow the x-ray beam to cover the image receptor at the given SID.
15. Inadvertent absorption of part of the useful beam resulting in unexposed of the image receptor. Cone cutting.
17. They represent the shadow of lines etched in the plastic cover of the collimator.
19. Never.

CHAPTER 18

1. a. The degree of difference between light and dark areas on an image.
   b. X-rays produced in the patient as a consequence of Compton interaction.
   c. Misalignment of the grid and x-ray source causing some transmitted x-rays to be absorbed in grid strips rather than transmitted through interspace material.
   d. The grid and x-ray source are mispositioned so that the central ray of the useful x-ray beam intersects the grid lateral to the center line of the grid.
   e. The ratio of primary radiation transmitted through the grid to scatter radiation transmitted

through the grid. The higher the selectively, the better image contrast and the higher the patient dose.
   f. Positioning the image receptor 10 to 15 cm from the object to reduce scatter radiation and enhance image contrast.
   g. A relative term describing the amount of the Compton-scattered x-rays that are absorbed in grid strip material.
   h. The ratio of image contrast of a radiograph made with the grid to the image contrast obtained without a grid.
3. Parallel grids, focused grids, and crossed grids.
5. 33 lines/cm.
7. 363 μm.
9. Generally, when air-gap technique is used, the mAs is increased about 10% for every centimeter of air-gap. The technique factors are usually about the same as those for an 8:1 grid.
11. It has high mass density and high atomic number, and it is easily shaped and relatively inexpensive.
13. 2.
15. See Figures 18-7 and 18-11.
17. It removes the possibility of grid lines appearing on the image.
19. kVp, degree of cleanup, patient dose, and size and shape of the anatomic part being radiographed.

CHAPTER 19

1. a. The electric potential applied to the x-ray tube; kVp controls radiographic contrast.
   b. The product of the x-ray tube current and the time over which it is applied.
   c. X-ray beam quality.
   d. Specialty tubes with very small effective focal spots for improved spatial resolution.
   e. The distance from the x-ray source to the image receptor formally target the film distance.
   f. A high-voltage generator designed that ensures shorter x-ray exposure by reducing x-ray tube mA during exposure.
   g. The factor by which mAs should be changed when SID is changed to maintain constant optical density on the image.
3. 50 mA, 100 mA, 200 mA, 400 mA, 600 mA, 800 mA, and 1000 mA.
5. When the SID is changed, the kVp should not be changed. The mA and exposure time (mAs) should be changed according to the square law. When the SID is changed from 100 to 180 cm, the mAs should be increased as follows: $180^2/100^2 = 3.24$.
7. An increase in mAs increases x-ray quantity proportionally. It has no effect on x-ray quality or contrast scale unless such increase is accompanied by a compensatory reduction in kVp. In such a case, x-ray quality is reduced, and the scale of contrast is shortened.

9. 40 mAs.

11. The mA simply changes the number of electrons flowing from cathode to the anode of an x-ray tube. The kinetic energy of the electrons is controlled by kVp.

13. 100 mA × 1s, 500 mA × 200 ms, 1000 × 100 ms. The shortest exposure time is always preferred to reduce motion blur.

15. Small and large. Many more x-rays can be produced with the large focal size. With the small focal spot, the capacity of x-ray production is limited. A small focal spot is reserved for fine-detail radiography, magnification radiography, and extremity radiography.

17. Less ripple of the high-voltage waveform results in higher x-ray quantity and quality.

19. More x-rays can be produced because a higher mA station can be used and therefore exposure times can be shortened, reducing motion blur.

CHAPTER 20

1. a. Measure of radiographic contrast. Gradient is the slope of the tangent at any point on the characteristic curve.
   b. A phenomenon in which the image of an inclined object can be smaller than the object itself.
   c. An undesirable blurred region on the radiograph that occurs caused by a large effective focal spot, a short SID, and a long OID; the most important factor in determining spatial resolution.
   d. A device that measures OD.
   e. Loss of radiographic quality that is the result of movement of either the patient or the x-ray tube.
   f. Unequal magnification of different portions of the same object.
   g. The random nature in which x-rays interact with the image receptor.
   h. The range of exposures over which the image receptor responds with ODs in the diagnostically useful range. Can also be thought of as the margin of error in technical factors.
   i. The ability to distinguish anatomic structures of similar subject contrast such as liver-spleen and gray matter–white matter.

3. A sensor, or optical step wedge, and a densitometer, which measures OD, are needed to construct the characteristic curve.

5. The answer will be worked out in class.

7. 2.5.

9. A is faster; A, 67; B, 22.

11. Most radiology departments use a standard SID of 180 cm for chest imaging, 100 cm for routine examinations, and 90 cm for special studies such as mobile radiography and skull radiography.

13. With foreshortening, an image of an inclined object appears to be smaller than the object itself; with elongation, the inclined object appears longer than it really is.

15. Standard film-processing techniques are absolutely necessary for consistent film contrast and good radiographic quality. Radiographic contrast can be greatly affected by changes in either image-receptor contrast or subject contrast. OD is affected by total exposure and mAs. Proper exposure is the best control the radiologic technologist can exercise.

17. 11 cm.

19. The reciprocity law states that the OD on a radiograph is proportional only to the total energy imparted to the radiographic film. Whether a radiograph is exposed over a very short period or over days, the OD will be the same if the total energy imparted, and therefore the mAs, is constant.

CHAPTER 21

1. a. If kVp is increased by 15%, mAs should be reduced to half its former value to maintain the same approximate OD on the finished radiograph.
   b. The general size, shape, and muscular condition of a patient.
   c. The combination of settings selected to produce a quality radiograph. Principal factors are kVp, mA, exposure time, and SID.
   d. The range of ODs from the whitest to blackest part of the radiograph.
   e. The chart developed by radiologic technologists to assist them in selecting proper radiographic technique so that a quality image is produced each time.
   f. Radiolucent tissue attenuates few x-rays and appears black on the radiograph. Radiopaque tissue absorbs x-rays and appears white on the radiograph.
   g. An increase of 5% in kVp should be accompanied by a 30% reduction in mAs to produce the same OD at a slightly reduced contrast scale.
   h. Computer-controlled selection of radiograph technique based on a description of an anatomic part.
   i. The detail of anatomic structures on a finished radiograph is best observed with good contrast resolution.
   j. Optical density, contrast, image detail, and distortion.

3. Increasing kVp results in a longer contrast scale.

5. 1200 mAs.

7. An OD less than approximately 0.5 is too light; an OD greater than approximately 3 is too dark. In between those ranges is just right.

9. kVp. kVp is the principal control of contrast; mAs is a secondary influence on contrast.

11. Patient factors, image-quality factors, and exposure-techniques factors.

13. Pathology that is destructive in nature results in radiolucent tissue, which requires less radiograph technique. On the other hand, other pathologies can constructively increase mass density, causing tissue to be more radiopaque; this tissue may require more radiographic technique.

15. By review of the patient's chart and interview of the patient if possible.

17. 0.2 to 4.0.

19. Contrast is the difference in OD between adjacent anatomic structures, or the variation in OD on the radiograph. A high contrast is black on white, whereas a low-contrast image has many shades of gray. Gray matter, white matter, the liver, and the spleen are low-contrast anatomic structures. The bone–soft tissue interface along the spinal column has a high contrast.

CHAPTER 22

1. a. The complete arc of swing of the x-ray tube during tomographic examination.
   b. Linear tomography with a tomographic angle of less than 10 degrees.
   c. Factor used to produce an enlarged image by increasing the object image receptor distance (OID). MF = SID/SOD.
   d. The imaginary pivot point about which the x-ray tube and image receptor move.
   e. The approximate thickness of tissue that is visible on a tomogram.

3. The larger the tomographic angle, the thinner the visibility of the tissue section.

5. If the overhead tube can be fixed to an arm that swings during exposure.

7. To improve contrast resolution.

9. The x-ray tube and image receptor must each be fastened to arms that rotate about a fixed fulcrum. The vertical position of the fulcrum must be selectable.

11. Abdomen and chest.

13. Grid lines must be positioned parallel to the x-ray tube slice image-receptor movement.

15. 24 mm.

CHAPTER 23

1. a. 0.5 mm of aluminum or 30 μm of molybdenum or 50 μm of rhodium.
   b. 4:1 or 5:1.
   c. Calcific deposits that appear as small grains of varying sizes on the x-ray.
   d. Charged coupled device.
   e. One of every 8 women.
   f. 60 to 80 cm.
   g. The accentuation of the interface between different tissues.

3. A low kVp must be used to maximize the photoelectric effect and therefore enhance differential absorption. As kVp is reduced, however, the penetrability of x-ray beam is also reduced, which in turn requires an increase in mAs. If kVp is too low, an inordinately high mAs may be required, resulting in an unacceptably high patient dose. Compromise must be reached between patient dose and image quality.

5. To reduce the size of the effective focal spot and therefore improve spatial resolution.

7. Because of the characteristics produced at 20 and 23 keV, respectively.

9. Low kVp is the technique required for soft tissue radiography.

11. Screening mammography is conducted on patients without symptoms and uses two views. Diagnostic mammography is conducted on patients with symptoms and may require several views per breast.

13. Improved spatial resolution, improved contrast resolution, uniform optical density, and reduced patient dose.

15. 0.3 mm/0.1 mm. To ensure good spatial resolution at a relatively short SID.

17. Ratio of 4:1 to 5:1; frequencies of 30 to 50 lines/cm are typical.

CHAPTER 24

1. a. An administrative program to ensure that the management of the patient, the operation of the imaging systems, and the interpretation and reporting of the results of examinations are of the highest quality and standards.
   b. Continuous quality improvement.
   c. Program designed to ensure that the radiologist is provided with the best possible image resulting from good equipment performance.
   d. Visible light emitted by a front screen that crosses the contiguous film emulsion and base and interacts with the far side emulsion.
   e. Mammography Quality Standards Act.

3. Maintaining darkroom cleanliness and performing processor QC.

5. The mammography technologists or the quality-control technologists in a larger facility.

7. Screens should be cleaned weekly, using the material and method suggested by the manufacturers. If liquid cleaner is used, screens should be allowed to air-dry. If compressed air is used, the air supply should be checked to ensure that no contaminants are present.

9. Surrounding the image to be examined by black paper to reduce, glare thereby improving visual conspicuity.

11. Scoring involves determining the number of fibers, speck groups, and masses visible in the photon image.

13. 0.05 OD.

15. 40 lb of compression.
17. Once the average ODs have been determined for each step from the five different sensitometer strips, the step that has an average OD closest to, but not less than, 1.2 should be found and marked as the mid-density step for future comparison. This is sometimes referred to as the *speed index*.
19. The normal clinical technique for a 50% fatty–50% dense, 4.5-cm breast.

CHAPTER 25

1. a. Technique to view a continuous image of the motion of internal structures while the x-ray tube is energized.
   b. Electronic feedback mechanism that maintains constant brightness of the fluoroscopic image.
   c. Flux gain is the multiplication of light photons at the output phosphor compared with x-rays at the input phosphor and the image minification from input to output phosphor. The minification gain is the ratio of the square of the diameter of the input phosphor to the square of the diameter of the output phosphor. Brightness gain = Minification gain (Flux gain.
   d. Imaging body vasculature and performing intravascular procedures to correct a normal defect or treat a diseased condition.
   e. A type of television-camera tube used in many fluoroscopic imaging systems.
   f. The emission of electrons after light stimulation.
   g. The engineering aspects of maintaining proper electron travel.
   h. A static image in a small-format image receptor.
   i. The magnitude of the video signal is directly proportional to the light intensity received by the television-camera tube.
3. The rods are located on the periphery of the retina and are the sensory cells responsible for scotopic or low-light vision. Cones are the sensory cells located centrally on the retina and are responsible for photopic or bright-light vision.
5. In photo emission, electrons are stimulated to be emitted by visible light. In thermionic emission, electrons are stimulated to be emitted by heat.
7. 67,500.
9. Because its spatial resolution, which is limited by the number of lines and the electronic bandwidth, is worse than that of any other part of the imaging chain.
11. Because we operate on 60-Hz electric power in the United States, each cycle is 33 ms, which results in 30 frames/s, the maximum frame rate available.
13. Yes, spatial resolution is improved.
15. See Figure 25-14.
17. See Figure 25-11.

CHAPTER 26

1. a. A barium or iodine-based solution introduced into vessels of the gastrointestinal tract to improve the contrast resolution of those structures.
   b. A fine wire introduced into a vessel over which a catheter is threaded and the guide wire removed before introduction of the contrast material.
   c. Visualization with a movie camera that records the image on film for later playback.
   d. Fluoroscopic imaging simultaneously or alternately with two imaging chains positioned at different angles to the patient.
   e. Feature of a patient table that rotates on a pivot so that the resting patient can be moved with head down or head up.
3. Uses a needle and catheter and makes cutdown of the vessel unnecessary.
5. Guidewires allow the catheter to be introduced safely into the vessel. Once the catheter is in place, the guidewire allows the radiologist to position the catheter.
7. To establish rapport and explain the procedure and its risks.
9. Interventional therapeutic procedures conducted in and through vessels.
11. 1.0 mm/0.3 mm. The small size is used for magnification radiation of the small vessels.
13. Up to four images per second can be made.
15. To help reduce a possible whiplash effect.
17. (CV).

CHAPTER 27

1. a. Decision-making function of the CPU; evaluates an immediate result and performs subsequent computations depending on the result.
   b. A device that modulates/demodulates signals to convert digital information into analog and allow data to be transmitted over a telephone line.
   c. Smallest unit on the screen that can be turned on or off or made different shades.
   d. The transfer of images and patient reports to remote sites.
   e. The computer program that organizes the course of data through the computer to solve a particular problem (for example, DOS, UNIX, and Windows).
   f. The process of transferring information into primary memory is input. Output is the process of transferring the results of a computation from primary memory to storage or the user.
   g. Basis of computer operation; uses only two digits, 0 and 1. Computer performs all functions by converting alphabetic characters, decimals, and logic functions to binary values.

3. A computer is faster and has more capacity but, in particular, it can perform logic functions while a calculator performs only arithmetic functions.

5. Hardware and software. One can see hardware; software consists of the many programs that operate the computer.

7. A bit is a single binary digit, a byte is 8 bits, and a word is 2 bytes.

9. FORTRAN, BASIC, COBOL, Pascal, C, and C++.

11. 2048 megabits.

13. FORTRAN.

15. The central processing unit is a microprocessor or computer on a chip. It contains a control unit and an arithmetic/logic unit. These two components are connected by an electrical conductor called a *bus*.

17. 10010011.

CHAPTER 28

1. a. An approach to digital radiography that uses a narrow fan beam of x-rays that intercepts a linear array of radiation defectors.

   b. Window level identifies the type of tissue to be imaged. Window width determines the gray-scale rendition of that tissue and therefore image contrast.

   c. Method of temporal subtraction that results in successive subtraction images of contrast-filled vessels.

   d. Method in which each subtracted image is made from a different mask and follow-up frame.

   e. The range of numbers that can be assigned to a given pixel. Usually described by 10-bit dynamic range (2^{10} = 1024 shades of gray) or 12-bit dynamic range (2^{12} = 4096 shades of gray).

   f. Time required for the x-ray tube to be switched on and reach the selected level of kVp and mA.

   g. Temporal subtraction refers to a number of computer-assisted techniques whereby an image obtained at one time is subtracted from an image obtained at a later time. Energy subtraction uses two x-ray beams alternately to provide a subtraction image resulting from differences in photoelectric interaction. Hybrid subtraction combines temporal- and energy-subtraction techniques.

3. Improved contrast resolution because of postprocessing procedures, instant access to spot films, signal-to-noise improvement by frame averaging, and instant image subtraction for contrast studies.

5. Windowing is a postprocessing procedure that allows one to view the entire dynamic range of the image even though the dynamic range of the human eye is only approximately 5 bits.

7. The acquisition of a series of images is followed by contrast administration, followed by another series of images. The precontrast and postcontrast images can be summed to improve the signal-to-noise ratio and then subtracted from one another to produce an angiogram or another such image of contrast-filled anatomy.

9. There are spurious electrical signals resulting from small stray electrical currents and thermally induced stray currents. Cooling electronics always reduces electronic noise.

11. Computed radiography uses an imaging plate coated with a photostimulable phosphor. On exposure a latent image is stored in electron traps in the phosphor. The phosphor is then read line by line with laser light stimulation. The intensity of stimulated light is digitized and formed into a digital image matrix.

13. Mammography, chest radiography, and fluoroscopy.

15. Contrast enhancement via postprocessing procedures.

17. That each pixel can contain up to 4096 values, each value representing a different shade of gray.

19. The spatial resolution of all digital images is pixel limited. We cannot image something smaller than a pixel. Theoretically, therefore, for digital fluoroscopy a limited spatial resolution is field of view divided by matrix size.

CHAPTER 29

1. a. The result of a CT scan; the image is perpendicular to the long axis of the body (axial).

   b. An intensity profile formed by the attenuation of the x-ray beam by the internal structures of the body.

   c. The time between the end of scanning and the appearance of an image.

   d. Beam collimation that precedes the patient and is principally designed to define the ghost profile and patient dose.

   e. A measure of spatial dimensions used to define the spatial resolution of many x-ray images (the number of line pairs per unit length). The units of line pair per centimeter and line pair per millimeter are directly related to the spatial units in centimeters and millimeters.

   f. Spatial frequency at an MTF equal to 0.1.

   g. Tissue volume, determined by multiplying the pixel size by the thickness of the CT scan slice.

   h. Modulation transfer function. A mathematical approach to evaluating the fidelity of imaging various-size objects, all at high contrast.

   i. One bar and its equal-width interspace.

   j. Mathematical equations adapted for computer processing.

3. The x-ray tube, the detector array, the high-voltage generator, the patient-support couch, and the mechanical support for each.

5. The higher the concentration of scintillation detectors, the better the image quality because of more image profiles will be generated. When detector spacing is increased, patient dose is increased because of the reduction in geometric efficiency.

7. Prepatient collimators to define dose profile. Predetector collimators to define sensitivity profile.

9. The multidata acquisition systems deliver enormous amounts of data to the computer. The computations using filtered backprojection of simultaneous equations require enormous computing power.

11. Predetector collimator.

13. *Filtered backprojection* is the term applied to the reconstruction mathematics. It involves the simultaneous solution to a number of equations equal to the matrix size.

15. 7.7 line pairs/cm.

17. 0.625 mm.

19. That the CT numbered displayed will be linearly related to the x-ray attenuation coefficient for the tissue in each voxel.

CHAPTER 30

1. a. A computer-controlled electronic amplifier and switching device to which the signal from each detector of a multislice spiral CT imaging system is connected.
   b. Resolution along the long axis of the body limited by collimation.
   c. Patient couch movement per 360 degrees of rotation divided by collimation.
   d. One measure of the multislice spiral CT scanner efficiency. SAR = Slices acquired per 360 degrees ÷ Rotation time.
   e. The width of the sensitivity profile at half its maximum value.
   f. Slip rings are electromechanical devices that allow the transfer of signal data and high voltage from a rotating cylinder to a stationary cylinder without a fixed conductor such as a cable.

3. Rather than interpolate values from one position on the spiral to the next similar position at 360 degrees, the interpolation is reduced to half that Z-axis distance.

5. 48 cm.

7. 3.0:1.

9. Exceptional heat capacity and high cooling rates.

11. Collimation, pitch, and image time.

13. Technique in which transverse images are stacked to form a three-dimensional data set that can be rendered as an image.

15. The volume of tissue that can be imaged.

17. 75 cm.

19. When pitch is increased, the section sensitivity profile is also increased. The effect is a thicker slice.

CHAPTER 31

1. a. QA concerns people. A QA program involves monitoring of the patient and the interpretation of the image.
   b. QC concerns instrumentation and equipment. It is more tangible and obvious than QA.
   c. A feature of the QC program that should be checked semiannually with an image of the AAPM five-pin insert.
   d. The follow-up of patient reports to see that the diagnosis was correct.
   e. Measurement used to ensure adequate filtration of the x-ray beam. It should be checked annually or at any time after a change in tube or tube housing.
   f. Council of Radiation Control Program Directors. This is the organization of the 50 directors of state radiation-control programs and their staffs. They formulate state radiation regulations.
   g. Measured with a specially designed phantom; should be performed semiannually.
   h. The ability of a radiographic unit to produce a constant radiation output for various combinations of mAs and exposure time.

3. (1) Acceptance testing should be performed on each new piece of radiographic equipment. (2) Routine performance monitoring of equipment is required periodically. (3) Maintenance of equipment will prevent the need for repair.

5. An experimental determination of half-value layer is obtained. Referring to Table 31-3, one can determine whether adequate filtration is present.

7. These are variously expressed but, basically, any misalignment must not exceed ± 2% of the SID along any edge.

9. ± 5%.

11. A soft, lint-free cloth and a cleaning solution provided by the manufacturer.

13. Approximately 3 to 5 R/min.

15. Noise and uniformity should be measured weekly. Semiannual measurements should be taken to check linearity, spatial resolution, contrast resolution, slice thickness, couch incrementation, and laser localizer. Patient dose and dose profile measurements should be taken annually.

17. The minimum HVL required to ensure adequate x-ray beam filtration varies depending on the operating kVp. See Table 31-3 for high-frequency values.

19. When there is a clear or obvious crack, hole, or other penetration through the protective lead.

CHAPTER 32

1. a. Any unwanted optical density on the image that does not represent an anatomic structure.

b. Marks that are found along the leading or trailing edge of the film; occur when the guide shoes in the turn-around assembly of the processor are sprung or improperly positioned.

c. An artifact produced in the processor when a dirty roller or other object peels off flecks of the emulsion.

d. A mark (for example. fingernail marks, pressure smudges) seen on the processed radiograph resulting from excess pressure of the emulsion before processing.

e. A pressure type mark produced when film is bent sharply before processing.

f. Yellow-brown stain on radiograph after long storage time. It indicates that not all the thiosulfide from the fixer was removed during washing.

g. The amber or red light in a darkroom that allows the radiologic technologists to see but does not expose unprocessed film.

h. When developer or fixer drains down a vertical film and some is improperly retained, the finished product may appear as though viewed through a curtain.

i. An artifact appearing at 3.1416-in intervals as a result of dirt or chemical stain on the 1-in diameter transport roller.

j. An image artifact produced during processing.

3. When the film is being exposed; when the film is being processed; when the film is being handled and stored.

5. Clearly communicate to the patient the importance of not breathing or moving during exposure.

7. Any three of the following: guide shoe marks, pi lines, emulsion pick-off, gelatin buildup, chemical fog, wet-pressure sensitization.

9. If the guide shoe is improperly positioned, if the pressure of the guide shoes on the roller assembly is too high, or if there is dirt trapped at the guide shoe, the ridges in the guide shoes press against the film and leave a mark.

11. Irregular or dirty rollers cause pressure during development and produce small, circular patterns of increased OD.

13. The buildup of electrons in the emulsion, most noticeably during periods of low humidity.

15. Artifacts may obscure pathology and reduce the opportunity for correct diagnosis. The cause of artifacts must be corrected.

17. The patient is placed under the x-ray tube when the tube is not centered to the table or Bucky tray.

19. Fading into a yellow-brown tone with time. This causes the image to lose contrast and appear clearly deteriorated.

CHAPTER 33

1. a. The idea that all plants and animals contain cells as their basic fundamental units, shown conclusively by Schneider and Schwann in 1838.

b. A metabolic activity that builds up large molecules from small ones.

c. A macromolecule associated with energy storage for the cell.

d. Phases of the cell cycle.

e. Tissue that covers an organ or body.

f. The largest part of the cell enclosed by the cell membrane.

g. A molecule necessary to allow biochemical reaction to continue, although it does not directly enter into the reaction. Acts as a catalyst in chemical interaction.

h. The constancy of the internal environment of the human body.

i. A response to radiation exposure that does not appear for months or perhaps years.

3. The ionization can disrupt molecular bonds and cause the large molecule to malfunction.

5. Robert Hooke.

7. Because water constitutes about 80% of human substance.

9. They store energy for subsequent use by the cell.

11. DNA.

13. 1 Mrad (10 kGy).

15. The cell undergoes a mitosis-like division, and each of those cells undergoes an additional like-like division without DNA replication. See Figure 33-13.

17. Nerve cells.

CHAPTER 34

1. a. Measure of the rate at which energy is transferred from a particular type of radiation to soft tissue. Approximately 3 keV/μm for diagnostic x-rays.

b. Orthovoltage x-radiation in the 200- to 250-kVp range.

c. A measure of the increased radiosensitivity of tissue in the presence of oxygen.

d. One mode of cellular recovery from radiation damage.

e. Radiation effect that kills cell before its next division.

f. Extending exposure to a total dose by delivering continuously but at a reduced rate.

g. Accounts for the relative radiosensitivity of various tissues and organs.

3. Patients receive the radiation dose at the same dose rate per minute but broken into equal fractions and given over time. A little today, a little next month, and perhaps a little next year. Radiation oncology patients receive prescribed doses daily.

5. OER = Dose necessary under anoxic conditions to produce a given effect divided by the dose necessary under aerobic oxygenated conditions to produce the same effect.

7. Methotrexate, actinomycin D, hydroxyurea, vitamin K, halogenated pyrimidines.

9. No. To be effective, they must be administered in toxic levels.

11. An equal amount of radiation dose will not necessarily produce an equal response.

13. Stem cells are most sensitive. Young tissue and organs are more radiosensitive than old tissues and organs. Tissue in a high state of metabolic activity also has high radiosensitivity. As cellular proliferation increases, so does cellular radiosensitivity.

15. 2.7.

17. With increasing LET, RBE increases to a maximum value of approximately 3 (see Figure 34-1).

19. OER is LET dependent. OER is highest for low-LET radiation and decreases for high-LET radiation (see Figure 34-2).

CHAPTER 35

1. a. Outside the body or outside the cell.
   b. Quantitative description of the relationship between the standard radiation and test radiation to produce a given effect.
   c. Radiation damage that consists of a molecular lesion of the DNA and causes genetic mutation.
   d. A short-lived, highly reactive, uncharged molecule containing a single unpaired electron in the outermost shell.
   e. The radiobiologic theory that says for a cell to die, after radiation exposure, its target molecule must be inactivated.
   f. The dose that will kill 63% of the cells after the single-hit single target model.
   g. Analogous to D_{37} and the single-hit single target model. *D0* refers to the single-hit multitarget model.
   h. Occurs when a radiation interaction occurs with the target.
   i. Sometimes called *target number*.
   j. Mean lethal dose.

3. Viscosity drops after a high dose of radiation of macromolecules. It is a measure of the degree of main-chain scission of macromolecules.

5. Synthesis (S) phase.

7. Refer to Figure 35-7.

9. They migrate within the cell, transferring energy to target molecules and ultimately join with another molecule to be neutralized.

11. Radiation exposure of tissue is rather uniform because tissue is large on the x-ray scale. However, radiation interaction with target molecules is random.

13. $S = N/N_0 = 1 - (1 - e^{+D/Do})^n$.

15. 5%.

17. A direct effect exist when the ionizing radiation interacts directly with the target-molecule DNA. An indirect effect occurs when the interaction is with some other molecule, resulting in free radical for-

mation which then transfers this energy to DNA. The indirect effect prevails in human radiobiology.

19. In vitro refers to irradiation that occurs outside the body or outside the cell; in vivo irradiation is irradiation of macromolecules in the living cell.

CHAPTER 36

1. a. Gastrointestinal syndrome occurs 3 to 5 days after exposure to 1000 to 5000 rad and results from the destruction of functional cells of the small intestine
   b. The period between radiation exposure and the appearance of a radiation response.
   c. The dose of radiation that will result in death in 50% of irradiated subjects within 60 days. $LD_{50/60}$ for humans is considered to be approximately 350 rad.
   d. A reddening of the skin such as a sunburn or an x-ray burn.
   e. Moist desquamation (ulceration and denudation of the skin) that follows a second wave of erythema with doses higher than 300 to 1000 rad.
   f. The sequence of events after high-level radiation exposure, leading to death within days or weeks.
   g. Red blood cell.
   h. The orderly arrangement of chromosomes into pairs according to size.
   i. Loss of hair.
   j. A chromosomal aberration resulting in a peculiar arrangement of somal material and representing severe chromosomal damage.

3. Period of acute clinical symptoms that occurs within hours of the exposure and continues for a day or two. It is the immediate response of radiation sickness.

5. If the dose is not lethal, recovery begins in 2 to 4 weeks, during the period of manifest illness.

7. Death occurs principally because of severe damage to the cells lining the intestines.

9. Stem cells of the ovaries (oogonia) multiply in number only during fetal life. During late fetal life, primordial follicles grow to encapsulate the oogonia, which become oocytes. This is the most radiosensitive phase. Prepuberty, when numbers of oocytes have been reduced, is also a radiosensitive period. Sensitivity then declines to a minimum in the 20- to 30-year range and then increases continually with age.

11. Basal cells of the skin are the stem cells; they transform to mature cells and migrate to the epidermis, the outer skin layer, and they are replaced at the rate of about 2% per day.

13. As whole-body radiation dose increases, the time of survival decreases, and the three stages of the acute radiation syndrome have characteristic survival times.

15. Erythrocytes (oxygen-carrying cells), lymphocytes (cells that are involved in immune response), granulocytes (scavenger cells that fight bacteria), and thrombocytes (platelets that clot blood to prevent hemorrhage).

17. A reduction in cell count (especially lymphocytes), increased risk of infection, and loss of electrolytes.

19. 1.29.

CHAPTER 37

1. a. The study of occurrence, distribution, and causes of disease in humankind.
   b. In the womb or during pregnancy.
   c. Atomic Bomb Casualty Commission, Radiation Effects Research Foundation.
   d. Effects that exhibit an increasing incidence, not severity, of response with increasing dose.
   e. A study of childhood malignancies in England, Scotland, and Wales, which investigated the effects of radiation in utero.
   f. The scientist who first described a linear non-threshold dose-response relationship based on genetic responses in fruit flies.
   g. The dose of radiation expected to double the normal incidence of genetic mutations; it is thought to be approximately 50 rad.
   h. A naturally occurring, alpha-emitting radioactive gas that is suspected of being a major contributor human lung cancer.

3. Approximately 10 days/rad.

5. Relative risk = Observed cases ÷ Expected cases.

7. When an investigation of human radiation response indicates the induction of some late effect.

9. Radiation control during the early years is suspected to have been better practiced by the British radiologic community than by their American counterpart.

11. Irradiation was used as a treatment for thymic enlargement shortly after birth. The late response of increased thyroid cancer was observed in that population.

13. Miners from a Colorado plateau in the 1950s and 1960s produced uranium oar in poorly ventilated mines and therefore were exposed to high levels of radon gas. The consequence was an increased incidence of lung cancer.

15. Low-dose chronic irradiation does not impair fertility.

17. 1.2.

19. Approximately 150 in the 100,000 person population.

CHAPTER 38

1. a. The scientific discipline of radiation protection.
   b. Tenth value layer.
   c. National Council on Radiation Protection and Measurement.
   d. Concept that attempts to specify the overall risk of harm to an organism by accounting for two variables with the use of appropriate weighting factors.
   e. As low as reasonably achievable.
   f. Tissue weighting factor. A numerical index of the relative radiosensitivity of various tissues.
   g. 500 mrem/9 mo, 50 mrem/mo.
   h. An occupational monitoring device worn on the wrist or finger.
   i. Policy that requires the radiologist to determine the start of the patient's previous menstrual cycle to ensure against irradiation of an unsuspected pregnancy.

3. To help ensure that the radiologist is aware of the fluoroscopic exposure time.

5. Minimize time, maximize distance, use shielding material.

7. With the use of wrist or ring badges.

9. Spontaneous abortion.

11. Review prior radiation exposure history, council the radiologic technologist on proper radiation-protection procedures, provide a second occupational radiation monitor identified as the *baby badge*.

13. 6 min.

15. 22 R.

17. Since most patient and personnel radiation exposure is received during fluoroscopy, keep fluoroscopic time to a minimum, back off from the patient couch when possible, and use protective apparel.

19. The Manhattan Project.

CHAPTER 39

1. a. Thermoluminescent dosimeter.
   b. The percentage of time during which the x-ray tube is on and diverted toward a particular wall.
   c. Instruments designed to detect radiation generally operate in pulse mode or rate mode. In pulse mode, the presence of radiation is indicated by a ticking, chirping, or beeping sound. In rate mode, the instrument response is in milliroentgen per hour (mR/hr) or roentgen per hour (R/hr).
   d. The response of a TLD as a function of temperature, displayed graphically.
   e. The image-intensifier assembly serves as a primary protective barrier. Secondary protective barriers are designed to shield areas from secondary radiation and are always less thick than primary barriers.
   f. Factor that takes into consideration the level of occupancy of a particular area being protected.
   g. The basis for the gamma camera in nuclear medicine and used in the detector arrays of many CT scanners.
   h. The measurement of the intensity of radiation.

3. Protective drapes, Bucky slot cover, 5-minute reset timer, exposure switch that fastens to the console.

5. 30 μm Mo or 50 μm Rh.

7. The protective curtain on the image-intensifier tower, the Bucky slot cover, the 5-minute reset timer.

9. Primary and secondary radiation.

11. Controlled areas are those primarily occupied by radiology personnel and patients. Normally, workers who enter a controlled area would be provided with an occupational radiation monitor. An uncontrolled area can be occupied by anyone; therefore the maximum exposure rate allowed is based on the recommended dose limit for the public.

13. The use factor of a room helps determine whether a given wall or the ceiling is a primary or secondary protective barrier.

15. Ionization chamber, proportional counter, Geiger-Mueller counter.

17. Nuclear medicine.

19. 1207.

CHAPTER 40

1. a. Genetically significant dose; the weighted-average gonad dose to the population gene pool.

   b. The most frequently reported measure of patient dose.

   c. A protective device that is suspended over the region of interest and casts a shadow over the patient's reproductive organs.

   d. The weighted average radiation dose to the bone marrow of a population.

   e. A measure of the radiation dose to glandular tissue.

   f. Shielding device (such as lens shield) that is positioned directly on the patient.

3. During cardiovascular and interventional procedures, fluoroscopy, and mobile radiography.

5. Entrance skin exposure (ESE), gonadal dose, and mean marrow dose.

7. These are used as an index of detriment to the gene pool and possible radiation response.

9. Both values are approximately the same order of magnitude; however, in CT, the dose is distributed rather uniformly across the a patient whereas in routine radiography, the dose is attenuated from 100% at the entrance skin to about 1% at the exit skin.

11. When there is any possibility that the radiation worker will receive in excess of 10% of the recommended dose limit.

13. The current exposure for that reporting period and the cumulative exposure for that year.

15. Radiologic personnel should never hold patients during an x-ray examination. If possible, mechanical restraining devices should be used. If that is not possible, someone accompanying the patient should restrain the patient during examination after having been provided with appropriate protective apparel and given necessary instructions.

17. Shaped crystals of aluminum sulfate store energy in the form of trapped electrons after x-ray exposure. When processed, this material is stimulated by laser light, and the trapped electrons return to the ground state with the emission of shorter-wavelength light. The intensity of this stimulated luminescence is directly proportional to the x-ray exposure received by the occupational radiation monitor.

Glossary

Abrasion layer   The protective covering of gelatin enclosing an emulsion.

Absolute age-response relationship   The increased incidence of a disease is a constant number of cases after a minimal latent period.

Absolute risk   The incidence of malignant disease in a population within 1 year for a given dose; it is expressed as number of cases/10^6 persons/rem.

Absorbed dose   **a.** The energy transferred from ionizing radiation per unit mass of irradiated material; expressed in rad (100 erg/g) or gray (1 J/kg). **b.** The thermalization of tissue by the absorption of ultrasound energy; expressed as a rise in temperature (°C).

Absorption   **a.** The transfer of energy from an electromagnetic field to matter. Removal of x-rays from a beam via the photoelectric effect. **b.** Process by which ultrasound transfers energy to tissue by the conversion of acoustic energy to heat.

Absorption blur   The characteristic of the subject affecting subject contrast.

Acceleration (a)   The rate of change of velocity with time.

Acceleration of gravity   The constant rate at which objects falling to the Earth accelerate.

Acetic acid   The chemical used in the stop bath.

Activator   Chemical, usually acetic acid in the fixer and sodium carbonate in the developer, used to neutralize the developer and swell the gelatin.

Active memory   Data can be stored or accessed at random from anywhere in main memory in approximately equal amounts of time, regardless of where the data are located.

Actual focal-spot size   The area on the anode target that is exposed to electrons from the tube current.

Units are shown in parenthesis: for example, (Joules), (mHz), (m/s).

Acute radiation syndrome Radiation sickness that occurs in humans after whole-body doses of 1 Gy (100 rad) or more of ionizing radiation delivered over a short time.

Adenine A nitrogenous organic base that attaches to a deoxyribose molecule.

Adhesive layer A protective covering of gelatin that encloses the emulsion.

Aerial oxidation Oxidation that occurs when air is introduced into the developer when it is mixed, handled, and stored.

Afterglow Phosphorescence in an intensifying screen.

Age-response function The pattern of change in radiosensitivity as a function of phase in the cell cycle.

Air-gap technique The practice of moving the image receptor 10 to 15 cm from the patient so that fewer scattered x-rays interact with the image receptor, enhancing contrast.

ALARA The principle that radiation exposure should be kept *as low as reasonably achievable*, economic and social factors being taken into account.

Algorithm A computer-adapted mathematical calculation applied to raw data during image reconstruction.

Alnico An alloy of aluminum, nickel, and cobalt; one of the more useful magnets produced from ferromagnetic material.

Alpha particle (α particle) The particulate form of ionizing radiation consisting of two protons and two neutrons. The nucleus of helium. Emitted from the nucleus of a radioactive atom.

Alternating current (AC) The oscillation of electricity in both directions in a conductor.

Amber filter A filter that transmits light with wavelengths longer than 550 nm, which is above the spectral response of blue-sensitive film.

American Association of Physicists in Medicine (AAPM) The scientific society of medical physicists.

American College of Medical Physicists (ACMP) The professional society of medical physicists.

American College of Radiology (ACR) The professional society of radiologists and medical physicists.

American Society of Radiologic Technologists (ASRT) The scientific and professional society of radiographers.

Ammeter A device that measures current.

Ampere (A) The SI unit of electric charge. 1A = 1C/s.

Amplitude The width of a waveform.

Anabolism The process of synthesizing smaller molecules into a larger macromolecule.

Anaphase The second phase of mitosis, during which chromatids repel one another and migrate along the mitotic spindle to opposite sides of the cell.

Anatomically programmed radiography (APR) Rather than have the technologist select a desired kVp and mAs, graphics on the console guide the technologist.

Angiography Fluoroscopy in which the x-ray examination is applied toward the visualization of vessels.

Angstrom (Ån) The unit of measure of wavelength. 1 Ån = 10^{-10} m.

Anode Positively charged side of an x-ray tube, which contains the target.

Anthropomorphic Human characteristics.

Antibodies Proteins produced by the body in response to the presence of foreign antigens, such as bacteria or viruses.

Antigen The molecular configuration of an antibody that attacks a particular type of invasive or infectious agent.

Aperture a. A circular opening for the patient in the gantry of a computed tomographic or magnetic resonance imaging system. b. The fixed collimation of a diagnostic x-ray tube, as in an aperture diaphragm. c. The variable opening before the lens of a cine or photospot camera.

Aperture diaphragm A simple beam-restricting device that attaches a lead-lined metal diaphragm to the head of the x-ray tube.

Archival quality Referring to the fact that the image does not deteriorate with age but remains in its original state.

Area beam The x-ray beam pattern that is usually shaped like a square or rectangle and that is used in conventional radiography and fluoroscopy.

Array processor The part of a computer that handles raw data and performs the mathematical calculations necessary to reconstruct a digital image.

Artifact An unintended optical density on a radiograph or another film-type image receptor.

Asthenic Referring to a body habitus of a patient who is small and frail.

Atom The smallest particle of an element that cannot be divided or broken by chemical means.

Atomic mass The relative mass of a specific isotope of an element.

Atomic mass number (A) The number of protons plus the number of neutrons in the nucleus.

Atomic mass unit (amu) The mass of a neutral atom of an element, expressed as one twelfth the mass of carbon, which has an arbitrarily assigned value of 12.

Atomic number (Z) The number of protons in the nucleus.

Atrophy The shrinking in size of a tissue or organ.

Attenuation The reduction in radiation intensity as a result of absorption and scattering.

Automatic brightness control (ABC) A feature on a fluoroscope that allows the radiologist to select an image-brightness level that is subsequently maintained automatically by varying the kVp. the mAs, or both.

Automatic exposure control (AEC) A feature that determines radiation exposure during radiography in most x-ray imaging systems.

Coolidge tube   A type of vacuum tube in use today that allows x-ray intensity and energy to be separately and accurately selected.

Cosmic rays   Particulate and electromagnetic radiation emitted by the sun and the stars.

Coulomb (C)   The SI unit of electric charge.

Coulomb per kilogram (C/kg)   The SI unit of radiation exposure. 2.58×10^{-4} C/kg = 1 R.

Coupling   The joining of magnetic fields produced by the primary and secondary coils.

Covalent bond   The chemical union between atoms formed by sharing one or more pairs of electrons.

Covering power   The more efficient use of silver in an emulsion to produce the same optical density per unit exposure.

Crookes tube   The forerunner of modern fluorescent, neon, and x-ray tubes.

Crossed grid   A grids that has lead strips running parallel to both the long and short axes.

Cross-linking   The process of side spurs created by irradiation and attaching to a neighboring macromolecule or to another segment of the same molecule.

Crossover   The process occurring during meiosis when chromatids exchange chromosomal material.

Crossover rack   A device in an automatic processor that transports film from one tank to the next.

Cryogen   An extremely cold liquid.

Crystal lattice   A three-dimensional, cross-linked structure of silver, bromine, and iodine atoms.

Curie (Ci)   The former unit of radioactivity. Expressed as 1 Ci = 3.7×10^{10} disintegrations per second = 3.7×10^{10} Bq.

Cutie pie   The nickname for an ionization chamber–type survey meter.

Cytoplasm   The protoplasm existing outside the cell's nucleus.

Cytosine   A nitrogenous organic base that attaches to a deoxyribose molecule.

Data acquisition system (DAS)   A computer-controlled electronic amplifier and switching device to which the signal from each radiation detector of a multislice spiral computed tomographic scanning system is connected.

Decimal system   A system of numbers based on multiples of 10.

Densitometer   Instrument that measures the optical density of exposed film.

Density difference (DD)   The difference between the step with an average optical density closest to 2.2 and the step with an average optical density closest to, but not less than, 0.5.

Deoxyribonucleic acid (DNA)   Molecule that carries the genetic information necessary for cell replication. The target molecule of radiobiology.

Derived quantities   Any secondary quantity derived from a combination of one or more of the three base quantities, such as mass, length, and time.

Desquamation   Ulceration and denudation of the skin.

Detail   The degree of sharpness of structural lines on a radiograph.

Detective quantum efficiency (DQE)   The percentage of x-rays absorbed by the screen.

Detector array   Group of detectors and interspace material used to separate them. The image receptor in computed tomography.

Deterministic effect   A biologic response whose severity varies with radiation dose. A dose threshold usually exists.

Developing   The stage of processing during which the latent image is converted to a manifest image.

Developing agent   A chemical, usually phenidone, hydroquinone, or Metol, that reduces exposed silver ions to atomic silver.

Development fog   An artifact that results from crystals that had not been exposed reducing to metallic silver as a result of the lack of a restrainer.

Diagnostic mammography   Examination performed on patients with symptoms or elevated risk factors for breast cancer.

Diagnostic-type protective tube housing   Lead-lined housing enclosing an x-ray tube that shields leakage radiation to less than 100 mR/hr at 1 m.

Diaphragm   A device that restricts an x-ray beam to a fixed size.

Dichroic stain   A two-colored stain that appears as a curtain effect on the radiograph.

Differential absorption   Different degrees of absorption in different tissues that results in image contrast and formation of the x-ray image.

Digital fluoroscopy (DF)   A digital x-ray imaging system that produces a series of dynamic images obtained with an area x-ray beam and an image intensifier.

Digital radiography (DR)   Static images produced with either a fan x-ray beam intercepted by a linear array of radiation detectors or an area x-ray beam intercepted by a photostimulable phosphor plate or a direct-capture solid-state device.

Dimagnetic   Nonmagnetic materials that are unaffected when brought into a magnetic field.

Dimensional stability   The property that allows the base of radiographic film to maintain its size and shape during use and processing so that it does not contribute to image distortion.

Diode   Vacuum tube with two electrodes, a cathode, and an anode.

Dipolar   Referring to a molecule with areas of opposing electric charges.

Direct current (DC)   The flow of electricity in only one direction in a conductor.

Direct-current motor   An electric motor in which many turns of wire are used for the current loop and many bar magnets are used to create the external magnetic field.

Direct effect Effect of radiation that occurs when the ionizing radiation interacts directly with a particularly radiosensitive molecule.

Direct-exposure film Film used without intensifying screens.

Disaccharide A sugar.

Dissociation The process of separating a whole into parts.

Distortion Unequal magnification of different portions of the same object.

Dose The amount of radiant energy absorbed by an irradiated object.

Dose equivalent (H) The radiation quantity that is used for radiation protection and that expresses dose on a common scale for all radiations. Expressed in rem or sievert (Sv).

Dose limit (DL) The maximum permissible dose.

Dosimeter An instrument that detects and measures exposure to ionizing radiation.

Dosimetry The practice of measuring the intensity of radiation.

Double-contrast examination An examination of the colon that uses air and barium for contrast.

Double-emulsion film Radiographic film that has an emulsion coating on both sides of the base and a layer of supercoat over each emulsion.

Double-helix The configuration of DNA that is shaped like a ladder twisted about an imaginary axis like a spring.

Doubling dose That dose of radiation expected to double the number of genetic mutations in a generation.

Duplicating film A single-emulsion film that is exposed to ultraviolet light or blue light through the existing radiograph to produce a copy.

Dynamic range The range of values that can be displayed by an imaging system; shades of gray.

Early effect A radiation response that occurs within minutes or days after radiation exposure.

Eddy current A current opposing the magnetic field that induced it, creating a loss of transformer efficiency.

Edge enhancement The accentuation of the interface between different tissues.

Edge-response function (ERF) The mathematical expression of the ability of the computed tomographic scanner to reproduce a high-contrast edge with accuracy.

Effective atomic number The weighted average atomic number for the different elements of a material.

Effective dose (E) The sum over specified tissues of the products of the equivalent dose in a tissue (H_T) and the weighting factor for the tissue (W_T).

Effective dose equivalent (H_E) The sum of the products of the dose equivalent to a tissue (H_T) and the weighting factors (W_T) applicable to each of the tissues irradiated. The values (W_T) are different for effective dose and effective dose equivalent.

Effective focal-spot size The area projected onto the patient and the image receptor.

Elective booking A safeguard against the irradiation of an unsuspected pregnancy.

Electrical energy The work that can be done when an electron or an electronic charge moves through an electric potential.

Electric circuit The path of the electron flow from the generating source through the various components and back again.

Electric current The flow of electrons.

Electric field The lines of force exerted on charged ions in the tissues by the electrodes that cause charged particles to move from one pole to another.

Electricity A form of energy created by the activity of electrons and other subatomic particles in motion.

Electrification The process of adding or removing electrons from a substance.

Electrified object An object that has too few or too many electrons.

Electrode An electrical terminal or connector.

Electromagnet A coil or wire wrapped around an iron core, which intensifies the magnetic field.

Electromagnetic energy The type of energy in x-rays, radio waves, microwaves, and visible light.

Electromagnetic radiation Oscillating electric and magnetic fields that travel in a vacuum with the velocity of light. Includes x-rays, gamma rays, and some nonionizing radiation (such as ultraviolet, visible, infrared, and radio waves).

Electromagnetic spectrum The continuum of electromagnetic energy.

Electromotive force Electric potential; measured in volts (V).

Electron Elementary particle with one negative charge. Electrons surround the positively charged nucleus and determine the chemical properties of the atom.

Electron binding energy The strength of attachment of an electron to the nucleus.

Electron optics The engineering aspects of maintaining proper electron travel.

Electron spin The momentum of a particle of an atom in a fixed pattern.

Electron volt (eV) The unit of energy equal to that which an electron acquires from a potential difference of 1 V.

Electrostatics Study of fixed or stationary electric charge.

Element An atom having the same atomic number and same chemical properties. A substance that cannot be broken down further without changing its chemical properties.

Elemental mass The characteristic mass of an element, determined by the relative abundance of isotopes and their respective atomic masses.

Elongation   An image made to appear longer than it really is because the inclined object is not located on the central x-ray beam.

Embryologic effect   Damage occurring as a result of an organism being exposed to ionizing radiation during its embryonic stage of development.

Emulsion   The material with which x-rays or light photons from screens interact and transfer information.

Endoplasmic reticulum   A channel or series of channels that allows the nucleus to communicate with the cytoplasm.

Energy   The ability to do work; measured in joules (J).

Energy levels   The orbits around the nucleus that contain a designated number of electrons.

Energy subtraction   A technique that uses the two x-ray beams alternately to provide a subtraction image resulting from differences in photoelectric interaction.

Entrance roller   A roller that grips the film to begin its trip through the processor.

Entrance skin exposure (ESE)   X-ray exposure to the skin; expressed in milliroentgen (mR).

Enzyme   A molecule that is necessary in small quantities to allow a biochemical reaction to continue even though it does not directly enter into the reaction.

Epidemiology   The study of the occurrence, distribution, and causes of disease in humans.

Epilation   The loss of hair.

Epithelium   The covering tissue that lines all exposed surfaces of the body, both exterior and interior.

Erg (Joule)   The unit of energy and work.

Erythema   A sunburnlike reddening of the skin.

Erythrocyte   A red blood cell.

EUR/OPE   Electrons *used* in *reduction/oxidation* procedure *electrons.*

Excess risk   The difference between the observed and the expected number of cases.

Excitation   The addition of energy to a system by raising the energy of electrons with the use of x-rays.

Exit radiation   The x-rays that remain after the beam exits through the patient.

Exponent   Superscript or power to which 10 is raised in scientific notation.

Exponential form   Power-of-10 notation.

Exposed matter   The matter that intercepts radiation and absorbs part or all of it; irradiated matter.

Exposure   The measure of the ionization produced in air by x-rays or gamma rays. The quantity of radiation intensity expressed in roentgen (R), Coulombs per kilogram (C/kg), or air kerma (Gy).

Exposure factors   The factors that influence and determine the quantity and quality of x-radiation to which the patient is exposed.

Exposure linearity   The ability of a radiographic unit to produce a constant radiation output for various combinations of mA and exposure time.

Extinction time   The time required to end an exposure.

Extrafocal radiation, off-focus radiation   Electrons that bounce off the focal spot and land on other areas of the target.

Extrapolation   The estimation of a value beyond the range of known values.

Falling-load generator   A design in which exposure factors are automatically adjusted to the highest mA at the shortest exposure time allowed by the high-voltage generator.

Fan beam   An x-ray beam pattern used in computed tomography and digital radiograph; projected as a slit.

Feed tray   The start of the transport system where the film to be processed is inserted into the automatic processor in the darkroom.

Ferromagnetic material   Material that is strongly attracted by a magnet and that can usually be permanently magnetized by exposure to a magnetic field.

Field   The interactions among different energies, forces, or masses that cannot be seen but can be described mathematically.

Field of view (FOV)   The image matrix size provided by digital x-ray imaging systems.

Fifteen-percent rule   A principle stating that if the optical density on a radiograph is to be increased using kVp, an increase in kVp by 15% is equivalent to doubling the mAs.

Filament   The part of the cathode that emits electrons, resulting in a tube current.

File   A collection of data or information that is treated as a unit by the computer.

Film badge   A pack of photographic film used for approximate measurement of radiation exposure to radiation workers. It is the most widely used and most economical type of personnel radiation monitor.

Film graininess   The distribution of silver halide grains in an emulsion.

Filtered back projection   The process by which an image acquired during computed tomography and stored in computer memory is reconstructed.

Filtration   The removal of low-energy x-rays from the useful beam with aluminum or another metal. It results in increased beam quality and reduced patient dose.

First-generation computed tomographic scanner   A finely collimated x-ray beam, single-detector assembly that translates across the patient and rotates between successive translations.

Five-percent rule   A principle stating that an increase of 5% in the kVp may be accompanied by a 30% reduction in the mAs to produce the same optical density at a slightly reduced contrast scale.

Fixing   The stage of processing during which the silver halide not exposed to radiation is dissolved and removed from the emulsion.

Fluorescence The emission of visible light only during stimulation.

Fluorescent screen The cycle in a television-picture tube when the electron beam creates the television optical signal and then immediately fades.

Fluoroscope A device used to image moving anatomic structures with x-rays.

Fluoroscopy An imaging modality that provides a continuous image of the motion of internal structures while the x-ray tube is energized. Real-time imaging.

Flux gain The ratio of the number of light photons at the output phosphor to the number of x-rays at the input phosphor.

Focal spot The region of anode target where electrons interact to produce x-rays.

Focal-spot blur A blurred region on the radiograph over which the technologist has little control.

Focused grid A radiographic grid constructed so that the grid strips converge on an imaginary line.

Focusing cup A metal shroud surrounding the filament.

Fog An unintended optical density on a radiograph that reduces contrast because of light or chemical contamination.

Fog density The development of silver grain that contains no useful information.

Force That which changes the motion of an object; a push or a pull. Expressed in newtons (N).

Foreshortening The reduction in image size; related to the angle of inclination of the object.

4% voltage ripple Three-phase, 12-pulse power whose voltage supplied to the x-ray tube never falls below 96% of the peak value.

14% ripple Three-phase, six pulse power whose voltage supplied to the x-ray tube never falls below 86% of the peak value.

Fourth-generation computed tomographic scanner A unit in which the x-ray source rotates but the detector assembly does not.

Fraction A numerical value expressed by dividing one number by another.

Fractionated A radiation dose delivered at the same dose in equal portions at regular intervals.

Free radical An uncharged molecule containing a single unpaired electron in the valence shell.

Frequency The number of cycles or wavelengths of a simple harmonic motion per unit time. Expressed in Hertz (Hz). 1 Hz = 1 cycle/s.

Fulcrum The imaginary pivot point about which the x-ray tube and the image receptor move.

Full-wave rectification A circuit in which the negative half-cycle corresponding to the inverse voltage is reversed so that a positive voltage is always directed across the x-ray tube.

Full width at half maximum (FWHM) The width of the profile at half its maximum value.

Fundamental laws of motion The three principles of inertia, force, and action/reaction established by Isaac Newton.

Fundamental particles The three primary constituents of an atom: electrons, photons, and neutrons.

Gantry The portion of the computed tomographic or magnetic resonance imaging system that accommodates the patient and source or the detector assemblies.

Gastrointestinal (GI) syndrome A form of acute radiation syndrome that appears in humans at a threshold dose of about 10 Gy (1000 rad). It is characterized by nausea, diarrhea, and damage to the cells lining the intestines.

Geiger-Muller (G-M) counter Radiation-detection and radiation-measuring instrument that detects individual ionizations. It is the primary radiation survey instrument for nuclear medicine facilities.

Gelatin The part of the emulsion that provides mechanical support for the silver halide crystals by holding them uniformly dispersed in place.

Generation time See **cell cycle time.**

Genetically significant dose (GSD) The average gonadal dose to members of the population who are of childbearing age.

Genetic cell The oogonium or the spermatogonium.

Genetic effect Effects of radiation that affects and individual and subsequent unexposed generations.

Germ cell A reproductive cell.

Glandular dose The average radiation dose to glandular tissue.

Glow curve A graph that shows the relationship of light output to temperature change.

Glycogen A human polysaccharide.

Gonadal dose The exposure to the reproductive organs.

Gradient The slope of the tangent at any point on the characteristic curve.

Granulocyte A scavenger cell used to fight bacteria.

Gray (Gy) Special name for the SI unit of absorbed dose and air kerma. 1 Gy = 1 J/kg = 100 rad.

Gray scale An image display in which intensity is recorded as variations in brightness.

Grid A device used to reduce the intensity of scatter radiation in the remnant x-ray beam.

Grid clean-up The ability of a grid to absorb scatter radiation.

Grid-controlled tube An x-ray tubes designed to be turned on and off very rapidly for situations requiring multiple exposures at precise exposure times.

Grid cutoff The absence of optical density on a radiograph because of unintended x-ray absorption in a grid.

Grid frequency The number of grid lines per inch or centimeter.

Grid lines A series of sections of radiopaque material.

Grid ratio The ratio of grid height to grid strip separation.

Guanine   A nitrogenous organic base that attaches to a deoxyribose molecule.

Guide shoe   A device in an automatic processor that is used for steering film around bends.

Guidewire   A device that allows the safe introduction of the catheter into the vessel.

Halation   The reflection of screen light transmitted through the emulsion and base.

Half-life   The time required for a quantity of radioactivity to be reduced to half its original value.

Half-valve layer (HVL)   The thickness of absorber necessary to reduce an x-ray beam to half its original intensity.

Half-wave rectification   A condition in which the voltage is not allowed to swing negatively during the negative half of its cycle.

Hard copy   A permanent image on film or paper, as opposed to an image on a cathode ray tube, disk, or magnetic tape.

Hardener   A chemical, usually potassium glutaraldehyde alum in the fixer, that is used to stiffen and shrink the emulsion.

Hard x-ray   An x-ray that has high penetrability and therefore is of high quality.

Hardware   The visible parts of the computer.

Health physics   The science concerned with the recognition, evaluation, and control of radiation hazards.

Heel effect   The absorption of x-rays in the heel of the target, resulting in reduced x-ray intensity to the anode side of the central axis.

Hematologic syndrome   A form of acute radiation syndrome after whole-body exposure to doses ranging from approximately 1 to 10 Gy (100 to 1000 rad). It is characterized by the reduction in white cells, red cells, and platelets in the circulating blood.

Hertz (Hz)   The unit of frequency; the number of cycles or oscillations each second of a simple harmonic motion.

Hexadecimal number system   Number system used by low-level applications to represent a set of four bits.

High-contrast resolution   The ability to image small objects having high subject contrast; spatial resolution.

High-voltage generator   One of three principal parts of an x-ray imaging system; it is always close to the x-ray tube.

Hit   A radiation interaction with the target.

Homeostasis   **a.** A state of equilibrium among tissue and organs. **b.** The ability of the body to return to normal function despite infection and environmental changes.

Hormone   A protein manufactured by various endocrine glands and carried by the blood to regulate body functions such as growth and development.

Horsepower (hp)   The British unit of power.

Houndsfield unit (HU)   The scale of computed tomographic numbers used to judge the nature of tissue.

Hybrid subtraction   A technique that combines temporal and energy subtraction.

Hydroquinone   The principal compound used in the chemical composition of film developers.

Hypersthenic   Referring to a body habitus of a patient who is big in frame and overweight.

Hypo   Sodium thiosulfate, a fixing agent that removes unexposed and undeveloped silver halide crystals from the emulsion.

Hypo retention   The undesirable retention of the fixer in the emulsion.

Hyposthenic   Referring to a body habitus of a patient who is thin but healthy looking.

Hysteresis   The additional resistance created by the alternate reversal of the magnetic field caused by the alternating current.

Image detail   The sharpness of small structures on the radiograph.

Image-forming x-ray   An x-ray that exits from the patient and enters the image receptor.

Image intensifier   An electronic vacuum tube that amplifies a fluoroscopic image to reduce patient dose.

Image matrix   A layout of cells in rows and columns.

Image noise   The deterioration of the radiographic image.

Image receptor (IR)   The medium that transforms the x-ray beam into a visible image; radiographic film or a phosphorescent screen.

Image receptor contrast   Contrast that is inherent in the film and is influenced by processing of the film. See also **subject contrast.**

Improper fraction   A fraction in which the quotient is greater than 1.

Indirect effect   The effect of radiation that results from the production of free radicals produced by the interaction of radiation with water.

Induction   The process of making ferromagnetic material magnetic.

Induction motor   An electric motor in which the rotor is a series of wire loops but the external magnetic field is supplied by several fixed electromagnets called *stators.*

Inertia   The property of matter that resists change in motion or at rest.

Infrared light   A light consisting of photons with wavelengths longer than those of visible light but shorter than those of microwaves.

Infrared radiation   Electromagnetic radiation just lower in energy than visible light, with a wavelength in the range of 0.7 to 1000 μm.

Inherent filtration   The filtration of useful x-ray beams provided by the permanently installed components of an x-ray tube housing assembly and the glass window of an x-ray tube.

Initiation time   The time required to start an exposure.

Input   The process of transferring information into primary memory.

Insulator   A material that inhibits the flow of electrons in a conductor or in heat transfer.

Integrate mode   A function of an instrument designed to measure the total accumulated intensity of radiation over a period of time.

Intensification factor (IF)   The ratio of exposure without screens to that with screens to produce the same optical density.

Intensifying screen   A sensitive phosphor that converts x-rays to light to shorten exposure time and reduce patient dose.

Intensity profile   The projection formed by the intensity of radiation detected according to the attenuation pattern.

Internally deposited radionuclide   A naturally occurring radionuclide in the human body.

International System of Units (SI)   Standard system of units based on the meter, kilogram, and second; it has been adopted by all countries and is used in all branches of science.

Interphase   The period of growth of the cell between divisions.

Interpolation   The estimation of a value between two known values.

Interrogation time   Time during which the signal from an image detector is sampled.

Interspace material   The sections of radiolucent material in a grid.

Interstitial   Referring to the area between cells.

Inverse square law   Law stating that the intensity of the radiation at a location is inversely proportional to the square of its distance from the source of radiation.

Inverse voltage   Current flowing from the anode to the cathode.

Inverter   High-speed switches that convert direct current into a series of square pulses.

In vivo   In the living cell.

Ion   An atom with too many or too few electrons; an electrically charged particle.

Ion chamber   An instrument that detects and measures the radiation intensity in areas outside of protective barriers.

Ionic bonds   A bonding that occurs because of an electrostatic force between ions.

Ionization   The removal of an orbital electron from an atom.

Ionization potential   The amount of energy (34 eV) necessary to ionize tissue atoms.

Ionized   Referring to an atom that has an extra electron or has had an electron removed.

Ionizing radiation   Radiation capable of ionization.

Ion pair   Two oppositely charged particles.

Irradiated   Referring to matter that intercepts radiation and absorbs part or all of it; exposed.

Isobars   Atoms having the same number of nucleons but different numbers of protons and neutrons.

Isochromatid   A fragment in a chromosome aberration.

Isomers   Atoms having the same number of protons and neutrons but a different nuclear energy state.

Isotones   Atoms having the same number of neutrons.

Isotopes   Atoms that have the same number of protons but a different number of neutrons.

Isotropic   Equal intensity in all directions; having the same properties in all directions.

Joule (J)   The unit of energy; the work done when a force of 1 N acts on an object along a distance of 1 m.

Karotype   A chromosome map.

Kerma (k)   The energy absorbed per unit mass from the initial kinetic energy released in matter of all the electrons liberated by x-rays or gamma rays. Expressed in gray (Gy). 1 Gy = 1 J/kg.

Kilo-   Prefix meaning "one thousand."

Kiloelectron volt (keV)   The kinetic energy of an electron equivalent to 1000 eV. 1 keV = 1000 eV.

Kilogram (kg)   The scientific unit of mass that is unrelated to gravitational effects; 1000 g.

Kilovolt (kV)   Electric potential equal to 1000 V.

Kinetic energy   The energy of motion.

Kilovolt peak (kVp)   A measure of the maximum electrical potential across an x-ray tube; expressed in kilovolts.

Lag   Phosphorescence.

Laser disk   A removable disk that uses laser technology to write and read data.

Late effect   A radiation response that is not observed for 6 months or more after the exposure.

Latent image   An unobservable image stored in the silver halide emulsion; it is made manifest by processing.

Latent image center   A sensitivity center that has many silver ions attracted to it.

Latent period   The period after the prodromal stage of the acute radiation syndrome during which there is no visible sign of radiation sickness.

Lateral decentering   The improper positioning of the grid that results in cutoff.

Latitude   The range of x-ray exposure over which a radiograph is acceptable.

Law of Bergonié and Tribondeau   The principle stating that the radiosensitivity of cells is directly proportional to their reproductive activity and inversely proportional to their degree of differentiation.

Law of conservation of energy   The principle stating that energy may be transformed from one form to another but cannot be created or destroyed; the total amount of energy is constant.

Law of conservation of matter   The principle stating that matter can be neither created nor destroyed.

Law of inertia   The principle stating that a body will remain at rest or continue to move with a constant velocity in a straight line unless acted on by an external force.

$LD_{50/60}$ Dose of radiation expected to cause death within 60 days to 50% of those exposed.

Leakage radiation   Secondary radiation emitted through the tube housing.

Limiting resolution   The spatial frequency at a modulation transfer function equal to 0.1.

Linear energy transfer (LET)   A measure of the rate at which energy is transferred from ionizing radiation to soft tissue. Expressed in kiloelectron volts per micrometer of soft tissue.

Linear, nonthreshold   Referring to the dose-response relationship that intersects the dose axis at or below zero.

Linear, threshold   Referring to the dose-response relationship that intercepts the dose axis at a value greater than zero.

Linear tomography   The imaging modality in which the x-ray tube is mechanically attached to the image receptor and moves in one direction as the image receptor moves in the opposite direction.

Line focus   The projection of an inclined line into a surface, resulting in a smaller size.

Line focus principle   A design incorporated into x-ray tube targets to allow a large area for heating while maintaining a small focal spot.

Line pair   One bar and its interspace of equal width.

Lodestone   A leading stone.

Logic function   A computer-recognized command that evaluates an intermediate result and performs subsequent computations depending on that result.

Log relative exposure (LRE)   The change in optical density over each exposure interval.

Long gray scale   A low-contrast radiograph that has many shades of gray.

Low-contrast resolution   The ability to image objects with similar subject contrast.

Luminescence   The emission of visible light.

Lymphocyte   The white blood cell that plays an active role in providing immunity for the body by producing antibodies; it is the most radiosensitive blood cell.

Lysosome   Cell that contains enzymes capable of digesting cellular fragments.

Magnetic dipole   Current flowing in an infinitesimally small loop.

Magnetic dipole moment   Vector with a magnitude equal to the product of the current flowing in a loop and the area of the current loop.

Magnetic domain   An accumulation of many atomic magnets with their dipoles aligned.

Magnetic permeability   The property of a material causing it to attract the imaginary lines of the magnetic field.

Magnetic susceptibility   The ease with which a substance can be magnetized.

Magnetite   The magnetic oxide of iron.

Magnetism   The polarization of a material.

Magnetization   The relative magnetic flux density in a material compared with that in a vacuum.

Magnification   The condition in which the images on the radiograph are larger than the object they represent.

Magnitude   A number representing a quantity.

Main-chain scission   The breakage of the long-chain macromolecule that divides the long, single molecule into smaller ones.

Mainframe computer   A fast, medium to large, large-capacity system that has multiple microprocessors.

Mammographer   A radiologic technologist specializing in breast x-ray studies.

Mammography   Radiographic examination of the breast using low kilovoltage.

Manifest illness   The stage of the acute radiation syndrome during which signs and symptoms are apparent.

Manifest image   The observable image formed when the latent image undergoes the proper chemical processing.

Man-made radiation   X-rays and artificially produced radionuclides used for nuclear medicine.

Mask image   The image obtained from mask mode.

Masking   The act of ensuring that no extraneous light from the viewbox enters the viewer's eyes.

Mask mode   The method of temporal subtraction that results in successive subtraction images of contrast-filled vessels.

Mass   A quantity of matter; expressed in kilograms.

Mass density   The quantity of matter per unit volume.

Mass-energy equivalence   Energy equals mass multiplied by the square of the speed of light.

Matrix   The rows and columns of pixels displayed on a digital image.

Matter   Anything that occupies space and has form or shape.

Maximum-intensity projection (MIP)   Reconstruction of an image by selecting the highest-value pixels along any arbitrary line through the data set and exhibiting only those pixels.

Maximum permissible dose (MPD)   The dose of radiation that would be expected to produce no significant radiation effects.

Mean lethal dose   A constant related to the radiosensitivity of a cell.

Mean marrow dose (MMD)   The average radiation dose to the entire active bone marrow.

Mean survival time   The average time between exposure and death.

Mechanical energy   The ability of an object to do work. See also **kinetic energy** and **potential energy.**

Medical physicist   A physicist who examines and monitors the performance of imaging equipment.

Meiosis   The process of germ cell division that reduces the chromosomes in each daughter cell to half the number of chromosomes in the parent cell.

Metabolism   Anabolism and catabolism.

Metaphase   The phase of cell division during which the chromosomes are divisible.

Metol   A secondary constituent used in the chemical composition of developing agents.

Microcalcifications   Calcific deposits that appear as small grains of varying sizes on the x-ray film.

Microcomputer   A personal computer or electronic organizer.

Microcontroller   A tiny computer installed in an appliance.

Microfocus tube   A tubes that has a very small focal spot and that is specifically designed for imaging very small microcalcifications at relatively short source-to-image distances.

Microwave   A short-wavelength radiofrequency.

Mid-density (MD) step   The step that has an average optical density closest to, but not less than, 1.2.

Milliampere (mA)   The measure of x-ray tube current.

Milliampere-second (mAs)   The product of exposure time and x-ray tube current; a measure of the total number of electrons.

Minification gain   The ratio of the square of the diameter of the input phosphor to the square of the diameter of the output phosphor.

Misregistration   Misalignment of two or more images because of patient motion between image acquisition.

Mitochondrion   A structure that digests macromolecules to produce energy for the cell.

Mitosis (M)   The process of somatic cell division wherein a parent cells divides to form two daughter cells identical to the parent cell.

Modem   A device that converts digital information into analog information.

Modulation   A changing of the magnitude of a video signal; the magnitude is directly proportional to the light intensity received by the television-camera tube.

Modulation transfer function (MTF)   A mathematical procedure for measuring resolution.

Molecule   A group of atoms of various elements held together by chemical forces; the smallest unit of a compound that can exist by itself and retain all its chemical properties.

Molybdenum   A target material for x-ray tubes that is used in mammography.

Momentum   The product of the mass of an object and its velocity.

Monoenergetic   A beam containing x-rays or gamma rays that all have the same energy.

Monosaccharide   A sugar.

Motherboard   The main circuit board in a system unit.

Motion blur   The blurring of the image that results from movement of either the patient or the x-ray tube during exposure.

Moving grid   A grid that moves while the x-ray exposure is being made.

Multiplanar reformation (MPR)   Process in which transverse images are stacked to form a three-dimensional data set.

Multislice computed tomography   An imaging modality that uses two detector arrays to produce two spiral slices at the same time.

Multitarget or single-hit model   A model of radiation dose-response relationship for more complicated biologic systems, such as human cells.

Muscle   A tissue capable of contracting.

Mutual induction   The process of producing electricity in a secondary coil by passing an alternating current through a nearby primary coil.

National Council on Radiation Protection and Measurement (NCRP)   The organization that continuously reviews the recommended dose limits.

Natural   A zero dose of radiation exposure.

Natural environmental radiation   Naturally occurring ionizing radiation, including cosmic rays, terrestrial radiation, and internally deposited radionuclides.

Natural magnet   A magnet that gets its magnetism from the Earth.

Nervous tissue   Tisue that consists of neurons and is the avenue through which electrical impulses are transmitted throughout the body for control and response.

Neuron   A cell of the nervous system that has long, thin extensions from the cell to distant parts of the body.

Neutron   Uncharged elementary particle, with a mass slightly greater than that of the proton, found in the nucleus of every atom heavier than hydrogen and in the nucleus of an atom.

Newton (N)   The unit of force in the SI system; $1 \text{ N} \approx$ ¼ lb.

Node   One of many stations or terminals of a computer network.

Noise   **a.** The grainy or uneven appearance of an image caused by an insufficient number of primary x-rays. **b.** A uniform signal produced by scattered x-rays.

Nonionizing radiation   Radiation for which the mechanism of action in tissue does not directly ionize atomic or molecular systems through a single interaction.

Nonlinear, nonthreshold   Referring to varied responses that are produced from varied doses, with any dose expected to produce a response.

Nonlinear, threshold   Referring to varied responses that are produced from varied doses, with a particular level below which there is no response.

Nonscheduled maintenance   Maintenance that becomes necessary because of a failure in the system that necessitates processor repair.

Nonstochastic effects   Biologic effects of ionizing radiation that demonstrate the existence of a threshold. The severity of the biologic damage increases with increased dose.

North pole   A magnetic pole that has a positive electrostatic charge.

Nuclear energy   The energy contained in the nucleus of an atom.

Nucleolus   A rounded structure that is often attached to the nuclear membrane and controls the passage of molecules, especially RNA, from the nucleus to the cytoplasm.

Nucleon   A proton or a neutron.

Nucleotide   The unit formed from a nitrogenous base, a five-carbon sugar molecule, and a phosphate molecule.

Nucleus   **a.** The center of a living cell; a spherical mass of protoplasm containing the genetic material (DNA), which is stored in its molecular structure. **b.** The center of an atom containing neutrons and protons.

Nuclide   General term referring to all know isotopes, both stable and unstable, of chemical elements.

Object plane   The plane in which the anatomic structures that are to be imaged lie.

Occupational dose   The dose received by an individual in a restricted area during the course of employment in which the individual's assigned duties involve exposure to radiation.

Occupational exposure   Radiation exposure received by radiation workers.

Off-focus radiation   X-rays produced in the anode but not at the focal spot.

Off-level grid   An artifact produced by having an improperly positioned radiographic tube, not by having an improperly positioned grid.

Object-to-image receptor distance (OID)   The distance from the image receptor to the object that is to be imaged.

1% voltage ripple   High-frequency generators that have higher x-ray quantity and quality.

100% voltage ripple   Single-phase power in which the voltage varies from zero to its maximum value.

Oocytes   Primordial follicles that grow to encapsulate oogonia.

Opaque   A surface that does not allow the passage of light.

Open filament   A condition that results when the filament becomes thinner and breaks.

Operating console   Console that allows the radiologic technologist to control the x-ray tube current and voltage so that the useful x-ray beam is of proper quantity and quality.

Operating system   The series of instructions that organizes the course of data through the computer to solve a particular problem.

Optical density   The degree of blackening of a radiograph.

Optical disk   A removable disk that uses laser technology to write and read data.

Ordered pairs   Notation for coordinates in which the first number of the pair represents a distance along the x-axis and the second number indicates a distance up the y-axis.

Origin   The point where two axes meet on a graph.

Organs   A collection of tissues of similar structure and function.

Organ system   A combination of tissues and organs that forms an overall integrated organization.

Organic molecule   A molecule that is life supporting and contains carbon.

Orthochromatic   Referring to blue- or green-sensitive film; usually exposed with rare earth screen.

Outcome analysis   Image interpretation that involves reconciling the patient's ultimate disease condition with the radiologist's diagnosis.

Output   The process of transferring the results of a computation from primary memory to storage or the user.

Overcoat   A protective covering of gelatin that encloses the emulsion.

Overexposed   Referring to a radiograph that is too dark because too much x-radiation reached the image receptor.

Ovum   The mature germ cell found in a female.

Oxidation   A reaction that produces an electron.

Oxygen enhancement ratio (OER)   The ratio of the dose necessary to produce a given effect under anoxic conditions to the dose necessary to produce the same effect under aerobic conditions.

Pair production   The interaction between the x-ray and the nuclear electric field that causes the x-ray to disappear and causes two electrons, one positive and one negative, to take its place.

Panchromatic   Referring to film that is sensitive to the entire visible light spectrum.

Parallel circuit   A circuit that contains elements that bridge conductors rather than lie in a line along a conductor.

Parallel grid   A simple grid in which all lead grid strips are parallel.

Paramagnetic   Referring to materials slightly attracted to a magnet and loosely influenced by an external magnetic field.

Parenchymal   Referring to part of the organ that contains tissues representative of that particular organ.

Partial volume effect   Distortion of the signal intensity from a tissue because it extends partially into an adjacent slice thickness.

Particle accelerator   An atom "smasher."

Particulate radiation   Radiation distinct from x-rays and gamma rays; examples are alpha particles, electrons, neutrons, and protons.

Penetrability   The ability of an x-ray to penetrate tissue; the range in tissue; x-ray quality.

Penetrometer   An aluminum step wedge.

Penumbra   Image blur result from the size of the focal spot; geometric unsharpness.

Permanent magnet   A magnet whose magnetism is artificially induced.

Phantom   A device that simulates some parameters of the human body for evaluating imaging system performance.

Phenidone   A secondary constituent used in the chemical composition of developing agents.

Phosphor   The active layer of the radiographic intensifying screen closest to the radiographic film.

Phosphorescence   The emission of visible light during and after stimulation.

Photoconductor   A material that conducts electrons when illuminated.

Photodiode   A solid-state device that converts light into an electric current.

Photodisintegration   The process by which very-high-energy x-rays can escape interaction with electrons and the nuclear electric field and can be absorbed directly by the nucleus.

Photoelectron   An electron that has been removed during the process of photoelectric absorption.

Photoelectric effect   The absorption of an x-ray by ionization.

Photoemission   Electron emission after light stimulation.

Photographic effect   The formation of the latent image.

Photometer   An instrument that measures light intensity.

Photomultiplier tube   An electron tube that converts visible light into an electrical signal.

Photon   Electromagnetic radiation that has neither mass nor electric charge but interacts with matter as though it is a particle; x-rays and gamma rays.

Photospot camera   A camera that exposes only one frame when active, receiving its image from the output phosphor of the image-intensifier tube.

Photostimulation   The emission of visible light after excitation by laser light.

Phototimer   A device that allows automatic exposure control.

Pitch   See **spiral pitch ratio.**

Pixel   A picture element; the cell of a digital image matrix.

Planck's constant (h)   A fundamental physical constant that relates the energy of radiation to its frequency.

Planetary rollers   Rollers positioned outside the master roller and guideshoes.

Pluripotential stem cell   A stem cell that has the ability to develop into several different types of mature cells.

Pocket ionization chamber (pocket dosimeter)   A personnel radiation-monitoring device.

Point lesion   Any change that results in the impairment or loss of function at the point of a single chemical bond.

Point mutation   A molecular lesion caused by the change or loss of a base that destroys the triplet code and may not be reversible.

Polarity   The existence of opposing negative and positive charges.

Pole   The magnetically charged end of a material.

Polyenergetic   Referring to radiation, such as x-rays, having a spectrum of energies.

Polysaccharide   A large carbohydrate that includes starches and glycogen.

Positive beam limiting (PBL)   A feature of radiographic collimators that automatically adjusts the radiation field to the size of the image receptor.

Potassium bromide   A compound used as a restrainer in the developer.

Potassium iodide   A compound used as a restrainer in the developer.

Potential energy   The ability to do work by virtue of position.

Power   Time rate at which work (W) is done. 1 W = 1 J/s.

Power-of-10 notation   Exponential form.

Precurser cell   An immature cell.

Predetector collimator   A collimator that restricts the x-ray beam viewed by the detector array.

Prepatient collimator   A collimator that consists of several sections so that a nearly parallel x-ray beam results.

Prereading voltmeter   A kVp meter that registers even though an exposure is not being made and no current is flowing in the circuit; this allows the voltage to be monitored before an exposure.

Preservative   A chemical additive, usually sodium sulfide, that maintains the chemical balance of the developer and fixer.

Preventative maintenance   A planned program of parts replacement at regular intervals.

Primary coil   The first coil through which the varying current in an electromagnet is passed.

Primary protective barrier   Any wall to which the useful beam can be directed.

Processing   Chemical treatment of the emulsion of a radiographic film to change a latent image to a manifest image.

Processor   The electronic circuitry that does the actual computations and the memory that supports it.

Prodromal period   The first stage of the acute radiation syndrome, which occurs within hours after radiation exposure.

Proper fraction   A fraction in which the quotient is less than 1.

Prophase   The phase of cell division during which the nucleus and the chromosomes enlarge and the DNA begins to take structural form.

Proportion   The relation of one part to another.

Proportional counter   A sensitive instruments used primarily as stationary laboratory instruments for the assay of small quantities of radioactivity.

Protective coating   The layer of the radiographic intensifying screen closest to the radiographic film.

Protective housing   A lead-lined metal container into which the x-ray tube is fitted.

Protein synthesis   The metabolic production of proteins.

Proton   An elementary particle with a positive electric charge equal to that of an electron and a mass approximately equal to that of a neutron. It is located in the nucleus of an atom.

Protracted dose   A dose of radiation delivered continuously but at a lower dose rate.

Pulse mode/rate mode   Instruments designed to detect the presence of radiation.

Quality assurance (QA)   All planned and systematic actions necessary to provide adequate confidence that a facility, system, or administrative component will perform safely and satisfactorily in service to a patient. It includes scheduling, preparation and promptness in the examination or treatment, reporting of results, and quality control.

Quality control (QC)   All actions necessary to control and verify the performance of equipment. It is included in quality assurance.

Quantum   An x-ray photon.

Quantum mottle   Radiographic noise produced by the random interaction of x-rays with an intensifying screen. This effect is more noticeable when very high rare-earth systems are used at a high kVp.

Quantum theory   The theory in the physics of matter smaller than an atom and of electromagnetic radiation.

Rad (radiation absorbed dose)   Special unit for absorbed dose and air kerma. 1 rad = 100 erg/g = 0.01 Gy.

Radiation   The energy emitted and transferred through matter.

Radiation biology   The branch of biology concerned with the effects of ionizing radiation on living systems.

Radiation exposure   X-ray quantity or intensity, measured in roentgens.

Radiation fog   Artifact caused by unintentional exposure to radiation.

Radiation hormesis   The theory that suggests that very low radiation doses may be beneficial.

Radiation quality   The relative penetrability of an x-ray beam determined by its average energy; usually measured by half-value layer or kilovolt peak.

Radiation quantity   The intensity of radiation; usually measured in milliroentgen (mR).

Radiation standards   The recommendations, rules, and regulations regarding permissible concentrations, safe handling, techniques, transportation, industrial control of radioactive material.

Radiation (thermal)   The transfer of heat by the emission of infrared electromagnetic radiation.

Radiation weighting factor (W_R)   The factor used for radiation-protection that accounts for differences in biologic effectiveness between different radiations. Formerly called *quality factor*.

Radioactive decay   A naturally occurring process whereby an unstable atomic nucleus relieves its instability through the emission of one or more energetic particles.

Radioactive disintegration   The process by which the nucleus spontaneously emits particles and energy and transforms itself into another atom to reach stability.

Radioactive half-life   The time required for a radioisotope to decay to half its original activity.

Radioactivity   The rate of decay or disintegration of radioactive material. Expressed in curie (Ci) or becquerel (Bq). 1 Ci = 3.7×10^{10} Bq.

Radiofrequency (RF)   Electromagnetic radiation having frequencies from 0.3 kHz to 300 GHz; magnetic resonance imaging uses RF in the range of approximately 1 to 100 mHz.

Radiographer   A radiologic technologist who deals specifically with x-ray imaging.

Radiographic contrast   The combined result of image receptor contrast and subject contrast.

Radiographic intensifying screen   A device that converts the energy of the x-ray beam into visible light to increase the brightness of an x-ray image.

Radiographic noise   The undesirable fluctuation in the optical density of the image.

Radiographic technique   The combination of settings selected on the control panel of the x-ray imaging system to produce a quality image on the radiograph.

Radiographic technique chart   A guide that describes standard methods for consistently producing high-quality images.

Radiography   An imaging modality that uses x-ray film and usually an x-ray tube mounted from the ceiling on a track that allows the tube to be moved in any direction and provides fixed images.

Radioisotopes   Radioactive atoms having the same number of protons. They are changed into a different atomic species by disintegration of the nucleus accompanied by the emission of ionizing radiation.

Radiological Society of North America (RSNA)   The scientific society of radiologists and medical physicists.

Radiologist   A physician specializing in medical imaging using x-rays, ultrasound, and magnetic resonance imaging.

Radiolucent   Referring to a tissue or material that transmits x-rays and appears dark on a radiograph.

Radiolysis of water   The dissociation of water into other molecular products as a result of irradiation.

Radionuclides   Any nucleus that emits radiation.

Radiopaque   Referring to a tissue or material that absorbs x-rays and appears bright on a radiograph.

Radiosensitivity   The relative susceptibility of cells, tissues, and organs to the harmful action of ionizing radiation.

Radon   A colorless, odorless, naturally occurring radioactive gas (^{222}Ra) that decays via alpha emission and has a half-life of 3.8 days.

RAID (redundant array of inexpensive disks) system   A system consisting of at least disk drives within a single cabinet that collectively act as a single storage system.

Random access memory (RAM) Data that can be stored or accessed at random from anywhere in main memory in approximately equal amounts of time, regardless of where they are located.

Rare earth element An element that is a transitional metal found in low abundance in nature.

Rare earth screen A radiographic intensifying screen made from rare earth elements, making it more useful for radiographic imaging.

Raster pattern The pattern produced on the screen of a television picture tube by the movement of electron beams.

Ratio The mathematical relationship between similar quantities.

Read-only memory (ROM) A data-storage device that contains information supplied by the manufacturer and cannot be written on or erased.

Real time A display for which the image is continuously renewed, often to view anatomic motion, in fluoroscopy and ultrasound.

Reciprocity law The principle stating that optical density on a radiograph is proportional only to the total energy imparted to the radiographic film.

Reconstruction The creation of an image from data.

Reconstruction time The time needed for the computer to present a digital image after an examination is completed.

Recorded detail The degree of sharpness of structural lines on a radiograph.

Recovery Repair and repopulation.

Rectification The process of converting alternating current to direct current.

Rectifier The electronic device that allows current flow in only one direction.

Red filter A filter that transmits light only above 600 nm; it is used with both green- and blue-sensitive film.

Redox Simultaneous reduction and oxidation reactions.

Reducing agent The chemical responsible for reduction.

Reduction The process by which an electron is given up by a chemical to neutralize a positive ion.

Reflection The return or reentry of an x-ray.

Reflective layer The layer of the intensifying screen that intercepts light headed in other directions and redirects it to the film.

Refraction The deviation of course when photons of visible light traveling in straight lines pass from one transparent medium to another.

Region of interest (ROI) The area of an anatomic structure on a reconstructed digital image as defined by the operator using a cursor.

Relative age-response relationship The increased incidence of a disease proportional to its natural incidence.

Relative biologic effectiveness (RBE) The ratio of the dose of standard radiation necessary to produce a given effect to the dose of test radiation needed for the same effect.

Relative risk The estimation of late radiation effects in large populations without having any precise knowledge of their radiation dose.

Relay An electrical device based on electromagnetic induction that serves as a switch.

Rem (radiation equivalent man) \he special unit for dose equivalent and effective dose. It has been replaced by the sievert (Sv) in the SI system. 1 rem = 0.01 Sv.

Remnant radiation The x-rays that pass through the patient and interact with the image receptor.

Replenishment The replacement of developer and of fixer in the automatic processing of film.

Repopulation Replication by surviving cells.

Resistance An opposition to a force.

Resolution A measure of the ability of a system to image two separate objects and visually distinguish one from the other.

Restrainer A compound that restricts the action of the developing agent to only irradiated silver halide crystals.

Ribonucleic acid (RNA) Molecules that are involved in the growth and development of a cell through a number of small, spherical cytoplasmic organelles that attach to the endoplasmic reticulum.

Ribosomes The site of protein synthesis.

Right-hand rule The rule by which the direction of the magnetic field lines can be determined.

Roller subassembly One of three principal film-transport subsystems in an imaging system.

Rotating anode Anode used in general-purpose x-ray tubes because the tubes must be capable of producing high-intensity x-ray beams in a short time.

Rotor The rotating part of an electromagnetic induction motor; it is located inside the glass envelope.

Saccharide A carbohydrate.

Safe industry An industry that has an associated annual fatality accident rate of no more than 1 per 10,000 workers.

Safelight An incandescent lamp with a color filter that provides sufficient illumination in the darkroom while ensuring that the film remains unexposed.

Sagittal plane Any anterior-posterior plane parallel to the long axis of the body.

Saturation current A filament current that has risen to its maximum value because all of the available electrons have been used.

Scalar Referring to a quantity or a measurement that has only magnitude.

Scanned projection radiography (SPR) Generalized method of making a digital radiograph; used in computed tomography for precision localization.

Scatter radiation X-rays scattered back in the direction of the incident x-ray beam.

Scheduled maintenance Procedures performed on a routine basis.

Scientific notation   Exponential form.

Scintillation detector   An instrument used in the detector arrays of many computed tomographic scanners.

Screen-film   The most commonly used film; used with intensifying screens.

Screening mammography   An imaging examination performed on the breasts of asymptomatic women using a two-view protocol to detect unsuspected cancer.

Screen lag   The phosphorescence in an intensifying screen.

Screen speed   A relative number used to identify the efficiency of conversion of x-rays into usable light.

Second (s)   The standard unit of time.

Secondary coil   The coil in which the induced current in an electromagnet flows.

Secondary electron   The ejected electron from the outer shell of an atom.

Secondary memory   Data stored on tape drives, diskettes, and hard disk drives.

Secondary protective barrier   Barriers designed to shield areas from secondary radiation.

Secondary radiation   Leakage and scatter reaction.

Second-generation computed tomographic scanner   A unit that incorporates the natural extension of the single-detector to a multiple-detector assembly intercepting a fan-shaped rather than a pencil-shaped x-ray beam.

Section thickness   The thickness of tissue that will not be blurred by tomography.

Selectivity   The ratio of primary radiation to scattered radiation transmitted through grid.

Self-induction   The magnetic field produced in a coil of wire that opposes the alternating current being conducted.

Self-rectified system   An imaging system in which the x-ray tube serves as the vacuum-tube rectifier.

Semiconductor   Material that can serve both as a conductor and as an insulator of electricity.

Sensitivity   The ability of an image receptor to respond to x-rays.

Sensitivity center   The physical imperfections in the lattice of the emulsion layer that occur during the film manufacturing process.

Sensitivity profile   The slice thickness.

Sensitizing agent   An agent that enhances the effect of radiation.

Sensitometer   An optical step wedge that is used to construct a characteristic curve.

Sensitometry   The study of the response of an image receptor to x-rays.

Sequestering agent   An agents introduced in the developer to form stable complexes with metallic ions and salts.

Shaded surface display (SSD)   A computer-aided technique that identifies a narrow range of values as belonging to the object to be imaged and displays that range.

Shadow dose equivalent (HS)   The dose of radiation to which the external skin or an extremity is exposed.

Shadow shield   A shields that is suspended over the region of interest and that casts a shadow over the patient's reproductive organs.

Shape distortion   A kind of distortion caused by elongation or foreshortening.

Shells   The orbital energy levels surrounding the nucleus of an atom.

Shell-type transformer   A transformer that confines more of the magnet field lines of the primary winding because there are essentially two closed cores.

Short gray scale   A high-contrast radiograph that exhibits black to white in just a few apparent steps.

Sievert (Sv)   Special name for the SI unit of dose equivalent and effective dose. 1 Sv = 1 Jkg^{-1} = 100 rem.

Sigmoid-type (S-type) dose-response relationship   A nonlinear, threshold radiation dose-response relationship.

Silver bromide   The material that makes up 98% of the silver halide crystals in a typical emulsion.

Silver halide crystals   The active ingredient of the radiographic emulsion. It is instrumental in creating a latent image on the radiograph.

Silver iodide   The material that makes up 2% of the silver halide crystals in a typical emulsion.

Sine wave   The variation of movement of photons in electrical and magnetic fields

Single-target hit model   A model of radiation dose-response relationships for enzymes, viruses, and bacteria.

Sinusoidal   Simple motion; a sine wave.

Skin erythema dose (SED)   A dose of radiation, usually about 200 rad or 2 Gy, that causes a redness of the skin.

Slice thickness   The thickness of the tissue being imaged.

Slice-acquisition rate (SAR)   A measure of the efficiency of a multislice spiral computed tomographic scanner.

Slip ring technology   Technology that allows the gantry to rotate continuously without interruption, making spiral computed tomography possible.

Sludge   Deposits on the film resulting from dirty or warped rollers, causing emulsion pick-off and gelatin buildup.

Sodium carbonate   An alkali compound contained in the developer.

Sodium hydroxide   An alkali compound contained in the developer.

Sodium sulfite   The preservative added to the developer that keeps it clear.

Soft copy   The output on a display screen.

Soft tissue radiography   Radiography in which only muscle and fat structures are imaged.

Software   The computer programs that tell the hardware what to do and how to store data.

Soft x-ray   An x-ray that has low penetrability and therefore is of low quality.

Solenoid Helical winding of current-carrying wire that produces a magnetic field along the axis of the helix.

Solid-state diode A diode that passes electric current in only one direction.

Solution A suspension of particles or molecules in a fluid.

Solvent A liquid into which various solids and powders can be dissolved.

Somatic cells All the cells of the body except the oogonium and spermatogonium.

Somatic effects Effects of radiation, such as cancer and leukemia, limited to an exposed individual. See also **genetic effect.**

Source-to-image receptor distance (SID) The distance from the x-ray tube to the image receptor.

Source-to-skin distance (SSD) The distance from the patient's skin to the fluoroscopic tube.

Space charge The electron cloud near the filament.

Space-charge effect The phenomenon of the space charge that makes it difficult for subsequent electrons to be emitted by the filament because of the electrostatic repulsion.

Spatial distortion The misrepresentation in the image of the actual spatial relationships among objects.

Spatial frequency The measure of resolution; usually expressed in line pairs per millimeter (lp/mm).

Spatial resolution The ability to image small objects that have high subject contrast.

Spatial uniformity The constancy of pixel values in all regions of the reconstructed image.

Special quantities Additional quantities designed to support measurement in specialized areas of science and technology.

Spectrum Graphic representation of the range over which a quantity extends.

Spectrum matching Use of rare earth screens only in conjunction with film emulsions that have light absorption characteristics matched to the light emission of the screen.

Speed Term used to loosely describe the sensitivity of film to x-rays.

Speed index The step that has an average optical density closest to, but not less than, 1.2.

Sperm See **spermatozoa.**

Spermatocyte A mature spermatogonia.

Spermatogonium The male germ cell.

Spermatozoa A functionally mature male germ cell.

Spindle fibers The fibers that connect a centromere and two chromatids to the poles of the nucleus during mitosis.

Spindles The poles of the nucleus.

Spinning top A device used to check exposure timers.

Spiral/helical The term given to computed tomography because it is the apparent motion of the x-ray tube during the scan.

Spiral pitch radio The relationship between the patient couch movement and x-ray beam collimation.

Spot film Static image in small-format image receptor taken during fluoroscopy.

Square law The principle stating that one can compensate for a change in the source-to-object distance by changing the mAs by the factor SID squared.

Starch A plant polysaccharide.

Stationary anode An anode used in imaging systems in which high tube current and power are not required.

Stator Stationary coil windings located in the protective housing but outside the x-ray tube glass envelope. It is part of the electromagnetic induction motor.

Stem cell An immature or a precursor cell.

Step-down transformer A transformer in which the voltage is decreased from the primary side to the secondary side.

Stepping A computer-controlled capability on a patient table that allows imaging from the abdomen to the feet after a single injection of contrast media.

Step-up transformer A transformer in which the voltage is increased from the primary side to the secondary side.

Step wedge A filter used when radiographing a body part, such as the foot, that varies in thickness from one end to the other.

Stereoradiography The practice of making two radiographs of the same object and viewing through a device which allows each eye to view a different radiograph.

Sthenic Referring to a body habitus of a patient who is strong and active; the average body habitus.

Stochastic effects The probability or frequency of the biologic response to radiation as a function of radiation dose. Disease incidence increases proportionally with dose, and there is no dose threshold.

Storage memory The main computer memory where the program and data files are stored.

Straight-line portion The portion of a sensitometric curve where the diagnostic or most useful range of density is produced.

Stromal Referring to part of an organ that is composed of connective tissue and vasculature that provides structure to the organ.

Structure mottle Distribution of phosphor crystals in an intensifying screen.

Subatomic particle A particle smaller than the atom.

Subject contrast The part of radiographic contrast determined by the size, shape, and x-ray attenuating characteristics of the subject being examined and the energy of the x-ray beam. See also **image receptor contrast.**

Substance Any drug, chemical, or biologic entity.

Subtraction technique A method of removing all unnecessary anatomic structures from an image and enhancing only those of interest.

Supercomputer   One of the fastest and highest-capacity computers, containing hundreds to thousands of microprocessors.

Superconductivity   The property of some materials to exhibit no resistance below a critical temperature.

Supporting tissue   Tissue that binds tissues and organs together.

Target   **a.** The region of an x-ray tube anode struck by electrons emitted by the filament. **b.** The molecule (DNA) that is most sensitive to radiation.

Target molecule   Molecule (DNA) that is few in number yet essential for cell survival and is particularly sensitive to the effects of ionizing radiation.

Target theory   The theory that a cell will die if of target molecules are inactivated as a result of radiation exposure.

Technique factors   The kVp and mA as selected for a given radiographic examination.

Teleradiology   The transfer of images and patient reports to remote sites.

Telophase   The final subphase of mitosis that is characterized by the disappearance of the structural chromosomes into a mass of DNA and the closing off of the nuclear membrane into two nuclei.

Temperature   A measure of heat and cold.

Temporal subtraction   Computer-assisted technique whereby an image obtained at one time is subtracted from an image obtained at a later time.

Temporary magnet   A magnet that retains the properties of a magnet only while its magnetism is being induced.

Tenth-value layer (TVL)   The thickness of absorber necessary to reduce an x-ray beam to one tenth its original intensity. 1 TVL = 3.3 half-value layers.

Terminal   An input and output device that uses a keyboard for input and a display screen for output.

Terrestrial radiation   The radiation emitted from deposits of uranium, thorium, and other radionuclides in the Earth.

Tesla (T)   The SI unit of magnetic field intensity. An older unit is the gauss (G). 1 T = 10,000 G.

Test object   **a.** A passive device that provides echoes and permits evaluation of one or more parameters of an ultrasound system but does not necessarily duplicate the acoustical properties of the human body. **b.** A passive device of geometric shapes designed to evaluate the performance of x-ray and magnetic resonance imaging systems. See also **phantom.**

Thermal energy   The energy of molecular motion; heat; infrared radiation.

Thermal radiation   The transfer of heat by infrared emission.

Thermaluminesecence dosimetry   The emission of light by a thermally stimulated crystal after irradiation.

Thermionic emission   The emission of electrons from a heated surface.

Thermometer   A device that measures temperature.

Thiosulfate   The fixing agent that removes unexposed and undeveloped silver halide crystals from the emulsion.

Three-phase electric power   The generation of three simultaneous voltage waveforms out of step with one another, thus never dropping the voltage to zero during exposure.

Threshold dose   The dose below which a person has a negligible chance of sustaining specific biologic damage or the dose at which a response to an increasing x-ray intensity first occurs.

Thrombocyte   A circular or oval disk called a *platelet* found in the blood that initiates blood clotting and prevents hemorrhage.

Thymine   A nitrogenous organic base that attaches to a deoxyribose molecule.

Time-interval-difference (TID) mode   Technique that produces subtracted images from progressive masks and the frames that follow.

Time-of-occupancy factor (T)   The amount of time the area being protected is used.

Tissue   A collection of cells of similar structure and function.

Tissue weighting factor (W_T)   The proportion of the risk of stochastic effects resulting from irradiation of the whole body when only an organ or tissue is irradiated. It accounts for the relative radiosensitivity of various tissues and organs.

Tomogram   An x-ray image of a coronal, sagittal, transverse, or oblique section through the body.

Tomography   Imaging modality that brings into focus only the anatomic structure lying in a plane of interest while blurring structures on either side of that plane.

Total effective dose (TED)   The recommendation by the National Council on Radiation Protection and Measurement that a radiation worker's lifetime effective dose be limited to the worker's age in years multiplied by 10 mSv.

Total filtration   Inherent filtration plus added filtration.

Transaxial   Across the body; transverse.

Transcription   The process of constructing mRNA.

Transfer   An addition of an amino acid during translation.

Transformer   An electrical device operating on the principle of mutual induction to change the magnitude of current and voltage.

Translation   The process of forming a protein molecule from messenger RNA.

Translucent   A surface that allows light to be transmitted but greatly alters and reduces its intensity.

Transmission   The passing of an x-ray beam through the anatomic part without any interaction with the atomic structures.

Transparent   A surface that allows light to be transmitted almost unaltered.

Transport roller   An agents that moves the film through the chemical tanks and dryer assembly.

Transverse   Across the body; axial.

Transverse image   An image perpendicular to the long axis of the body.

Tungsten   A metal element that is the principal component of the cathode and the anode.

Turnaround assembly   A device in the automatic processor for reversing the direction of the film.

Turns ratio   The quotient of the number of turns in the secondary coil to the number of turns in the primary coil.

Ultraviolet light   Light that is located at the short end of the electromagnetic spectrum between visible light and ionizing x-rays; it is beyond the range of human vision.

Uncontrolled area   Area occupied by anyone; the maximum exposure rate allowed in this area is based on the recommended dose limit for the public.

Underexposed   Referring to a radiograph that is too light because too little x-radiation reached the image receptor.

Undifferentiated cell   An immature or a nonspecialized cell.

Unified field theory   The theoretical combination of magnetic, electric, gravitational, and strong nuclear forces along with weak interaction to explain the physical laws of magnetism.

Unit   A standard of measurement.

Use factor (U)   The proportional amount of time during which the x-ray beam is energized or directed toward a particular barrier.

Useful beam   The primary radiation used to form the image.

Valence electron   an electron in the outermost shell.

Variable aperture collimator   A box-shaped device containing a radiographic beam-defining system. It is the device most often used to decline the size and shape of a radiographic beam.

VDT   Abbreviation for **video display terminal.**

Vector   A quantity or measurement that has magnitude, unit, and direction.

Velocity (v)   The rate of change of an object's position with time; speed.

Video display terminal   A monitor similar to a television screen.

Vidicon   The television-camera tube most often used in television fluoroscopy.

Vignetting   A reduction in brightness at the periphery of the image.

Visible light   The radiant energy in the electromagnetic spectrum that is visible to the human eye.

Volt (V)   The SI unit of electric potential and potential difference.

Voltage ripple   A way to characterize voltage waveforms.

Voltaic pile   A stack of copper and zinc plates that produces an electric current; a precursor of the modern battery.

Voxel   A three-dimensional pixel; volume element.

Washing   The stage of processing during which any remaining chemicals are removed from the film.

Watt (W)   One ampere of current flowing through an electric potential of one volt.

Wave equation   The formula stating that velocity equals frequency multiplied by wavelength.

Waveform   The graphic representation of a wave.

Wavelength   The distance between similar points on a sine wave; the length of one cycle.

Wave-particle duality   The principle stating that both wave and particle concepts must be retained, since wavelike properties are exhibited in some experiments and particle-like are exhibited properties in others.

Wave theory   The theory that electromagnetic energy travels through space in the form of waves.

Weight   The force on a mass caused by the acceleration of gravity. Properly expressed in newtons (N), but commonly expressed in pounds (lb).

Wetting   A process that makes the emulsion film swell so that subsequent chemical baths can reach all parts of the emulsion uniformly.

Wetting agent   The agent, usually water, that treats the radiograph so that the chemicals can penetrate the emulsion.

Whole body   For purposes of external exposure, the head, trunk (including gonads), arms above the elbow, and leg above the knee.

Whole-body exposure   A radiographic exposure in which the whole body, rather than an isolated part, is irradiated.

Window   A thin section of glass envelope through which the useful beam emerges.

Windowing   The technique that allows one to see only a "window" of the entire dynamic range.

Window level   The location on a digital image number scale where the levels of grays are assigned. It regulates the optical density of the displayed image and identifies the type of tissue to be imaged.

Window width   A specific number of gray levels or digital image numbers assigned to an image. It determines the gray-scale rendition of the imaged tissue and therefore the image contrast.

Word   Two bytes of information.

Work (W)   The product of the force on an object and the distance over which the force acts. Expressed in Joules (J). $W = F \times d$.

Workload (W)   The product of the maximum milliamperage (mA) and the number of x-ray examinations performed per week. Expressed in milliamperes per minute per week (mA/min/wk).

Workstation   A powerful desktop system, often connected to larger computer systems so that users can transfer and share information.

X-axis   The horizontal line of a graph.

X-ray   Penetrating, ionizing electromagnetic radiation having a wavelength much shorter than that of visible light.

X-ray imaging system   An x-ray system designed for radiography, tomography, or fluoroscopy.

X-ray quality   The penetrability of an x-ray beam.

X-ray quantity   The output intensity of an x-ray imaging system, measured in roentgens (R).

X-ray tube rating charts   Charts that guide the technologist in the use of x-ray tubes.

Y-axis   The vertical line of a graph.

Zonography   Thick-slice tomography with a tomographic angle of less than 10 degrees.

PHOTO CREDITS

Figure 1-7   From Eisenberg RL: *Radiology: an illustrated history,* St Louis, 1992, Mosby.
Figure 9-5   From *Mosby's radiographic instructional series: radiographic imaging,* St Louis, 1998, Mosby.
Figure 17-14   From *Mosby's radiographic instructional series: radiographic imaging,* St Louis, 1998, Mosby.
Figure 17-18   From Bontrager KL: *Textbook of radiographic positioning and related anatomy,* ed 4, St Louis, 1997, Mosby.
Figure 18-13   From McQuillan-Martensen K: *Radiographic critique,* Philadelphia, 1996, WB Saunders.
Figure 20-1   From Fauber T: *Radiographic imaging and exposure,* St Louis, 2000, Mosby.
Figure 21-7   From Fauber T: *Radiographic imaging and exposure,* St Louis, 2000, Mosby.
Figure 28-9   Seeram E: *Computed tomography: physical principals, clinical applications, and quality control,* ed 2, Philadelphia, 2000, WB Saunders.
Figure 32-3   From Papp J: *Quality management in the imaging sciences,* St Louis, 1998, Mosby.
Figure 32-4   From Papp J: *Quality management in the imaging sciences,* St Louis, 1998, Mosby.
Figure 32-5   From *Mosby's radiographic instructional series: radiographic imaging,* St Louis, 1998, Mosby.
Figure 32-6   From *Mosby's radiographic instructional series: radiographic imaging,* St Louis, 1998, Mosby.
Figure 40-12   From *Mosby's radiographic instructional series: radiographic imaging,* St Louis, 1998, Mosby.
Figure 40-13, A   Sherer MA: *Radiation protection in medical radiology,* ed 3, St Louis, 1998, Mosby.

Index

Conversion Tables

Length

Unit	Equivalent in Meters
1 centimeter (cm)	10^{-2}
1 micron (μm)	10^{-6}
1 nanometer (nm)	10^{-9}
1 angstrom (Å)	10^{-10}
1 mile (mi)	1609

Mass-energy*

Electron Volts	Joules	Kilograms	Atomic Mass Units
1.0	1.60×10^{-19}	1.78×10^{36}	1.07×10^{-9}
6.24×10^{18}	1.0	1.11×10^{17}	6.69×10^{9}
5.61×10^{32}	8.99×10^{13}	1.0	6.02×10^{23}
9.32×10^{8}	1.49×10^{-10}	1.66×10^{27}	1.0

*(1 J = 10^7 ergs; 4.19 J = 1 calorie; 1 BTU = 1.06×10^{10} ergs.)

Time

Years	Days	Hours	Minutes	Seconds
1	365	8.75×10^3	5.26×10^5	3.15×10^7
	1	24	1.44×10^3	8.64×10^4
		1	60	3.6×10^3
			1	60